Biotoxins in Food

Biotoxins are naturally occurring substances present in living organisms as a way of conferring biological defense or protection on such organisms. But their presence in food has been found to be a threat to unsuspecting food consumers. While they are exploited as biocontrol agents and as a biological defense mechanism against pests and predators in the field, biotoxins are implicated in foodborne illness in humans if consumed. Naturally occurring substances present in food include glycoalkaloids found in potatoes and lectins (phytohemagglutinin) in green beans and red kidney beans. *Biotoxins in Food: Threats and Benefits* discusses the natural poisons present in food, the threats posed, and the possible detection methods. This book assesses the implications of these biotoxins in food by evaluating the threats posed by the consumption of these naturally occurring poisons and the various emerging detection procedures available in the food industry. Several reports from contributing authors focus on the various threats linked to various food products and offer solutions in terms of removal. Early detection of these biotoxins to prevent food illnesses is well documented.

Key Features:

- Discusses the emerging concepts of types, sources, and distribution of biotoxins in food
- Addresses the prevalence and applications of biotoxins in food products
- Analyzes the current detection technology of biotoxins in foods

Biotoxins in Food
Threats and Benefits

Edited by
Sesan Abiodun Aransiola,
Bunmi Comfort Kotun,
and Naga Raju Maddela

CRC Press
Taylor & Francis Group
Boca Raton London New York

CRC Press is an imprint of the
Taylor & Francis Group, an **informa** business

Cover credit: http://images.tandf.co.uk/common/jackets/agent
jpg/978100350/9781003500605.jpg

First edition published 2025
by CRC Press
2385 NW Executive Center Drive, Suite 320, Boca Raton FL 33431

and by CRC Press
4 Park Square, Milton Park, Abingdon, Oxon, OX14 4RN

CRC Press is an imprint of Taylor & Francis Group, LLC

ISBN: 978-1-032-80670-9 (hbk)
ISBN: 978-1-032-81624-1 (pbk)
ISBN: 978-1-003-50060-5 (ebk)

DOI: 10.1201/9781003500605

Typeset in Palatino LT Std
by Apex CoVantage, LLC

Contents

Foreword

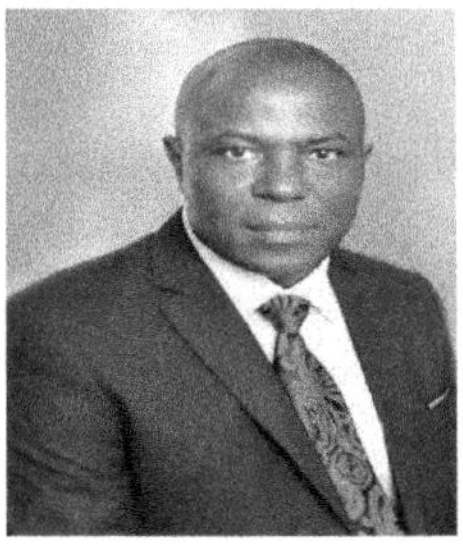

This book, titled *Biotoxins in Food: Threats and Benefits*, discusses natural poisons in food, their threats, benefits, and detection methods. Our food, essential for survival, can also contain biotoxins. These naturally occurring substances in organisms such as bacteria, fungi, algae, and viruses provide biological defense. Biotoxins help repel predators, protecting the producing organisms. However, their presence in food poses threats to consumers, as they can be found at various stages of food production. Documented biotoxins include bacterial toxins (Salmonella, *E. coli*), mycotoxins (ochratoxins, aflatoxins), zootoxins (oral toxins, crinotoxins), and phytotoxins (lectins in beans, cyanogenic glycosides in root plants).

Biotoxins pose severe and widespread threats, causing an estimated 600 million foodborne illnesses and 420,000 fatalities yearly, according to the World Health Organization (WHO). This book outlines these threats, including foodborne illnesses, food poisoning, liver damage, neurological problems, and immune system suppression. Biotoxins can lead to economic and social hazards, such as costly product recalls, loss of consumer trust, and disease outbreaks, especially affecting vulnerable populations. Despite these threats, biotoxins offer medical benefits. For instance, botulinum toxin treats pain and muscle disorders and shows potential for cancer and neurodegenerative disease treatments. In the pharmaceutical industry, biotoxins aid in drug development and antibiotic production. They also benefit environmental monitoring, pollution management, pest control, and biological research. Detecting biotoxins is essential to mitigate their risks and harness their benefits.

This book explores various methods for detecting biotoxins in food, from traditional culture-based assays to advanced techniques such polymerase chain reaction (PCR), chromatography, enzyme-linked immunosorbent assay (ELISA), biosensors, mass spectrometry, and lateral flow devices. These advanced methods offer more reliable and rapid detection compared to traditional ones. Proper food handling, storage, preparation to avoid contamination, and regular testing and monitoring of food samples are essential for the prevention of biotoxin threats. Upon detecting biotoxins, immediate recall of contaminated products and public warnings about symptoms and treatment options are crucial. Treatments range from supportive care (hydration, symptom management) to hospitalization for severe cases, with ongoing research into targeted treatments using biomarkers and antidotes. Biotoxins pose challenges due to their widespread presence and detection difficulties, being mostly odorless and tasteless. New biotoxins and the costly, time-consuming nature of detection add to these challenges. Thus, effective prevention strategies, including good farm practices, proper storage, and regular testing, are vital. Enhancing detection methods can improve food safety, prevent outbreaks, and protect consumer health while reducing the need for costly recalls.

This book is designed for students, researchers, and professionals seeking to understand food biotoxins, their types, classification, societal impact, potential threats, and detection methods. It is also useful for regulatory bodies involved in food safety. With comprehensive coverage, the book aims to enhance knowledge on food safety and raise public awareness. Collaborative efforts from food processors, farmers, regulators, and public health officials are essential for effectively managing biotoxins and protecting consumer health.

Professor John Danjuma Mawak, Ph.D., FNSM
Professor of Microbiology
University of Jos
July 7, 2024

Preface

Biotoxins are bioactive molecules that can be obtained as metabolites of living organisms or by the exploitation of microorganisms in degradation leading to the release of toxic products. These molecules are produced by microorganisms; animal and plant examples include Diphtheria toxin, pertussis toxin, snake venom, aflatoxin, fumonisins, and others. These biotoxins can be categorized based on their sources into phytotoxins (plant origin), zoo toxins (animal origin), mycotoxins (fungi origin), enterotoxins (bacterial origin), and phycotoxins (microalgae origin). Biotoxins are considered harmful substances produced to prevent predation on the producing organism or as a biological defense mechanism which confers protection on the producer. These compounds could also be harnessed for pharmaceutical uses as antitumor agents, chemotherapeutic agents, and biological research probes.

In this book, the implications of these biotoxins in food was assessed by evaluating the threats posed by the consumption of these naturally occurring poisons and the various emerging detection procedures available in the food industry. Several reports from authors focusing on the various threats linked to various food products are highlighted, and solutions in terms of removal and early detection of these biotoxins to prevent food illnesses are documented.

In addition, this book has three sections, with 6, 8, and 7 chapters in Sections 1, 2, and 3, respectively, making up 19 chapters. The first section is an introduction, which looks at the *concepts of biotoxins* and covers the following topics: types, sources, and effects of biotoxins; distributions of microbial toxins in foods; mycotoxins in children's foods; global perspectives; general evaluation of bacterial toxins in food products; mycotoxins and global food safety; and the challenges and benefits of marine biotoxins in seafoods. The second section covers the *applications of biotoxins,* which include plant-based biotoxins: applications and controls, industrial applications of biotoxins, applications of animal toxins: traditional and modern techniques, the potential of biotoxins for drug discovery and development, harmful algal blooms: threat to marine life, therapeutic application of mycotoxins and phytotoxins in cancer management, applications of edible marine green biotoxins, and exploring the therapeutic potential of snake venom biotoxins. The final section enlightens on *biotoxin detection in food,* with topics on the mode of transmission of biotoxins to humans, emerging applications of biotoxin detection in food, availability of biotoxins in foods: animal and plant sources, extraction techniques of biotoxins in food, exploring the origin and epidemiology of biotoxins in foods and feeds: an updated perspective, emerging trends in cyanotoxins: unravelling threats and discovering benefits in food safety, and mycotoxins in feed and feeding: promising detoxification strategies and mechanism of action in food all treated in this section.

The chapters were contributed by 69 academicians, scientists, and researchers from 15 different countries (the United Kingdom, Nigeria, India, the United States, South Africa, China, Pakistan, Egypt, Czech Republic, Republic of Korea, Australia, Indonesia, Botswana, Turkey, and Malaysia) across the world.

Sesan Abiodun Aransiola, Ph.D.,
Department of Microbiology, University of Abuja, Nigeria
National Biotechnology Research and Development Agency (NRBDA),
Ogbomoso, Nigeria

Bunmi Comfort Kotun, Ph.D.,
Department of Biological Sciences and Biotechnology,
College of Pure and Applied Science,
Caleb University Imota,
Lagos State, Nigeria

Naga Raju Maddela, Ph.D.,
Departamento de Ciencias Biológicas,
Facultad de Ciencias de la Salud,
Universidad Técnica de Manabí,
Portoviejo 130105,
Ecuador

Acknowledgments

We are deeply grateful for the support of all the contributors to this volume, whose valuable input and prompt responses have been instrumental in the success of this book. We appreciate each contributor's enthusiasm and generous support in ensuring that this piece was completed on time. Their collaboration and partnership are truly commendable. We also extend our gratitude to the anonymous reviewers whose constructive feedback helped enhance the quality of this book by inviting additional expert contributions. We would like to acknowledge the invaluable support of the CRC Press and production team, whose guidance was crucial in ensuring the timely completion of this project. Working with them has been an honor and a privilege. Last, we would like to express our sincere thanks to the management and colleagues at the University of Abuja (Nigeria); National Biotechnology Research Development Agency (Nigeria); Caleb University, Imota, Lagos (Nigeria); and Universidad Técnica de Manabí (Ecuador) for their unwavering support throughout the book proposal and preparation process.

Sesan Abiodun Aransiola, Ph.D.
Department of Microbiology
University of Abuja, Nigeria
National Biotechnology Research and Development Agency (NRBDA)
Ogbomoso, Nigeria

Bunmi Comfort Kotun, Ph.D.
Department of Biological Sciences and Biotechnology
College of Pure and Applied Science
Caleb University Imota
Lagos State, Nigeria

Naga Raju Maddela, Ph.D.
Departamento de Ciencias Biológicas
Facultad de Ciencias de la Salud
Universidad Técnica de Manabí
Portoviejo, Equador

The Editors

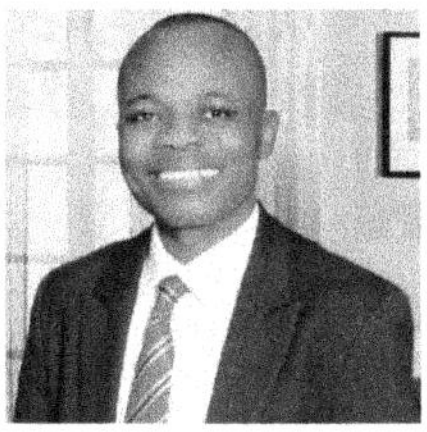

Sesan Abiodun Aransiola is a Ph.D. holder in environmental microbiology in the Department of Microbiology, Federal University of Technology, Minna, Nigeria. He obtained his first degree (B.Tech.) and master's degree (M.Tech.) from the same department in 2009 and 2014, respectively. He has demonstrated his research expertise in the production of vermicasts from vermicoposting (vermitechnology) of organic wastes to assist plants in the remediation of soil polluted with heavy metals. Currently, he is a lecturer at the Department of Microbiology, University of Abuja, Nigeria. His area of interest is environmental microbiology, with research areas in phytoremediation, vermicomposting, biosorption, and bioremediation of contaminated soil environments. He is an award-winning researcher and has over 80 publications, including book chapters and research and review articles of good international repute with a high impact factor. He has co-edited scientific books of global interest, which include *Microbial Biotechnology for Bioenergy* (Elsevier); *Ecological Interplays in Microbial Enzymology, Prospects for Soil Regeneration and Its Impact on Environmental Protection* (Springer); *Microbial Biofilms—Applications and Control; Marine Greens: Environmental, Agricultural, Industrial and Biomedical Applications;* and *Emerging Contaminants in Food and Food Products, Phytoremediation in Food Safety: Risks and Prospects* (CRC Press), with many more in process. Also, has worked up to the rank of an assistant chief scientific officer at Bioresources Development Centre, National Biotechnology Research and Development Agency, Nigeria, where he was involved in the uses of vinasse (a byproduct of ethanol) as bio-fertilizer to reclaim polluted soil for agricultural purposes. Abiodun is a member of the Nigerian Society for Microbiology and American Society for Microbiology, among others.

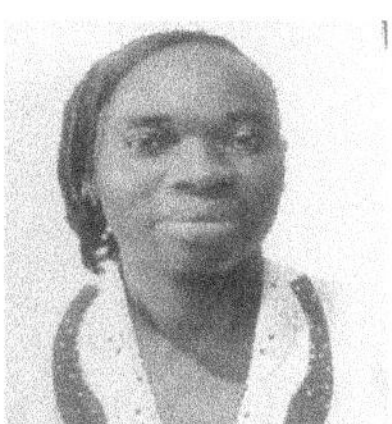

Bunmi Comfort Kotun is a graduate of microbiology (B.Sc.), University of Lagos, Akoka, Nigeria, in 2004, received her master's degree (M.Sc.) in food microbiology in 2008, and obtained her (Ph.D.) in food mycology in 2017, both from the University of Ibadan, Ibadan, Oyo state, Nigeria. Her Ph.D. research was focused on investigating the presence of toxigenic mold present in sampled millet grains from the southwestern states of Nigeria. Bunmi is presently with Caleb University, Imota, Lagos, Nigeria, as a lecturer in the Department of Biological Sciences and Biotechnology. She is an upcoming researcher with book chapters and publications in scientific conferences and journals. Her research interest is in food microbiology and has covered areas which include mycology, mycotoxicology, food safety, molecular characterization, and microbial-related research. She is a member of the Nigerian Society for Microbiology, Mycology Society, and also Mycotoxicology Society of Nigeria.

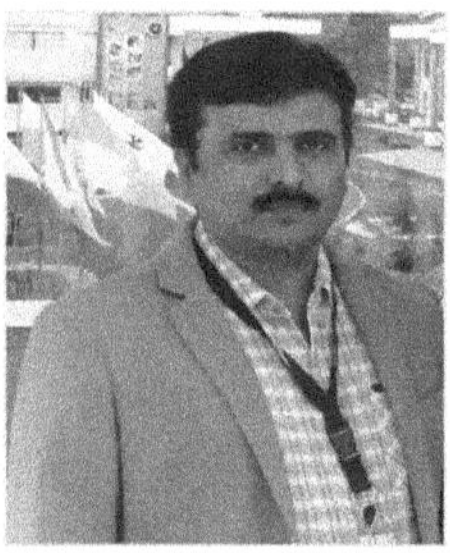

Naga Raju Maddela received his M.Sc. (1996–1998) and Ph.D. (2012) in microbiology from Sri Krishnadevaraya University, Anantapuramu, India. During his doctoral program in the area of environmental microbiology, he investigated the effects of industrial effluents/insecticides on soil microorganisms and their biological activities. He has worked as Faculty in Microbiology since 1998, teaching undergraduate and postgraduate students. He worked as a Prometeo Investigator (fellowship received from SENESCYT) at Universidad Estatal Amazónica, Ecuador during 2013–15, and received a postdoctoral fellowship (2016–2018) from Sun Yat-sen University, China. He also received external funding from the China Postdoctoral Science Foundation in 2017 and internal funding from Universidad Técnica de Manabí in 2020. He has participated in national/international conferences and presented research data in China, Cuba, Ecuador, India, and Singapore. Currently, he is working as a full professor at the Facultad de Ciencias de la Salud, Universidad Técnica de Manabí, Portoviejo, Ecuador. He has been actively publishing scientific articles, books (authored and edited), and chapters since 2007. As of now, he published 105 articles, 22 books, and 50 book chapters.

Contributors

Grace Onyukwo Abakpa
Department of Microbiology
Federal University of Health Sciences
Otukpo, Benue, Nigeria

David Oyeyemi Aboyeji
Department of Microbiology
Federal University of Technology
Minna, Nigeria

Oyewole Oluwafemi Adebayo
Department of Microbiology
Federal University of Technology
Minna, Nigeria

Adebayo-Olajide, T.C
Department of Biological Sciences and Biotechnology
Caleb University
Lagos State, Nigeria

Adedola Adeboye
African Food Research Network
Gauteng, South Africa

Moyosore Joseph Adegbeye
Department of Animal Production and Health
University of Africa Toru-Orua
Bayelsa, Nigeria

Adegoke, C.O.
Department of Medical Laboratory Science
Ladoke Akintola University of Technology
Ogbomosho, Oyo State, Nigeria

Adeleke A.J.
Department of Microbiology
Modibbo Adamawa University
Yola, Nigeria

Isiaka Adedayo Adelere
Department of Microbiology
Federal University of Technology
Minna, Nigeria

Omolara Adenaike
TOMS Laboratory
Evangelist & Mrs. Job Alabi Crescent
Itedo Alafia-Are Ago
Ogbomoso, Nigeria

Eric M. Adetutu
Department of Environmental Health
Mt. Barker District Council
Mt. Barker, SA, Australia

Oluwatosin Adefunke Adetuyi
Department of Chemistry and Biochemistry
Texas Tech University
Lubbock, Texas, USA

Babatunde Oluwafemi Adetuyi
Department of Natural Sciences Faculty of Pure and Applied Sciences
Precious Cornerstone University
Ibadan, Oyo State, Nigeria

Maria M. Adeyemi
Department of Chemistry and Biochemistry
Caleb University
Lagos, Nigeria

Victoria Olufunmi Adeyemo-Eleyode
Department of Biological Sciences
College of Agriculture and Natural Sciences
Joseph Ayo Babalola University
Ikeji, Nigeria

Aziz Ahmed
Faculty of Marine Sciences Lasbela
University of Agriculture
Water & Marine Sciences
Uthal, Balochistan, Pakistan

Akinboboye O.A.
Department of Biological Sciences
Southwestern University
Okun-Owa, Ogun State, Nigeria

Asiat Na'Allah
Department of Biochemistry
Faculty of Pure and Applied Sciences
Kwara State University
Malete, Kwara State, Nigeria

Simon Ameh
Department of Biochemistry
Federal University of Technology
Minna, Nigeria

Abraham Olufemi Asuku
Bioresources Development Centre
National Biotechnology Development Agency
Ogbomoso, Nigeria
and
Department of Physiology
Faculty of Basic Medical Sciences
College of Health Sciences
University of Ilorin
Ilorin, Nigeria

Helen Shnada Auta
Department of Microbiology and African Centre of Excellence for Mycotoxins and Food Safety
Federal University of Technology
Minna, Nigeria

Ayobami Ifeoluwa Awe
Department of Biology
Catholic University of America
Washington, DC, USA

Ayedun J.
Department of Biological Sciences and Biotechnology
Caleb University
Imota, Lagos, Nigeria

Olalekan Blessing Balogun
Department of Microbiology
College of Agriculture and Natural Sciences
Joseph Ayo Babalola University
Ikeji, Nigeria

Jayanthi Barasarathi
Faculty of Health and Life Sciences (FHLS)
Inti International University
Nilai, Negeri Sembilan, Malaysia

Gaber El-Saber Batiha
Department of Pharmacology and Therapeutics
Faculty of Veterinary Medicine
Damanhour University
AlBeheira, Egypt

Sharon Bose
School of Pharmaceutical Technology
School of Health and Medical Sciences
Adamas University
Kolkata, India

Doofan Bur
Department of Medical Biotechnology
National Biotechnology Development Agency
Abuja, Nigeria

Arundhuti Chatterjee
School of Pharmaceutical Technology
School of Health and Medical Sciences
Adamas University
Kolkata, India

Charles Chinazaekpele Chidume
Department of Natural Sciences
Faculty of Pure and Applied Sciences
Precious Cornerstone University
Ibadan, Oyo State, Nigeria

Ibrahim Dabai
Queen's University
Belfast, United Kingdom

Prity Das
School of Pharmaceutical Technology
School of Health and Medical Sciences
Adamas University
Kolkata, India

P. Gnana Deepu
Center for Biotechnology
University College of Engineering Science and Technology
JNTUH
Hyderabad, Telangana, India

Egbeagu, U.U.
College of Resource and Environment
Northeast Agricultural University
Harbin, China

Lorretha Emenyeonu
Bioresources Development Centre
Owode National Biotechnology Development Agency
Abuja, Nigeria

Fagbemi K.
Department of Microbiology
Babcock University
Ilishan-Remo, Ogun State, Nigeria

Olutayo, I. Falodun
Department of Microbiology, Faculty of Science
University of Ibadan
Idaban, Oyo State, Nigeria

Mariyam Fatima
Center for Biotechnology
University College of Engineering Science and Technology, JNTUH
Hyderabad, Telangana, India

Evelyn N. Fatokun
Department of Biological Science and Biotechnology
College of Pure and Applied Sciences
Caleb University
Imota, Nigeria

Folorunso, O.A.
Department of Biological Sciences and Biotechnology
Caleb University
Lagos State, Nigeria

Mordecai Gana
Department of Microbiology
Federal University of Technology
Minna, Nigeria

Jogipeta Harihara
Center for Biotechnology
University College of Engineering Science and Technology, JNTUH
Hyderabad, Telangana, India

Kathroju Harikrishna
Center for Biotechnology
University College of Engineering Science and Technology, JNTUH
Hyderabad, Telangana, India

Gordon Ibeanu
Department of Pharmaceutical Science
North Carolina Central University
Durham, North Carolina, USA

Anem I. Igirigi
Department of Animal Production and Health
University of Africa Toru-Orua
Bayelsa Nigeria

Ikhimiukor, O.O.
University at Albany State University of New York
Albany, New York, USA

Makinde, O.M.
Department of Biological Sciences and Biotechnology
Caleb University
Imota, Lagos, Nigeria

Sandip Mondal
Amity Institute of Pharmacy
Amity University
Kolkata, West Bengal, India

Anjaneyulu Musini
Center for Biotechnology
University College of Engineering Science and Technology JNTUH
Hyderabad, Telangana, India

Blessing I. Nwadike
Department of Microbiology Faculty of Science
University of Ibadan
Idaban, Nigeria

Ezinne Janefrances Nwonu
Department of Medical Biotechnology
National Biotechnology Development Agency
Abuja, Nigeria

Ogunbanwo, S.T.
Department of Microbiology
University of Ibadan
Ibadan, Nigeria

Gbonjubola Oyinlola Ogungbanagbe
Department of Physiology
Faculty of Basic Medical Sciences
College of Health Sciences
University of Ilorin
Ilorin, Nigeria

Adeniyi A. Ogunjobi
Department of Microbiology
Faculty of Science
University of Ibadan
Idaban, Nigeria

Felix Oladele Okunlola
Department of Natural Sciences Faculty of Pure and Applied Sciences
Precious Cornerstone University
Ibadan, Oyo State, Nigeria

Peace Abiodun Olajide
Department of Biological Sciences and Biotechnology
Caleb University
Lagos State, Nigeria

Ifeoluwa O. Olayemi
Department of Chemistry and Biochemistry
Caleb University
Lagos, Nigeria

Oluwaseun Iyadunni Oluwasogo
Soil Science Laboratory, School of Applied Biosciences
Kyungpook National University
Daegu, Republic of Korea

Peter Gbenga Oni
Department of Chemistry and Biochemistry
Worchester Polytechnic Institute
Worchester, Massachusetts, USA

Edward Kwame Opata
Department of Biochemistry
Molecular Drug Metabolism and Toxicology Unit
University of Idaban
Ibadan, Nigeria

Amarachi Rosemary Osi
Ningbo Institute of Material Technology and Engineering
Chinese Academy of Sciences
Zhejiang province, P.R. China

Abolade A. Oyelade
New Jersey Department of Health
Public Health and Environmental Laboratories
Ewing, New Jersey, USA

Valiollah Palangi
Visiting Researcher at Department of Life Sciences
Western Caspian University
Baku, Azerbaijan

Olalekan Blessing Balogun
Department of Microbiology
College of Agriculture and Natural Sciences
Joseph Ayo Babalola University
Ikeji-Arakeji, Ilesha, Nigeria

Adekunle Rowaiye
Department of Agricultural Biotechnology
National Biotechnology Development Agency
Abuja, Nigeria
and
Department of Pharmaceutical Science
North Carolina Central University
Durham, North Carolina, USA

Isaiah Woru Sabinari
Department of Physiology
Faculty of Science
Charles University
Prague, Czech Republic

Salam Babatunde Saliu
Department of Physiology
Faculty of Basic Medical Sciences
College of Health Sciences
University of Ilorin
Ilorin, Nigeria

Sardaman Sardaman
Department of Animal Science
Faculty of Agriculture and Animal Science
Universitas Islam Negeri Sultan Syarif Kasim Riau
Pekanbaru, Indonesia

Susan N. Thera-Sekgweng
African Food Research Network
Gauteng, South Africa
and
Plethora Consulting
Gaborone, Botswana

Section 1

Concepts of Biotoxins

1

Types, Sources, and Effects of Biotoxins

Mordecai Gana, Oyewole Oluwafemi Adebayo, Simon Ameh, Amarachi Rosemary Osi, and Ibrahim Dabai

1.1 Introduction

The term "biotoxins" refers to naturally occurring harmful compounds that are produced by living organisms. These substances pose substantial risks to the public's health and the safety of the food people consume. It is possible to find these toxins in a wide variety of dietary sources, and they have the potential to have severe acute and chronic impacts on human biology. In order to develop successful measures to limit the impact of biotoxins and assure the safety of the food supply, it is vital to have a solid understanding of the many types of biotoxins, their origins, and the impacts they have.

The study of biotoxins found in food involves a wide range of fields, such as microbiology, toxicology, environmental science, and food safety. In terms of detection, control, and regulation, every type of biotoxin, regardless of whether it originates from fungi, algae, bacteria, or plants, poses individual issues that are distinct from one another (Aransiola et al., 2024). According to Bennett and Klich (2003), mycotoxins are secondary metabolites that are produced by specific species of fungi. These fungi are responsible for the contamination of crops such as maize, wheat, and peanuts due to their presence. According to Wu (2010), when these poisons are taken in high quantities or over an extended length of time, they have the potential to pose significant health risks, including the development of cancer and immunological deficiencies.

Phycotoxins, produced by algae, are another group of biotoxins that can contaminate seafood. The accumulation of toxic toxins in marine species, which poses a risk to human consumers, is caused by algal blooms, which are frequently made worse by environmental changes and pollution (Hallegraeff, 2003). Bacterial toxins, such as those generated by *Clostridium botulinum* and *Staphylococcus aureus*, are especially significant because they have the ability to induce foodborne diseases that could potentially result in death (Schmid-Hempel & Frank, 2007).

DOI: 10.1201/9781003500605-2

The various nature of biotoxins and the potential dangers they pose are further highlighted by the presence of plant toxins, such as ricin, which is derived from castor beans, and alkaloids, which are derived from specific medicinal plants. As stated by Colegate and Dorling (1994), the presence of these poisons in food can be the result of natural contamination, inappropriate farming methods, or inadequate conditions for the processing and storage of food.

The purpose of this chapter is to provide a complete overview of the several types of biotoxins found in food, as well as their sources and consequences. It is possible to gain a better understanding of the impact of these toxins and to develop measures to manage and prevent their presence in the food supply if we investigate their origins and the health implications they have. It is essential for policymakers, professionals in the field of food safety, and the general public to have this knowledge in order to secure a food environment that is both safe and nutritious.

1.2 Types of Biotoxins

Biotoxins are a wide range of naturally occurring compounds that are produced by different species, such as fungi, algae, bacteria, and plants. Every variety of biotoxin presents distinct hazards to both food safety and human well-being. This section offers a comprehensive examination of the primary classifications of biotoxins: mycotoxins, phycotoxins, bacterial toxins, and plant toxins. It contains detailed information about their properties, origins, and the impact they have on human health.

1.3 Mycotoxins

Mycotoxins are toxic secondary metabolites produced by certain species of fungi. They are common contaminants in food crops and pose significant health risks when ingested. Key types of mycotoxins include:

1.3.1 Aflatoxins

Aspergillus flavus and *Aspergillus parasiticus*, which are bacteria that are widely found in crops like peanuts, maize and tree nuts, are the primary organisms responsible for the production of aflatoxins. There is a considerable potential for carcinogenicity in aflatoxins, with aflatoxin B1 being the most potent. Children who are exposed to the substance for an extended period of time may develop liver cancer, immunosuppression, and stunted growth (Wild & Gong, 2010).

1.3.2 Ochratoxins

Ochratoxins are produced by *Aspergillus* and *Penicillium* species, frequently contaminating cereals, coffee, dried fruits, and wine. Ochratoxin A is nephrotoxic, causing kidney damage and increasing the risk of urinary tract tumours. It is also immunotoxic and teratogenic (Stoev, 2013).

1.3.3 Fusarium Toxins

The *Fusarium* species that produce these toxins are responsible for the contamination of cereals including wheat, barley, and maize almost all of the time. Fumonisins, trichothecenes, and zearalenone are known to be among the most important *Fusarium* toxins. Fumonisins have been linked to tumours of the oesophagus as well as the neural tube abnormalities. Trichothecenes, which include deoxynivalenol, are responsible for immunosuppression as well as symptoms of gastrointestinal diseases. According to Marin et al. (2013), zearalenone has estrogenic effects, which result in disruptions to reproductive health.

1.4 Phycotoxins

Phycotoxins are toxins produced by algae, particularly during harmful algal blooms (HABs). These toxins can accumulate in seafood, posing a risk to human health when consumed.

1.4.1 Saxitoxins

Produced by dinoflagellates in the genus *Alexandrium*, these toxins are associated with paralytic shellfish poisoning (PSP). Saxitoxins block sodium channels, leading to paralysis. In severe cases, PSP can be fatal due to respiratory failure (Etheridge, 2010).

1.4.2 Ciguatoxins

The toxins are derived by dinoflagellates belonging to the genus *Gambierdiscus* and build up in the tissues of reef fish. Ciguatera fish poisoning (CFP), resulting from the ingestion of ciguatoxins, manifests as symptoms affecting the gastrointestinal, neurological, and cardiovascular systems. The consequences can be severe and enduring (Friedman et al., 2017).

1.4.3 Brevetoxins

Neurotoxic shellfish poisoning (NSP) is caused by toxins produced by *Karenia brevis*. Brevetoxins exert an impact on nerve cells, resulting in symptoms such as nausea, vomiting, and neurological disruptions. Respiratory irritation can occur when brevetoxins are inhaled in the form of aerosols (Flewelling et al., 2005).

1.5 Bacterial Toxins

Bacterial toxins are produced by pathogenic bacteria and can contaminate food, leading to foodborne illnesses.

1.5.1 Botulinum Toxin

Botulinum toxin, which is produced by *Clostridium botulinum*, is recognised as one of the most powerful neurotoxins in existence. Botulism, which is caused by the ingestion of botulinum toxin, leads to muscle paralysis and can be lethal if the breathing muscles are impacted. Common symptoms of this condition encompass dysphagia, muscular debility, and respiratory insufficiency (Peck, 2009).

1.5.2 Staphylococcal Enterotoxins

Staphylococcus aureus produces these toxins, which are frequently found in inadequately preserved foods. Staphylococcal food poisoning presents with symptoms such as nausea, vomiting, and abdominal cramps. The symptoms appear quickly, usually within a few hours of consuming the substance (Argudín et al., 2010).

1.6 Plant Toxins

Plant toxins are naturally occurring chemicals found in certain plants, which can be harmful if ingested.

1.6.1 Ricin

Ricin is a potent toxin derived from the seeds of the castor oil plant (*Ricinus communis*). Ricin inhibits protein synthesis, leading to cell death. Ingestion of ricin causes severe abdominal pain, vomiting, diarrhoea, and can be fatal without prompt treatment (Audi et al., 2005).

1.6.2 Alkaloids

Alkaloids are found in various plants, including nightshade (Solanaceae) family members such as potatoes, tomatoes, and eggplants. Some alkaloids, like solanine and chaconine, can cause gastrointestinal distress and neurological symptoms. Chronic exposure may lead to long-term health issues (Friedman & Levin, 2009).

1.7 Sources of Biotoxins

Several different kinds of organisms, such as fungi, algae, bacteria, and plants, are responsible for the production of biotoxins. Their presence in food is influenced by a wide variety of environmental and human factors, which include the conditions of the climate, farming techniques, and the methods used to store food. In this section, we will explore the natural sources of biotoxins, the environmental factors that have an impact on their development, and the precise conditions that can lead to contamination in the food supply.

1.8 Natural Sources of Biotoxins

1.8.1 Fungal Contamination in Crops and Stored Food Products

Fungi, and more specifically species of *Aspergillus*, *Fusarium*, and *Penicillium*, are notable contributors to the production of mycotoxins. It is possible for these organisms to infect crops both while they are in the field and while they are being stored. They thrive in particular environmental conditions. Cereals (wheat, barley, and maize), nuts (peanuts and almonds), and dried fruits (figs and raisins) are among the crops that are most frequently impacted by this disease. The supply chain is susceptible to contamination at a number of different locations, ranging from the pre-harvest stage to the post-harvest storage stage (Bryden, 2012). Spores of fungi can be found either in the soil, in the air, or on the surfaces of plants. According to Magan and Aldred (2007), ineffective agricultural methods, such as insufficient drying and incorrect storage, can encourage the growth of fungi and also lead to the creation of toxins.

1.8.2 Algal Blooms in Aquatic Environments

Harmful algal blooms arise from the excessive growth of algae colonies in aquatic environments, resulting in the production of phycotoxins. These harmful substances have the ability to build up in marine species, including shellfish and fish, and are subsequently ingested by humans. Phycotoxins that are frequently encountered include saxitoxins, ciguatoxins, and brevetoxins. The presence of these toxins is linked to different symptoms related to shellfish poisoning, including paralytic shellfish poisoning (PSP) and neurotoxic shellfish poisoning (NSP) (Landsberg, 2002). The expansion of harmful algal blooms is largely influenced by nutrient pollution resulting from agricultural runoff, climate change, and the rise in water temperature (Anderson et al., 2002).

1.8.3 Bacterial Contamination in Food Processing and Storage

Pathogenic microorganisms, such as *Clostridium botulinum* and *Staphylococcus aureus*, release powerful toxins that can contaminate food during its preparation and storage. Botulinum toxin can be produced in inadequately canned or stored foods, where the absence of oxygen creates an environment that allows *Clostridium botulinum* spores to develop and generate toxins. Improper handling and storage of food at room temperature can lead to the contamination of Staphylococcal enterotoxins, which promotes bacterial development (Lindström et al., 2010). Frequently impacted food items include preserved vegetables, cured seafood, and prepared foods like deli meats and salads (Peck, 2009).

1.8.4 Toxic Plants and Plant Products

Some plants synthesise natural toxins as a means of self-protection against herbivorous organisms. These substances can pose a risk to human health if consumed. *Ricinus communis*, commonly known as the castor oil plant, is capable of producing ricin, a protein with extremely potent toxicity. Plants belonging to the Solanaceae family, such as potatoes and tomatoes, contain glycoalkaloids such solanine and chaconine (Wink, 2009). Human exposure may arise from consuming inadequately prepared plant products or unintentionally ingesting poisonous plant components. Adhering to appropriate techniques for processing and preparing food is crucial in order to minimise these dangers (Friedman & Levin, 2009).

1.9 Environmental Factors Influencing Biotoxin Production

1.9.1 Climate Conditions

Temperature and Humidity: Warmth and high humidity promote fungal growth and the synthesis of mycotoxins. Climatic regions characterised by tropical and subtropical conditions are especially vulnerable to the occurrence of fungal contamination in crops (Paterson & Lima, 2010).

Climate Change: Climate change can alter the geographic distribution of biotoxin-producing organisms. For example, rising sea temperatures and changing ocean currents can expand the habitats of harmful algal species, increasing the incidence of algal blooms (Glibert et al., 2014; Gimba et al., 2024).

1.9.2 Agricultural Practices

Crop Management: Implementing techniques such as crop rotation, utilisation of resistant cultivars, and appropriate watering methods can mitigate the likelihood of fungal infestation. On the other hand, the practice of growing only one type of crop and relying heavily on chemical fertilisers can make plants more vulnerable to fungal diseases (Leslie & Summerell, 2006).

Pesticide Use: Applying fungicides can effectively manage fungal infections, while excessive usage might result in the development of resistant strains. Implementing integrated pest management (IPM) strategies is crucial for achieving sustained control of mycotoxins (Munkvold, 2003; Abioye et al., 2021).

1.9.3 Food Storage and Handling Conditions

Post-Harvest Practices: Proper drying and storage of crops are crucial to prevent fungal growth and mycotoxin production. High moisture levels in stored grains can lead to rapid fungal colonisation (Sauer et al., 1992).

Temperature Control: Maintaining appropriate storage temperatures is vital for preventing the growth of toxin-producing bacteria in foods. Refrigeration and proper canning techniques can inhibit bacterial growth and toxin formation (Lindström et al., 2010).

1.10 Specific Conditions Leading to Contamination

1.10.1 Pre-Harvest Contamination

Field Conditions: Crops can be contaminated with mycotoxins in the field due to environmental conditions favourable for fungal growth. Rainfall, temperature, and insect damage are key factors influencing pre-harvest contamination (Miller, 1995).

Soil Quality: Soil health and composition can impact the susceptibility of crops to fungal infections. Healthy soil with balanced nutrients and microbial diversity can reduce the risk of mycotoxin contamination (Larkin & Griffin, 2007).

1.10.2 Post-Harvest Contamination

Storage Facilities: The design and maintenance of storage facilities play a critical role in preventing mycotoxin contamination. Ventilation, moisture control, and regular inspection are essential practices (Magan & Aldred, 2007).

Processing Techniques: Food processing methods, such as milling, cooking, and fermentation, can reduce or inactivate certain biotoxins. However, some toxins are resistant to heat and processing, necessitating careful monitoring and control measures (Bryden, 2012).

1.10.3 Distribution and Retail

Supply Chain Management: The integrity of the food supply chain, from farm to table, is crucial for preventing biotoxin contamination. Regular monitoring, testing, and adherence to food safety standards are essential to ensure food safety (Hell & Mutegi, 2011).

Consumer Practices: Educating consumers about proper food handling, storage, and preparation techniques can help reduce the risk of biotoxin exposure. Public awareness campaigns and food safety guidelines play a significant role in minimising risks (Lynch et al., 2006).

1.11 Effects of Biotoxins on Human Health

Biotoxins, due to their varied sources and chemical structures, can have a wide range of toxic effects on human health. These effects depend on several factors including the type of biotoxin, the dose, the route of exposure, and the individual's health status. The primary routes of exposure to biotoxins are through ingestion, inhalation, and skin contact. This section will explore the acute and chronic health effects of various biotoxins, as well as the mechanisms through which they exert their toxic effects.

1.12 Acute Health Effects

Mycotoxins

a. Aflatoxins: Produced by *Aspergillus* species, aflatoxins are potent carcinogens. Acute exposure can lead to aflatoxicosis, characterised by liver damage, haemorrhage, oedema, and possibly death. Symptoms of aflatoxicosis include abdominal pain, vomiting, convulsions, and jaundice (Liu & Wu, 2010).

b. Ochratoxin A: Produced by *Aspergillus* and *Penicillium* species, ochratoxin A can cause acute kidney damage. Symptoms of ochratoxin A poisoning include nausea, vomiting, and abdominal pain. Severe cases can lead to nephropathy and renal failure (Bennett & Klich, 2003).

c. Trichothecenes: Produced by *Fusarium* species, trichothecenes like T-2 toxin can cause a condition known as alimentary toxic aleukia, which is characterised by gastrointestinal haemorrhage, skin inflammation, and severe leukopenia. Symptoms include vomiting, diarrhoea, and bleeding (Pestka, 2010).

Phycotoxins

a. Saxitoxins: These neurotoxins, produced by certain marine dinoflagellates and cyanobacteria, cause paralytic shellfish poisoning. Symptoms include tingling, numbness, headache, dizziness, nausea, and muscular paralysis. In severe cases, respiratory failure and death can occur (Wiese et al., 2010).

b. Ciguatoxins: Produced by *Gambierdiscus toxicus*, ciguatoxins accumulate in fish and cause ciguatera fish poisoning. Symptoms include gastrointestinal distress, cardiovascular abnormalities, and neurological symptoms such as hot-cold temperature reversal, numbness, and muscle pain (Friedman et al., 2008).

c. Brevetoxins: Produced by *Karenia brevis*, these toxins cause neurotoxic shellfish poisoning. Symptoms include gastrointestinal and neurological effects, such as nausea, vomiting, diarrhoea, tingling, and ataxia (Backer et al., 2003).

Bacterial Toxins

a. Botulinum Toxin: Produced by *Clostridium botulinum*, this toxin causes botulism, a potentially fatal illness. Symptoms include muscle paralysis, difficulty swallowing, blurred vision, and respiratory failure. Without treatment, botulism can lead to death due to respiratory muscle paralysis (Peck, 2009).

b. Staphylococcal Enterotoxins: Produced by *Staphylococcus aureus*, these toxins can cause staphylococcal food poisoning. Symptoms include severe nausea, vomiting, abdominal cramps, and diarrhoea. Symptoms typically appear within a few hours of ingestion and last for about a day (Argudín et al., 2010).

1.13 Chronic Health Effects

Mycotoxins

a. Aflatoxins: Chronic exposure to low levels of aflatoxins is a major risk factor for liver cancer, particularly in individuals with hepatitis B or C infections. Aflatoxins can also cause immunosuppression and stunted growth in children (Wild & Gong, 2010).

b. Ochratoxin A: Long-term exposure can lead to chronic kidney disease and an increased risk of urinary tract cancers. Ochratoxin A is also suspected to be a teratogen, potentially causing birth defects (Turner et al., 2009).

c. Fumonisins: Produced by *Fusarium* species, fumonisins are linked to oesophageal cancer in humans. Chronic exposure is also associated with neural tube defects in developing embryos, making them a concern for pregnant women (Marasas et al., 2004).

Phycotoxins

a. Domoic Acid: Produced by *Pseudo-nitzschia* species, domoic acid causes amnesic shellfish poisoning (ASP). Chronic exposure can lead to persistent neurological symptoms such as memory loss and cognitive deficits (Pulido, 2008).

b. Ciguatoxins: Long-term effects of ciguatera poisoning can include chronic fatigue, myalgias, and neurological symptoms that can persist for months or even years after initial exposure (Friedman et al., 2008).

Bacterial Toxins

a. Botulinum Toxin: Although botulism primarily causes acute effects, recovery can be prolonged, requiring extended respiratory support and rehabilitation to regain muscle function (Hughes et al., 1981).

b. Staphylococcal Enterotoxins: While generally causing acute effects, repeated exposure to these toxins can contribute to chronic conditions such as autoimmune diseases and chronic inflammatory conditions due to their superantigen properties (Fraser & Proft, 2008).

1.14 Mechanisms of Toxicity

Mycotoxins

a. Aflatoxins: These toxins are metabolised in the liver to a reactive epoxide form that binds to DNA and proteins, causing mutations and cell death. This mechanism underlies their carcinogenic and hepatotoxic effects (Kensler et al., 2011).

b. Ochratoxin A: Ochratoxin A inhibits protein synthesis and induces oxidative stress, leading to cell damage and death, particularly in kidney cells (Reddy & Bhoola, 2010).

c. Trichothecenes: These toxins inhibit protein synthesis by binding to ribosomes, leading to cell apoptosis and immune suppression (Pestka, 2010).

Phycotoxins

a. Saxitoxins: Saxitoxins block voltage-gated sodium channels in nerve cells, preventing the transmission of nerve impulses, which results in paralysis (Bricelj & Shumway, 1998).

b. Ciguatoxins: These toxins activate voltage-gated sodium channels, causing excessive neuronal firing and neurotransmitter release, leading to neurological and cardiovascular symptoms (Lewis, 2006).

c. Brevetoxins: Brevetoxins also bind to sodium channels, but they cause prolonged channel opening, leading to neuronal hyperexcitability and associated symptoms (Baden et al., 2005).

Bacterial Toxins

a. Botulinum Toxin: This neurotoxin inhibits the release of acetylcholine at neuromuscular junctions by cleaving SNARE proteins, essential for neurotransmitter vesicle fusion, resulting in muscle paralysis (Simpson, 2004).

b. Staphylococcal Enterotoxins: These act as superantigens, activating a large proportion of T-cells non-specifically, leading to massive cytokine release and toxic shock (Balaban & Rasooly, 2000).

1.15 Vulnerable Populations

1.15.1 Infants and Young Children

Infants and young children are particularly vulnerable to biotoxin exposure due to their developing immune and detoxification systems. Mycotoxins, such as aflatoxins, can cause growth retardation and developmental delays in this population (Gong et al., 2004).

1.15.2 Pregnant Women and Developing Fetuses

Pregnant women and their developing fetuses are at increased risk from biotoxins like fumonisins, which can cause neural tube defects, and ochratoxin A, which is teratogenic (Marasas et al., 2004; Turner et al., 2009).

1.15.3 Individuals with Pre-Existing Health Conditions

People with pre-existing liver conditions, such as hepatitis, are more susceptible to the carcinogenic effects of aflatoxins. Similarly, those with weakened immune systems may experience more severe effects from biotoxin exposure (Wild & Gong, 2010).

1.16 Prevention and Mitigation Strategies

1.16.1 Regulatory Standards and Monitoring

Establishing and enforcing regulatory standards for permissible levels of biotoxins in food is crucial. Regular monitoring of food products for biotoxin contamination can help prevent outbreaks (Codex Alimentarius Commission, 2014).

1.16.2 Good Agricultural Practices

Implementing good agricultural practices, such as crop rotation, use of resistant crop varieties, and proper irrigation techniques, can reduce the incidence of biotoxin contamination in the field (Leslie & Summerell, 2006).

1.16.3 Proper Food Handling and Storage

Ensuring proper drying, storage, and handling of food products can prevent the growth of biotoxin-producing organisms. For example, keeping grains dry and stored in well-ventilated conditions can reduce mycotoxin contamination (Magan & Aldred, 2007).

1.16.4 Public Awareness and Education

Educating farmers, food handlers, and consumers about the risks of biotoxins and the importance of preventive measures can help reduce exposure and health impacts (Lynch et al., 2006).

1.17 Detection and Management of Biotoxins

As a result of their potential toxicity and the fact that they are found in a wide variety of food products, biotoxins pose serious challenges to the fields of food safety and public health. When it comes to preventing illnesses that are caused by foodborne pathogens and protecting public health, the detection and management of biotoxins are essential tasks. In the next section, we will explore the methods that are used to identify biotoxins, the regulatory frameworks that govern their management, and the tactics that are utilised to manage and mitigate the dangers that are connected with biotoxins.

1.18 Detection of Biotoxins

1.18.1 Analytical Methods

The detection of biotoxins involves sophisticated analytical methods to identify and quantify these compounds in food and environmental samples. The primary methods include:

a. High-Performance Liquid Chromatography (HPLC): HPLC is extensively utilised for the identification of mycotoxins, including aflatoxins, ochratoxins, and fumonisins. It employs a stationary phase and a mobile phase to separate chemicals, enabling accurate quantification (Zheng et al., 2018).

b. Liquid Chromatography-Mass Spectrometry (LC-MS): LC-MS is a technique that combines the ability to separate substances using liquid chromatography with the ability to detect and analyse them using mass spectrometry. The device has a high level of sensitivity and is capable of detecting numerous biotoxins at the same time. This makes it well suited for analysing complicated matrices (Turner et al., 2009).

c. Gas Chromatography-Mass Spectrometry (GC-MS): Gas chromatography-mass spectrometry is employed to analyse volatile and semi-volatile biotoxins. It is especially beneficial for identifying marine biotoxins such as domoic acid and saxitoxin (Yasumoto & Murata, 1993).

d. Enzyme-Linked Immunosorbent Assay (ELISA): ELISA is a widely used immunoassay technique for identifying biotoxins. It is favoured for its simplicity, specificity, and capacity to handle huge sample quantities. It is frequently employed for the detection of mycotoxins and phycotoxins (Usleber et al., 2002).

1.18.2 Biosensors

a. Biosensors: Biosensors are analytical devices that combine a biological sensing element with a transducer to detect biotoxins. They offer rapid, on-site detection with high sensitivity. Common biosensors include those based on antibodies, nucleic acids, and enzymes (Perez et al., 2013).

b. Surface Plasmon Resonance (SPR): SPR biosensors detect changes in refractive index near the sensor surface when biotoxins bind to immobilised ligands. SPR is used for real-time, label-free detection of biotoxins such as mycotoxins and marine toxins (Rich & Myszka, 2008).

1.18.3 Molecular Techniques

a. Polymerase Chain Reaction (PCR): PCR-based methods are used to detect genes encoding biotoxin production in microorganisms. Real-time PCR (qPCR) allows for quantitative detection and monitoring of toxin-producing organisms in food and environmental samples (Niessen, 2007).
b. Next-Generation Sequencing (NGS): NGS technologies can provide comprehensive profiles of microbial communities, identifying potential biotoxin-producing species and their abundance in various samples (Tournas et al., 2016).

1.18.4 Rapid Test Kits

a. Lateral Flow Assays (LFA): LFAs are simple, portable devices for the rapid detection of biotoxins. They are based on immunochromatographic principles and are widely used for mycotoxins and bacterial toxins in field settings (Brandon et al., 2003).

1.19 Management and Mitigation Strategies

1.19.1 Pre-Harvest Interventions

a. Agricultural Practices: Implementing good agricultural practices (GAP) can significantly reduce biotoxin contamination in crops. These practices include crop rotation, proper irrigation, use of resistant varieties, and timely harvesting to prevent fungal growth and mycotoxin production (Leslie & Summerell, 2006).
b. Biological Control: Utilising biological control agents, such as non-toxigenic strains of fungi, can inhibit the growth of toxigenic fungi and reduce mycotoxin contamination. For example, non-toxigenic strains of *Aspergillus flavus* can outcompete toxigenic strains and reduce aflatoxin levels (Dorner & Cole, 2002).

1.19.2 Post-Harvest Interventions

a. Storage Conditions: Proper storage conditions, including low moisture levels, adequate ventilation, and temperature control, are critical in preventing the growth of biotoxin-producing organisms. Storage facilities should be regularly inspected and maintained to prevent contamination (Magan & Aldred, 2007).

b. Decontamination Techniques: Various physical, chemical, and biological methods can be used to decontaminate food products. These include sorting and cleaning, thermal treatment, irradiation, and the use of adsorbents and detoxifying agents (Kabak et al., 2006).

1.19.3 Food Processing Interventions

a. Processing Methods: Certain food processing methods can reduce biotoxin levels in food products. These methods include milling, fermentation, roasting, and extrusion. Processing parameters should be optimised to maximise biotoxin reduction while maintaining food quality (Karlovsky et al., 2016).

b. Additives and Preservatives: The use of additives and preservatives can inhibit the growth of biotoxin-producing organisms and reduce biotoxin levels. For example, organic acids and antifungal agents can be used to control mould growth in stored grains (Bullerman & Bianchini, 2007).

1.19.4 Regulatory and Public Health Interventions

a. Regulatory Compliance: Ensuring compliance with regulatory standards for biotoxins through regular inspections and testing is crucial for food safety. Regulatory agencies should work closely with food producers and processors to enforce standards and provide guidance on best practices (van Egmond & Jonker, 2004).

b. Public Health Education: Educating farmers, food handlers, and consumers about the risks of biotoxins and the importance of preventive measures can reduce exposure and health impacts. Public health campaigns and training programs can raise awareness and promote safe practices (Lynch et al., 2006).

1.19.5 Emerging Technologies and Future Directions

a. Nanotechnology: Nanotechnology offers innovative solutions for the detection and mitigation of biotoxins. Nanomaterials can be used to develop highly sensitive biosensors, enhance food packaging materials, and create novel decontamination methods (He et al., 2019).

b. Genomic and Metabolomic Approaches: Advances in genomics and metabolomics can provide deeper insights into the mechanisms of biotoxin production and the interactions between biotoxins and their hosts. These approaches can lead to the development of new strategies for detecting and controlling biotoxins (Tang et al., 2018).

1.20 Conclusion

The widespread occurrence of biotoxins in food is a substantial obstacle to worldwide food safety and public health. These naturally occurring poisonous chemicals, produced by diverse organisms such as fungi, algae, and bacteria, can cause severe harm to human health, encompassing acute poisoning and chronic diseases, including cancer, over an extended period of time. A comprehensive approach is required to detect, monitor, and mitigate the complexity and diversity of biotoxins in order to assure food safety.

Effectively addressing the threat of biotoxins necessitates a collaborative and coordinated endeavour involving researchers, politicians, industry partners, and public health specialists. Cooperation and the exchange of information are crucial for enhancing our understanding and capacities in the management of biotoxins. Education and awareness campaigns play a crucial role in empowering farmers, food handlers, and consumers to implement measures that reduce the likelihood of biotoxin contamination.

Ensuring food safety in the context of biotoxins is an ongoing and dynamic process. It demands continuous vigilance, innovation, and adaptation to evolving challenges. By integrating scientific advancements with practical interventions and regulatory oversight, we can mitigate the risks associated with biotoxins and safeguard public health for future generations.

References

Abioye, O. P., Ijah, U. J. J., Aransiola, S. A., Auta, S. H., & Ojeba, M. I. (2021). Bioremediation of toxic pesticides in soil using microbial products. In R. Prasad, S. C., Nayak, R. N., Kharwar, & N. K. Dubey (Eds.), *Mycoremediation and Environmental Sustainability*. Fungal Biology. Springer. https://doi.org/10.1007/978-3-030-54422-5_1.

Anderson, D. M., Glibert, P. M., & Burkholder, J. M. (2002). Harmful algal blooms and eutrophication: Nutrient sources, composition, and consequences. *Estuaries*, 25(4), 704–726. https://doi.org/10.1007/BF02804901

Aransiola, S. A., Akinsola, R. O., Abioye, O. P., & Maddela, N. R. (Eds.). (2024). *Emerging Contaminants in Food and Food Products* (1st ed.). CRC Press. Taylor and Francis Group. https://www.routledge.com/Emerging-Contaminants-in-Food-and-Food-Products/Aransiola-Akinsola-Abioye-Maddela/p/book/9781032556307

Argudín, M. A., Mendoza, M. C., & Rodicio, M. R. (2010). Food poisoning and Staphylococcus aureus enterotoxins. *Toxins*, 2(7), 1751–1773 https://doi.org/10.3390/toxins2071751

Audi, J., Belson, M., Patel, M., Schier, J., & Osterloh, J. (2005). Ricin poisoning: A comprehensive review. *JAMA*, 294(18), 2342–2351. https://doi.org/10.1001/jama.294.18.2342

Backer, L. C., Fleming, L. E., Rowan, A., Cheng, Y. S., Benson, J., Pierce, R. H.,. . . Baden, D. G. (2003). Recreational exposure to aerosolized brevetoxins during Florida red tide events. *Harmful Algae*, 2(1), 19–28. https://doi.org/10.1016/S1568-9883(03)00005-2

Balaban, N., & Rasooly, A. (2000). Staphylococcal enterotoxins. *International Journal of Food Microbiology*, 61(1), 1–10. https://doi.org/10.1016/S0168-1605(00)00377-9

Bennett, J. W., & Klich, M. (2003). Mycotoxins. *Clinical Microbiology Reviews*, 16(3), 497–516. https://doi.org/10.1128/CMR.16.3.497-516.2003

Brandon, D. L., & Price, R. L. (2003). Use of immunoassays in food testing. *Food Control*, 14(6), 419–423. https://doi.org/10.1016/S0956-7135(03)00014-4

Bricelj, V. M., & Shumway, S. E. (1998). Paralytic shellfish toxins in bivalve molluscs: Occurrence, transfer kinetics, and biotransformation. *Reviews in Fisheries Science*, 6(4), 315–383. https://doi.org/10.1080/10641269891314294

Bryden, W. L. (2012). Mycotoxin contamination of the feed supply chain: Implications for animal productivity and feed security. *Animal Feed Science and Technology*, 173(1–2), 134–158. https://doi.org/10.1016/j.anifeedsci.2011.12.014

Bullerman, L. B., & Bianchini, A. (2007). Stability of mycotoxins during food processing. *International Journal of Food Microbiology*, 119(1–2), 140–146. https://doi.org/10.1016/j.ijfoodmicro.2007.07.035

Codex Alimentarius Commission. (2014). *Codex Alimentarius: General Standard for Contaminants and Toxins in Food and Feed*. FAO/WHO.

Colegate, S. M., & Dorling, P. R. (1994). *Plant-Associated Toxins: Agricultural, Phytochemical and Ecological Aspects*. CAB International.

Dorner, J. W., & Cole, R. J. (2002). Effect of application of nontoxigenic strains of Aspergillus flavus and A. parasiticus on subsequent aflatoxin contamination of peanuts in storage. *Journal of Stored Products Research*, 38(4), 329–339. https://doi.org/10.1016/S0022-474X(01)00038-1

Etheridge, S. M. (2010). Paralytic shellfish poisoning: Seafood safety and human health perspectives. *Toxicon*, 56(2), 108–122. https://doi.org/10.1016/j.toxicon.2009.12.013

Flewelling, L. J., Naar, J. P., Abbott, J. P., Baden, D. G., Barros, N. B., Doucette, G. J.,. . . Van Dolah, F. M. (2005). Red tides and marine mammal mortalities. *Nature*, 435(7043), 755–756. https://doi.org/10.1038/nature435755a

Fraser, J. D., & Proft, T. (2008). The bacterial superantigen and superantigen-like proteins. *Immunological Reviews*, 225(1), 226–243. https://doi.org/10.1111/j.1600-065X.2008.00681.x

Friedman, M., & Levin, C. E. (2009). Analysis and biological activities of potato glycoalkaloids, calystegine alkaloids, phenolic compounds, and anthocyanins. *Advances in Potato Chemistry and Technology*, 247–270. https://doi.org/10.1016/B978-0-12-374349-7.00010-8

Friedman, M. A., Fernandez, M., Backer, L. C., Dickey, R. W., Bernstein, J., Schrank, K.,. . . Azziz-Baumgartner, E. (2008). An updated review of ciguatera fish poisoning: Clinical, epidemiological, environmental, and public health management. *Marine Drugs*, 6(3), 456–479. https://doi.org/10.3390/md6030456

Friedman, M. A., Fernandez, M., Backer, L. C., Dickey, R. W., Bernstein, J., Schrank, K.,. . . Hemphill, J. B. (2017). An updated review of ciguatera fish poisoning: Clinical, epidemiological, environmental, and public health management. *Marine Drugs*, 15(3), 72. https://doi.org/10.3390/md15030072

Gimba, U. A., Aransiola, S. A., Oyewole, O. A., & Maddela, N. R. (2024). Marine Greens: Roles in climate change and global warming mitigations. In S. A. Aransiola, O. A. Oyewole, N. R. Maddela, U. J. J. Ijah, & B. Manjunatha (Eds.), *Marine Greens: Environmental, Agricultural, Industrial and Biomedical Applications*. CRC Press. ISBN: 9781032438856. https://www.routledge.com/Marine-Greens-Environmental-Agricultural-Industrial-and-Biomedical-Applications/Aransiola-Oyewole-Maddela-Josiah-Ijah-Manjunatha/p/book/9781032438856

Glibert, P. M., Icarus Allen, J., Artioli, Y., Beusen, A. H., Bouwman, L., Harle, J.,. . . Holmes, R. (2014). Vulnerability of coastal ecosystems to changes in harmful algal bloom distribution in response to climate change: Projections based on model analysis. *Global Change Biology*, 20(12), 3845–3858. https://doi.org/10.1111/gcb.12662

Gong, Y. Y., Hounsa, A., Egal, S., Turner, P. C., Sutcliffe, A. E., Hall, A. J.,. . . Wild, C. P. (2004). Postweaning exposure to aflatoxin results in impaired child growth: A longitudinal study in Benin, West Africa. *Environmental Health Perspectives*, 112(13), 1334–1338. https://doi.org/10.1289/ehp.6954

Hallegraeff, G. M. (2003). Harmful algal blooms: A global overview. In G. M. Hallegraeff, D. M. Anderson, & A. D. Cembella (Eds.), *Manual on Harmful Marine Microalgae* (pp. 25–49). UNESCO.

He, Q., Zhang, Z., & Li, L. (2019). Nanomaterials for the removal of biotoxins from food and water: A review. *Nanomaterials*, 9(8), 1110. https://doi.org/10.3390/nano9081110

Hell, K., & Mutegi, C. (2011). Aflatoxin control and prevention strategies in maize for sub-Saharan Africa. *Journal of Plant Pathology*, 93(4), 1–10. https://www.jstor.org/stable/41998665

Hughes, J. M., Blumenthal, J. R., Merson, M. H., Lombard, G. L., Dowell, V. R., & Gangarosa, E. J. (1981). Clinical features of types A and B food-borne botulism. *Annals of Internal Medicine*, 95(4), 442–445. https://doi.org/10.7326/0003-4819-95-4-442

Kabak, B., Dobson, A. D., & Var, I. (2006). Strategies to prevent mycotoxin contamination of food and animal feed: A review. *Critical Reviews in Food Science and Nutrition*, 46(8), 593–619. https://doi.org/10.1080/10408390500436185

Karlovsky, P., Suman, M., Berthiller, F., Meester, J., Miraglia, M., Dong, M. W.,. . . Binder, E. M. (2016). Impact of food processing and detoxification treatments on mycotoxin contamination. *Mycotoxin Research*, 32(4), 179–205. https://doi.org/10.1007/s12550-016-0257-7

Kensler, T. W., Roebuck, B. D., Wogan, G. N., & Groopman, J. D. (2011). Aflatoxin: A 50-year odyssey of mechanistic and translational toxicology. *Toxicological Sciences*, 120(Suppl 1), S28–S48. https://doi.org/10.1093/toxsci/kfq283

Landsberg, J. H. (2002). The effects of harmful algal blooms on aquatic organisms. *Reviews in Fisheries Science*, 10(2), 113–390. https://doi.org/10.1080/20026491051695

Larkin, R. P., & Griffin, T. S. (2007). Control of soilborne potato diseases using Brassica green manures. *Crop Protection*, 26(7), 1067–1077. https://doi.org/10.1016/j.cropro.2006.10.004

Leslie, J. F., & Summerell, B. A. (2006). *The Fusarium Laboratory Manual*. Blackwell Publishing.

Lewis, R. J. (2006). Ciguatera: Australian perspectives on a global problem. *Toxicon*, 48(7), 799–809. https://doi.org/10.1016/j.toxicon.2006.07.016

Lindström, M., Korkeala, H., & Lindström, M. (2010). Laboratory diagnostics of botulism. *Clinical Microbiology Reviews*, 23(2), 298–314. https://doi.org/10.1128/CMR.00070-09

Liu, Y., & Wu, F. (2010). Global burden of aflatoxin-induced hepatocellular carcinoma: A risk assessment. *Environmental Health Perspectives*, 118(6), 818–824. https://doi.org/10.1289/ehp.0901388

Lynch, M. F., Tauxe, R. V., & Hedberg, C. W. (2006). The growing burden of foodborne outbreaks due to contaminated fresh produce: Risks and opportunities. *Epidemiology and Infection*, 134(3), 551–560. https://doi.org/10.1017/S0950268806005408

Magan, N., & Aldred, D. (2007). Post-harvest control strategies: Minimizing mycotoxins in the food chain. *International Journal of Food Microbiology*, 119(1–2), 131–139. https://doi.org/10.1016/j.ijfoodmicro.2007.07.034

Marasas, W. F. O., Riley, R. T., Hendricks, K. A., Stevens, V. L., Sadler, T. W., Gelineau-van Waes, J.,. . . Merrill Jr, A. H. (2004). Fumonisins disrupt sphingolipid metabolism, folate transport, and neural tube development in embryo culture and in vivo: A potential risk factor for human neural tube defects among populations consuming fumonisin-contaminated maize. *The Journal of Nutrition*, 134(4), 711–716. https://doi.org/10.1093/jn/134.4.711

Marin, S., Ramos, A. J., Cano-Sancho, G., & Sanchis, V. (2013). Mycotoxins: Occurrence, toxicology, and exposure assessment. *Food and Chemical Toxicology*, 60, 218–237. https://doi.org/10.1016/j.fct.2013.07.047

Miller, J. D. (1995). Fungi and mycotoxins in grain: Implications for stored product research. *Journal of Stored Products Research*, 31(1), 1–16. https://doi.org/10.1016/0022-474X(94)00039-W

Munkvold, G. P. (2003). Cultural and genetic approaches to managing mycotoxins in maize. *Annual Review of Phytopathology*, 41(1), 99–116. https://doi.org/10.1146/annurev.phyto.41.052002.095510

Paterson, R. R., & Lima, N. (2010). How will climate change affect mycotoxins in food? *Food Research International*, 43(7), 1902–1914. https://doi.org/10.1016/j.foodres.2009.07.010

Peck, M. W. (2009). Biology and genomic analysis of Clostridium botulinum. *Advances in Microbial Physiology*, 55, 183–265. https://doi.org/10.1016/S0065-2911(09)05503-9

Perez, J. G., Bazin, I., & Jouanneau, S. (2013). Aptamer-based surface plasmon resonance biosensors for highly sensitive detection of mycotoxins in food. *Analytical Chemistry*, 85(11), 5077–5082. https://doi.org/10.1021/ac400601f

Pestka, J. J. (2010). Deoxynivalenol: Toxicity, mechanisms and animal health risks. *Animal Feed Science and Technology*, 163(3–4), 74–79. https://doi.org/10.1016/j.anifeedsci.2010.07.003

Pulido, O. M. (2008). Domoic acid toxicologic pathology: A review. *Marine Drugs*, 6(2), 180–219. https://doi.org/10.3390/md6020180

Reddy, L., & Bhoola, K. D. (2010). Ochratoxins—Food contaminants: Impact on human health. *Toxins*, 2(4), 771–779. https://doi.org/10.3390/toxins2040771

Sauer, D. B., Meronuck, R. A., & Christensen, C. M. (1992). Microflora. In D. B. Sauer (Ed.), *Storage of Cereal Grains and Their Products* (pp. 313–340). American Association of Cereal Chemists.

Schmid-Hempel, P., & Frank, S. A. (2007). Pathogenesis, virulence, and infective dose. *PLOS Pathogens*, 3(10), e147. https://doi.org/10.1371/journal.ppat.0030147

Simpson, L. L. (2004). Identification of the major steps in botulinum toxin action. Annual *Review of Pharmacology and Toxicology*, 44, 167–193. https://doi.org/10.1146/annurev.pharmtox.44.101802.121554

Stoev, S. D. (2013). Food safety and mycotoxins. In A. N. M. Iqbal & M. S. M. Khalid (Eds.), *Mycotoxin and Food Safety in Developing Countries* (pp. 1–30). InTech. https://doi.org/10.5772/52980

Tang, J., Liu, R., Zhang, Y., & Li, J. (2018). The role of omics technologies in food safety: Metabolomics and beyond. *Food Reviews International*, 34(1), 63–80. https://doi.org/10.1080/87559129.2016.1225025

Turner, N. W., Subrahmanyam, S., & Piletsky, S. A. (2009). Analytical methods for determination of mycotoxins: A review. *Analytica Chimica Acta*, 632(2), 168–180. https://doi.org/10.1016/j.aca.2008.11.010

van Egmond, H. P., & Jonker, M. A. (2004). Worldwide regulations on aflatoxins—the situation in 2002. *Journal of Toxicology—Toxin Reviews*, 23(2–3), 273–293. https://doi.org/10.1081/TXR-200027844

Wiese, M., D'Agostino, P. M., Mihali, T. K., Moffitt, M. C., & Neilan, B. A. (2010). Neurotoxic alkaloids: Saxitoxin and its analogs. *Marine Drugs*, 8(7), 2185–2211. https://doi.org/10.3390/md8072185

Wild, C. P., & Gong, Y. Y. (2010). Mycotoxins and human disease: A largely ignored global health issue. *Carcinogenesis*, 31(1), 71–82. https://doi.org/10.1093/carcin/bgp264

Wink, M. (2009). Mode of action and toxicology of plant toxins and poisonous plants. *Mitteilungen Klosterneuburg*, 59, 39–48.

Wu, F. (2010). Mycotoxin reduction in Bt corn: Potential economic, health, and regulatory impacts. *Transgenic Research*, 19(1), 123–140. https://doi.org/10.1007/s11248-009-9301-6

Yasumoto, T., & Murata, M. (1993). Marine toxins. *Chemical Reviews*, 93(5), 1897–1909. https://doi.org/10.1021/cr00022a008

Zheng, M., Yin, H., Li, Z., Zhong, L., Zhang, J., Yu, L.,. . .Tang, Z. (2018). Development and application of a multi-mycotoxin method for the determination of mycotoxins in cereal grains by liquid chromatography-tandem mass spectrometry. *Food Chemistry*, 245, 1233–1242. https://doi.org/10.1016/j.foodchem.2017.11.081

2

Distribution of Microbial Toxins in Foods

Makinde O.M., Ayedun J., Akinboboye O.A., Fagbemi K., and Ikhimiukor O.O.

2.1 Introduction

Toxins generated by bacteria, fungus, and other microorganisms are known as microbial toxins. They represent serious risks to agriculture, the environment, and human health. These poisons can cause acute poisoning as well as long-term health problems. Exotoxins, which are produced by Gram-positive bacteria as well as Gram-negative ones, and endotoxins, which are usually produced by Gram-negative bacteria, are the two main categories of bacterial toxins (Alizadeh et al., 2018). However, fungi like *Aspergillus, Fusarium,* and *Penicillium* can create fungal toxins, sometimes referred to as mycotoxins, which can contaminate a variety of crops and endanger human health and food safety (Eltariki et al., 2018; Ezekiel et al., 2013; Makinde et al., 2023).

During infections, microbes use toxins as weapons to harm hosts and get past their defenses. Because they interfere with host cells and immunological responses, toxins are essential in the pathophysiology of many microbial diseases (Brown et al., 2021). For instance, Candidalysin, a cytolytic peptide toxin secreted by *Candida albicans*, damages host cells and eludes immune recognition, adding to the fungus's pathogenicity (Chen et al., 2021b; Richardson et al., 2022). Creating efficient plans to fight microbial illnesses requires an understanding of the mechanisms of action of these toxins.

One class of fungal toxin that is well known for its detrimental impact on the well-being of humans and animals is mycotoxin. These poisons, which are produced by molds like *Fusarium* and *Aspergillus*, can contaminate feed and food supplies and have detrimental effects on human health (Awuchi et al., 2021; Plewa-Tutaj et al., 2024). *Aspergillus* species produce aflatoxins, one of the most widely recognized mycotoxins that pose a serious threat to food safety due to their strong carcinogenic properties (Afolabi et al., 2015; Dahal et al., 2021; Ezekiel et al., 2020; Sombie et al., 2018; Amobonye et al., 2023). To protect the public's health, contamination by mycotoxin in agricultural products must be controlled and minimized.

DOI: 10.1201/9781003500605-3

Microbial toxins not only have direct toxic effects but also have the ability to alter host immune responses and make infectious pathogens more dangerous. Certain toxins generated by fungus, such *Aspergillus fumigatus*'s gliotoxin, have been connected to increased virulence and harm to host cells (Guruceaga et al., 2021). These toxins demonstrate the complex relationship between microbial toxins as well as host defenses since they have the ability to alter immune signaling pathways in the host, elude immune surveillance, and encourage the spread of infections.

The variety of fungal toxins and their intricate relationships with host species highlight how crucial it is to understand the biosynthetic processes and regulatory mechanisms involved in toxin synthesis. Toxins and pharmaceuticals are examples of fungal secondary metabolites that are controlled by transcription factors as well as biosynthetic gene clusters (Wang et al., 2021). Gaining knowledge of these regulatory networks can help create new antifungal treatments and shed light on how fungus produce toxins over time.

Crop resistance to mycotoxin contamination and fungal infections can be influenced by environmental factors including temperature and CO_2 levels. A frequent mycotoxin present in cereals, deoxynivalenol, is produced by fungi like *Fusarium graminearum*, and its growth can be impacted by changes in climate (Hay et al., 2021; Mesterhazy et al., 2022). Food security and sustainable agriculture depend on tracking and forecasting how fungal infections and mycotoxin contamination will be affected by climate change.

Certain strains of Streptomyces, for example, have demonstrated potential as biocontrol agents because they can stop plant diseases like *Fusarium graminearum* from growing and can lower the amount of mycotoxin contamination in cereals (Colombo et al., 2020). These advantageous microbes have the ability to outcompete harmful fungus, generate antifungal substances, and strengthen plant defenses against fungal diseases. Utilizing biocontrol agents' potential provides environmentally friendly and long-lasting ways to lessen the effects of microbial toxins on agricultural crops.

Additionally, microbial toxins can influence the composition of microbial communities and ecosystems. Bacteriophages, often known as phages, are viruses that infect bacteria and have the ability to affect community dynamics and microbial interactions (Grigson et al., 2023). Clarifying the intricate interactions between microbes in diverse settings requires an understanding of the function of microbial toxins in microbial ecology.

In fact, microbial poisons pose a serious threat to human health, agriculture, and food safety, among other areas. Creating efficient plans to lessen the effects of these toxins requires an understanding of their diversity, mechanisms of action, detection techniques, and regulatory pathways. The protection of public health and the environment can be ensured by improving the capacity to identify, prevent, and manage microbial toxins through the utilization of cutting-edge technology, multidisciplinary research methodologies, and sustainable practices.

2.2 Microbial Toxins in Food

Due to their potential to cause foodborne diseases and outbreaks, microbial toxins in food pose a serious threat to public health. Because it is linked to food contamination and foodborne illnesses, one subset of bacteria called Shiga toxin-producing *Escherichia coli* (STEC) is especially dangerous (Kotun et al., 2024; Makinde et al., 2022; Petrucci et al., 2022). Numerous foodborne illnesses are caused by these bacteria as well as other microbial toxins, including those generated by *Clostridium botulinum, Bacillus cereus,* and *Clostridium perfringens* (Bowe et al., 2022; Fayyaz et al., 2022; Mellou et al., 2019). These bacteria are a constant concern in the food supply chain because their toxins may survive the harsh conditions involved in food processing (Moi et al., 2022). A primary source of infections and foodborne illnesses is foodborne microorganisms, especially those that release toxins as a virulence factor (Banerji et al., 2021). Hospitalization and financial losses are among the serious health effects that can arise from eating tainted food that contains pathogenic bacteria and associated toxins (Yousef et al., 2021).

Controlling the dangers related to microbial toxins in food requires effective detection and management methods. Assessing the pathogenic potential and dangers associated with bacteria such as *Bacillus cereus* in foodborne disorders requires an understanding of their genetic diversity and capacity to produce toxins (Miller et al., 2018).

Clinical recommendations are necessary for the diagnosis and treatment of foodborne botulism, which is a serious hazard that arises from consuming contaminated foods (Rao, 2021). The possibility of bioterrorism incidents involving the deliberate tainting of food to expose toxicants emphasizes the significance of alertness and readiness in handling such risks (Rao, 2021). In order to better understand the trends and patterns of foodborne illnesses and to help develop strategies for their prevention and management, epidemiological research on foodborne outbreaks offer useful data (Franklin et al., 2020).

Food safety and public health are complicatedly challenged by microbial poisons in food. In order to reduce the hazards associated with these poisons, it is essential to comprehend their sources, detection techniques, genetic variety, and management strategies. Reducing the frequency of foodborne illnesses brought on by microbial toxins and guaranteeing the safety of the food supply chain require ongoing research, technical developments, and surveillance activities.

2.3 Common Sources of Microbial Toxins

Numerous organisms and substances that can seriously endanger human health and the natural environment are common sources of microbial toxins.

1. **Bacterial toxins**: Pathogenic bacteria like *Escherichia coli* as well as *Clostridium botulinum* frequently produce bacterial toxins including Shiga and botulinum toxins (Sivamaruthi et al., 2018). It is crucial to keep an eye out for and take precautions against bacterial toxin contamination in food and water supplies since these toxins have the potential to cause serious illnesses, such as foodborne illnesses and botulism (Franklin et al., 2020; Gavage et al., 2021).
2. **Mycotoxins** are another common source of microbial toxins present in a variety of food products. They are produced by fungi such as *Aspergillus* and *Fusarium* species (Awuchi et al., 2021; Ezekiel et al., 2018; Ezekiel, Kraak, et al., 2020; Wang et al., 2021). Among the common mycotoxins that can contaminate crops and seriously endanger consumer health are aflatoxins, fumonisins, and ochratoxin A (Plewa-Tutaj et al., 2024). To protect public health and food safety, mycotoxin contamination in agricultural products must be controlled (Liu et al., 2022).
3. **Algal toxins**: According to Kumar et al. (2019), algae can also create toxins called phycotoxins, which can infect seafood and be harmful to human health. One phycotoxin that can result in paralytic shellfish poisoning is tetrodotoxin, a strong neurotoxin present in some marine creatures (Biessy et al., 2020). In order to safeguard customers and avoid foodborne illnesses, it is essential to monitor and control the amounts of phycotoxins in seafood.
4. **Cyanotoxins**: In freshwater environments, cyanobacteria produce cyanotoxins, which can be produced and distributed by microbial toxins depending on environmental conditions (Kumar et al., 2019). Drinking water sources can become contaminated with microcystins, hepatotoxins that are produced by cyanobacteria during toxic algal blooms, which can be damaging to human health (Manheim et al., 2018). Ensuring public health requires regular monitoring of water quality and the implementation of initiatives aimed at mitigating the effects of cyanotoxin contamination.

Microbial toxins can come from a range of sources and affect human health and the environment in different ways. Toxins have sources, mechanisms of action, and detection techniques that must be understood in order to create strategies that effectively reduce their effects and protect public health.

2.4 Importance of Microbial Toxins in Food

Microbial toxins in food are a serious concern because of their capacity to cause diseases as well as deaths (Fletcher & Netzel, 2020). These toxins, arising from different sources such as bacteria, fungi, algae, and plants, represent a hazard to food safety as well as public health (Bartholomew et al., 2021). Foodborne epidemics have been linked to the presence of microbial toxins in food, which has raised attention on monitoring and tracking of these toxins (Russini et al., 2022). It is crucial to identify and control microbial toxins since some of them have strong toxic effects even when at low concentrations, and when they coexist in the environment, they can cause additive or synergistic toxicity (Li et al., 2019).

Microorganisms also release toxins during handling of food, which can withstand processing and endanger consumers (Silva et al., 2020). Foodborne outbreaks linked to a variety of food categories, including poultry, meats, fruits, vegetables, fish, milk, and dairy products, are caused by major foodborne pathogens such as *Salmonella enterica, Listeria monocytogenes*, and *Escherichia coli* (Abdelhaseib et al., 2019).

Food and feed can get contaminated with mycotoxins, a type of microbial toxin generated by fungi that can be harmful to the health of humans as well as animals. These toxins, which include alternariol, patulin, and aflatoxin, can lower the overall quality of agricultural products and have negative health impacts (Bartholomew et al., 2021).

Ecosystems, water quality, and human health can all be impacted by harmful algal bloom toxins produced by cyanobacteria, such as microcystin as well as anatoxin (Lad et al., 2022). Food safety organizations and businesses need to exercise caution because these poisons are found in seafood and waterways (Gaiani et al., 2019).

Microbial toxins can have significant impacts beyond food safety, altering different aspects of health. Toxins such as β-N-methylamino-L-alanine (BMAA) have been associated with diseases such as Parkinson's disease, which emphasizes the importance of keeping an eye on their presence in food (Esteves et al., 2023). Furthermore, food-derived uremic toxins have been linked to chronic kidney illness, which emphasizes how critical it is to understand the origins and effects of these toxins (Lauriola et al., 2023). The intricate relationship among gut microbiota, microbial toxins, and human health is demonstrated by the way in which toxins such as triclosan modify gut microbial communities and may have an impact on the health of the host (Mahalak et al., 2020). Eating food contaminated with bacteria such as *Salmonella* spp., *Shigella* spp., *Escherichia coli*, and *Staphylococcus aureus* can cause serious diseases and even death, which highlights the urgent need for efficient detection and preventive methods (Odo et al., 2021). Toxin exposure is linked to both animal and human health, as evidenced by the serious risks that domestic animals face from toxins found in vegetation, feed, including water sources (Nagy, 2024).

Furthermore, using microbial pesticides and toxins for agricultural purposes can have an adverse effect on ecosystems and the health of the environment, which highlights the need of sustainable pest management techniques (Oliveira-Filho & Grisolia, 2022). A deeper understanding of these communities of microbes and their influences is imperative in light of the potential health effects of environmental pollutants, such as airborne microbial aerosols (Rao et al., 2020).

It is essential to understand the mechanisms of action, detection techniques, and management of microbial toxins in food to guarantee food safety, safeguard the public's health, and reduce the hazards connected with toxin exposure. Through investigating the origins, consequences, and interplay of these pollutants, scientists can devise approaches to reduce their influence on the well-being of people, animals, and the ecosystem. To address the issues raised by microbial toxins within the food chain and elsewhere, vigilance, research, and regulatory actions are crucial.

2.5 Mechanisms of Toxin Production

Examining the complex systems that control the synthesis as well as release of these toxic compounds is crucial to comprehending the mechanisms of toxin generation in different organisms. Toxin production is the result of a complex interaction between environmental, genetic, and regulatory factors that eventually lead to the expression of virulent factors. According to Wydau-Dematteis et al. (2018), *Clostridium difficile* uses a TcdE-dependent secretion mechanism to guarantee ample toxin synthesis while maintaining cell viability. This tactic emphasizes how infections have evolved to maximize the release of toxins in order to survive and proliferate inside their host environment.

The genetic factors that influence toxin production have been clarified by the identification of a set of core genes that are directly involved in toxin production in cyanobacteria, as well as tailor genes implicated in toxin transformation (Zhang et al., 2018). The identification of these genes sheds light on the molecular mechanism that these organisms use to produce toxins. Additionally, the variation in toxin production between strains of *Alexandrium minutum* as well as *Alexandrium pacificum* can be attributed to the presence of genetic isoforms of toxin-related genes as well as their control via transcriptional along with post-transcriptional mechanisms (Geffroy et al., 2021).

The intricate relationship between light, photosynthesis, phosphate availability, and toxin formation is essential for toxin manufacture in dinoflagellates, including *Alexandrium catenella* (Tse et al., 2020). This highlights how important environmental variables are in controlling these species' generation of toxins. Further elucidating the molecular mechanisms underpinning toxin manufacturing in poisonous strains is the overexpression of particular proteins, such as the peridinin-chlorophyll a-binding protein, under various conditions (Lee et al., 2023).

The generation of β-toxin in *Staphylococcus aureus* is controlled through an active lysogeny mechanism, underscoring the complex regulatory systems that govern the development of toxins in bacteria (Tran et al., 2019). This regulatory system emphasizes how crucial it is to comprehend how bacterial physiology as well as toxin production interact. The RNA-binding protein CsrA regulates the release of the toxin ColicinE2 in *Escherichia coli*, highlighting the significance of post-transcriptional regulation in toxin production (Götz et al., 2018).

The control over the synthesis of toxins is not exclusive to bacteria; it also applies to fungi. The inhibition of toxin synthesis in *Macrophomina phaseolina*, the fungus that causes charcoal rot disease in soybeans, under specific circumstances points to the existence of a regulatory mechanism that modifies toxin expression in response to environmental cues (Abbas et al., 2019). Through this adaptive reaction, the fungus is able to adjust the amount of poison it produces in response to the environment, which increases its likelihood of survival and pathogenicity.

The generation of toxins is regulated by a complex interplay of genetic, regulatory, and environmental factors, which determine the synthesis and excretion of toxins in different organisms. Comprehending these complex mechanisms is essential to formulating focused approaches to reduce the deleterious consequences of toxins and combat the pathogenicity of toxin-producing organisms.

2.6 Current Trends and Emerging Concerns with Microbial Toxins

2.6.1 Mycotoxins

Future plans must focus on the need to control fungal contamination and mycotoxin generation throughout the whole food chain, beginning from manufacturing until the food reaches the consumers, due to the prevalence of mycotoxin contamination. It is important to consider the potential existence of hidden mycotoxins as well as the combined harmful effects of many mycotoxins present at the same time in food (Ezekiel et al., 2019; Penagos-Tabares et al., 2023; Yu & Pedroso, 2023). The development of techniques that quantify masked mycotoxins is crucial, and conventional screening approaches that are dependable, practical, quick, and affordable are required (Agriopoulou et al., 2020). The potential toxicity of masked mycotoxins and mycotoxin by-products has to be further investigated via exposure assessments, safety evaluations, and research. To remove mycotoxins from food as much as possible, techniques that incorporate an integrated decontamination strategy must be developed, along with further study on the safety of physical, chemical, and biological decontamination approaches (Peivasteh-Roudsari et al., 2022). It is essential to carry out studies that quantify the effects of climate change on mycotoxins and fungus. Future study, according to Daou et al. (2021), should concentrate on figuring out how the development of climate change will affect mycotoxin production patterns and how certain secondary mycotoxins may become major ones. Research has to be done on how mycotoxin contamination varies by location and how well the present crop management methods work to reduce mycotoxin under altered climatic circumstances.

According to Bhat et al. (2010) and Imran et al. (2020), consuming goods contaminated with mycotoxin is linked to a number of acute and chronic illnesses in both humans and animals. The illnesses or physiological anomalies brought on by mycotoxin exposure are referred to as "mycotoxicosis" (Awuchi et al., 2021).

According to Ekwomadu et al. (2022), these hazardous compounds may cause cancer (aflatoxin B1, ochratoxin A, and fumonisin B1), estrogenic reactions (zearalenone), neurotoxicity (fumonisin B1), nephrotoxicity (ochratoxin), demartotoxicity (trichothecenes), or immunosuppression (aflatoxin B1, ochratoxin A, and T-2 toxin).

Mycotoxins are low molecular weight toxic metabolites of fungal origin that, when ingested, inhaled, or absorbed through the skin, cause lowered performance, illness, or death in humans and animals.

Mycotoxins are very dangerous substances that are found in nature and have garnered international interest recently due to this. Aflatoxigenic hepatitis in Kenya (2004–2005) and India, enteric ergotism in India, vascular erogitsm in Ethiopia, and deoxynivalenol mycotoxicosis in India and China are a few acute diseases with evidence of association with mycotoxins (Imran et al., 2020; Mamo et al., 2020). A commonality among these illnesses was the use of stable food (such as maize, wheat, millet, etc.). Mycotoxins are among the dietary pollutants that have the worst effects on animal and human health, as well as the economy, according to Muhialdin et al. (2020). Fumonisins may be a possible risk factor for neural tube defects in societies where maize is a staple food, according to experimental and epidemiological studies (Gelineau-van Waes et al., 2009). *Aspergillus turbingensis* and *A. ruber, Fusarium verticilioides, A. flavus, A. ochraceus, A. parasiticus,* and *A. nominus* are fungi that exhibit toxic strains (Chen et al., 2021a). Mycotoxin use has often led to major health issues such pulmonary hemorrhage, incoordination, irregular menstrual cycles, and infertility (Adeyeye et al., 2022).

Opajobi (2011) reported that the use of house-made beer prepared from moldy cobs, which contain high amounts of fumonisin, was typically linked to the greater prevalence of esophageal cancer among the male population in KwaZulu Natal, South Africa. Furthermore, in China, Italy, Iran, and South Africa, fumonisin production by *Fusarium verticillioides* has been statistically linked to esophageal cancer in people (Mamo et al., 2020; Zhou et al., 2022). In addition to their potential to cause animals to become less resistant to infectious agents, reproduce less successfully, or refuse food, mycotoxins have also been linked to a number of human disorders. These poisons find their way into milk and foods made with milk, where they endanger both people and animals (Mavrommatis et al., 2021). According to Yu and Pedroso (2023), cereals and grain-based products are typically the primary sources of mycotoxins in human and animal nutrition. The appearance of fungal growth is not a reliable indicator of the presence of mycotoxins.

Aflatoxin, especially aflatoxins, seems to be more of an issue in the tropics than in temperate regions generally, but because different food items are transported around the world, no region of the world can be deemed mycotoxin free (Sankaranarayanan et al., 2021). Certain fungi provide a possible health danger because their toxins may linger long after the mold dies, even after the vegetative development has stopped (Guo et al., 2020). These naturally occurring toxins are very stable and diverse chemically and structurally. The most common methods used to estimate human exposure to these toxins are data on food consumption patterns and contamination levels of raw food or agricultural raw materials, which are the main sources of toxin exposure (Li et al., 2021). The European Union (EU) and the United States Food and Drug Administration (FDA) established regulatory limits on the allowable levels of aflatoxins and ochratoxins as well as guidelines for deoxynivalenol, fumonisins, and patulin due to concerns about their high toxicity (Marrez & Ayesh, 2022).

When contaminated food or feed is consumed or comes into contact with mycotoxins, it may be harmful to both human and animal health. According to estimates from the Food and Agricultural Organisation (FAO) of the United Nations, mycotoxins contaminate 25% of the world's food crops annually (Daou et al., 2021). Ochratoxin, which is produced by several *Aspergillus* and *Penicillium* species, is thought to be primarily found in cereals and foods derived from them.

Depending on the animal, sex, breed, and dose, fungus toxins may result in either acute or chronic intoxications (El-Sayed et al., 2022). There is some evidence that people living in sub-Saharan Africa are heavily exposed to aflatoxin and fumonisins, two types of food-borne mycotoxins, via their diets. The NMA and the 1993 World Development Report both state that mycotoxin-related illnesses shorten life expectancy, particularly in impoverished nations (Mamo et al., 2020).

The global media has focused emphasis on mycotoxin contamination that is ubiquitous. There are several approaches to remove mycotoxins, but biological decomposition is thought to be the most secure. Probiotics, which have many advantageous qualities, are said to be helpful in the clearance of mycotoxins. One interesting approach to the efficient co-degradation of many mycotoxins is the use of microbial consortiums. Furthermore, recombinant degrading enzymes are becoming more and more popular in biological detoxification due to the advancement of genetic engineering technology (Liu et al., 2022). The development of recombinant degrading enzymes that can break down several poisons is essential. However, due to a lack of a complete knowledge of the degradation routes and possible health implications of the degradation products, most biological detoxification solutions have not yet been developed for commercial use. Future research should concentrate on elucidating the specific breakdown processes, carrying out metabolite toxicological studies, and creating innovative analytical techniques in order to support the commercial deployment of these strategies (Nešić et al., 2021). More study is advised to emphasize the field-applicable degrading methods for the control of mycotoxins, given the wide variety of complicated matrices. Future research should focus on investigating mycotoxin biodegradation systems that are economical, very effective, instrument simple, and simple to use for industrial use on a wide scale (Yadavalli et al., 2023).

2.7 Infrequently Isolated Bacteria Toxin Identification

The toxins that are covered here have all undergone extensive research and are crucial elements of foodborne illness; without them, organisms are either rendered incapable of causing disease or are attenuated. Since many of the bacteria are seldom-isolated pathogens, reference labs are usually where toxin detection is carried out. Toxin identification using toxigenicity tests is often necessary for a conclusive diagnosis; hence identifying the toxins is still crucial (Ahmad-Mansour et al., 2021).

2.7.1 Cholera Toxin

Diarrhea is caused by *Vibrio cholerae*, namely serogroups O1 and O139. When *V. cholerae* is found in non-endemic areas, the disease tends to spread quickly, while in cholera-endemic nations, the prevalence of the illness follows a seasonal distribution. Notably, for more than 60 years, two key virulence components of *V. cholerae* associated with toxin generation have been identified. They are the toxin-co-regulated pilus and cholera toxin (CT). The ctxAB operon, which is incorporated into the *V. cholerae* chromosome and corresponds to the genome of CTXF, encodes CT (Leard et al., 2023). Specifically, cholera toxin works by triggering adenylyl cyclase, which raises cAMP. This, in turn, causes a number of metabolic alterations, including intestinal lumen electrolyte imbalances and ion channel activation, which may result in secretory diarrhea (Kenworthy et al., 2021). The most reliable way to identify *V. cholerae* is still to isolate the organism from clinical (often stool) and environmental specimens. Consequently, it has been shown that selective media, including thiosulfate citrate bile salt or chromID Vibrio, are helpful for identification (Huq et al., 2012).

2.7.2 Botulinum Toxin

Among the most powerful toxins known is the clostridial neurotoxins generated by *Clostridium botulinum* (BoNT), the 50% fatal toxin dosage of which is 0.001 g/kg body weight in BoNT. The SNARE (soluble N-ethylmaleimide-sensitive fusion protein attachment receptor) complex, which is crucial for synaptic transmission, is the target of these metalloprotease poisons (Dong & Stenmark, 2021). Although the majority of the time, clostridial botulism diagnoses are made clinically, based on the patient's history and symptoms, a laboratory test is necessary to confirm the diagnosis. Finding the poison is more important for a conclusive diagnosis than isolating the bacterium. As a result, the best toxin detection techniques include mouse neutralization tests, PCR, and environmental imaging assays (Daou et al., 2021). Numerous kinds of biological specimens may provide BoNT, serum, feces, stomach contents or vomiting, wounds, autopsy specimens, and dietary samples are among them. Fluid and wound specimens should be sent (to reference labs) via an anaerobic transport system; if a refrigerant is not present, this method is advised. It is necessary to package any additional specimens submitted for BoNT testing with a refrigerant (Centurioni et al., 2022).

2.7.3 Anthrax Toxin

The first bacterial pathogen to be identified was *Bacillus anthracis*, which causes anthrax. Koch's hypotheses were supported by early research on *B. anthracis*. Pasteur also developed the first antibacterial vaccination by exposing sheep to virulent strains of *B. anthracis* that had been attenuated (Cote et al., 2024). *B. anthracis* endospores enter the body by three different mechanisms: cutaneous, pulmonary, and gastrointestinal. These are the three recognized primary types of the illness. Meningeal anthrax, a very frequent consequence of inhalational and gastrointestinal anthrax, and injection-related illness, which is mostly linked to intravenous drug use, are two further, less common types of disease. Encoding poisons, spores quickly proliferate and divide, allowing the organism to elude the host's immune system (Wang et al., 2021).

Two plasmids, pXO1 and pXO2, which encode protective antigen (PA), lethal factor (LF), and edema factor (EF), are necessary for the formation of toxins and capsules. These three toxin components, or tripartite, are necessary for *B. anthracis* virulence. Together, they create two toxins: PA and EF make edema toxin, while PA and LF form fatal toxin. Translocation of LF and EF to the host cell cytosol, where they mediate cellular damage via distinct pathways, is facilitated by PA's binding to the anthrax toxin receptors, TEM8 (tumor endothelium marker 8) and CMG2 (capillary morphogenesis protein 2) (Mondange et al., 2022). LF is a zinc metalloprotease that cleaves and inactivates mitogen-activated protein kinases, interfering with signal transduction activities in a calmodulin-dependent manner. EF is an adenylate cyclase that increases cAMP concentrations to disrupt cell wall function, which in turn promotes fluid accumulation and oedema (Rougeaux et al., 2020).

2.7.4 New Bacterial Toxins as Well as Other Toxins

Although they are not included in this overview, there are many more toxins that exist and are crucial to illness. Pneumolysin (*Streptococcus pneumoniae*),

Bacillus fragilis enterotoxin, cytotoxic necrotizing factors (*E. coli*), and ExoY (*Pseudomonas aeruginosa*) are a few examples. Molecular detection techniques, including PCR, have now been established for a wide variety of poisons. But in many instances, knowing whether a strain is toxic has little bearing on treatment. Toxin genes, however, provide targets for molecular tests for particular species, which may be crucial for establishing a conclusive diagnosis (Amjad, 2020).

Novel toxin identification and the ability to detect new species are made possible by advances in sequencing and analytics. This is especially true for metagenomics and whole-genome sequencing. For instance, it was recently shown that *Weissella oryzae*, *Chryseobacterium piperi*, and *Enterococcus faecium* all had botulinum-like toxins (Grenda et al., 2023). The use of metagenomics has great promise since it offers a direct sequencing method from specimens, which can detect all toxins present. However, if clinical metagenomics were used, confirmatory toxigenicity testing would be necessary because to the inability to identify toxin expression (D'Humières et al., 2021).

2.8 Distribution Patterns of Microbial Toxins in Food

2.8.1 Mycotoxins in Cereals and Grains

Mycotoxins are predominant contaminants of cereals and grains, as they are more susceptible to contamination by field fungi. Prominent mycotoxins reported in these products include aflatoxins, ochratoxins, and fumonisins. Aflatoxins are predominant in corn and peanuts in humid regions (Kamala et al., 2017), with 60% of corn samples from sub-Saharan Africa reported to exceed the European Union acceptable limits. Ochratoxins are prominent in wheat- and barley-based products especially in Europe due to seasonal changes which significantly predispose them to contamination (Loi et al., 2023). Fumonisins, especially Fumonisin B_1, have been detected in corn, especially in regions that experience high humidity in Asia and Africa (Khodaei et al., 2021; Koskei et al., 2020).

2.8.2 Bacterial Toxins in Dairy Products

Dairy products are prone to contamination by bacterial toxins produced by *Staphylococcus aureus* and *Bacillus cereus*. Staphylococcal enterotoxins are heat stable and can survive pasteurization processes. Dairy products such as cheese and powdered milk have been implicated with high levels and 15% of dairy samples contaminated with staphylococcal toxins from various countries (Huang et al., 2021). *Bacillus cereus* toxins such as emetic and diarrheal toxins are common contaminants of milk- and cream-based dairy products. A survey of milk-based products in Switzerland indicated that 10% of samples were contaminated with *Bacillus cereus* toxins (Heini et al., 2018).

2.8.3 Marine Toxins in Seafood

Algae are the major producers of marine toxins in seafoods such as fish and shellfish. Ciguatoxins are predominantly found in the reef fish of the tropical and subtropical regions. The barracuda and grouper of the Pacific and Caribbean regions are the most contaminated with ciguatoxins (Chinain et al., 2021). Dinoflagellates and shellfish produce the paralytic shellfish toxins (PSTs) that commonly occur in shellfish. Shellfish harvested from coastal waters of North America, Europe, and Asia revealed the prevalence of PST in shellfish (Turner et al., 2021).

2.8.4 Microbial Toxins in Fruits and Vegetables

Microbial toxins are also found in fruits and vegetables but in trace amounts compared to cereals, grains, and seafoods. Patulin is a mycotoxin commonly found in apples and apple-based products. The prevalence of patulin in apple juices has been linked to poor storage conditions (Bacha et al., 2023). Alternaria toxins are predominantly found in fruits and vegetables such as tomatoes, peppers, and citrus fruits. Organic vegetables and fruits have been implicated in contamination by Alternaria toxins due to the absence of fungicides (Bartholomew et al., 2021).

2.9 Detection and Quantification of Microbial Toxins in Food

The detection and quantification of microbial toxins is of the utmost importance for ensuring food safety. The detection of microbial toxins in food has progressed through traditional methods such as chromatography and immunoassays to high-throughput technologies such as next-generation sequencing technology.

Chromatographic techniques that make extensive use of high-performance liquid chromatography (HPLC) and gas chromatography (GC) have been the cornerstone of microbial toxin detection in food. The introduction of mass spectrometry (MS) has further improved on the sensitivity and specificity of this technique. Liquid chromatography tandem mass spectrometry (LCMS/MS) and HPLC-MS/MS have been reported to detect multiple mycotoxins in cereals with a lower detection limit in a short time compared to traditional methods (Iqbal, 2021; Yilmaz Eker et al., 2023).

Immunoassay techniques, notably the enzyme-linked immunosorbent assay (ELISA) technique, have been further refined for better accuracy and efficiency. The development and application of multiplex immunoassays to simultaneously detect various microbial toxins have been reported. The use of the lateral flow immunoassay to detect aflatoxins, ochratoxins, and zearalenone simultaneously in food is an example of this application (Wang et al., 2022; Xing et al., 2020; Zhao et al., 2021).

The use of biosensors is an emerging tool that is effective in the detection of microbial toxins in food. Its possesses high sensitivity, specificity, and rapid response and can be used for on-site testing. The application of electrochemical biosensors that employ nanomaterials has been employed in the detection of mycotoxins in food with a high level of sensitivity and specificity (Gupta et al., 2021; Jiang et al., 2024; Sohrabi et al., 2022).

The use of next-generation sequencing (NGS) has been able to aid the detection of toxin-producing microorganisms with the aim of further elucidating possible sources of contamination. Profiling the microbiome of food products to identify specific species capable of producing toxins has been reported (Fayyaz et al., 2022; Ferone et al., 2020; Rajkovic et al., 2020).

To achieve effective risk assessment, accurately quantifying microbial toxins in food is of the utmost importance, with an emphasis on enhanced precision and specificity of methods.

Quantitative PCR (qPCR) has been extensively used in the detection and quantification of microbial toxins in food. Enhancing qPCR with digital technology produced droplet digital PCR (ddPCR), which has improved its precision and specificity. ddPCR has been employed in the quantification of genes responsible for the production of microbial toxins in foodborne microorganisms, an improved alternative to qPCR (Aladhadh, 2023; Capobianco et al., 2020).

The integration of mass spectrometry with chromatography remains the gold standard for microbial toxin quantification. The use of tandem mass spectrometry (MS/MS) for more accurate quantification of multiple microbial/biotoxins from various food samples has achieved high precision and low detection limits in cereals, nuts and ready-to-eat (RTE) foods (Ezekiel et al., 2019, 2023; Makinde et al., 2023).

The advent of fluorescence-based detection and quantification methods has enhanced the use of fluorescent nanoparticles and dyes in detection of microbial toxins in food. This method has been employed in the quantification of ochratoxin A in wine (Li et al., 2023; Liang et al., 2023).

The aforementioned methods of detection and quantification of microbial toxins have a significant impact on public health and food safety as they aid in more precise detection of these contaminants and consequently reduce the risk of foodborne diseases. These technologies will also support regulatory agencies in implementing stricter safety standards that will improve the safety of food consumed. There is also need for continuous funding for research into technologies that will aid in tracking microbial toxins in food matrixes.

2.10 Prevention and Control of Microbial Toxin Contamination in Food

Microbial toxins are secondary metabolites produced by microorganisms such as bacteria, fungi, and algae. These toxins can contaminate food at various stages of production, processing, and storage, leading to foodborne illnesses. To prevent contamination by microbial toxins in food, the following strategies can be explored:

Good agricultural practices (GAP): These practices include crop rotation, proper irrigation, and the use of resistant crop varieties, which when implemented prevents mycotoxin contamination by field fungi. GAP have been reported to reduce aflatoxin contamination in maize (Neme & Mohammed, 2017).

Biocontrol methods: This involves the use of predators or antagonistic microbes to control toxin-producing fungi on the field. A typical example is the application of non-toxigenic *Aspergillus flavus* (Aflasafe) to outcompete toxigenic field fungi, which consequently reduces aflatoxin levels in maize-grown fields (Atehnkeng et al., 2022).

Genetic engineering: This will help improve the resistance of field crops to toxin-producing pathogens. Genetically modified corn resistant to *Fusarium* species has reported low fumonisin levels (Magarini et al., 2023).

To control contamination by microbial toxins, hazard analysis and critical control points (HACCP), physical and chemical treatment, and post-harvest handling and storage of food crops are of the utmost importance (Motarjemi, 2023; Nada et al., 2022; Ráduly et al., 2020).

In addition, the application of rapid detection methods, predictive modeling, and blockchain technology for traceability along the supply chain are innovative approaches to tracking, preventing, and controlling microbial toxins in food (Castano-Duque et al., 2022; Kong et al., 2023; Yu et al., 2024). Regulatory frameworks and policies at the international and national levels must be harmonized and enforced to ensure proper control of microbial toxins in food products.

2.11 Relevance of Microbial Toxins to Public Health and Food Safety

The consumption of food contaminated with microbial toxins can lead to mild and severe health conditions among consumers. The public health impact is usually enormous, as effects can range from food poisoning symptoms such as vomiting, nausea, and diarrhea to more severe conditions like liver cancer and immunosuppression. The global burden from aflatoxin-related cancer in high-risk regions is well documented (Wild & Gong, 2010). In addition, children, immunocompromised individuals, and the elderly are vulnerable populations constantly plagued with the effects of consuming food contaminated by microbial toxins (Gong et al., 2002; Turner & Snyder, 2021). Continuous research and innovation are critical to developing and innovating new methods to aid detection, control, and mitigation of microbial toxins in food.

2.12 Conclusion

Microbial toxins in food present significant risks to public health and food safety. This chapter has provided an extensive overview of the common sources and types of microbial toxins, including bacterial, fungal, and algal toxins, which are prevalent in various food items. The importance of these toxins is underscored by their potential to cause severe illnesses and fatalities, highlighting the critical need for robust food safety measures.

The mechanisms of toxin production by microorganisms are complex and influenced by various factors such as environmental conditions and food handling practices. Recent trends and emerging concerns, including the impact of climate change on toxin distribution and the identification of new toxin types, underscore the evolving nature of microbial toxin threats. Advanced detection and quantification methods have significantly improved our ability to monitor and manage food safety, enabling more effective identification of high-risk foods and regions.

Understanding the distribution patterns of microbial toxins is crucial for implementing targeted prevention and control strategies. These strategies are essential to mitigate contamination risks and ensure the safety of the food supply. The relevance of microbial toxins to public health and food safety cannot be overstated, necessitating ongoing research and the development of improved regulatory measures to protect consumers.

In conclusion, the fight against microbial toxin contamination in food is an ongoing battle that requires continuous vigilance, research, and collaboration among scientists, regulatory bodies, and the food industry. By enhancing our understanding of microbial toxins and implementing effective control measures, we can better safeguard public health and ensure the safety of our food systems.

References

Abbas, H. K., Bellaloui, N., Accinelli, C., Smith, J. R., & Shier, W. T. (2019). Toxin production in soybean (Glycine max L.) plants with charcoal rot disease and by Macrophomina phaseolina, the fungus that causes the disease. *Toxins*, *11*(11), 645.

Abdelhaseib, M. U., Singh, A. K., & Bhunia, A. K. (2019). Simultaneous detection of Salmonella enterica, Escherichia coli and Listeria monocytogenes in food using a light scattering sensor. *Journal of Applied Microbiology, 126*(5), 1496–1507.

Adeyeye, S. A. O., Ashaolu, T. J., & Idowu-Adebayo, F. (2022). Mycotoxins: Food safety, consumer health and Africa's food security. *Polycyclic Aromatic Compounds, 42*(8), 5779–5795.

Afolabi, C. G., Ezekiel, C. N., Kehinde, I. A., Olaolu, A. W., & Ogunsanya, O. M. (2015). Contamination of groundnut in South-Western Nigeria by aflatoxigenic fungi and aflatoxins in relation to processing. *Journal of Phytopathology, 163*(4), 279–286. https://doi.org/10.1111/jph.12317

Agriopoulou, S., Stamatelopoulou, E., & Varzakas, T. (2020). Advances in occurrence, importance, and mycotoxin control strategies: Prevention and detoxification in foods. *Foods, 9*(2), 137.

Ahmad-Mansour, N., Loubet, P., Pouget, C., Dunyach-Remy, C., Sotto, A., Lavigne, J.-P., & Molle, V. (2021). Staphylococcus aureus toxins: An update on their pathogenic properties and potential treatments. *Toxins, 13*(10), 677.

Aladhadh, M. (2023). A review of modern methods for the detection of foodborne pathogens. *Microorganisms, 11*(5), 1111.

Alizadeh, N., Memar, M. Y., Mehramuz, B., Abibiglou, S. S., Hemmati, F., & Samadi Kafil, H. (2018). Current advances in aptamer-assisted technologies for detecting bacterial and fungal toxins. *Journal of Applied Microbiology, 124*(3), 644–651.

Amjad, M. (2020). An overview of the molecular methods in the diagnosis of gastrointestinal infectious diseases. *International Journal of Microbiology, 2020*(1), 8135724.

Amobonye, A., Aruwa, C., Aransiola, S. A., John, O., Alabi, T. D., & Lalung, J. (2023). Exploring the potential of fungi in the bioremediation of pharmaceutically active compounds. *Frontiers in Microbiology, 14,* 1207792. https://doi.10.3389/fmicb.2023.1207792

Atehnkeng, J., Ojiambo, P. S., Ortega-Beltran, A., Augusto, J., Cotty, P. J., & Bandyopadhyay, R. (2022). Impact of frequency of application on the long-term efficacy of the biocontrol product Aflasafe in reducing aflatoxin contamination in maize. *Frontiers in Microbiology, 13,* 1049013.

Awuchi, C. G., Ondari, E. N., Eseoghene, I. J., Twinomuhwezi, H., Amagwula, I. O., & Morya, S. (2021). Fungal growth and mycotoxins production: Types, toxicities, control strategies, and detoxification. *Fungal Reproduction and Growth, 100207.*

Bacha, S. A. S., Li, Y., Nie, J., Xu, G., Han, L., & Farooq, S. (2023). Comprehensive review on patulin and Alternaria toxins in fruit and derived products. *Frontiers in Plant Science, 14,* 1139757.

Banerji, R., Karkee, A., Kanojiya, P., & Saroj, S. D. (2021). Pore-forming toxins of foodborne pathogens. *Comprehensive Reviews in Food Science and Food Safety, 20*(3), 2265–2285.

Bartholomew, H. P., Bradshaw, M., Jurick, W. M., & Fonseca, J. M. (2021). The good, the bad, and the ugly: Mycotoxin production during postharvest decay and their influence on tritrophic host—Pathogen—Microbe interactions. *Frontiers in Microbiology, 12,* 611881.

Bhat, R., Rai, R. V, & Karim, A. A. (2010). Mycotoxins in food and feed: Present status and future concerns. *Comprehensive Reviews in Food Science and Food Safety, 9*(1), 57–81.

Biessy, L., Pearman, J. K., Smith, K. F., Hawes, I., & Wood, S. A. (2020). Seasonal and spatial variations in bacterial communities from tetrodotoxin-bearing and non-tetrodotoxin-bearing clams. *Frontiers in Microbiology, 11,* 1860.

Bowe, B. K., Wentz, T. G., Gregg, B. M., Tepp, W. H., Schill, K. M., Sharma, S., & Pellett, S. (2022). Genomic diversity, competition, and toxin production by Group I and II Clostridium botulinum strains used in food challenge studies. *Microorganisms, 10*(10), 1895.
Brown, R., Priest, E., Naglik, J. R., & Richardson, J. P. (2021). Fungal toxins and host immune responses. *Frontiers in Microbiology, 12*, 643639.
Capobianco, J. A., Clark, M., Cariou, A., Leveau, A., Pierre, S., Fratamico, P., Strobaugh Jr, T. P., & Armstrong, C. M. (2020). Detection of Shiga toxin-producing Escherichia coli (STEC) in beef products using droplet digital PCR. *International Journal of Food Microbiology, 319*, 108499.
Castano-Duque, L., Vaughan, M., Lindsay, J., Barnett, K., & Rajasekaran, K. (2022). Gradient boosting and bayesian network machine learning models predict aflatoxin and fumonisin contamination of maize in Illinois—First USA case study. *Frontiers in Microbiology, 13*, 1039947.
Centurioni, D. A., Egan, C. T., & Perry, M. J. (2022). Current developments in diagnostic assays for laboratory confirmation and investigation of botulism. *Journal of Clinical Microbiology, 60*(4), e00139–20.
Chen, X., Landschoot, S., Detavernier, C., De Saeger, S., Rajkovic, A., & Audenaert, K. (2021a). Cross-talk between Fusarium verticillioides and Aspergillus flavus in vitro and in planta. *Mycotoxin Research, 37*(3), 229–240.
Chen, Y.-Q., Li, Q., Zhang, T.-Y., & Liu, N.-N. (2021b). Candidalysin: From mechanism of action to biomarker development and therapeutic response. *Innovations in Digital Health, Diagnostics, and Biomarkers, 1*(2), 41–44.
Chinain, M., Gatti, C. M. I., Darius, H. T., Quod, J.-P., & Tester, P. A. (2021). Ciguatera poisonings: A global review of occurrences and trends. *Harmful Algae, 102*, 101873.
Colombo, E. M., Kunova, A., Gardana, C., Pizzatti, C., Simonetti, P., Cortesi, P., Saracchi, M., & Pasquali, M. (2020). Investigating useful properties of four Streptomyces strains active against Fusarium graminearum growth and deoxynivalenol production on wheat grains by qPCR. *Toxins, 12*(9), 560.
Cote, C. K., Heffron, J. D., Bailey, S. O., Welkos, S. L., & Bozue, J. A. (2024). Bacillus anthracis and other Bacillus species. *Molecular Medical Microbiology*, 1681–1742.
D'Humières, C., Salmona, M., Dellière, S., Leo, S., Rodriguez, C., Angebault, C., Alanio, A., Fourati, S., Lazarevic, V., Woerther, P.-L., & others. (2021). The potential role of clinical metagenomics in infectious diseases: Therapeutic perspectives. *Drugs, 81*(13), 1453–1466.
Dahal, A., Lamichhane, A., & Karna, A. (2021). Metabolic pathways and pathological outcomes of aflatoxins: A review. *Nepal Journal of Health Sciences, 1*(2), 63–68.
Daou, R., Joubrane, K., Maroun, R. G., Khabbaz, L. R., Ismail, A., & El Khoury, A. (2021). Mycotoxins: Factors influencing production and control strategies. *AIMS Agriculture and Food, 6*(1), 416–447.
Dong, M., & Stenmark, P. (2021). The structure and classification of botulinum toxins. *Botulinum Toxin Therapy*, 11–33.
Ekwomadu, T., Mwanza, M., & Musekiwa, A. (2022). Mycotoxin-linked mutations and cancer risk: A global health issue. *International Journal of Environmental Research and Public Health, 19*(13), 7754.
El-Sayed, R. A., Jebur, A. B., Kang, W., & El-Demerdash, F. M. (2022). An overview on the major mycotoxins in food products: Characteristics, toxicity, and analysis. *Journal of Future Foods, 2*(2), 91–102.

Eltariki, F. E. M., Tiwari, K., Ariffin, I. A., & Alhoot, M. A. (2018). Genetic diversity of fungi producing mycotoxins in stored crops. *Journal of Pure & Applied Microbiology, 12*(4).

Esteves, A. R., Munoz-Pinto, M. F., Nunes-Costa, D., Candeias, E., Silva, D. F., Magalhães, J. D., Pereira-Santos, A. R., Ferreira, I. L., Alarico, S., Tiago, I., & others. (2023). Footprints of a microbial toxin from the gut microbiome to mesencephalic mitochondria. *Gut, 72*(1), 73–89.

Ezekiel, C. N., Kraak, B., Sandoval-Denis, M., Sulyok, M., Oyedele, O. A., Ayeni, K. I., Makinde, O. M., Akinyemi, O. M., Krska, R., Crous, P. W., & Houbraken, J. (2020). Diversity and toxigenicity of fungi and description of Fusarium madaense sp. nov. from cereals, legumes and soils in north-central Nigeria. *MycoKeys, 67*, 95–124. https://doi.org/10.3897/mycokeys.67.52716

Ezekiel, C. N., Ogbonna, P. N., Williams, G. Y., Sulyok, M., & Krska, R. (2023). Occurrence of mycotoxins, phytoestrogens and other fungal metabolites in Ready-to-Use Therapeutic Foods for severely and acutely malnourished children. *Food Control*, 110191.

Ezekiel, C. N., Oyedele, O. A., Kraak, B., Ayeni, K. I., Sulyok, M., Houbraken, J., & Krska, R. (2020). Fungal diversity and mycotoxins in low moisture content ready-to-eat foods in Nigeria. *Frontiers in Microbiology, 11*, 615.

Ezekiel, C. N., Somorin, Y. M., Sulyok, M., & Krska, R. (2018). Fate of aflatoxins during traditional melon cake and sauce processing. *African Journal of Food Science, 12*(10), 283–287. https://doi.org/10.5897/ajfs2016.1552

Ezekiel, C. N., Sulyok, M., Frisvad, J. C., Somorin, Y. M., Warth, B., Houbraken, J., Samson, R. A., Krska, R., & Odebode, A. C. (2013). Fungal and mycotoxin assessment of dried edible mushroom in Nigeria. *International Journal of Food Microbiology, 162*(3), 231–236. https://doi.org/10.1016/j.ijfoodmicro.2013.01.025

Ezekiel, C. N., Sulyok, M., Ogara, I. M., Abia, W. A., Warth, B., Šarkanj, B., Turner, P. C., & Krska, R. (2019). Mycotoxins in uncooked and plate-ready household food from rural northern Nigeria. *Food and Chemical Toxicology, 128*(November 2018), 171–179. https://doi.org/10.1016/j.fct.2019.04.002

Fayyaz, K., Nawaz, A., Olaimat, A. N., Akram, K., Farooq, U., Fatima, M., Siddiqui, S. A., Rana, I. S., Shahbaz, H. M., & others. (2022). Microbial toxins in fermented foods: Health implications and analytical techniques for detection. *Journal of Food and Drug Analysis, 30*(4), 523.

Ferone, M., Gowen, A., Fanning, S., & Scannell, A. G. M. (2020). Microbial detection and identification methods: Bench top assays to omics approaches. *Comprehensive Reviews in Food Science and Food Safety, 19*(6), 3106–3129.

Fletcher, M. T., & Netzel, G. (2020). Food safety and natural toxins. *Toxins, 12*(4), 236.

Franklin, N., Hope, K., Glasgow, K., & Glass, K. (2020). Describing the epidemiology of foodborne outbreaks in New South Wales from 2000 to 2017. *Foodborne Pathogens and Disease, 17*(11), 701–711.

Gaiani, G., O'Sullivan, C. K., & Campàs, M. (2019). Magnetic beads in marine toxin detection: A review. *Magnetochemistry, 5*(4), 62.

Gavage, M., Delahaut, P., & Gillard, N. (2021). Suitability of high-resolution mass spectrometry for routine analysis of small molecules in food, feed and water for safety and authenticity purposes: A review. *Foods, 10*(3), 601.

Geffroy, S., Lechat, M.-M., Le Gac, M., Rovillon, G.-A., Marie, D., Bigeard, E., Malo, F., Amzil, Z., Guillou, L., & Caruana, A. M. N. (2021). From the sxtA4 gene to saxitoxin production: What controls the variability among Alexandrium minutum and Alexandrium pacificum strains? *Frontiers in Microbiology, 12*, 613199.

Gelineau-van Waes, J., Voss, K. A., Stevens, V. L., Speer, M. C., & Riley, R. T. (2009). Maternal fumonisin exposure as a risk factor for neural tube defects. *Advances in Food and Nutrition Research*, *56*, 145–181.

Gong, Y. Y., Cardwell, K., Hounsa, A., Egal, S., Turner, P. C., Hall, A. J., & Wild, C. P. (2002). Dietary aflatoxin exposure and impaired growth in young children from Benin and Togo: Cross sectional study. *British Medical Journal*, *325*(7354), 20–21. https://doi.org/10.1136/bmj.325.7354.20

Götz, A., Lechner, M., Mader, A., von Bronk, B., Frey, E., & Opitz, M. (2018). CsrA and its regulators control the time-point of ColicinE2 release in Escherichia coli. *Scientific Reports*, *8*(1), 6537.

Grenda, T., Jarosz, A., Sapała, M., Stasiak, K., Grenda, A., Domaradzki, P., & Kwiatek, K. (2023). Molecular diversity of BoNT-producing clostridia a still-emerging and challenging problem. *Diversity*, *15*(3), 392.

Grigson, S. R., Giles, S. K., Edwards, R. A., & Papudeshi, B. (2023). Knowing and naming: Phage annotation and nomenclature for phage therapy. *Clinical Infectious Diseases*, *77*(5), 352–359.

Guo, K., Qian, H., Zhao, D., Ye, J., Zhang, Y., Kan, H., Zhao, Z., Deng, F., Huang, C., Zhao, B., & others. (2020). Indoor exposure levels of bacteria and fungi in residences, schools, and offices in China: A systematic review. *Indoor Air*, *30*(6), 1147–1165.

Gupta, R., Raza, N., Bhardwaj, S. K., Vikrant, K., Kim, K.-H., & Bhardwaj, N. (2021). Advances in nanomaterial-based electrochemical biosensors for the detection of microbial toxins, pathogenic bacteria in food matrices. *Journal of Hazardous Materials*, *401*, 123379.

Guruceaga, X., Perez-Cuesta, U., Pellon, A., Cendon-Sanchez, S., Pelegri-Martinez, E., Gonzalez, O., Hernando, F. L., Mayayo, E., Anguita, J., Alonso, R. M., & others. (2021). Aspergillus fumigatus fumagillin contributes to host cell damage. *Journal of Fungi*, *7*(11), 936.

Hay, W. T., McCormick, S. P., & Vaughan, M. M. (2021). Effects of atmospheric CO2 and temperature on wheat and corn susceptibility to Fusarium graminearum and deoxynivalenol contamination. *Plants*, *10*(12), 2582.

Heini, N., Stephan, R., Ehling-Schulz, M., & Johler, S. (2018). Characterization of Bacillus cereus group isolates from powdered food products. *International Journal of Food Microbiology*, *283*, 59–64.

Huang, Z., Yu, X., Yang, Q., Zhao, Y., & Wu, W. (2021). Aptasensors for Staphylococcus aureus risk assessment in food. *Frontiers in Microbiology*, *12*, 714265.

Huq, A., Haley, B. J., Taviani, E., Chen, A., Hasan, N. A., & Colwell, R. R. (2012). Detection, isolation, and identification of Vibrio cholerae from the environment. In *Current Protocols in Microbiology* (Vol. 1, Issue Suppl. 26). https://doi.org/10.1002/9780471729259.mc06a05s26

Imran, M., Cao, S., Wan, S. F., Chen, Z., Saleemi, M. K., Wang, N., Naseem, M. N., & Munawar, J. (2020). Mycotoxins—a global one health concern: A review. *Agrobiological Records*, *2*, 1–16.

Iqbal, S. Z. (2021). Mycotoxins in food, recent development in food analysis and future challenges; a review. *Current Opinion in Food Science*, *42*, 237–247.

Jiang, Y., Sima, Y., Liu, L., Zhou, C., Shi, S., Wan, K., Chen, A., Tang, N., He, Q., & Liu, J. (2024). Research progress on portable electrochemical sensors for detection of mycotoxins in food and environmental samples. *Chemical Engineering Journal*, 149860.

Kamala, A., Kimanya, M., Lachat, C., Jacxsens, L., Haesaert, G., Kolsteren, P., Ortiz, J., Tiisekwa, B., & De Meulenaer, B. (2017). Risk of exposure to multiple mycotoxins from maize-based complementary foods in Tanzania. *Journal of Agricultural and Food Chemistry, 65*(33), 7106–7114.

Kenworthy, A. K., Schmieder, S. S., Raghunathan, K., Tiwari, A., Wang, T., Kelly, C. V, & Lencer, W. I. (2021). Cholera toxin as a probe for membrane biology. *Toxins, 13*(8), 543.

Khodaei, D., Javanmardi, F., & Khaneghah, A. M. (2021). The global overview of the occurrence of mycotoxins in cereals: A three-year survey. *Current Opinion in Food Science, 39*, 36–42.

Kong, Y., Zhu, Y., Song, J., Liu, Q., Song, L., Fei, X., & Li, X. (2023). A novel multi-mode biosensor for sensitive detection of AFB1 in food based on Mxenes nano enzymes. *Food Chemistry, 426*, 136645.

Koskei, P., Bii, C., Musotsi, P., & Karanja, S. (2020). Presence of fusarium species and fumonisin contamination of maize in Sub-Saharan Africa: A Systematic review. *African Journal of Education, Science and Technology, 5*(4), 132–146.

Kotun, B., Adewara, O., Ayedun, J. S., Makinde, O. M., Oda, O., Adeleke, A. J., Ajunwa, O., & Ogunbanwo S. T. (2024). Distribution, prevention and control of emerging food contaminations. In *Emerging Contaminants in Food and Food Products* (pp. 216–235). CRC Press.

Kumar, P., Hegde, K., Brar, S. K., Cledon, M., & Kermanshahi-Pour, A. (2019). Potential of biological approaches for cyanotoxin removal from drinking water: A review. *Ecotoxicology and Environmental Safety, 172*, 488–503.

Lad, A., Breidenbach, J. D., Su, R. C., Murray, J., Kuang, R., Mascarenhas, A., Najjar, J., Patel, S., Hegde, P., Youssef, M., & others. (2022). As we drink and breathe: Adverse health effects of microcystins and other harmful algal bloom toxins in the liver, gut, lungs and beyond. *Life, 12*(3), 418.

Lauriola, M., Farré, R., Evenepoel, P., Overbeek, S. A., & Meijers, B. (2023). Food-derived uremic toxins in chronic kidney disease. *Toxins, 15*(2), 116.

Leard, E., Carmichael, R. H., Ortmann, A. C., & Jones, J. L. (2023). Environmental drivers of Vibrio cholerae abundances in Mobile Bay, Alabama. *Microbiology Spectrum, 11*(1), e01733–22.

Lee, T. C.-H., Lai, K. K.-Y., Xu, S. J.-L., & Lee, F. W.-F. (2023). Upregulation of peridinin-chlorophyll A-binding protein in a toxic strain of Prorocentrum hoffmannianum under normal and phosphate-depleted Conditions. *International Journal of Molecular Sciences, 24*(2), 1735.

Li, J., Liu, B., Liu, L., Zhang, N., Liao, Y., Zhao, C., Cao, M., Zhong, Y., Chai, D., Chen, X., Zhang, D., Wang, H., He, Y., & Li, Z. (2023). Fluorescence-based aptasensors for small molecular food contaminants: From energy transfer to optical polarization. *Spectrochimica Acta Part A: Molecular and Biomolecular Spectroscopy, 285*, 121872.

Li, X., Ma, W., Ma, Z., Zhang, Q., & Li, H. (2021). The occurrence and contamination level of ochratoxin A in plant and animal-derived food commodities. *Molecules, 26*(22), 6928.

Li, Z., Li, X., Jian, M., Geleta, G. S., & Wang, Z. (2019). Two-dimensional layered nano-material-based electrochemical biosensors for detecting microbial toxins. *Toxins, 12*(1), 20.

Liang, Y., Gong, Y., Yu, Y., Jiang, Q., Zhao, J., Zou, H., & Zhang, J. (2023). Fluorescence resonance energy transfer-based analytical methods for determination of food contaminants: A review. *Food Control, 152*, 109892.

Liu, L., Xie, M., & Wei, D. (2022). Biological detoxification of mycotoxins: Current status and future advances. *International Journal of Molecular Sciences, 23*(3), 1064.

Loi, M., Logrieco, A. F., Pusztahelyi, T., Leiter, É., Hornok, L., & Pócsi, I. (2023). Advanced mycotoxin control and decontamination techniques in view of an increased aflatoxin risk in Europe due to climate change. *Frontiers in Microbiology, 13*, 1085891.

Magarini, A., Passera, A., Ghidoli, M., Casati, P., & Pilu, R. (2023). Genetics and environmental factors associated with resistance to fusarium graminearum, the causal agent of gibberella ear rot in maize. *Agronomy, 13*(7), 1836.

Mahalak, K. K., Firrman, J., Lee, J.-J., Bittinger, K., Nuñez, A., Mattei, L. M., Zhang, H., Fett, B., Bobokalonov, J., Arango-Argoty, G., & others. (2020). Triclosan has a robust, yet reversible impact on human gut microbial composition in vitro. *Plos One, 15*(6), e0234046.

Makinde, O. M., Sulyok, M., Adeleke, R. A., Krska, R., & Ezekiel, C. N. (2023). Bacteriological Quality and Biotoxin Profile of Ready-to-Eat Foods Vended in Lagos, Nigeria. *Foods, 12*(6), 1224.

Makinde, O. M., Wyk, D. Van, Ikhimiukor, O. O., Bezuidenhout, C., Adeleke, R. A., & Ezekiel, C. N. (2022). Draft genome sequences of multidrug-resistant shiga toxin-producing Escherichia coli O116:H25 strains from ready-to-eat foods sold in Lagos, Nigeria. *Microbiology Resource Announcements, 11*(8), e00314–22.

Mamo, F. T., Abate, B. A., Tesfaye, K., Nie, C., Wang, G., & Liu, Y. (2020). Mycotoxins in Ethiopia: A review on prevalence, economic and health impacts. *Toxins, 12*(10), 648.

Manheim, D., Cheung, Y.-M., & Jiang, S. (2018). The effect of organic carbon addition on the community structure and kinetics of microcystin-degrading bacterial consortia. *Water, 10*(11), 1523.

Marrez, D. A., & Ayesh, A. M. (2022). Mycotoxins: The threat to food safety. *Egyptian Journal of Chemistry, 65*(1), 353–372.

Mavrommatis, A., Giamouri, E., Tavrizelou, S., Zacharioudaki, M., Danezis, G., Simitzis, P. E., Zoidis, E., Tsiplakou, E., Pappas, A. C., Georgiou, C. A., & others. (2021). Impact of mycotoxins on animals' oxidative status. *Antioxidants, 10*(2), 214.

Mellou, K., Kyritsi, M., Chrysostomou, A., Sideroglou, T., Georgakopoulou, T., & Hadjichristodoulou, C. (2019). Clostridium perfringens foodborne outbreak during an athletic event in northern Greece, June 2019. *International Journal of Environmental Research and Public Health, 16*(20), 3967.

Mesterhazy, A., Szieberth, D., Toldine, E. T., Nagy, Z., Szabó, B., Herczig, B., Bors, I., & Tóth, B. (2022). Updating the methodology of identifying maize hybrids resistant to ear rot pathogens and their toxins artificial inoculation tests for kernel resistance to Fusarium graminearum, F. verticillioides, and Aspergillus flavus. *Journal of Fungi, 8*(3), 293.

Miller, R. A., Jian, J., Beno, S. M., Wiedmann, M., & Kovac, J. (2018). Intraclade variability in toxin production and cytotoxicity of Bacillus cereus group type strains and dairy-associated isolates. *Applied and Environmental Microbiology, 84*(6), e02479–17.

Moi, I. M., Ibrahim, Z., Abubakar, B. M., Katagum, Y. M., Abdullahi, A., Yiga, G. A., Abdullahi, B., Mustapha, I., Ali, J., Mahmud, Z., & others. (2022). *Properties of Foodborne Pathogens and Their Diseases*. IntechOpen.

Mondange, L., Tessier, É., & Tournier, J.-N. (2022). Pathogenic Bacilli as an emerging biothreat? *Pathogens, 11*(10), 1186.

Motarjemi, Y. (2023). Whistleblowing: An essential element of public health and food safety management. In *Food Safety Management* (pp. 1089–1107). Academic Press.

Muhialdin, B. J., Saari, N., & Meor Hussin, A. S. (2020). Review on the biological detoxification of mycotoxins using lactic acid bacteria to enhance the sustainability of foods supply. *Molecules, 25*(11), 2655.

Nada, S., Nikola, T., Bozidar, U., Ilija, D., & Andreja, R. (2022). Prevention and practical strategies to control mycotoxins in the wheat and maize chain. *Food Control, 136,* 108855.

Nagy, A.-L. (2024). Animal poisoning: Toxins from plants or feed an important chemical risk for domestic animals. *Toxins, 16*(1), 39.

Neme, K., & Mohammed, A. (2017). Mycotoxin occurrence in grains and the role of postharvest management as a mitigation strategies. A review. *Food Control, 78,* 412–425.

Nešić, K., Habschied, K., & Mastanjević, K. (2021). Possibilities for the biological control of mycotoxins in food and feed. *Toxins, 13*(3), 198.

Odo, S. E., Uchechukwu, C. F., & Ezemadu, U. R. (2021). Foodborne diseases and intoxication in Nigeria: Prevalence of Escherichia coli 0157: H7, Salmonella, Shigella and Staphylococcus aureus. *Journal of Advances in Microbiology, 20*(12), 84–94.

Oliveira-Filho, E. C., & Grisolia, C. K. (2022). The ecotoxicology of microbial insecticides and their toxins in genetically modified crops: An overview. *International Journal of Environmental Research and Public Health, 19*(24), 16495.

Opajobi, A. O. (2011). Changes in serum triacylglycerol level and blood pressure measures induced by varying doses of alcohol in man. *Continental Journal of Biomedical Sciences, 5*(1), 1–4.

Peivasteh-Roudsari, L., Pirhadi, M., Shahbazi, R., Eghbaljoo-Gharehgheshlaghi, H., Sepahi, M., Mirza Alizadeh, A., Tajdar-Oranj, B., & Jazaeri, S. (2022). Mycotoxins: Impact on health and strategies for prevention and detoxification in the food chain. *Food Reviews International, 38*(sup1), 193–224.

Penagos-Tabares, F., Sulyok, M., Artavia, J. I., Flores-Quiroz, S. I., Garzón-Pérez, C., Castillo-Lopez, E., Zavala, L., Orozco, J. D., Faas, J., Krska, R., & Zebeli, Q. (2023). Mixtures of mycotoxins, phytoestrogens, and other secondary metabolites in whole-plant corn silages and total mixed rations of dairy farms in Central and Northern Mexico. *Toxins, 15*(2), 1–26. https://doi.org/10.3390/toxins15020153

Petrucci, S., Dikici, E., Daunert, S., & Deo, S. K. (2022). Isothermal amplification and lateral flow nucleic acid test for the detection of Shiga toxin-producing bacteria for food monitoring. *Chemosensors, 10*(6), 210.

Plewa-Tutaj, K., Twarużek, M., Kosicki, R., & Soszczyńska, E. (2024). Analysis of mycotoxins and cytotoxicity of airborne molds isolated from the zoological garden screening research. *Pathogens, 13*(4), 294.

Ráduly, Z., Szabó, L., Madar, A., Pócsi, I., & Csernoch, L. (2020). Toxicological and medical aspects of Aspergillus-derived mycotoxins entering the feed and food chain. *Frontiers in Microbiology, 10,* 2908.

Rajkovic, A., Jovanovic, J., Monteiro, S., Decleer, M., Andjelkovic, M., Foubert, A., Beloglazova, N., Tsilla, V., Sas, B., Madder, A., & others. (2020). Detection of toxins involved in foodborne diseases caused by Gram-positive bacteria. *Comprehensive Reviews in Food Science and Food Safety, 19*(4), 1605–1657.

Rao, A. K. (2021). Clinical guidelines for diagnosis and treatment of botulism, 2021. *MMWR. Recommendations and Reports, 70.*

Rao, Y., Li, H., Chen, M., Huang, K., Chen, J., Xu, J., & Zhuang, G. (2020). Community structure and influencing factors of airborne microbial aerosols over three Chinese cities with contrasting social-economic levels. *Atmosphere, 11*(4), 317.

Richardson, J. P., Brown, R., Kichik, N., Lee, S., Priest, E., Mogavero, S., Maufrais, C., Wickramasinghe, D. N., Tsavou, A., Kotowicz, N. K., & others. (2022). Candidalysins are a new family of cytolytic fungal peptide toxins. *MBio, 13*(1), e03510–21.

Rougeaux, C., Becher, F., Goossens, P. L., & Tournier, J.-N. (2020). Very early blood diffusion of the active lethal and edema factors of Bacillus anthracis after intranasal infection. *The Journal of Infectious Diseases, 221*(4), 660–667.

Russini, V., Corradini, C., De Marchis, M. L., Bogdanova, T., Lovari, S., De Santis, P., Migliore, G., Bilei, S., & Bossù, T. (2022). Foodborne toxigenic agents investigated in central Italy: An overview of a three-year experience (2018–2020). *Toxins, 14*(1), 40.

Sankaranarayanan, A., Amaresan, N., Sharma, A., & Khalifa, A. Y. Z. (2021). Mycotoxins associated food safety concerns of agricultural crops, prevention and control. In *Fungi Bio-Prospects in Sustainable Agriculture, Environment and Nano-Technology* (pp. 357–374). Elsevier.

Silva, A., Silva, S. A., Lourenço-Lopes, C., Jimenez-Lopez, C., Carpena, M., Gullón, P., Fraga-Corral, M., Domingues, V. F., Barroso, M. F., Simal-Gandara, J., & others. (2020). Antibacterial use of macroalgae compounds against foodborne pathogens. *Antibiotics, 9*(10), 712.

Sivamaruthi, B. S., Kesika, P., & Chaiyasut, C. (2018). Toxins in fermented foods: Prevalence and preventions–a mini review. *Toxins, 11*(1), 4.

Sohrabi, H., Arbabzadeh, O., Khaaki, P., Majidi, M. R., Khataee, A., & Woo Joo, S. (2022). Emerging electrochemical sensing and biosensing approaches for detection of Fumonisins in food samples. *Critical Reviews in Food Science and Nutrition, 62*(31), 8761–8776.

Sombie, J. I., Ezekiel, C. N., Sulyok, M., Ayeni, K. I., Jonsyn-Ellis, F., & Krska, R. (2018). Survey of roasted street-vended nuts in Sierra Leone for toxic metabolites of fungal origin. *Food Additives and Contaminants—Part A Chemistry, Analysis, Control, Exposure and Risk Assessment, 35*(8), 1573–1580. https://doi.org/10.1080/19440049.2018.1475753

Tran, P. M., Feiss, M., Kinney, K. J., & Salgado-Pabón, W. (2019). φSa3mw prophage as a molecular regulatory switch of Staphylococcus aureus β-toxin production. *Journal of Bacteriology, 201*(14), 10–1128.

Tse, S. P., Lee, F. W., Mak, D. Y., Kong, H., Chan, K. K., Lo, P., & Lo, S. C. (2020). Production of paralytic shellfish toxins (PSTs) in toxic Alexandrium catenella is intertwined with photosynthesis and energy production. *Toxins, 12*(8), 477.

Turner, A. D., Lewis, A. M., Bradley, K., & Maskrey, B. H. (2021). Marine invertebrate interactions with harmful algal blooms—implications for one health. *Journal of Invertebrate Pathology, 186*, 107555.

Turner, P. C., & Snyder, J. A. (2021). Development and limitations of exposure biomarkers to dietary contaminants mycotoxins. *Toxins, 13*(5), 314.

Wang, D.-B., Cui, M.-M., Li, M., & Zhang, X.-E. (2021). Biosensors for the detection of Bacillus anthracis. *Accounts of Chemical Research, 54*(24), 4451–4461.

Wang, Y., Wang, X., Wang, S., Fotina, H., & Wang, Z. (2022). A novel lateral flow immunochromatographic assay for rapid and simultaneous detection of aflatoxin b1 and zearalenone in food and feed samples based on highly sensitive and specific monoclonal antibodies. *Toxins, 14*(9), 615.

Wild, C. P., & Gong, Y. Y. (2010). Mycotoxins and human disease: A largely ignored global health issue. *Carcinogenesis, 31*(1), 71–82. https://doi.org/10.1093/carcin/bgp264

Wydau-Dematteis, S., El Meouche, I., Courtin, P., Hamiot, A., Lai-Kuen, R., Saubaméa, B., Fenaille, F., Butel, M.-J., Pons, J.-L., Dupuy, B., & others. (2018). Cwp19 is a novel lytic transglycosylase involved in stationary-phase autolysis resulting in toxin release in Clostridium difficile. *MBio, 9*(3), 10–1128.

Xing, K.-Y., Shan, S., Liu, D.-F., & Lai, W.-H. (2020). Recent advances of lateral flow immunoassay for mycotoxins detection. *TrAC Trends in Analytical Chemistry, 133*, 116087.

Yadavalli, R., Valluru, P., Raj, R., Reddy, C. N., & Mishra, B. (2023). Biological detoxification of mycotoxins: Emphasizing the role of algae. *Algal Research, 71*, 103039.

Yilmaz Eker, F., Muratoglu, K., Ozturk, M., Cetin, B., & Buyukunal, S. K. (2023). Determination of multimycotoxin in cereal-based products sold in open-air markets. *Foods, 12*(14), 1–13. https://doi.org/10.3390/foods12142744

Yousef, N. M. H., Abd El-Aziz, D. M., & Mansour, M. A. (2021). Molecular characterization of foodborne pathogenic bacteria recovered from fermented meat products. *Journal of Multidisciplinary Sciences, 3*(2), 1–10.

Yu, J., & Pedroso, I. R. (2023). Mycotoxins in cereal-based products and their impacts on the health of humans, livestock animals and pets. In *Toxins* (Vol. 15, Issue 8, p. 480). https://doi.org/10.3390/toxins15080480

Yu, Q., Zhang, M., & Mujumdar, A. S. (2024). Blockchain-based fresh food quality traceability and dynamic monitoring: Research progress and application perspectives. *Computers and Electronics in Agriculture, 224*, 109191.

Zhang, S.-F., Zhang, Y., Lin, L., & Wang, D.-Z. (2018). iTRAQ-based quantitative proteomic analysis of a toxigenic dinoflagellate Alexandrium catenella at different stages of toxin biosynthesis during the cell cycle. *Marine Drugs, 16*(12), 491.

Zhao, X., Jin, X., Lin, Z., Guo, Q., Liu, B., Yuan, Y., Yue, T., & Zhao, X. (2021). Simultaneous rapid detection of aflatoxin B1 and ochratoxin a in spices using lateral flow immuno-chromatographic assay. *Foods, 10*(11), 2738.

Zhou, L., Kori, D. S., Sibanda, M., & Nhundu, K. (2022). An analysis of the differences in vulnerability to climate change: A review of rural and urban areas in south Africa. *Climate, 10*(8), 118.

3

Mycotoxins in Children's Food: Global Perspectives

Ogunbanwo, S.T., Adegoke, C.O., and Folorunso, O.A.

3.1 Global Perspective of Mycotoxins in Children's Food

In Africa, the contamination of food products with mycotoxins presents a significant challenge, impacting human health, animal well-being, and economic stability. Aflatoxin-related liver diseases have been documented across various African nations, while ochratoxin and fumonisin-related toxicities are prevalent among both humans and animals. In contrast, Europe faces increasing plant disease issues linked to toxic fungal species and their metabolites (Leslie & Summerell, 2006). These fungi are capable of producing a vast array of secondary metabolites, including mycotoxins—small toxic compounds that pose serious health risks globally (Hussein & Brasel, 2001). Cereals, being staple foods for a large segment of the global population, are particularly vulnerable, making mycotoxins a significant food safety concern.

Mycotoxins are naturally occurring compounds found throughout the life cycle of food-producing plants, exhibiting various chemical and physical properties that can have toxic effects on both humans and animals (Hussein & Brasel, 2001). They are viewed as one of the most critical contaminants in the food supply chain due to their long-term adverse health effects and economic implications. Often referred to as the "great threat" of the 21st century, mycotoxins are linked to a range of diseases and clinical symptoms, including nasal bleeding, eye inflammation, respiratory issues, vomiting, and in severe cases, pulmonary hemorrhage and bone marrow suppression (Darwish et al., 2014).

Awareness of these symptoms can help healthcare professionals identify potential exposures to mycotoxins, thereby protecting children from various sources of contamination (Iheshiulor et al., 2011). These sources include contaminated food, clothing, indoor air, and furniture. Early exposure to mycotoxins during infancy may significantly influence long-term health

 DOI: 10.1201/9781003500605-4

outcomes, with in utero exposure also being a critical factor. Numerous conditions, including neural tube defects and certain cancers, have been linked to the consumption of foods contaminated with mycotoxins (Bennett & Klich, 2003). Understanding the history of exposure to mycotoxins can aid pediatricians in diagnosing and treating affected children and their families. This chapter aims to address issues related to the presence of common mycotoxins in children's food and explore potential strategies for mitigation.

Cereals are fundamental ingredients in infants' and children's diets, providing essential nutrients for growth and development. They are also easily digestible, making them ideal for transitioning infants to solid foods (Bennett & Klich, 2003). Children are generally more vulnerable than adults to toxic food contaminants, such as mycotoxins, which are common in cereal products. While some mycotoxins are regulated by food safety agencies in Nigeria, knowledge about others, particularly emerging mycotoxins, remains limited, and many are not yet subject to regulation. This chapter will highlight the impact of mycotoxins in cereal-based foods for infants and children.

Research has indicated that both regulated and emerging mycotoxins can be found together in cereal products intended for children, underscoring the need for clear guidelines (Bonel et al., 2011). Despite ongoing efforts to eliminate mycotoxins from food and agricultural products, these initiatives have not yielded the desired results. Methods such as biological purification, chemical treatments, and nutritional strategies have been explored (Kabak et al., 2006). People may be exposed to mycotoxins through the consumption of contaminated plant-based foods, including vegetables, eggs, and meat (Bonel et al., 2011). Additionally, exposure can occur via contaminated air, moisture, and dust (Jarvis, 2002; Niculita-Hirzel et al., 2016).

The risk of mycotoxin exposure is heightened in regions with inadequate pest control practices for crops and poor storage facilities. This issue is particularly acute in low-income communities, where people may have limited food choices and consume whatever is available rather than what is optimal (Zain, 2011). Regular exposure to mycotoxins is also prevalent where there are insufficient regulations to safeguard public food consumption. In developed countries, especially in areas with substandard food handling practices, there remains a risk of mycotoxin exposure, making the general population susceptible to contamination. While the presence of mycotoxins in food is a known risk (Zinedine et al., 2009), it often cannot be entirely avoided.

Mycotoxins have been a significant factor in epidemics affecting both humans and animals over the past decades. Notably, the ergotism outbreak in Europe resulted in thousands of deaths during that time. Additionally, gastrointestinal toxic aleukia was responsible for approximately 100,000 fatalities in Russia between 1942 and 1948 (John & Miller, 2017). These toxins can lead to various health issues, including abdominal pain, vomiting, and diarrhea (FAO/WHO, 2011; John & Miller, 2017).

3.2 Occurrence of Mycotoxins in Children's Food: Global Perspectives

Mycotoxin contamination of food can occur throughout the growing season, encompassing pre-harvest, post-harvest, and storage phases (Begum & Samajpati, 2000). Different fungi are responsible for toxin production at various stages; for instance, species like *Fusarium*, *Claviceps*, and *Alternaria* thrive before harvest, while *Aspergillus* and *Penicillium* species are more prevalent during storage (Tsitsigiannis et al., 2010).

Cereals intended for infant food undergo rigorous quality control before reaching consumers. However, these crops remain vulnerable to toxigenic fungi during both pre- and post-harvest periods, which can generate harmful mycotoxins. The primary fungal genera involved in mycotoxin production include *Aspergillus*, *Penicillium*, and *Fusarium*. Identifying the specific fungi responsible for contamination can be challenging, as a single species may produce multiple mycotoxins, and conversely, a specific mycotoxin can originate from various species. For example, *Aspergillus* species can produce aflatoxins, ochratoxins, and citrinin, while *Fusarium* species often generate trichothecenes, zearalenone, and emerging mycotoxins like beauvericin (Mallebrera et al., 2018; Dorninger-Gruber et al., 2017).

Mycotoxins in animal feed pose significant risks to livestock health and can subsequently enter the human food chain. The prevalence of mycotoxins in agricultural products is influenced by various factors, including the specific fungal species involved, environmental conditions such as humidity and temperature, and agricultural practices (Paterson & Lima, 2010; Jouany, 2007). Each region faces unique challenges regarding mycotoxin contamination based on its climate and agricultural practices. While mycotoxin levels in many regions align with EU regulatory standards, significant contamination is still observed, particularly in sub-Saharan Africa and South Asia, where concentrations can exceed safe limits, posing risks to both animal and human health (Pereira et al., 2014).

Infants and young children are particularly vulnerable to the harmful effects of mycotoxins due to their lower body weight and developing detoxification systems (IARC, 2015). Despite the evident risks, regulations regarding mycotoxin levels in complementary foods are lacking in Nigeria, with only aflatoxins being subject to regulation based on EU standards. This gap in regulation jeopardizes the health of vulnerable populations and hinders progress toward achieving United Nations Sustainable Development Goal 3, which focuses on good health and well-being (Bentley & Nulty, 2020).

Mycotoxin contamination remains a pressing issue in many sub-Saharan African countries, notably Nigeria, where it significantly impacts human and animal health and poses challenges for international trade (Gong et al., 2016). Common mycotoxins such as aflatoxins and fumonisins are found in various crops, including maize and groundnuts, making exposure to contaminated food likely. Therefore, establishing effective regulations similar to those in developed countries is crucial for ensuring food safety (Cascant et al., 2015).

In many low- and middle-income countries, including Nigeria, there is a notable lack of awareness and information regarding the risks associated with mycotoxin contamination and its effects on health and the economy. This chapter aims to summarize the current state of mycotoxin presence in Nigerian food and feed in relation to global regulatory standards. Despite the variations in contamination factors, the effects of mycotoxin exposure are universally concerning (Ladeira et al., 2017). Both short- and long-term exposure can lead to severe toxic effects, primarily through direct consumption or through animal products contaminated with mycotoxin metabolites (Abdallah et al., 2020).

Recently, the global issue of food and feed contamination by mycotoxins has escalated, resulting in serious outbreaks that affect public health and economic stability. It is estimated that approximately 25% of the world's food crops are contaminated with mycotoxins produced by fungi, leading to substantial financial losses in both domestic and international agricultural markets (Doughari, 2015).

3.3 Sources of Mycotoxins in Children's Food: A Global Perspective

Mycotoxins are toxic compounds produced by certain molds and fungi and can be found in various food items. These molds thrive on a wide range of crops, including cereals, dried fruits, nuts, spices, apples, and coffee beans, particularly in warm and humid environments. Mycotoxins represent a diverse group of naturally occurring toxins that have been linked to health risks in both humans and animals (Pereira et al., 2014; Sun et al., 2017). The health implications of mycotoxin contamination arise from their ubiquitous presence in food supplies, leading to potential exposure across all age groups. Instances of acute intoxication due to consumption of heavily contaminated food have been reported in various populations.

Chronic health issues, including cancer, can result from even low-level exposure to mycotoxins. Avoiding human exposure is challenging because it is difficult to prevent fungal growth in food (CAST, 2003). The health impacts of mycotoxin exposure can vary significantly in severity and clinical significance, with laboratory studies showing that toxicity can differ based on factors like species, age, and sex. In humans, mycotoxins can lead to serious health conditions, as evidenced by sporadic outbreaks of acute mycotoxicosis (CDCP, 2004; Zain, 2011). There have also been reported cases of infant fatalities associated with mold exposure in living environments (Jarvis, 2002). Mycotoxins disrupt various cellular processes and can have a range of toxic effects.

The production of mycotoxins, particularly in cereals, heavily depends on environmental conditions before and after harvest, such as moisture and temperature. Weather plays a crucial role in the incidence of mycotoxins and fungi, but other factors can also influence their prevalence, including the availability of micronutrients and damage from insects (Milani et al., 2013). Mycotoxin exposure can lead to several chronic and acute health issues in humans and animals, including hepatotoxicity, immunosuppression, and carcinogenic effects (Da Rocha et al., 2014). Moreover, mycotoxins are not completely eliminated during food processing, leading to contamination of finished products (Streit et al., 2013; Clarke et al., 2014).

Globally, mycotoxin contamination in food and feed poses a significant threat to human and animal health, resulting in substantial economic losses (Bryden, 2012). Although quantifying these financial impacts is challenging, the U.S. Food and Drug Administration (FDA) estimates that the economic costs associated with crop losses due to mycotoxin contamination in the USA average around $932 million annually (CAST, 2003).

Among the various fungal metabolites, only a few mycotoxins are of major concern from safety and economic perspectives. Key groups include aflatoxins (AFs), primarily produced by *Aspergillus* species; ochratoxin A (OTA), produced by both *Aspergillus* and *Penicillium* species; and fumonisins (FUM), particularly deoxynivalenol (DON) and trichothecenes (TCTs), which are mainly produced by various *Fusarium* species (Binder et al., 2007; Streit et al., 2013; Clarke et al., 2014). Additionally, some *Fusarium* species can produce other mycotoxins with toxicological properties, including moniliformin (MON), enniatins (ENNs), and beauvericin (BEA), which are categorized as emerging mycotoxins (Williams et al., 2004; Jestoi, 2008).

Children are particularly vulnerable to the harmful effects of mycotoxins, as their health can be impacted differently than that of adults (WHO, 2006). The serious consequences of exposure to these toxins in children are a significant concern.

3.4 Major Mycotoxins and Identification of Fungi-Producing Mycotoxins in Children's Food

Mycotoxins are secondary metabolites produced by certain molds, and they are a naturally occurring phenomenon. Currently, between 300 and 400 mycotoxins are recognized, with key examples including aflatoxins, ochratoxins, fumonisins, trichothecenes, and others (Esam et al., 2022). While the production of mycotoxins is not essential for fungal growth, it is believed to serve as a defense mechanism against predators and environmental changes (Fox & Howlett, 2008; Amobonye et al., 2023).

Crops that are most sensitive to mycotoxin contamination include cereals such as maize, millet, wheat, and sorghum, as well as oilseeds like soybean and peanut. Foods such as moldy bread, spices, and industrial by-products can also contain mycotoxins (Coppock et al., 2018). It is important to note that mycotoxin contamination can occur at multiple stages of crop development, from planting to harvesting, storage, and processing.

The global incidence of fungal metabolites in food is a pressing concern, particularly regarding the levels of these toxins. Certain species of fungi, such as *Alternaria, Fusarium,* and *Claviceps,* are more active during the pre-harvest phase, while *Aspergillus and Penicillium* species thrive during storage (Magan et al., 2003; Tsitsigiannis et al., 2012). In temperate and polar regions, *Penicillium* Ojuriis frequently identified as a common mycotoxin producer, while *Aspergillus* is more prevalent in tropical and subtropical regions. In contrast, *Fusarium* and *Alternaria* are found globally, with specific fungi dominating at various growth stages. Human exposure to mycotoxins can occur through inhalation, ingestion, or contact with contaminated food (Bryden, 2007).

Mycotoxin contamination in food remains a significant public health issue, with mechanisms of action that link it to a variety of health disorders. This contamination poses a serious challenge to food safety, especially in economically developing areas like sub-Saharan Africa (SSA) (IARC, 2015). A single crop, such as maize, can be exposed to multiple mycotoxins, including aflatoxins, citrinin, fumonisins, ochratoxins, and trichothecenes (Ojuri et al., 2019). Consequently, many individuals in high-risk regions, including children, are likely to encounter a combination of mycotoxins through their diets.

Infants' and young children's diets typically consist of breast milk and complementary foods based on cereals and nuts (Gong et al., 2016). There is considerable concern regarding the presence of these toxins in foods designed for infants and young children, as well as the potential for these toxins to be present in breast milk due to maternal exposure. Pregnant women in many low-income countries, particularly in Africa and Asia, face a heightened risk of aflatoxin exposure (International Agency for Research on Cancer, 2002).

Research by Tesfamariam et al. (2022) indicates that chronic maternal exposure to aflatoxins is associated with reduced fetal growth in rural Ethiopia. These findings underscore the importance of nutrition-sensitive strategies to reduce dietary aflatoxin exposure and the need for improved food safety measures in low-income settings, particularly during critical periods of fetal development.

3.5 Mycotoxins Commonly Found in Infants' and Young Children's Food

3.5.1 Aflatoxins

Aflatoxins are highly toxic secondary metabolites produced by certain molds, particularly *Aspergillus flavus* and *A. parasiticus*. The most notable naturally occurring aflatoxins include B1, B2, G1, G2, M1, M2, GM1, B2a, and G2a (El-Kerdasy et al., 2019). These compounds are recognized as some of the most carcinogenic mycotoxins. Aflatoxin M1 (AFM1) can be transferred into the milk of lactating mothers who consume contaminated food (Polychronaki et al., 2006; Prandini et al., 2009). AFM1 is classified as both carcinogenic (Luongo et al., 2014) and mutagenic (IARC, 2015). Research indicates that aflatoxins may contribute to increased neonatal mortality, stillbirths, and greater susceptibility to conditions like neonatal jaundice (Ladeira et al., 2017). Additionally, they are thought to play a role in the development of Kwashiorkor and heighten children's vulnerability to infections and malignant diseases (El-Kerdasy et al., 2019). Studies conducted in Portugal (Alvito et al., 2010), Spain (Beltrán et al., 2011), and Italy (Juan et al., 2014) reported low levels of aflatoxins in infant foods and cereals.

3.5.2 Ochratoxin

Ochratoxin is produced by several *Aspergillus* and *Penicillium* species and is a common contaminant in food. This toxin can affect grains, legumes, and various food products globally. Ochratoxin A is typically generated during the storage of crops and is known to have multiple toxic effects on animals, primarily leading to kidney damage. Although evidence of ochratoxin A's association with kidney toxicity and cancer in animals is well established, its effects in humans are less clear, although kidney damage has been observed (Meucci et al., 2010). In Sierra Leone, studies found that 35% of breast milk samples contained Ochratoxin A at concentrations between 200 and 337 ng/ml, suggesting potential risks to kidney function and the development of urinary tumors in infants and young children. In Denmark, ochratoxin was detected in barley and oats, with 72% of the 185 samples analyzed containing levels ranging from 35.1 to 689.5 ng/l (Meucci et al., 2010).

3.5.3 Fumonisins

Fumonisins are metabolites produced by *Fusarium* species, particularly *F. verticillioides*. These fungi, typically found in soil, generate various toxins, including trichothecenes such as deoxynivalenol (DON), nivalenol (NIV), T-2, and HT-2 toxins, as well as zearalenone (ZEN) and fumonisins in maize (corn). Fumonisins have been linked to esophageal cancer in humans and can be toxic to the liver and kidneys (Marasas, 2001). *F. verticillioides* has been prominently isolated from corn and is associated with a disease known as leukoencephalomalacia (ELEM) that has affected livestock in South Africa (Marasas, 2001).

3.5.4 Zearalenone

Zearalenone is another toxin produced by *Fusarium* species, commonly found on crops like sesame, corn, wheat, oats, sorghum, and barley. In children, zearalenone primarily affects the reproductive system, potentially leading to hyperestrogenism and altering the structure and function of reproductive organs (Sherif et al., 2009; Zheng et al., 2016).

3.5.5 Patulin

Patulin is produced by various molds, mainly from the genera *Aspergillus, Penicillium,* and *Byssochlamys* (Boussabbeh et al., 2016). It is often found in spoiled apples and apple products but can also occur in other moldy fruits, grains, and foods. Patulin levels in commercial apple juice and children's apple products have been recorded at concentrations between 10 and 170 ppb (Battilani et al., 2008). It poses health risks due to its potential to cause nausea, gastrointestinal disturbances, and vomiting. In animals, acute exposure can lead to damage in the liver, spleen, and kidneys, and though it is considered genotoxic, its carcinogenic potential has not yet been established.

3.6 Identification of Mycotoxigenic Fungi in Infants' and Young Children's Food

Infants' and young children's foods are particularly susceptible to fungal contamination when conditions are conducive to fungal growth. Fungi are multicellular organisms with long filamentous structures called hyphae. Unlike plants, they lack chlorophyll and possess a filamentous structure (Adeyeye, 2016). Fungi can be categorized into two groups: field fungi and storage fungi. Field fungi, such as *Alternaria, Fusarium,* and *Cladosporium,* typically invade crops in the field (Hashem & Alamri, 2010). In contrast, storage fungi thrive in stored crops when humidity, temperature, and moisture levels are favorable (Hashem & Alamri, 2010). According to Yogendrarajah et al. (2014), *Aspergillus* and *Penicillium* are prevalent storage fungi that contaminate stored crops. These genera are known as mycotoxigenic fungi due to their ability to produce harmful secondary metabolites known as mycotoxins.

The presence of multiple mycotoxins in foods for children underscores the need for continuous monitoring and evaluation to protect this vulnerable demographic. Timely detection of fungal contaminants and identification of the main mycotoxigenic species are essential for assessing food safety and developing effective control measures (Suanthie et al., 2009). Fungal identification can be performed through cultural and morphological analyses, utilizing both macroscopic and microscopic techniques to evaluate colony growth patterns, conidial morphology, pigmentation, and hyphal structures (Tafinta et al., 2013).

The method described by Oyeleke and Manga (2008) involves using cotton blue in lactophenol stains for identification. A drop of the stain is placed on a clean slide, followed by a small sample of aerial mycelia from the fungal culture. The mycelium is spread evenly, and a cover slip is applied to minimize air bubbles before examining under a microscope with varying magnifications. Observing the morphology of the fungi allows for the identification of spore arrangements (Gaddeyya et al., 2012). However, morphological and biochemical identification can be time consuming and may require specialized skills, as well as the potential for different morphotypes within a single species. Molecular techniques, such as PCR, can provide alternatives to traditional methods for detecting mycotoxigenic fungi.

Molecular identification methods that involve extracting total fungal DNA allow for precise identification of various fungal isolates at the species level (Landeweert et al., 2003; Sohail et al., 2017). These molecular methods have become crucial tools for mycologists studying fungal taxonomy, molecular evolution, and interactions between fungi and plants. Fungal identification through molecular techniques often relies on sequencing PCR-amplified regions of 18S rRNA genes using universal primers (Monod et al., 2006), comparing sequences with databases like NCBI-BLAST (Sohail et al., 2017). Multiplex PCR assays that can amplify multiple species-specific genes related to mycotoxin biosynthesis have been successfully implemented to detect mycotoxigenic fungi in various foods and feeds (Kim et al., 2011; Ramana et al., 2011; Rashmi et al., 2013). Such genomic methods have proven to be rapid and accurate alternatives for the early detection of toxic and spoilage molds in food products (Rodríguez et al., 2015). However, there have been limited instances of using multiplex PCR for differentiating mycotoxin-producing fungi in food and feed. Wang and colleagues developed a multiplex PCR assay for the simultaneous detection of genes responsible for type B trichothecene mycotoxins found in food, focusing on the genetic identification of specific mycotoxin chemotypes within *Fusarium* species (Wang et al., 2012).

3.7 Mycotoxin Bioavailability in Cereal and Cereal-Derived Foods

Research indicates that mycotoxins are present in cereals and cereal-derived products intended for children; however, there is limited knowledge regarding their bioavailability and bioaccessibility after ingestion (Gonzalez-Arias et al., 2013; Cardoso et al., 2015; Arce-Lopez et al., 2020). Bioavailability refers to the fraction of mycotoxins that enters the bloodstream through the intestinal lining, while bioaccessibility is influenced by the food matrix and the specific characteristics of the mycotoxins themselves (Gonzalez-Arias et al., 2013; Cardoso et al., 2015; Rebellato et al., 2021). The bioactivity of mycotoxins involves their transport to target tissues, interaction with biomolecules, and the resultant physiological and biochemical effects. This bioavailability indicates the proportion of mycotoxins present in target tissues that can exert effects once they have entered those tissues (Pereira et al., 2022).

While some studies have explored mycotoxin bioaccessibility in children, it is understood that children may be more susceptible to injury in intestinal cells due to higher toxin levels in their digestive fluids compared to adults (Raiola et al., 2012; Rebellato et al., 2021).

Research employing an in vitro static digestion model has assessed the bioaccessibility of patulin and ochratoxins in processed cereal-based foods. Findings indicate that ochratoxins exhibited significantly higher bioaccessibility than patulin. However, when patulin was evaluated alone or in combination with ochratoxins, no significant differences were noted. In contrast, ochratoxins showed markedly higher bioaccessibility when assessed alone or in combination with patulin, potentially due to interactions among the mycotoxins, digestive fluids, and food matrices (Assuncao et al., 2016).

In another study using an in vitro static digestion model, the influence of probiotic bacteria on the bioaccessibility of ochratoxins and aflatoxin B1—both individually and together—was examined in infant formula. Aflatoxins demonstrated greater bioaccessibility than ochratoxins. The type of probiotic bacteria used also significantly affected mycotoxin bioaccessibility; for instance, *Lactobacillus casei* and *Lactobacillus acidophilus* lowered the bioaccessibility of aflatoxin B1 but had no effect on ochratoxins (Kabak et al., 2009).

The bioaccessibility of various enniatins (A, A1, B, and B1) was studied in different breakfast foods spiked with concentrations of 1.5 and 3.0 μmol/g of mycotoxins. Food samples containing 1.5 μmol/g of Enniatin B1 showed the highest bioaccessibility, while no significant differences were found among food samples with different mycotoxin concentrations. The highest bioaccessibility was recorded for Enniatin A1, followed by Enniatin B1, B, and A. Variations in bioaccessibility among similar food types may be attributed to their matrix composition and the chemical structures of the mycotoxins (Prosperini et al., 2013).

When comparing different cereals, those with higher fiber content exhibited lower bioaccessibility of mycotoxins. This interaction suggests that dietary fiber can help mitigate the toxic effects of mycotoxins. Additionally, food products with higher fat content demonstrated reduced mycotoxin bioaccessibility, likely due to incomplete release of the mycotoxins during digestion (Prosperini et al., 2013).

3.8 Techniques for Mycotoxin Assessment in Food and Bioaccessibility Studies

3.8.1 Mycotoxin Assessment Techniques

Quantifying mycotoxins is crucial for managing their presence in food, facilitating proper regulation, quality control, and informed research (Whitaker, 2006). The analytical techniques employed must be precise and effective, as mycotoxins are complex compounds that vary chemically and exist in diverse matrices, typically at low concentrations (Zheng et al., 2006). Co-occurrence of different mycotoxins is a significant consideration during analysis (Pereira et al., 2022).

The methods for mycotoxin analysis involve several critical steps: sampling, extraction, cleanup, and detection (Pereira et al., 2014; Alshannaq & Yu, 2017).

3.8.1.1 Sampling

Sampling is the initial step in the quantification process, which involves collecting a representative sample from a larger batch, based on the assumption that the mycotoxin concentration in the sample reflects that of the entire batch (Whitaker, 2006). Sampling poses challenges due to the uneven distribution of mycotoxins within food products (Rahmani et al., 2009; Alshannaq & Yu, 2017; Shanakhat et al., 2018).

Therefore, a standard sampling method for regulating mycotoxins, including patulin, aflatoxins, *Fusarium* toxins, and ochratoxin in children's cereals and cereal-based foods, has been established by the European Union under Community Regulation No. 401/2006, as shown in Table 3.1.

3.8.1.2 Extraction of Mycotoxins

The extraction and purification of mycotoxins from contaminated food aim to isolate these toxins using appropriate solvents and to produce a purified extract free from interfering matrix components. Various methods are utilized for this purpose, including the following.

3.8.1.2.1 QuEChERS

This stands for quick, easy, cheap, effective, rugged, and safe. The method employs a mixture of acetonitrile and water for extraction, along with inorganic salts for liquid–liquid partitioning. Mycotoxins typically migrate to the organic phase, while many matrix components remain in the aqueous phase. Subsequent dispersive solid phase extraction helps to further purify the extract. This technique has proven effective for extracting fumonisins B1 and B2 from cereals aimed at children (Assuncao et al., 2015) and for isolating *Alternaria* mycotoxins from infant cereals (Gotthardt et al., 2019).

TABLE 3.1

Mycotoxin Bioaccessibility in Children's Cereal and Cereal-Based Foods (Pereira et al., 2022)

Country	Mycotoxins	Food Sample	Total Number of Foods Sampled	Bioaccessibility (%)	References
Italy	DON	Commercial pasta	6	2.12 – 41.5	Raiola et al., 2012
Portugal	PAT OTA PAT + OTA OTA + PAT	Cereal-based food	6	30 ± 3 – 77 ± 2 95 ± 0 – 105 ± 2 33 ± 1 – 64 ± 2 (PAT) 103 ± 1 – 109 ± 0 (OTA)	Assuncao et al., 2016
The Netherlands	AFB1 OTA	Infant formula (spaghetti Bolognese)	2	88 ± 16 – 94 ± 8 29 ± 6 – 32 ± 4	Kabak et al., 2009
Spain	ENA ENA1 ENB ENB1	Breakfast cereals Cookies Bread	14	50 ± 3 – 80 ± 3 40 ± 2 – 64 ± 2 43 ± 3 – 70 ± 3 46 ± 3 – 74 ± 2	Prosperini et al., 2013

Key: DON – Deoxynivalenol; PAT – Patulin; OTA – Ochratoxin; AFB1 – Aflatoxin B1; ENA – Enniatin A; ENA1 – Enniatin A1; ENB – Enniatin B; ENB1 – Enniatin B1

1. For samples exceeding 50 tons, 100 incremental samples should be collected, resulting in a total of 10 kg for the aggregated sample.
2. For samples below 50 tons, between 10 and 100 incremental samples should be taken, leading to an aggregated sample of 1 to 10 kg.
3. For samples at the retail level, a minimum of 1 kg should be collected (European Commission Regulation, 2006).

3.8.1.2.2 Liquid–Liquid Extraction (LLE)

This method leverages the differing solubilities of mycotoxins in organic and aqueous phases. At the conclusion of the extraction, the target mycotoxins are found in one solvent layer, while the matrix components reside in another (Turner et al., 2009). LLE has been successfully applied to extract aflatoxins and ochratoxins from breast milk (Andrade et al., 2013a).

3.8.1.2.3 Solid–Liquid Extraction (SLE)

This straightforward method involves mixing the sample with extraction solvents (such as acetonitrile/water or methanol/water) and agitating the mixture. This approach is often used for extracting various mycotoxins from solid food matrices (Rubert et al., 2012).

3.8.1.2.4 Pressurized Liquid Extraction (PLE)

Similar to SLE, this technique uses a pressure-resistant container, applying high pressure (1500–2000 psi) and elevated temperatures (100–180°C) to facilitate extraction (Razzazi-Fazeli & Reiter, 2011; Rico-Yuste et al., 2018; Miklos et al., 2020). It has been effective in detecting mycotoxins from *Alternaria alternata*.

3.8.1.2.5 Supercritical Fluid Extraction (SFE)

This method is particularly useful for extracting non-polar organic compounds using supercritical CO_2, which can often eliminate the need for organic solvents (Xie et al., 2016). SFE has been employed to detect zearalenone mycotoxins in maize flour (Zougagh & Rios, 2008).

3.8.1.3 Clean-Up of Mycotoxins

Clean-up methods are designed to minimize matrix interferences and enhance the specificity of mycotoxin quantification. The most commonly used techniques include solid phase extraction and immunoaffinity column methods (Razzazi-Fazeli & Reiter, 2011; Alshannaq & Yu, 2017).

3.8.1.3.1 Solid Phase Extraction

This technique employs solid adsorbents contained in cartridges, which are washed to remove impurities and isolate mycotoxins (Huertas-Perez et al., 2017). Common absorbents include amino-propyl, octadecyl silyl, silica gel, and hydrophilic-lipophilic balance materials. Recently, stronger adsorbents like magnetic carbon nanotubes have been utilized for enhanced performance in detecting trichothecenes A in various grains (Dong et al., 2015; Han et al., 2017; Dong et al., 2016). While this method is efficient, its effectiveness may be influenced by sample pH, ionic strength, and the solvent used (Pereira et al., 2014).

3.8.1.3.2 Immunoaffinity Column Technique

This method utilizes monoclonal antibodies that specifically bind to the target mycotoxin while removing water-soluble contaminants. The mycotoxins are subsequently eluted using pure acetonitrile or methanol. This technique conserves solvent usage; however, it may fail for mycotoxins that exceed the column's binding capacity, leading to unreliable results (Castegnaro et al., 2006). It has been applied to analyze ochratoxins, zearalenone, and aflatoxins in various cereal products (Irakli et al., 2017; Lattanzio et al., 2007; Lattanzio et al., 2014).

3.8.1.4 Detection of Mycotoxins

Numerous analytical techniques are used to detect mycotoxins in food and feed, including chromatographic methods such as thin layer chromatography, high-performance liquid chromatography (HPLC), and gas chromatography coupled with mass spectrometry (Turner et al., 2015; Zhang et al., 2018). Rapid detection methods include immunoassays like enzyme-linked immunosorbent assays (ELISA) and lateral flow immunoassays (Urusov et al., 2010; Lattanzio et al., 2019), as well as the use of biosensors (Evtugyn et al., 2017).

3.8.1.4.1 Chromatographic Methods

3.8.1.4.1.1 Thin Layer Chromatography This technique involves a stationary phase (such as cellulose or silica) and a mobile phase (composed of solvent mixtures) to separate mycotoxins (Wacoo et al., 2014). This technique is used in the quantitative and qualitative analysis of mycotoxins such as patulin and aflatoxin (Odhav & Naicker, 2002; Andrade et al., 2013a). The detection of mycotoxins using this method is associated with poor precision and low sensitivity (Singh & Mehta, 2020); also, the preparation of sample and the clean-up technique depends on the mycotoxin kind and properties (Yang et al., 2014). While it can analyze mycotoxins like patulin and aflatoxin, it may suffer from low precision and sensitivity (Singh & Mehta, 2020).

3.8.1.4.1.2 Liquid Chromatography This versatile method can effectively separate thermal-labile and polar mycotoxins. HPLC, which may utilize UV-visible or fluorescent detectors, allows for simultaneous detection of various mycotoxins (Turner et al., 2009). HPLC with fluorescence detection has been used for ochratoxin detection in different matrices (Zinedine et al., 2007).

3.8.1.4.1.3 Gas Chromatography This method is useful for detecting mycotoxins in processed grain products, involving the stx1eparation of analytes in the stationary phase with subsequent detection by mass spectrometry (Rodriguez-Carrasco et al., 2012; Rodriguez-Carrasco et al., 2014).

3.8.1.4.2 Rapid Methods

3.8.1.4.2.1 ELISA This immunochemical method allows for quick testing of multiple samples and is based on antigen–antibody interactions, measured spectrophotometrically (Li et al., 2009; Urusov et al., 2010; (Al-Jaal et al., 2019; Oplatowska-Stachowiak et al., 2018). It has been successfully used for detecting mycotoxins in various grains, although it can be affected by cross-reactivity with structurally similar compounds (Zheng et al., 2005; Pleadin et al., 2012; Thway & Salimi-Moosavi, 2014; Omar et al., 2020, Singh & Mehta, 2020).

3.8.1.4.2.2 Lateral Flow Immunoassay This strip test utilizes labeled antibodies to provide a visual signal indicating the presence of mycotoxins (Anfossi et al., 2013; Song et al., 2014). It employs capillary action similar to absorbent paper (Wang et al., 2009; Zhang et al., 2017; Anfossi et al., 2018; Li et al., 2020) and has been utilized for various mycotoxins in cereals (Ren et al., 2015; Li et al., 2019).

3.8.1.4.2.3 Biosensors These devices integrate biological sensing elements with transducers to convert biological signals into electrical signals (Perumal & Hashim, 2014; Santana Oliveira et al., 2019). Various transducer types, such as optical and electrochemical, can enhance sensitivity through the use of nanomaterials (Dora et al., 2012; Altintas et al., 2017).

The methods for analyzing mycotoxins in cereal-based foods for children from 2014 to 2021 are detailed in Table 3.2.

3.8.2 Bioaccessibility and Bioavailability Studies of Mycotoxins

Bioaccessibility studies of mycotoxins can be performed using either in vivo or in vitro methods.

In vivo studies are categorized into two main types: those focused on determining metabolites and those examining overall balance. These studies are complex, involving various analytical and ethical considerations. Additionally, they require significant time for planning and resource acquisition, as well as stringent experimental controls (Cardoso et al., 2015).

In vitro studies, on the other hand, can be divided into dynamic and static models. The static model simulates the digestive process by exposing food substances to conditions resembling those in the stomach and small intestine. In contrast, the dynamic model replicates the sequential movement of food through the digestive system, providing a more precise representation of digestion. Some models mimic the digestive processes found in animal stomachs and intestines, while others represent the large intestine, including its microbial community (Cardoso et al., 2015).

The physiological components of in vitro digestion models typically include saliva (often simulated as a fluid containing α-amylase, electrolytes, and urea), gastric fluids (a mixture of pepsin, water, and electrolytes at a low pH), and intestinal juices (which consist of bile salts, electrolytes, and pancreatin). Factors such as incubation time, temperature, peristalsis, and the presence of microorganisms are also considered (Gonzalez-Arias et al., 2013). Numerous studies have investigated the bioaccessibility of mycotoxins, focusing on their extraction and detection in food (Gil-Izquierdo et al., 2002; Versantvoort et al., 2005; Kabak et al., 2009; Raiola et al., 2012; Prosperini et al., 2013; Minekus et al., 2014; Assuncao et al., 2016).

3.9 Global Regulations and Limitations of Mycotoxin Exposure in Children's Food

Mycotoxins produced by fungi pose significant health risks, particularly in food products intended for children. The objective of global regulations concerning mycotoxin limits in children's food is to reduce these risks and protect young consumers, although there are still research gaps regarding the prevalence and health impacts of these toxins.

TABLE 3.2

Methods for Mycotoxin Analysis in Children's Cereal-Based Foods from 2014–2021

		Sample Pretreatment		Methods		
Matrix	Mycotoxin	Extraction	Cleanup	Derivatization	Detection Methods	Reference
Infant formula and baby food	DON, NIV, FUS-X, DAS, 15acDON, 3acDON, NEO, HT2, T2	ACN:water; 84:16 v/v	–	–	LC-MS/MS	Juan et al., 2014
	ZON, ENB(ENB1/4), ENA(ENA1), BEA	ACN:MeOH; 60:40 v/v				
Infant formula and baby food	OTA	ACN:water 60:40 (v/v)	Ochratest IAC	–	HPLC-FD	Juan et al., 2014
	AFB1	NaCl, MeOH:water 80:20 v/v	Aflatest IAC			
	AFM1	NaCl Dichloromethane:acetone 1:1 v/v	Aflatest IAC			
	PAT	Na_2SO_4 + $NaHCO_3$ + ethylacetate/ hexane 60:40 (v/v)	Strata SPE C18-E		HPLC-UV	
Cereal baby food	VER, DON. FUS-X, DAS, 3acDON, 15acDON, NIV, T2-Tetrol, NEO, T2-Triol, HT2, T2	QuEChERS d-SPE		Tri-SilTBT BSA + TMSI + TMCS (3:3:2)	GS-MS	Pereira et al., 2015
Breakfast food	AFB1, AFB2, AFG1, AFG2, AFM1, OTA	MeOH:water (80:20)	IAC (AflaOchra, Vicam)	–	RP-HPLC-FD	Martins et al., 2018
	DON, NEO, DAS, FUS-X, 15acDON, T-2 Triol, NIV T-2, HT-2, 3acDON, VER T2-Tetrol	QuEChERS d-SPE		BSA + TMCS + TMSI (3:2:3)	GS-MS	
	FB1, FB2, ZEA	MeOH:water(75:25)	–	–	UPLC-MS/MS	
Cereal-based food	AFB1, AFB2, AFG1, AFG2, AFM1, OTA	MeOH:water(80:20)	IAC (AflaOchra, Vicam)	–	RP-HPLC-FD	Assuncao et al., 2018
	DON, NIV, T-2, HT-2	QuEChERS d-SPE		BSA + TMCS + TMSI (3:2:3)	GS-MS	
	FB1, FB2, ZEA	MeOH:water(75:25)	–	–	UPLC-MS/MS	

(Continued)

TABLE 3.2 ***(Continued)***

Methods for Mycotoxin Analysis in Children's Cereal-Based Foods from 2014–2021

		Sample Pretreatment		Methods		
Matrix	**Mycotoxin**	**Extraction**	**Cleanup**	**Derivatization**	**Detection Methods**	**Reference**
Cereal-based baby food	AOH, AME, TEN, ATX1, ATLP, TA	ACN:water(84:16) + formic acid ACN:MeOH:water(50:25:25) + formic acid	SPE	–	UPLC-MS/MS	Gotthardt et al., 2019
Breakfast cereals, sweet snacks	OTA	Dichloromethane	–	–	ELISA (I'screen Ochracod. OR360	Capei et al., 2019
Cereal-based baby food	AFB1, AFB2, AFG1, AFG2	MeOH:water(80:20)	IAC (AflaTest, Vicam)	–	HPLC-FD	Herrera et al., 2019
	DON	MeOH	IAC (Don est, Vicam)	–	HPLC-DAD	
Cereal-based infant and children's food	DON, NIV, ZEA, OTA, HT-2, T-2, FB1, FB2	MeCN:acetic acid:water (80:1:19)	–	–	HPLC-MS/MS	Postupolski et al., 2019
Cereal-based infant food	AFL, AFB1, STG, ZEN, DON, NIV, T-2, BEA, ENA, ENA1, ENB, ENB1, FB1, AME, TA, TTX, ATLP	MeOH: H_2O: acetic acid (79:20:1)	–	–	LC-MS/MS	Braun et al., 2021

Key: DON: Deoxynivalenol, NIV: Nivalenol, FUS-X: Fusarenon-X, DAS: Diacetoxyscirpenol, 15acDON: 15-Acetyldeoxynivalenol, 3acDON: 3-Acetyldeoxynivalenol, NEO: Neosolaniol, HT-2: HT-2 Mycotoxin, T-2: T-2 Mycotoxin, ACN: Acetonitrile, LC-MS/MS: Liquid Chromatography-Tandem Mass Spectrometry, ZON: Zearalenone, ENB: Enniatin B, ENA: Enniatin A, BEA: Beauvericin, MeOH: Methanol, OTA: Ochratoxin, AFB1: Aflatoxin B1, AFM1: Aflatoxin M1, IAC: Immunoaffinity Column, HPLC-FD: High-Performance Liquid Chromatography with Fluorescence Detection, HPLC-UV: High-Performance Liquid Chromatography with Ultraviolet Detection, T2-Tetrol: T2-Tetrol Mycotoxin, PAT: Patulin, T2 Triol: Trichothecene Mycotoxin, QuEChERS: Quick, Easy, Cheap, Effective, Rugged, and Safe, d-SPE: Dispersive Solid-Phase Extraction, Tri-SilTBT: TMSI:BSA; TMCS Reagent, BSA: N,O-Bis(trimethylsilyl)acetamide, TMSI: N-Trimethylsilylimidazole, TMCS: Trimethylchlorosilane, GC-MS: Gas Chromatography-Mass Spectrometry, AFB2: Aflatoxin B2, AFG1: Aflatoxin G1, AFG2: Aflatoxin G2, RP-HPLC-FD: Reversed-Phase High-Performance Liquid Chromatography with Fluorescence Detection, FB2: Fumonisin B2, FB1: Fumonisin B1, UPLC-MS/MS: Ultra-Performance Liquid Chromatography-Tandem Mass Spectrometry, AOH: Alternariol, AME: Alternariol Monomethyl Ether, TEN: Tentoxin, ATLP: Alterperylenol, ATX I: Altertoxin 1, SPE: Solid-Phase Extraction, TA: Tenuazonic Acid, AFL: Aflatoxicol, STG: Sterigmatocystin, ZEN: Zearalenone, ENA: Enniatin A, ENA1: Enniatin A1, ENB1: Enniatin B1, ELISA: Enzyme-Linked Immunosorbent Assay, TTX: Tetrodotoxin, RP-HPLC-DAD: Reversed-Phase High-Performance Liquid Chromatography with Diode Array Detection, NaCl: Sodium Chloride, UPLC-MS: Ultra-Performance Liquid Chromatography-Mass Spectrometry.

3.9.1 Regulatory Framework for Mycotoxin Exposure in Children's Food

International regulatory agencies such as the Food and Agriculture Organization (FAO) and the World Health Organization (WHO), along with various national authorities, set limits on mycotoxin levels in food for children. These regulations aim to safeguard public health, focusing on vulnerable populations like children. For example, the European Union (EU) has established maximum allowable limits for mycotoxins in cereals and related products to minimize exposure (European Commission, 2021). Additionally, the Codex Alimentarius Commission offers guidelines on mycotoxin restrictions for globally traded food products, ensuring safety across national borders (Codex Alimentarius, 2020).

3.9.2 Limitations of Mycotoxin Exposure in Children's Food

Children, due to their developing immune systems and relatively high food intake based on body weight, are particularly susceptible to mycotoxins. Chronic exposure to contaminants such as aflatoxins, ochratoxin A, and fumonisins can lead to serious health issues, including impaired growth, weakened immune function, and potential carcinogenic effects (Smith et al., 2022; Gong et al., 2024). Regulatory efforts focus on minimizing these toxins in foods specifically designed for children, like infant cereals and baby foods, ensuring compliance with strict safety standards.

3.10 Research Gaps in Mycotoxin Exposure in Children's Food

Despite existing regulations, notable research gaps persist regarding mycotoxin contamination in children's cereal-based foods. Recent findings identify several critical areas needing attention:

3.10.1 Diversity of Mycotoxin Analysis

Current regulations primarily address a limited number of well-known mycotoxins. However, there is less understanding of emerging mycotoxins and their potential synergistic effects with established toxins (Braun et al., 2021). Comprehensive screening methods are essential to evaluate the full range of mycotoxin contamination in foods for children.

3.10.2 Exposure Assessment

There is a scarcity of thorough exposure assessments specifically designed for children, especially concerning simultaneous exposure to multiple mycotoxins from various dietary sources (Assuncao et al., 2018; Martins et al., 2018). Longitudinal studies are necessary to assess the cumulative effects of exposure over time.

3.10.3 Impact on Vulnerable Groups

Research on how different ages, health conditions, and geographic locations affect children's susceptibility to mycotoxins is limited (Assuncao et al., 2018). More focused studies are required to evaluate health outcomes across diverse demographics.

3.10.4 Mitigation Strategies

There is an ongoing need for research into effective strategies aimed at reducing mycotoxin levels in children's foods, including better agricultural practices, development of mycotoxin-resistant crop varieties, and advancements in food processing technologies (Gong et al., 2024).

3.10.5 Regulatory Harmonization

Although international guidelines exist, variations in mycotoxin regulations among different regions impede global harmonization and complicate food trade and safety (European Commission, 2021).

3.11 Conclusions

Addressing mycotoxin contamination in children's food is a complex issue requiring coordinated efforts among regulatory bodies, industry players, and researchers. Global perspectives highlight the necessity of stringent regulations set by organizations like the FAO and WHO to protect vulnerable groups from the adverse health effects of mycotoxins. These regulations provide essential guidelines for acceptable mycotoxin levels in cereals and cereal-based products, which are vital for ensuring children's health. However, the challenges posed by mycotoxin contamination necessitate ongoing research to bridge existing gaps. Recent studies underscore the importance of robust monitoring systems capable of detecting a variety of mycotoxins and assessing trends in exposure over time. Furthermore, developing targeted mitigation strategies that consider the unique vulnerabilities of children is crucial, involving improvements in agricultural practices and processing technologies.

Collaboration among researchers, regulators, and food industry stakeholders is essential to enhance understanding, improve detection methodologies, and align regulatory frameworks globally. This collaborative effort is key to ensuring reliable safety standards for children's food products and effectively mitigating the risks associated with mycotoxin contamination. Through continued innovation and evidence-based approaches, we can work towards creating safer and healthier food environments for children around the world.

References

Abdallah, M. F., Audenaert, K., Lust, L., Landschoot, S., Bekaert, B., Haesaert, G., De Boevre, M., & De Saeger, S. (2020). Risk characterization and quantification of mycotoxins and their producing fungi in sugarcane juice: A neglected problem in a widely-consumed traditional beverage. *Food Control, 108.*

Adeyeye, S. A. O. (2016). Fungal mycotoxins in foods: A review. *Cogent Food & Agriculture,* 2(1), 1213127.

Al-Jaal, B., Salama, S., Al-Qasmi, N., & Jaganjac, M. (2019). Mycotoxin contamination of food and feed in the Gulf Cooperation Council countries and its detection. *Toxicon, 171,* 43–50.

Alshannaq, A., & Yu, J. H. (2017). Occurrence, toxicity and analysis of major mycotoxins in food. *International Journal of Environmental Research and Public Health,* 14(6), 632.

Altintas, Z., Davis, F., & Scheller, F. W. (2017). Applications of quantum dots in biosensors and diagnostics. *Biosensors and Bioelectronics, 3,* 185–199.

Alvito, P. C., Sizoo, E. A., Almeida, C. M. M., & van Egmond, H. P. (2010). Occurrence of aflatoxins and ochratoxin A in baby foods in Portugal. *Food Analytical Methods, 3,* 22–30.

Amobonye, A., Aruwa, C., Aransiola, S. A., John, O., Alabi, T. D., & Lalung, J. (2023). Exploring the potential of fungi in the bioremediation of pharmaceutically active compounds. *Frontiers in Microbiology, 14,* 1207792, https://doi.10.3389/fmicb.2023.1207792

Andrade, P. D., da Silva, J. L. G., & Caldas, E. D. (2013a). Simultaneous analysis of aflatoxins B1, B2, G1, G2, M1 and ochratoxin A in breast milk by high-performance liquid chromatography/fluorescence after liquid-liquid extraction with low temperature purification (LLE-LTP). *Journal of Chromatography A, 1304,* 61–68. https://doi.org/10.1016/j.chroma.2013.06.049

Anfossi, L., Baggiani, C., Giovannolu, C., D'Arco, G., & Giraudi, G. (2013). Lateral-flow immunoassays for mycotoxins and phycotoxins: A review. *Analytical and Bioanalytical Chemistry, 405,* 467–480.

Anfossi, L., Di Nardo, F., Cavalera, S., Giovannoli, C., Spano, G., Speranskaya, E. S., Goryacheva, I. Y., & Baggiani, C. (2018). A lateral flow immunoassay for straightforward determination of fumonisin mycotoxins based on the quenching of the fluorescence of CdSe/ZnS quantum dot by gold and silver nanoparticles. *Microchimica Acta, 185,* 94.

Arce-Lopez, B., Lizarraga, E., Vettorazzi, A., & Gonzalez-Penas, E. (2020). Human biomonitoring of mycotoxins in blood, plasma and serum in recent years: A review. *Toxins, 12,* 147.

Assuncao, R., Martins, C., Dupont, D., & Alvito, P. (2016). Patulin and ochratoxin A co-occurrence and their bioaccessibility in processed cereal-based foods: A combination for Portuguese children risk assessment. *Food and Chemical Toxicology, 96,* 205–214.

Assuncao, R., Martins, C., Vasco, E., Jager, A., Oliveira, C., Cunha, S. C., Fernandes, J. O., Nunes, B., Loureiro, S., & Alvito, P. (2018). Portuguese children dietary exposure to multiple mycotoxins-An overview of risk assessment under MYCOMIX project. *Food and Chemical Toxicology, 118,* 399–408.

Assuncao, R., Vasco, E., Nunes, B., Loureiro, S., Martins, C., & Alvito, P. (2015). Single compound and cumulative risk assessment of mycotoxins present in breakfast cereals consumed by children from Lisbon region, Portugal. *Food and Chemical Toxicology, 86*, 274–281.

Battilani, P., Barbano, C., & Logrieco, A. (2008). Risk assessment and safety evaluation of mycotoxins in fruits. In R. Barkai-Golan & N. Paster (Eds.), *Mycotoxins in fruits and vegetables* (pp. 1–26). Academic Press.

Begum, F., & Samajpati, N. (2000). Mycotoxin production on rice, pulses and oilseeds. *Naturwissenschaften, 87*, 275–277.

Beltrán, E., Ibáñez, M., Sancho, J. V., Cortés, M. Á., Yus, V., & Hernández, F. (2011). UHPLC-MS/MS highly sensitive determination of aflatoxins, the aflatoxin metabolite M1 and ochratoxin A in baby food and milk. *Food Chemistry, 126*, 737–744.

Bennett, J. W., & Klich, M. (2003). Mycotoxins. *Clinical Microbiology Reviews, 16*, 497–516. https://doi.org/10.1128/CMR.16.3.497-516.2003

Bentley, M. E., & Nulty, A. K. (2020). When does it all begin: What, when, and how young children are fed. *Nestle Nutrition Institute Workshop Series, 93*, 15–24.

Binder, E. M., Tan, L. M., Chin, L. J., Handl, J., & Richard, J. (2007). Worldwide occurrence of mycotoxins in commodities, feeds and feed ingredients. *Animal Feed Science and Technology, 137*, 265–282.

Bonel, L., Vidal, J. C., Duato, P., & Castillo, J. R. (2011). An electrochemical competitive biosensor for ochratoxin A based on a DNA biotinylated aptamer. *Biosensors & Bioelectronics, 26*, 3254–3259.

Boussabbeh, M., Ben Salem, I., Belguesmi, F., Neffati, F., Najar, M. F., Abid-Essefi, S., & Bacha, H. (2016). Crocin protects the liver and kidney from patulin-induced apoptosis in vivo. *Environmental Science and Pollution Research International, 23*(10), 9799–9808.

Braun, D., Eiser, M., Puntscher, H., Marko, D., & Warth, B. (2021). Natural contaminant in infant food: The case of regulated and emerging mycotoxins. *Food Control, 123*, 107676.

Bryden, W. L. (2007). Mycotoxins in the food chain: Human health implications. *Asia Pacific Journal of Clinical Nutrition, 16*, 95–101.

Bryden, W. L. (2012). Mycotoxin contamination of the feed supply chain: Implications for animal productivity and feed security. *Animal Feed Science and Technology, 173*, 134–158.

Capei, R., Pettini, L., Mando Tacconi, F. (2019). Occurrence of ochratoxin A in breakfast cereals and sweet snacks in Italy: Dietary exposure assessment. *Annali di Igiene, 31*, 130–139.

Cardoso, C., Afonso, C., Lourenco, H., Costa, S., & Nunes, M. L. (2015). Bioaccessibility assessment methodologies and their consequences for the risk-benefit evaluation of food. *Trends in Food Science & Technology, 41*, 5–23.

Cascant, M. M., Garrigues, S., & de la Guardia, M. (2015). Direct determination of major components in human diets and baby foods. *Analytical and Bioanalytical Chemistry, 407*, 1961–1972.

CAST. (2003). Mycotoxins: Risks in plant, animal, and human systems. Task force report no. 139.

Castegnaro, M., Tozlovanu, M., Wild, C., Molinie, A., Sylla, A., & Leszkowicz, A. (2006). Advantages and drawbacks of immunoaffinity columns in analysis of mycotoxins in food. *Molecular Nutrition & Food Research, 50*(6), 480–487.

Centers for Disease Control and Prevention (CDCP). (2004). Outbreak of aflatoxin poisoning eastern and central provinces, Kenya. *Morbidity and Mortality Weekly Report (MMWR), 53*(34), 790–793.

Clarke, R., Connolly, L., Frizzell, C., & Elliott, C. T. (2014). Cytotoxic assessment of the regulated, co-existing mycotoxins aflatoxin B1, fumonisin B1 and ochratoxin, in single, binary and tertiary mixtures. *Toxicon, 90,* 70–81.

Codex Alimentarius Commission. (2020). General standard for contaminants and toxins in food and feed. Codex STAN 193–1995. Rome, Italy: FAO/WHO.

Coppock, R. W., Christian, R. G., & Jacobsen, B. J. (2018). Aflatoxins in veterinary toxicology: Basic and clinical principles. In R. C. Gupta (Ed.), *Aflatoxins in veterinary toxicology* (pp. 983–994). Academic Press.

Da Rocha, M. E. B., da Freire, F. C. O., Maia, F. E. F., Guedes, M. I. F., & Rondina, D. (2014). Mycotoxins and their effects on human and animal health. *Food Control, 36,* 159–165.

Darwish, W. S., Ikenaka, Y., Nakayama, S. M. M., & Ishizuka, M. (2014). An overview on mycotoxin contamination of foods in Africa. *Journal of Veterinary Medical Science, 76,* 789–797.

Dong, M., Si, W., Jiang, K., Nie, D., Wu, Y., Zhao, Z., . . . Han, Z. (2015). Multi-walled carbon nanotubes as solid-phase extraction sorbents for simultaneous determination of type A trichothecenes in maize, wheat and rice by ultra-high performance liquid chromatography-tandem mass spectrometry. *Journal of Chromatography A, 1423,* 177–182.

Dong, M., Si, W., Wang, W., Bai, B., Nie, D., Song, W., . . . Han, Z. (2016). Determination of type A trichothecenes in coix seed by magnetic solid-phase extraction based on magnetic multi-walled carbon nanotubes coupled with ultra-high performance liquid chromatography-tandem mass spectrometry. *Analytical and Bioanalytical Chemistry, 408*(25), 6823–6831.

Dora, G., Conde, J., Veigas, B., Giestas, L., Almeida, C., Assuncao, M., Rosa, J., & Baptista, P. V. (2012). Noble metal nanoparticles for biosensing applications. *Sensors, 12,* 1657–1687.

Dorninger-Gruber, C., Novak, B., Nagl, V., & Berthiller, F. (2017). Emerging mycotoxins: Beyond traditionally determined food contaminants. *Journal of Agricultural and Food Chemistry, 65,* 7052–7070.

Doughari, J. H. (2015). The occurrence, properties and significance of citrinin mycotoxin. *Journal of Plant Pathology & Microbiology, 6,* 11.

El-Kerdasy, A. F., Fathalla, S. I., & Abdel-Aziz, A. Mosaad. (2019). Effect of probiotic (lactobacillus& saccaromyces) on the immunological, biochemical and haematological changes of broiler chicken fed on ochratoxicated ration. *World Journal of Pharmaceutical Sciences, 7*(3), 137–141.

Esam, R. M., Hafez, R. S., Khafaga, N. I. M., Fahim, K. M., & Ahmed, L. I. (2022). Assessment of aflatoxin M1 and B1 in some dairy products with referring to the analytical performances of enzyme-linked immunosorbent assay in comparison to high-performance liquid chromatography. *Veterinary World, 15*(1), 91–101. https://doi.org/10.14202/vetworld.2022.91-101

European Commission. (2006). Regulation (EC) No 401/2006 of 23 February 2006 laying down the methods of sampling and analysis for the official control of the levels of mycotoxins in foodstuffs. *Official Journal of the European Union, 70*(12), 12–34.

European Commission. (2021). *Mycotoxins*. Retrieved from https://ec.europa.eu/food/safety/chemical_safety/contaminants/catalogue/mycotoxins_en
Evtugyn, G. A., Shamagsumova, R. V., & Hianik, T. (2017). Biosensors for detection mycotoxins and pathogenic bacteria in food. In A. M. Grumezescu (Ed.), *Nanobiosensors* (pp. 35–92). Academic Press.
Fox, E. M., & Howlett, B. J. (2008). Secondary metabolism: Regulation and role in fungal biology. *Current Opinion in Microbiology, 11*, 481–487.
Gaddeyya, G., Niharika, P. S., Bharathi, P., & Kumar, P. K. R. (2012). Isolation and identification of soil mycoflora in different crop fields at Salur Mandal. *Advances in Applied Science Research, 3*, 2020–2026.
Gil-Izquierdo, A., Zafrilla, P., & Tomas-Barberan, F. A. (2002). An in vitro method to simulate phenolic compound release from the food matrix in the gastrointestinal tract. *European Food Research and Technology, 214*, 155–159.
Gong, Q., Zhang, Z., Huang, P., Wang, B., & Zheng, X. (2024). Assessment of fungal and contamination of ochratoxin A and patulin in foods susceptible to contamination in the Yangzhou Market, China. *Foods, 13*(19), 3205.
Gong, Y. Y., Watson, S., & Routledge, M. N. (2016). Aflatoxin exposure and associated human health effects, a review of epidemiological studies. *Food Safety, 4*, 14–27.
Gonzalez-Arias, C. A., Marin, S., Sanchis, V., & Ramos, A. J. (2013). Mycotoxin bioaccessibility/absorption assessment using in vitro digestion models: A review. *World Mycotoxin Journal, 6*, 167–184.
Gotthardt, M., Asam, S., Gunkel, K., Moghaddam, A. F., Baumann, E., Kietz., R., & Rychlikm, M. (2019). Quantitation of six Alternaria toxins in infant foods applying stable isotope labeled standards. *Frontiers in Microbiology, 10*, 109–109.
Han, Z., Jiang, K., Fan, Z., Diana Di Mavungu, J., Dong, M., Guo, W., . . . Wu, Y. (2017). Multi-walled carbon nanotubes-based magnetic solid-phase extraction for the determination of zearolenone and its derivatives in maize by ultra-high performance liquid chromatography-tandem mass spectrometry. *Food Control, 79*, 177–184.
Hashem, M., & Alamri, S. (2010). Contamination of common spices in Saudi Arabia markets with potential mycotoxin-producing fungi. *Saudi Journal of Biological Sciences, 17*(2), 167–175.
Herrera, M., Bervis, N., Carraminana, J. J., Juan, T., Herrera, A., Arino, A., & Loran., S. (2019). Occurrence and assessment of aflatoxins and deoxynivalenol in cereal-based baby foods for infants. *Toxins (Basel), 11*, 3.
Huertas-Perez, J. F., Arroyo-Manzanares, N., Garcia-Campana, A. M., & Gamiz-Gracia, L. (2017). Solid phase extraction as sample treatment for the determination of ochratoxin A in foods: A review. *Critical Reviews in Food Science and Nutrition, 57*(15), 3405–3420.
Hussein, H. S., & Brasel, J. M. (2001). Toxicity, metabolism, and impact of mycotoxins on humans and animals. *Toxicology, 167*, 101–134.
Iheshiulor, O. O. M., Esonu, B. O., Chuwuka, O. K., Omede, A. A., Okoli, I. C., & Ogbuewu, I. P. (2011). Effects of mycotoxins in animal nutrition. *Asian Journal of Animal Science, 5*, 19–33.
International Agency for Research on Cancer (IARC). (2002). Some traditional herbal medicines, some mycotoxins, naphthalene and styrene. In *International Agency for Research on Cancer Monographs on the evaluation of carcinogenic risks to humans* (Vol. 82, p. 590). Lyon, France: IARC Press.
International Agency for Research on Cancer (IARC). (2015). Mycotoxin control in low- and middle-income countries. In C. P. Wild, J. D. Miller, & J. D. Groopman (Eds.), *Working group report*. Lyon, France: IARC.

Irakli, M. N., Skendi, A., & Papageorgiou, M. D. (2017). HOLC-DAD-FLD methods for simultaneous determination of mycotoxins in wheat bran. *Journal of Chromatographic Science, 55*(7), 690–696.
Jarvis, B. B. (2002). Chemistry and toxicology of molds isolated from water damaged buildings. In J. W. deVries, M. W. Trucksess, & L. S. Jackson (Eds.), *Mycotoxins and food safety* (pp. 43–52). Kluwer Academic/Plenum Publications.
Jestoi, M. (2008). Emerging Fusarium mycotoxins fusaproliferin, beauvericin, enniatins, and moniliformin-A review. *Critical Reviews in Food Science and Nutrition, 48,* 21–49.
John, I. P., & Miller, J. D. (2017). A concise history of mycotoxin research. *Journal of Agricultural and Food Chemistry, 65,* 7021–7033.
Jouany, J. P. (2007). Methods for preventing, decontaminating and minimizing the toxicity of mycotoxins in feeds. *Animal Feed Science and Technology, 137,* 342–362.
Juan, C., Raiola, A., Mañes, J., & Ritieni, A. (2014). Presence of mycotoxin in commercial infant formulas and baby foods from Italian market. *Food Control, 39,* 227–236.
Kabak, B., Brandon, E. F. A., Var, I., Blokland, M., & Sips, A. J. A. M. (2009). Effects of probiotic bacteria on the bioaccessibility of aflatoxin B1 and ochratoxin A using an in vitro digestion model under fed conditions. *Journal of Environmental Science and Health Part B, 44,* 472–480.
Kabak, B., Dobson, A. D., & Var, I. (2006). Strategies to prevent mycotoxin contamination of food and animal feed: A review. *Critical Reviews in Food Science and Nutrition, 46*(8), 593–619.
Kim, D. M., Chung, S. H., & Chun, H. S. (2011). Multiplex PCR assay for the detection of aflatoxigenic and non-aflatoxigenic fungi in meju, a Korean fermented soybean food starter. *Food Microbiology, 28,* 1402–1408.
Ladeira, C., Frazzoli, C., & Orisakwe, O. E. (2017). Engaging one health for non-communicable diseases in Africa: Perspective for mycotoxins. *Frontiers in Public Health, 5,* Article 266. https://doi.org/10.3389/fpubh.2017.00266
Landeweert, R., Leeflang, P., Kuyper, T. W., Hoffland, E., Rosling, A., Wernars, K., & Smit, E. (2003). Molecular identification of ectomycorrhizal mycelium in soil horizons. *Applied and Environmental Microbiology, 69,* 327–333.
Lattanzio, V. M. T., Ciasca, B., Powers, S., & Visconti, A. (2014). Improved method for the simultaneous determination of aflatoxins, ochratoxin A and Fusarium toxins in cereals and derived products by liquid chromatography/tandem mass spectrometry after multitoxin immunoaffinity cleanup. *Journal of Chromatography A, 1354,* 139–143.
Lattanzio, V. M. T., Solfrizzo, M., Powers, S., & Visconti, A. (2007). Simultaneous determination of aflatoxins, ochratoxin A and Fusarium toxins in maize by liquid chromatography/tandem mass spectrometry after multitoxin immunoaffinity column cleanup. *Rapid Communications in Mass Spectrometry, 21*(19), 3253–3261.
Lattanzio, V. M. T., von Holst, C., Lippolis, V., De Girolamo, A., Logrieco, A. F., Mol, H. G. J., & Pascale, M. (2019). Evaluation of mycotoxin screening tests in a verification study involving first time users. *Toxins, 11*(3), Article 129.
Leslie, J. F., & Summerell, B. A. (2006). *The Fusarium Laboratory Manual.* Blackwell Publishing. https://doi.org/10.1002/9780470278376
Li, P., Zhnag, Q., & Zhang, W. (2009). Immunoassays for aflatoxins. *TrAC Trends in Analytical Chemistry, 28,* 1115–1126.
Li, R., Meng, C., Wen, Y., Fu, W., & He, P. (2019). Fluorometric lateral flow immunoassay for simultaneous determination of three mycotoxins (aflatoxin B1, zearalenone and deoxynivalenol) using quantum dot microbeads. *Microchimica Acta, 186,* 748.

Li, Y., Liu, L., Kuang, H., & Xu, C. (2020). Visible and eco-friendly immunoassays for the detection of cyclopiazonic acid in maize and rice. *Journal of Food Science, 85*, 105–113.
Luongo, D., Russo, R., Balestrieri, A., Marzocco, S., Bergamo, P., & Severino, L. (2014). In vitro study of AFB1 and AFM1 effects on human lymphoblastoid Jurkat T-cell model. *Journal of Immunotoxicology, 11*, 353–358.
Magan, N., Sanchis, V., & Aldred, D. (2003). The Role of Spoilage Fungi in Seed Deterioration. In D. K. Aurora (Ed.), *Fungal biotechnology in agriculture, food and environmental application* (pp. 311–323). Marcel Dekker, Inc.
Mallebrera, B., Prosperini, A., Font, G., & Ruiz, M. J. (2018). In vitro mechanisms of beauvericin toxicity: A review. *Food and Chemical Toxicology, 111*, 537–545.
Marasas, W. F. O. (2001). Discovery and occurrence of the fumonisins: A historical perspective. *Environmental Health Perspectives, 109*(Supplement 2), 239–243.
Martins, C., Assuncao, R., Cunha, S. C., Fernandes, J. O., Jager, A., Petta, T., Oliveira, C. A., & Alvito, P. (2018). Assessment of multiple mycotoxins in breakfast cereals available in the Portuguese market. *Food Chemistry, 239*, 132–140. https://doi.org/10.1016/j.foodchem.2017.06.147
Meucci, V., Razzuoli, E., Soldani, G., & Massart, F. (2010). Mycotoxin detection in infant formula milks in Italy. *Food Additives & Contaminants Part A, 27*, 64–71.
Miklos, G., Angeli, C., Ambrus, A., Nagy, A., Kardos, V., Zentai, A., . . . Bartok, T. (2020). Detection of aflatoxins in different matrices and food-chain positions. *Frontiers in Microbiology, 11*, Article 1916.
Milani, J. M. (2013). Ecological conditions affecting mycotoxin production in cereals: A review. *Veterinarni Medicina, 58*, 405–411.
Minekus, M., Alminger, M., Alvito, P., Balance, S., Bohn, T., Bourlieu, C., . . . Brodkorb, A. (2014). Standardised static in vitro digestion method suitable for food-an international consensus. *Food and Function, 5*, 1113–1124.
Monod, M., Bontems, O., Zaugg, C., Chenne, B. L., Fratti, M., & Panizzon, R. (2006). Fast and reliable PCR/sequencing/RFLP assay for identification of fungi in onychomycoses. *Journal of Medical Microbiology, 55*, 1211–1216.
Niculita-Hirzel, H., Hantier, G., Storti, F., Plateel, G., & Roger, T. (2016). Frequent occupational exposure to Fusarium mycotoxins of workers in the Swiss grain industry. *Toxins, 8*, 370.
Odhav, B., & Naicker, V. (2002). Mycotoxins in South Africa traditionally brewed beers. *Food Additives & Contaminants, 19*(1), 55–61.
Ojuri, O. T., Ezekiel, C. N., Eskola, M. K., Šarkanj, B., Babalola, A. D., Sulyok, M., Hajšlová, J., Elliott, C. T., & Krska, R. (2019). Mycotoxin co-exposures in infants and young children consuming household- and industrially-processed complementary foods in Nigeria and risk management advice. *Food Control*, 98, 312–322. https://doi.org/10.1016/j.foodcont.2018.11.049
Omar, S. S., Haddad, M. A., & Parisi, S. (2020). Validation of HPLC and Enzyme-Linked Immunosorbent Assay (ELISA) techniques for quantification of aflatoxins in different food samples. *Foods, 9*, 661.
Oplatowska-Stachowiak, M., Reiring, C., Sajic, N., Haasnoot, W., Brabet, C., Campbell, K., Elliott, C. T., & Salden, M. (2018). Development and in-house validation of a rapid and simple to use ELISA for detection and measurement of the mycotoxin sterigmotocystin. *Analytical and Bioanalytical Chemistry, 410*, 3017–3023.
Oyeleke, A., & Manga, S. B. (2008). *Essentials of laboratory practice* (3rd ed.). Minna, Niger state, Nigeria: Tobest Publisher.

Paterson, R. R. M., & Lima, N. (2010). How will climate change affect mycotoxins in food? *Food Research International, 43*(7), 1902–1914. https://doi.org/10.1016/j.foodres.2009.07.010

Pereira, C., Cunha, S. C., & Fernandes, J. O. (2022). Mycotoxins of concern in children and infant cereal food at European level: Incidence and bioaccessibility. *Toxins (Basel), 14*(7), 488.

Pereira, C., Fernandes, J. O., & Cunha, S. C. (2014). Mycotoxins in cereals and related foodstuffs: A review on occurrence and recent methods of analysis. *Trends in Food Science & Technology, 36*(2), 96–136.

Pereira, V. L., Fernandes, J. O., & Cunha, S. C. (2015). Comparative assessment of three cleanup procedures after QuEChERS extraction for determination of trichothecenes (type A and type B) in processed cereal-based baby foods by GC-MS. *Food Chemistry, 182*, 143–149.

Perumal, V., & Hashim, U. (2014). Advances in biosensors: Principles, architecture and applications. *Journal of Applied Biomedicine, 12*, 1–15.

Pleadin, J., Persi, N., Zadravec, M., Sokolovic, M., Vulic, A., Jaki, V., & Mitak, M. (2012). Correlation of deoxynivalenol and fumonisin concentration determined in maize by ELIZA methods. *Journal of Immunoassay and Immunochemistry, 33*, 414–421.

Polychronaki, N., Hannu, M., Paul, T. C., Yunyun, G., Amra, H., Abdel-Wahhab, M. A., & El-Nezami, H. (2006). Determinants of AFM1 in breast milk of Egyptian mothers. *Food Additives & Contaminants, 23*(7), 700–708.

Postupolski, J., Starski, A., Ledzion, E., Kurpinska-Jaworska, J., & Szczesna, M. (2019). Exposure assessment of infant and young children on selected Fusarium toxins. *Roczniki Panstwowego Zakladu Higieny, 70*, 5–14.

Prandini, A., Tansini, G., Sigolo, S., Filippi, L., Laporta, M., & Piva, G. (2009). On the occurrence of aflatoxin M1 in milk and dairy products. *Food and Chemical Toxicology, 7*, 984–991.

Prosperini, A., Meca, G., Font, G., & Ruiz, M. J. (2013). Bioaccessibility of enniatins A, A1, B, B1 in different commercial breakfast cereals, cookies and breads of Spain. *Journal of Agricultural and Food Chemistry, 61*, 456–461.

Rahmani, A., Jinap, S., & Soleimany, F. (2009). Qualitative and quantitative analysis of mycotoxins. *Comprehensive Reviews in Food Science and Food Safety, 8*(3), 202–251.

Raiola, A., Meca, G., Manes, J., & Ritieni, A. (2012). Bioaccessibility of deoxynivalenol and its natural co-occurrence with ochratoxin A and aflatoxin B1 in Italian commercial pasta. *Food and Chemical Toxicology, 50*, 280–287.

Ramana, M. V., Balakrishna, K., Murali, H. C., & Batra, H. V. (2011). Multiplex PCR-based strategy to detect contamination with mycotoxigenic Fusarium species in rice and finger millet collected from southern India. *Journal of the Science of Food and Agriculture, 91*, 1666–1673.

Rashmi, R., Ramana, M. V., Shylaja, R., Uppalapati, S. R., Murali, H. S., & Batra, H. V. (2013). Evaluation of a multiplex PCR assay for concurrent detection of four major mycotoxigenic fungi from foods. *Journal of Applied Microbiology, 114*, 819–827.

Razzazi-Fazeli, E., & Reiter, E. (2011). Sample preparation and clean up in mycotoxin analysis: Principles, applications and recent development. In E. Razzazi-Fazeli & A. R. Reiter (Eds.), *Determination of mycotoxins and mycotoxigenic fungi in food and feed* (pp. 37–70). Nova Science Publishers.

Rebellato, A. P., dos Santos Carames, E. T., Pallone, J. A. L., & de Oliveira Rocha, L. (2021). Mycotoxin bioaccessibility in baby food through in vitro digestion: An overview focusing on risk assessment. *Current Opinion in Food Science, 41*, 107–115.

Ren, W., Huang, Z., Xu, Y., Li, Y., Ji, Y., Su, B, (2015). Urchin-like gold nanoparticles-based immunochromatographic strip test for rapid detection of fumonisin B1 in grains. *Analytical and Bioanalytical Chemistry, 407,* 7341–7348.

Rico-Yuste, A., Gomez-Arribas, L. N., Perez-Conde, M. C., Urraca, J. L., & Moreno-Bondi, M. C. (2018). Rapid determination of Alternaria mycotoxins in tomato samples by pressurized liquid extraction coupled to liquid chromatography with fluorescence detection. *Food Additives & Contaminants Part A, 35*(11), 2175–2182.

Rodríguez, A., Rodríguez, M., Andrade, M. J., & Córdoba, J. J. (2015). Detection of filamentous fungi in foods. *Current Opinion in Food Science, 5,* 36–42. https://doi.org/10.1016/j.cofs.2015.07.007

Rodriguez-Carrasco, Y., Berrada, H., Font, G., & Manes, J. (2012). Multi-mycotoxin analysis in wheat semolina using an acetonitrile-based extraction procedure and gas chromatography-tandem mass spectrometry. *Journal of Chromatography A, 1270,* 28–40.

Rodriguez-Carrasco, Y., Molto, J. C., Berrada, H., & Manes, J. (2014). A survey of trichothecenes, zearalenone and patulin in milled grain-based products using GC-MS/MS. *Food Chemistry, 146,* 212–219.

Rubert, J., Dzuman, Z., Valclavikova, M., Zachariasova, M., Soler, C., & Hajslova, J. (2012). Analysis of mycotoxins in barley using ultra high liquid chromatography high resolution mass spectrometry: Comparison of efficiency and efficacy of different extraction procedures. *Talanta, 99,* 712–719.

Santana Oliveira, I., da Silva Junior, A. G., De Andrade, C. A. S., & Lima Oliveira, M. D. (2019). Biosensors for early detection of fungi spoilage and toxigenic and mycotoxins in food. *Current Opinion in Food Science, 29,* 64–79.

Shanakhat, H., Sorrentino, A., Raiola, A., Romano, A., Masi, P., & Cavella, S. (2018). Current methods for mycotoxins analysis and innovative strategies for their reduction in cereals: An overview. *Journal of the Science of Food and Agriculture, 98*(11), 4003–4013.

Sherif, S. O., Salama, E. E., & Abdel-Wahhab, M. A. (2009). Mycotoxins and child health: The need for health risk assessment. *International Journal of Hygiene and Environmental Health, 212,* 347–368.

Singh, J., & Mehta, A. (2020). Rapid and sensitive detection of mycotoxins by advanced and emerging analytical methods: A review. *Food Science & Nutrition, 8*(5), 2183–2204.

Smith, J. W., Matchado, A. J., Wu, L. S., Arnold, C. D., Burke, S. M., Maleta, K. M., . . . Schulze, K. J. (2022). Longitudinal assessment of prenatal, perinatal, and early-life aflatoxin b1 exposure in 828 mother–child dyads from Bangladesh and Malawi. *Current Developments in Nutrition, 6*(2), nzab153.

Sohail, A. A., & Bani-Hasan, B. M. (2017). Morphological and molecular identification of fungi isolated from different environmental sources in the Northern Eastern Desert of Jordan. *Jordan Journal of Biological Sciences, 11,* 329–337.

Song, S., Liu, N., Zhao, Z., Njumbe Ediage, E., Wu, S., Sun, C., De Saeger, S., & Wu, A. (2014). Multiplex lateral flow immunoassay for mycotoxin determination. *Analytical Chemistry, 86,* 4995–5001.

Streit, E., Naehrer, K., Rodrigues, I., & Schatzmayr, G. (2013). Mycotoxin occurrence in feed and feed raw materials worldwide: Long-term analysis with special focus on Europe and Asia. *Journal of the Science of Food and Agriculture, 93,* 2892–2899.

Suanthie, Y., Cousin, M. A., & Woloshuk, C. P. (2009). Multiplex real-time PCR for detection and quantification of mycotoxigenic Aspergillus, Penicillium, and Fusarium. *Journal of Stored Products Research, 45*, 139–145.

Sun, X. D., Su, P., & Shan, H. (2017). Mycotoxin contamination of rice in China. *Journal of Food Science, 82*, 573–584.

Tafinta, I. Y., Shehu, K., Abdulganiyyu, H., Rabe, A. M., & Usman, A. (2013). Isolation and identification of fungi associated with the spoilage of sweet orange (*Citrus sinensis*) fruits in Sokoto State. *Nigerian Journal of Basic and Applied Sciences, 21*(3), 193–196.

Tesfamariam, K., Gebreyesus, S. H., Lachat, C., Hanley-Cook, G. T., Roro, M., Mengistu, Y. G., Endris, B. S., Belachew, T., Kolsteren, P., De Saeger, S., De Boevre, M., & Argaw, A. (2022). Chronic aflatoxin exposure during pregnancy is associated with lower fetal growth trajectories: A prospective cohort from the Butajira Nutrition, Mental Health, and Pregnancy (BUNMAP) Study in rural Ethiopia. *American Journal of Clinical Nutrition, 116*, 1634–1641.

Thway, T., Salimi-Moosavi, H. (2014). Evaluating the impact of matrix effects on biomarker assay sensitivity. *Bioanalysis, 6*, 1081–1091.

Tsitsigiannis, D. I., Georgiadou, M., Agoritsis, S., Zakynthinos, G., Varzakas, T. H., Tjamos, S. E., Antoniou, P. P., Dimakopoulou, M., Karnavas, G., Paplomatas, E., Gianniotis, S., & Tjamos, E. C. (2010). Ecology, epidemiology and control of *Aspergillus* spp. in pistachio orchards in Greece. *Petria, 20*(2), 67–633.

Tsitsigiannis, D. I., Mirto, D., Antoniu, P. P., & Tjamos, E. C. (2012). Biological control strategies of mycotoxigenic fungi and associated mycotoxins in Mediterranean basin crops. *Phytopathologia Mediterranea, 51*, 158–174.

Turner, N. W., Bramhmbhatt, H., Szabo-Vezse, M., Poma, A., Coker, R., & Piletsky, S. A. (2015). Analytical methods for determination of mycotoxins: An update (2009–2014). *Analytica Chimica Acta, 901*, 12–33.

Turner, N. W., Subrahmanyam, S., & Piletsky, S. A. (2009). Analytical methods for determination of mycotoxins: A review. *Analytica Chimica Acta, 632*(2), 168–180.

Urusov, A. E., Zherdev, A. V., & Dzantiev, B. B. (2010). Immunochemical methods of mycotoxin analysis (review). *Applied Biochemistry and Microbiology, 46*(3), 253–266.

U.S. Food and Drug Administration. (2021). *Mycotoxins*. Retrieved from [FDA] https://www.fda.gov/food/chemical-contaminants-food/mycotoxins

Versantvoort, C. H. M., Oomen, A. G., Van de Kamp., E., Rompelberg, C. J. M., Sips, A. J. A. M (2005). Applicability of an in vitro digestion model in assessing the bioaccessibility of mycotoxins from food. *Food and Chemical Toxicology, 43*, 31–40.

Wacoo, A. P., Wendiro, D., Vuzi, P. C., & Hawumba, J. F. (2014). Methods for detection of aflatoxins in agricultural food crops. *Journal of Applied Chemistry, 2014*, Article 706291.

Wang, J. H., Zhang, J. B., Chen, F. F., Li, H. P., Ndoye, M., & Liao, Y. C. (2012). A multiplex PCR assay for genetic chemotyping of toxigenic Fusarium graminearum and wheat grains for 3-acetyldeoxynivalenol, 15-acetyldeoxynivalenol and nivalenol mycotoxin. *Journal of Food, Agriculture & Environment, 10*, 505–511.

Wang, Y., Xu, H., Wei, M., Gu, H., Xu, Q., & Zhu, W. (2009). Study of superparamagnetic nanoparticles as labels in the quantitative lateral flow immunoassay. *Materials Science and Engineering: C, 29*, 714–718.

Whitaker, T. B. (2006). Sampling foods for mycotoxins. *Food Additives and Contaminants, 23*, 50–61.

Williams, J. H., Phillips, T. D., Jolly, P. E., Stiles, J. K., Jolly, C. M., & Aggarwal, D. (2004). Human aflatoxicosis in developing countries: A review of toxicology, exposure, potential health consequences, and interventions. *American Journal of Clinical Nutrition, 80*, 1106–1122.
World Health Organization (WHO). (2006). *Evaluation of certain contaminants in food: Eighty-third report of the Joint FAO/WHO Expert Committee on Food Additives* (83rd ed.). Geneva, Switzerland: World Health Organization.
World Health Organization, & Food and Agriculture Organization of the United Nations. (2011). *FAO/WHO guide for application of risk analysis principles and procedures during food safety emergencies*. Rome: Food and Agriculture Organization of the United Nations.
Xie, L., Chen, M., & Ying, Y. (2016). Development of methods for determination of aflatoxins. *Critical Reviews in Food Science and Nutrition, 56*(16), 2642–2664.
Yang, J., Li, J., Jiang, Y., Duan, X., Qu, H., Yang, B., . . . Sivakumar, D. (2014). Natural occurrence, analysis and prevention of mycotoxins in fruits and their processed products. *Critical Reviews in Food Science and Nutrition, 54*(1), 64–83.
Yogendrarajah, P., Deschuyffeleer, N., Jacxsens, L., Sneyers, P. J., Maene, P., De Saeger, S., Devlieghere, F., & De Meulenaer, B. (2014). Mycological quality and mycotoxin contamination of Sri Lankan peppers (*Piper nigrum* L.) and subsequent exposure assessment. *Food Control, 41*(1), 219–230.
Zain, M. E. (2011). Impact of mycotoxins on humans and animals. *Journal of Saudi Chemical Society, 15*, 129–144.
Zhang, L., Dou, X. W., Zhang, C., Logrieco, A. F., & Yang, M. H. (2018). A review of current methods for analysis of mycotoxins in herbal medicines. *Toxins, 10*(2), Article 65.
Zhang, X., Yu, X., Wen, K., Li, C., Mujtaba Mari, G., Jiang, H., Shi, W., Shen, J., Wang, Z (2017). Multiple lateral flow immunoassays based on amorphous carbon nanoparticles for detecting three Fusarium mycotoxins in maize. *Journal of Agricultural and Food Chemistry, 65*, 8063–8071.
Zheng, M. Z., Richard, J. L., & Binder, J. A. (2006). A review of rapid methods for the analysis of mycotoxins. *Mycopathologia, 161*, 261–273.
Zheng, W., Pan, S., Wang, G., Wang, Y. J., Liu, Q., Gu, J., Yuan, Y., Liu, X. Z., Liu, Z. P., & Bian, J. C. (2016). Zearalenone impairs the male reproductive system functions via inducing structural and functional alterations of Sertoli cells. *Environmental Toxicology and Pharmacology, 42*, 146–155.
Zheng, Z., Hanneken, J., Houchins, D., King, R. S., Lee, P., & Richard, J. L. (2005). Validation of an ELISA test kit for the detection of ochratoxin A in several food commodities by comparison with HPLC. *Mycopathologia, 159*, 265–272.
Zinedine, A., & Mañes, J. (2009). Occurrence and legislation of mycotoxins in food and feed from Morocco. *Food Control, 20*, 334–344.
Zinedine, A., Soriano, J. M., Juan, C., Mojemmi, B., Mplti, J. C., Bouklouze, A., . . . Manes, J. (2007). Incidence of ochratoxin A in rice and dried fruits from Rabat and Sale area, Morocco. *Food Additives & Contaminants, 24*(3), 285–291.
Zougagh, M., & Rios, A. (2008). Supercritical fluid extraction of macrocyclic lactone mycotoxins in maize flour samples for rapid amperometric screening and alternative liquid chromatographic method for confirmation. *Journal of Chromatography A, 1177*(1–2), 50–57.

4

General Evaluation of Bacterial Toxins in Food Products

Blessing I. Nwadike, Olutayo, I. Falodun, Eric M. Adetutu, and Adeniyi A. Ogunjobi

4.1 Overview of Bacterial Toxins

Toxins are a wide range of substances biologically produced within living cells or organisms that are harmful to other organisms while benefiting their own survival. They are inanimate and not capable of reproducing themselves. Toxins can be small molecules, peptides or proteins that are capable of causing disease on contact with or absorption by body tissues interacting with biological macromolecules such as enzymes or cellular receptors. Bacterial toxins are broadly grouped into two main types, lipopolysaccharides (LPS) and proteins. Lipopolysaccharide are associated with the cell wall of Gram-negative bacteria, while proteins are released from bacterial cells and may act at tissue sites removed from the site of bacterial growth. Cell-associated toxins are referred to as endotoxins, while extracellular diffusible toxins are referred to as exotoxins or protein toxins. While exotoxins can be named after organisms generating the toxin or after susceptible tissue/organ types, protein toxins can be further divided according to modes of action: (1) targeting host membrane receptors; (2) targeting the host membrane lipid bilayer; and (3) targeting host cytosolic proteins, either through uptake by host endocytosis of paired bacterial proteins called AB toxins or by direct delivery through a molecular syringe of a bacterial injection apparatus.

Protein toxins can also be characterized based on their secretion systems. To exert virulence, bacterial toxins produced in the cytosol must be transported across the bacterial membranes through co-translational and post-translational mechanisms to reach their targets. These transports are mediated through various secretion systems, which now include nine different mechanisms, types I–IX. Gram-positive bacteria utilize only types I and VII, and Gram-negative bacteria exploit all but type VII, while one bacterial species can possess multiple secretion systems. Finally, toxins

DOI: 10.1201/9781003500605-5

are also classified based on virulence mechanisms targeting the following: cytoskeleton components, ubiquitin/proteasomal system, cell translational machinery, neurotransmission system, cAMP production and MAP kinase signalling and DNA and inducing endoplasmic reticulum stress responses, some of which may be highly relevant to carcinogenesis. Subsequent sections provide more details about individual bacterial toxins with which potential links to human cancers have been increasingly recognized.

4.2 Sources of Food Contamination with Bacterial Toxins

Microbes can enter into food from humans, kitchen tools and their surfaces adulterated by raw food products. Different types of contamination mechanisms are involved in food contamination. Some factors that can cause foodborne illness are storage and cooking temperatures, insufficient hand washing and animal waste. Other sources of bacterial toxins in food include foods contaminated with species of *Staphylococcus* that produce enterotoxin, such as *Staphylococcus aureus*, *Staphylococcus hyicus* and *Staphylococcus intermedius*, which produce one or more heat-stable proteins that behave as enterotoxins (SET). Also, enterohemorrhagic *E. coli* (EHEC) produce verotoxin or shiga toxin and are known as verotoxin-producing *E. coli* (VTEC) or Shiga toxin–producing *E. coli* (STEC) and cause most common food-related bacterial diseases. These bacteria can contaminate foods through raw meat and unpasteurized dairy products. The botulinum toxin produced by *Clostridium botulinum* is the most toxic substance. *Listeria monocytogenes*, associated with foodborne illnesses, specifically targets cholesterol by producing a pore-forming toxin protein, listeriolysin O.

4.3 Mode of Bacterial Toxin Production

Bacterial toxins are important for the survival of bacteria in different environments, including the food matrix, and this is because toxins allow them to outcompete other microbial groups, ensuring their dominance in the food matrix. Unfortunately, toxins can cause food poisoning or foodborne diseases with morbidities such as gastroenteritis, toxic shock syndrome, fever and fatality in severe instances when human beings consume such contaminated foods (Hernandez-Cortez et al., 2017). Therefore, toxins are not only important for bacterial survival but are one of the key factors responsible for the maintenance of bacterial virulence (Rajkovic et al., 2020).

Foodborne diseases associated with bacterial contamination of food items (toxins and other metabolites) remain one of the key public health issues of concern worldwide, causing a global 600 million illnesses annually (Hernandez-Cortez et al., 2017). It is, therefore, important to understand the mode by which bacteria produce toxins prior to developing therapeutic approaches to mitigate their effect or eliminate them in the food matrix. There are two types of toxins, exotoxins and endotoxins (Edae and Wabalo, 2019; Ghazaei, 2022), and each one is evaluated in the next sections.

4.4 Endotoxins

Endotoxins are endogenous toxins associated with LPS cell walls of Gram-negative bacteria, which are released into the food matrix because of bacterial metabolic activities or the lysis of bacteria by host cells or antimicrobial compounds (Ghazaei, 2022; Popoff, 2024). Although the cell walls of these bacterial groups are composed of LPS and phospholipids, it is the lipid portion of the LPS (Lipid A) that is the endotoxin (Ghazaei, 2022). This LPS is hydrophobic and consists of the O-antigen, core polysaccharides, disaccharide diphosphate and fatty acids (Sampath, 2018). Lipid A attaches the LPS to the outer cell wall membrane, while the core oligosaccharide plays key roles in maintaining membrane integrity. The O-antigen polysaccharide, attached to the core polysaccharide, variable amongst bacteria, is hydrophilic in nature and composed of glycosidic residues. This antigen is in direct contact with the external environment, such as the food matrix (Sampath, 2018; Farhana and Khan, 2023) (Figure 4.1).

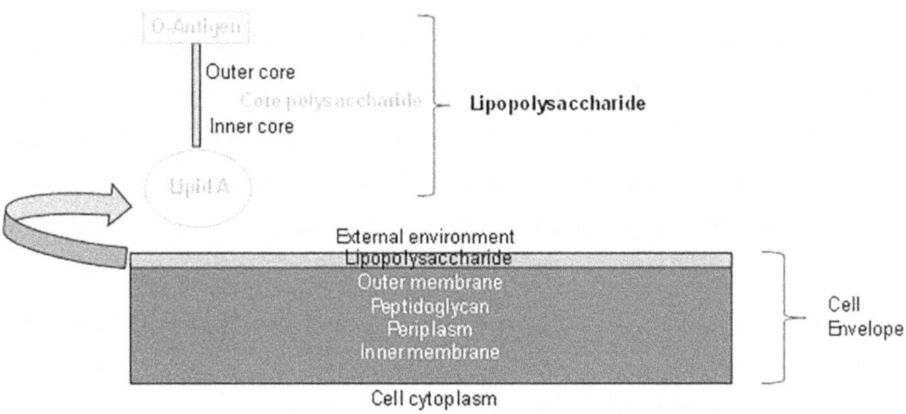

FIGURE 4.1
Gram-negative bacterial cell envelope showing a simplified structure of lipopolysaccharide produced by *E. coli* (adapted from Bertani and Ruiz, 2018).

As endotoxins are part of the cell wall of the Gram-negative bacteria, they are produced whenever bacteria multiply and or produce cell wall components. This process is initiated by bacterial genes as part of the metabolic processes of the different bacterial species. The synthesis of LPS is thought to involve the Raetz pathway and is well-characterized in *E. coli* and *Salmonella* sp. (Putker et al., 2015).

The synthesis of LPS occurs in the cytoplasm, inner membrane and periplasm, mediated by different pathways. Lipid A synthesis takes place at the inner membrane via the Raetz pathway. It involves the convergence of two pathways: the oligosaccharide pathway and the Kdo residue pathway (Bertani and Ruiz, 2018; Sperandeo et al., 2017). The oligosaccharide pathway mediated by Raez enzymes involves the initial acylation of nucleotide UDP-N-acetyglucosamine (UDP-GlcNAc) mediated by the LpxA enzyme to form UDP-3-O-(acyl)-GlcN. The latter compound is deacylated by the zinc metalloenzyme LpxC to form UDP-3-O-(acyl)-GlcN. After this process, another enzyme, LpxD, acylates the compound again, resulting in the formation of UDP-2,3-diacyl-GlcN. Three enzymes, LpxH, LpxB and LpxK, act sequentially on generated compounds, ultimately resulting in the formation of a compound designated Lipid IV_A (Sperandeo et al., 2017). The other pathway, the Kdo pathway, involves the conversion of Ru5P to Ara-5P by the enzyme KdsD (an arabinose 5 P isomerase), with Ara-5P then being converted to Kdo8P by KdsA, Kdo8P to Kdo by KdsC and Kdo transformation into CMP-Kdo (2X) by KdsB. The two compounds, CMP-Kdo and Lipid IV_A, then combine to form Lipid IV_A-Kdo_2 in a reaction mediated by KdtA, and further sequential reactions mediated by LpxL and LpxM lead to the formation of Lipid A-Kdo_2. This Lipid A compound is then anchored to the inner membrane (Sperandeo et al., 2017).

The synthesis of the core oligosaccharide also involves sequential reactions mediated by various enzymes and has been extensively reviewed (Bertani and Ruiz, 2018). Briefly, two heptose residues are added to the Lipid A-Kdo2 molecule sequentially by WaaC and WaaF enzymes, and the final steps of the inner core saccharide synthesis are completed and mediated sequentially by WaaP, WaaQ and WaaY enzymes (Bertani and Ruiz, 2018). The outer core saccharide synthesis involves the addition of glucose, galactose and heptose molecules by various enzymes such as WaaG, WaaB, WaaO, WaaJ and WaaU (Bertani and Ruiz, 2018). The O antigen consisting of multiple oligosaccharide units (1–8 glycosidic units) is highly variable in size and composition in different bacterial species. The biogenesis of the O antigen occurs independently, not on the core-lipid A nor the rest of the LPS molecule but on undecaprenyl phosphate (Und-P), a lipid carrier molecule (Sperandeo et al., 2017). After synthesis, it is transferred to the inner membrane and the outer-core oligosaccharide (Bertani and Ruiz, 2018). The O antigen biosynthesis which is highly variable in different bacterial groups is in three designated pathways: (1) the synthase-dependent pathways, (2) the ABC-dependent pathway and (3) the Wzy pathway (Bertani and Ruiz, 2018).

4.5 Exotoxins

Bacterial exotoxins, on the other hand, are small peptides (proteins) with different structures, chemical characteristics, solubility and toxicological profiles, which are produced by both Gram-positive and Gram-negative bacteria. Although they are often named after the secreting bacteria, exotoxins can further be classified into three types: superantigens or Type 1, membrane-disrupting toxins or Type II and A-B toxins or Type III (Hernandez-Cortez et al., 2017; Rajkovic et al., 2020; Ghazaei, 2022). Exotoxin production is initiated by genes in the bacterial genome or on mobile genetic elements such as plasmids and bacteriophages. They are produced endogenously and secreted into the external matrix through the Sec pathway (Popoff, 2024).

Pathogenic microbes apply their destructive impacts on the host through a course of destructive factors: exotoxins, endotoxins, intrusion proteins and so on. Different poisons emitted by various microorganisms subvert the host intracellular flagging pathways and have one-of-a-kind partiality for explicit host cells. Data has been gathered throughout the years concerning the sanitization, synthetic portrayal, chemical activity and design of different bacterial toxins. Toxins' capacity to tie to explicit target cells makes them a great contender for medication conveyance and in disease therapeutics (Sengupta and Austin, 2011; Edae and Wabalo, 2019).

Type I toxins disrupt host cells without the need to enter the cells. Few intracellular targets of Type I toxins have been identified, possibly due to the difficult nature of analysing proteins that are poisonous to their bacterial hosts. These include superantigens (SAgs) produced by *S. aureus* and *S. pyogenes*.

Type II toxins, such as hemolysins and phospholipases, destroy host cell membranes to invade and interrupt host defence processes within the cell. Damaged host cells release danger-associated molecular patterns (DAMPs) that bind to pattern-recognition receptors (PRRs), causing the release of inflammatory cytokines.

Type III toxins, also known as A/B toxins due to their binary structure, disrupt host cell defences to allow dissemination to remote organs. The B component of these toxins binds to the host cell surface, while the A component has enzymatic activity to damage the cell (Pimbley, 1998; Michel, 2018).

Each toxin possesses a unique mechanism of action, which is responsible for the elicitation of a specific pathology. The role of toxins in microbial pathogenesis is a long-known phenomenon (Barbieri, 2009). Much less is known about reasons a microorganism produces particular toxins, as for most of the toxins, there is no final proof of ecological or evolutionary advantages that have been established. Bacterial toxins damage host cells by directly modifying intracellular targets, which may lead to cell death. Bacterial toxins traffic within host cells and recognize host proteins that are targeted for modification. The toxin produced by *Pseudomonas aeruginosa* is responsible for many hospital-acquired infections and infections of compromised individuals, including children with cystic fibrosis, and tetanus toxin, a neurotoxin that elicits spastic paralysis in humans. Characterization of these bacterial toxins provides information on how bacteria damage the host and may lead to translational products to detect, prevent and treat bacterial infections.

4.6 Factors Responsible for Bacterial Toxin Production in Food Products

Production of bacterial toxins usually results from excessive growth and may also occur at any stage of the food production chain. Importantly, it must be noted that there is a possibility for produced toxins to remain in downstream food processing and still be active biologically even when the bacteria that produce the toxin have been inactivated (Rajkovic, 2014). The factors that influence toxin production in food could either be intrinsic or extrinsic. The intrinsic factors include pH, water activity and nutrients, while the extrinsic factors include temperature, humidity and atmosphere. Other factors that could influence bacterial toxin production are density of bacterial cell, growth phase, cell stress and injury. However, the conditions required for bacterial growth may be different from those responsible for the production of toxins (Rajkovic et al., 2020). In other word, a bacteria possessing toxin-encoding genes or the genes that are responsible for the regulation of toxin production may not imply production of the toxin (Wang et al., 2012; Rajkovic et al., 2020). Hence, the growth conditions for pathogens might be different from the conditions that influence toxin production. For instance, it was discovered in a study that the minimum water activity required for *Staphylococcus aureus* growth was 0.83, while it was 0.86 for enterotoxin production (Ross and Nichols, 2014; Rajkovic et al., 2020). Many bacteria of the same species usually demonstrate qualitative toxin profiles that are similar this and therefore corroborate the assertion that production of toxins by microorganisms, including bacteria, is genetic. The intrinsic factors that affect the production of toxins by bacteria have a connection to the internal characteristics of the food and food products alongside the way these characteristics contribute to maintaining and/or affecting microbial growth. Such intrinsic factors include water activity, pH, oxidation-reduction potential, content and type of nutrients, inhibiting substances and biological structures (Dashdorj et al., 2015; Hernández-Cortez et al., 2017).

Water activity: This is the amount of water that is available for microbial growth. In the event that there is a reduction in the available water for the growth of microbes, the rate at which the microbes proliferate will also be substantially reduced. The water made available to bacteria to carry out their metabolic activities also has a great impact on the rate at which the bacteria grow and proliferate. The required water for bacteria growth is measured as water activity (Aw) and is calculated by comparing the water vapour pressure of the food substrate and the water vapour pressure of pure water under the same temperature condition. This perception is related to relative humidity (RH). It can therefore be expressed as: $RH = 100 \times Aw$. The optimum Aw required for growth by most microbes is approximately 0.99; moreover, the required Aw by most bacteria for their optimum growth is usually greater than 0.91. However, the requirement for growth by Gram-negative bacteria is higher than that required by Gram-positive strains. The Aw of most available natural foods and their products is usually greater than or equal to 0.99. Among microorganisms, bacteria require the highest level of Aw, while the bacteria that are involved in the decomposition of food will not grow at Aw that is less than 0.91. Nevertheless, an Aw of 0.75 has been reported for bacteria in food; this is the lowest and is for halophilic bacteria (Akhtar et al., 2014; Hernández-Cortez et al., 2017).

pH: This is the negative logarithm of hydronium ion concentration. It is the measure of the acidic and alkalinity level of a material, such as food and food products. Enzyme cell functioning and the transportation of nutrients to the cell are adversely affected by pH. Hence, the surrounding medium of bacteria and the value of its pH play a critical role in development and toxin production; the cell surface of the bacteria could be affected directly or indirectly through nutrient availability. Bacteria that find themselves in an environment with either lower or higher than neutral pH will proliferate if such an organism is able to cause a change in the pH of the environment to a more suitable range. This is because the key components, such as DNA and ATP, require a medium of neutral pH (Akhtar et al., 2014). For many microorganisms, the optimum growth pH requirement is usually between 6.6 and 7.5, that is, about neutral pH, which is also the pH that favours the growth of bacteria, except for acidophiles that can grow at a pH of 5.2. This is one of the reasons most meat and sea products that have a pH of 5.6 or more are decomposed by bacteria (Carrasco et al., 2011).

Oxidation-reduction potential: This is an indicator of the power of a substrate to be oxidize or reduced. Food product oxidation occurs when it loses electrons but is reduced when electrons are gained; hence, the food or food products that release electrons indicate a good reducing agent, while those that accept electrons indicate a good oxidizing agent. The optimum growth requirements for some are reducing conditions, while in others, it is oxidized conditions. If a substance is oxidized, the electrical potential will be positive, and if it is reduced, the electrical potential will be negative, but an equal concentration of both oxidant and reducer will lead to zero electrical potential (Madigan et al., 2010). Aerobic bacteria require oxidized conditions, while anaerobic bacteria require reduced conditions, but facultative bacteria can withstand any conditions. In addition, microaerophilic bacteria such as *Lactobacillus* and *Campylobacter* grow optimally under a slight reduced condition.

Nutrient content: All microbes have their own nutritional requirements, and many need external sources of nitrogen, energy, minerals, and vitamins as well as related growth factors to proliferate. Food and food products contain these requirements and aid the development of microorganisms. The nutrient requirement for Gram-negative bacteria is lower compared to Gram-positive bacteria (Wildman, 2016). The principal sources of nitrogen that are used by heterotrophic bacteria are amino acids, a simple compound that is first used before more complex compounds like high molecular weight proteins such as polysaccharides and lipids (Midgan et al., 2010). Some bacteria are also capable of synthesizing enough vitamin B to meet their needs, but some may also depend on external sources such as food and food products. Gram-negative bacteria have the ability to synthesize most of their nutrient needs and can thrive in food products with low vitamin B content.

Extrinsic parameters: These are also called external factors, which refers to environmental factors that affect the rate of microbial growth one way or the other. These factors include the following: temperature, oxygen availability, relative humidity and the presence and activities of other microorganisms (Hernández-Cortez et al., 2017).

Temperature: For all microorganisms, there is usually an optimum, minimum and maximum temperature range required for growth. Temperature not only affects the rate of proliferation of bacteria but their development and activities including toxin production. Temperature changes are very important, to the extent that a few degrees of change can lead to the growth of different organisms as well as different types of food decomposition, food intoxication and foodborne illness.

Oxygen availability: The presence of oxygen as well as other gases is a determinative factor for the organisms that will grow and be active. The oxygen requirement for some bacteria is absolute (aerobic), while some require the complete absence of oxygen (anaerobic), and some can grow whether oxygen is present or absent (facultative) (Peelman et al., 2016).

Relative humidity: The importance of relative humidity can be seen in the light of water activity in food and food products as well as bacterial growth within and on the surface of food. This factor affects bacterial growth and can be influenced by temperature. High water is required for the growth and maximum activity of all bacteria, including the production of their metabolites. When the relative humidity is high, it can lead to humidity condensation in food, equipment used, walls and ceilings, which can eventually lead to wet surfaces, causing growth of bacteria and food decomposition. However, low relative humidity is inhibitory to microbes. The relative humidity required by bacteria (greater than or equal to 92%) is higher compared to yeasts and fungi (85 to 90%).

Presence and activities of other microorganisms: Some food microflora may produce inhibitory and lethal substances such as antibiotics, bacteriocins, hydrogen peroxide and organic acids that can affect other organisms. For example, lactic acid-producing bacteria from various food and food products like meat produce bacteriocin that are of interest. Gram-positive bacteria produce biologically active bacteriocin that has a bactericidal effect. Also, some of the bacteria-produced bacteriocins have an inhibitory effect on a number of food pathogens such as *B. cereus, C. perfringens, Listeria* spp., *A. hydrophila* and *S. aureus* (Madigan, 2010).

4.7 Effects of Bacterial Toxins in Food and Food Products

Most foods serve as the best media for the growth of diverse microorganisms. Bacterial growth in foods may cause changes in appearance, flavour, odour and other features of the foods. Some of the degradative changes produced by bacteria such as putrefaction, fermentation and rancidity, in addition to degradation, cause changes in food quality. Bacteria can also synthesize substances such as pigments and slimes, and these also affect the food quality. The presence of bacterial toxins in food and food products can lead to food deterioration and other changes in the food like spoilage by decay and food poisoning. When toxin-producing bacteria grow on food and food products, they release these toxins and other metabolites into the surroundings and absorb the products of external digestion, thus causing food spoilage, which lowers the nutritional value and causes well-known ill effects (Udebuani and Abara, 2018). Food can serve as medium to transmit a wide range of diseases to humans, as the food serves as a vehicle for the transfer of pathogens to the consumer in whom the pathogen grows and causes disease in a food infection. The pathogen can grow and produce toxins that can affect the consumer, leading to food intoxication (Willey et al., 2008). One of the effects of bacterial toxins in food and food products is food spoilage, a metabolic process that causes foods to be undesirable or unacceptable for human consumption due to changes in sensory characteristics of the foods. Foodborne disease is one of the main problems in public health and can cause disabilities. Foodborne diseases can be caused by consuming foods contaminated with bacterial toxins or microorganisms that produce them. Some of the bacteria that cause foodborne diseases include *V. cholera, S. aureus, B. cereus, C. perfringens, C. botulinum* and *L. monocytogens*. Replications of pathogens present in food can cause diseases. Some species of bacteria produce toxins, and when foods contaminated with these bacterial toxins are ingested, they cause food poisoning.

4.8 Public Health Challenges Associated with Bacterial Toxins in Foods

One of the important global issues that greatly affects the health of the public is food safety. This is a serious factor to be considered in the health of the public because many countries of the world, especially developing countries, are interdependent in terms of food availability and supply to their citizens. Contaminated foods with microbial pathogens such as bacteria, viruses, parasites and fungi or chemical substances have been implicated in well over 200 illnesses which range from diarrhoea to cancer. It is estimated that about 600 million people all over the world fall ill after they have consumed microbial contaminated foods, out of which about 420,000 die annually. The burden of foodborne infections is higher in children under the age of five years, accounting for about 40%, out of which about 125,000 die yearly (Gizaw, 2019). Toxins are poisonous substances that are produced within the living cells of organisms and can comprise different classes of small molecules or proteins that are responsible for disease when there is contact with them. The adverse effects and the type of the diseases which may be due to toxins can range from just trivial to severely deadly effects. The release of bacterial toxins usually leads to metabolic pathway disruption, notwithstanding the time they are released into the surrounding environment. Metabolic pathway disruption includes cell membrane damage, protein synthesis disruption, inhibition of the release of neurotransmitters and host immune system activation. There are a number of species of both Gram-negative and Gram-positive bacteria that produce toxins. Some bacteria may only be able to produce a single toxin, while some may possess the capability to produce multiple toxins. Some examples of bacteria that produce multitoxins include *B. cereus, C. botulinum, C. perfringens* and *S. aureus*. However, each toxin, whether produced singly or in multiple, has a unique mode of action, eliciting specific pathological characteristics (Rajkovic et al., 2020).

The manner in which the produced toxins cause disruption of eukaryotes cell processes greatly depends on the target. For instance, the target of *Listeria monocytogenes*, a bacterial pathogen implicated in foodborne infections, is cholesterol through the production of a pore-forming toxin protein called listeriolysin O. The exotoxin produced by these bacteria negatively affects the intracellular processes of the host by creating unregulated pores within the cell membranes. In addition, *S. aureus* can produce enterotoxin, a type of exotoxin; the staphylococcal enterotoxin B is linked to intestinal disorder that leads to the promotion of immune system activation. The outcome of immune system activation is that cytokines, inflammatory-related molecules, will be released in large amounts, leading to significant inflammation. Also, Gram-negative bacteria produce endotoxins, including protein lipopolysaccharide, which is a component of the outer membranes of bacteria that are involved in the promotion of the structural integrity of bacteria. When the membrane is destroyed by the host immune response, the protein lipopolysaccharide will be released and will serve as a toxin.

The bacterial potential to produce toxins and the possibility of the produced toxins to cause disease symptoms depends on a number of factors, including the following: strain of the pathogen, quantity of the produced toxins, toxin physico-chemical properties, interaction of the toxin with food components and other microbial metabolites, interplay with food components and other microbial metabolites, how stable the toxins are in food as well as the human gastrointestinal tract, the possibility of metabolizing the toxin molecules and the resulting characteristics of the metabolites, the dose of the innate (sub)clinical toxin, the toxin mode of action, the noticeable effect of acute and (sub)chronic exposure and targets and receptors in the human body. The three most important bacterial pathogens that are responsible for causing foodborne diseases as a result of bacterial exotoxin are *S. aureus, B. cereus* and *C. perfringens*, and it was estimated that out of the 9.4 million foodborne illnesses that were caused by known pathogens annually, 1.3 million were ascribed to these three pathogens in the United States. Also, in the European Union in 2010, bacterial toxins were reported to be the second most important agent implicated among those hospitalized (Rajkovic et al., 2020). Foodborne outbreaks have been linked to toxins produced by bacteria such as *Clostridium perfringens, Staphylococcus aureus* and *Bacillus cereus*. Although these are preventable causes of both morbidity and mortality, they are very important in foodborne infections. However, because of the short incubation time and the period of the illnesses caused by these bacterial toxins, most of the outbreaks go unreported (May et al., 2016).

Bacterial toxins find their way into fermented food products when the substrate of the foods is contaminated with the bacteria that produce the toxins, thereby constituting a food safety risk. The presence and detection of bacterial toxins has been reported from meat and vegetable-based fermented foods (Adekoya et al., 2019). There are studies of the high risk of contamination due to indirect microbial infestation of the raw substrate used for the production of many vegetable-based fermented foods such as cucumbers, young melons, mustard greens, cabbage, bamboo shoots and papayas. Also, a substantial bacterial load of toxin-producing bacteria such as *Bacillus cereus*, *Proteus mirabilis* and *Clostridium botulinum* has been recovered from samples of soybean, fish and pork-based fermented foods (Keisam et al., 2019).

Furthermore, another public health challenge of bacteria-produced toxins in foods by bacteria such as *C. perfringens* and *B. cereus* is that they are resistant to heat even after the foods are cooked. The risk of illness still remains if such food is consumed because the heat-resistant spores that would have been produced can subsist the period of heating, regerminate after cooking and produce toxins in the food. Although the vegetative cells of the bacteria would have been killed (FDA, 2012; Mary et al., 2016).

A recent development is the demand for and increased consumption of fermented foods because they are safe and have nutritional value as well as health-promoting properties. Nevertheless, because of the use of unsuitable starter cultures, processing conditions and inappropriate storage, some toxins such as bacterial toxins, including endotoxins, enterotoxins and emetic toxins, may be produced. The public health challenges that can be associated with the production of these toxins are foodborne illnesses, which can also lead to cardiovascular abnormalities and gastrointestinal symptoms (Fayyaz et al., 2022). Bacteria can cause illness either by invasion and inflammation or production of toxins. Toxins produced by bacteria are biological elements that are toxic, and they provide pathogenic features to the produced microorganisms. However, the effect of toxins depends on the type of toxins, the toxin concentration and the affected cells. Moreover, the consequences of bacterial toxin production may include the following: failure of a single cell, tissue or organ; manipulation of the innate and adaptive immune responses; and impairment of the nervous system. The ability of some microorganisms, including bacteria, to produce toxins is referred to as toxigenicity and is responsible for the negative effects that lead to various disease conditions called toxinoses. The transportation of these toxins through the blood and lymph could lead to the manifestation of some symptoms of diseases such as fever, diarrhoea, shock and cardiovascular disorder. Furthermore, bacterial toxins can also lead to the following: protein synthesis being inhibited; destruction of blood cells and vessels; and disruption of nervous system, which can thereafter lead to spasms. The presence of toxins in the blood, termed termetoxemia, is a factor of toxins called the virulence factor; it is a molecular component that is released by bacteria and interferes with the mechanisms of the immune system and leads to the promotion of colonization that is injurious to the host. In combination with endotoxins, some of the surface molecules produced by Gram-positive bacteria have also been implicated in septic shock (Ghazaei, 2022).

4.9 Selected Bacteria Pathogens That Produce Toxins of Public Health Concern

Bacillus cereus: A bacterial pathogen responsible for two different types of food poisoning (emetic or vomiting and diarrhoea forms). The emetic form emanates from food intoxication due to the presence of emetic toxin; it is also referred to as cereulide in foods. This toxin is both heat and acid resistant. Intoxication is usually characterized by a rapid onset of symptoms such as nausea and vomiting. It may also sometimes be characterized with symptoms like abdominal cramps and/or diarrhoea that typically resolve within a period of 24 hours. However, this intoxication has been reported to be associated with fatality (Dierick et al., 2005). Examples of some of the foods involved in intoxication include rice, pasta and potato-based meals. Secondly, the diarrhoea form usually occurs when the vegetative cells and/or spores and viable cells of *B. cereus* are consumed, and the protein enterotoxins are produced and released into the small intestine. The following are the toxins that are involved in the diarrhoea type: hemolysin BL, nonhemolytic enterotoxin and cytotoxin K. Unlike the emetic type, this form of food poisoning is heat, acid and protease sensitive.

Clostridium botulinum: The bacteria and its toxins are a food safety and public health threat because the toxins are highly toxic, the bacterial spores are heat stable and the spores and bacteria are capable of growing at low temperatures. There are two forms of the *C. botulinum* group, groups I and II. Group I spores are resistant to heat; they constitute a serious safety concern in canned food production, while group II is capable of growing and producing neurotoxins at a very low temperature, even at 3°C, and is a concern in processed refrigerated foods. Severe neuroparalytic disease is associated with foodborne botulism, which usually results from consuming preformed neurotoxins, and about 10% of foodborne botulism is fatal, with full recovery taking longer than several months (Peck, 2005). The foods involved in botulism include fruits, vegetables, meats and fish

Clostridium perfringens: Several toxins resulting in both histotoxic and enterotoxic diseases in humans and animals are produced by *C. perfringens*. Lately, *C. perfringens* toxins are grouped into seven types, A to G, but type F carries the α-toxin gene but lacks the structural genes for β-toxin, ε-toxin or ι-toxin. Foodborne toxico-infection due to *C. perfringens* is the second most common foodborne ailment in developed nations (Rood et al., 2018). The most common foods that serve as means of transmission of this foodborne infection are meats and poultry products (Mi et al., 2018; Rood et al., 2018)

Staphylococcus aureus: This is one of the most notable foodborne pathogens that produce staphylococcal enterotoxins, mostly associated with the virulence factor of *S. aureus*. Staphylococcal enterotoxins are part of the family of staphylococcal and streptococcal pyrogenic exotoxins. It is connected with gastrointestinal toxins that trigger emesis and stimulation of nonspecific T-cell proliferation. Among the foods that are commonly implicated in staphylococcal intoxication are meat, meat products, poultry, egg products, milk and dairy products, salads and bakery products (Rajkovic et al., 2020).

Campylobacter jejuni: These bacteria produce both cytotoxins and enterotoxins. *Campylobacter jejuni* toxin, an enterotoxin, has a resemblance to a cholera-like toxin in structure and functions and can cause watery diarrhoea. Although it can be inactivated using cholera antitoxin, it is genetically different from cholera toxin (Dolgun et al., 2020). This toxin can cause Guillain-Barré syndrome, and the foods involved include cheese made with raw milk and chicken meat.

Clostridium difficile: Toxin A (enterotoxin) and toxin B (cytotoxin) produced by *C. difficile* are responsible for the pathogenesis of its disease. The toxigenic strains of these bacteria produce both toxins. The mode of action of both toxins is entrance into the intestinal epithelial cells through endocytosis. It can thereafter lead to cell death by affecting the actin skeleton of the cell. Another problem associated with these toxins is that certain cytokines can be secreted, thereby leading to inflammatory response developing in addition to pseudomembranes being formed (Dolgun et al., 2020).

***Vibrio cholerae*:** This is the causative agent of diarrheal disease. The two major virulence factors associated with *V. cholerae* are cholera toxin (CT) and toxin-co-regulated pilus. Cholera toxin functions by activating adenylyl cyclase, thus leading to cAMP increase and then causing several metabolic changes, including activation of ion channels and imbalances in the lumen electrolyte of the intestine, called secretory diarrhoea (Rivera-Chávez and Mekalanos, 2019).

4.10 Preventive and Control Measures for Bacterial Toxins

Thes following are preventive measures to be employed against bacterial toxin–related illnesses: (1) controlling the initial number of bacteria present, (2) preventing a small number from growing, (3) destroying the bacteria by proper cooking and (4) avoiding re-contamination. Poor personal hygiene, improper cleaning of storage and preparation areas and unclean utensils cause contamination of raw and cooked foods. Since food-poisoning bacteria are often present on many foods, knowing the characteristics of such bacteria is essential to an effective control program. Control of enteropathogenic *E. coli* and other foodborne pathogens such as *Salmonella* and *Staphylococcus aureus* can be achieved. Precautions should include adequate cooking and avoidance of recontamination of cooked meat by contaminated equipment, water or infected food handlers. Food service establishments should monitor adequacy of cooking, holding times and temperatures as well as the personal hygiene of food handlers. The first step in preventing food poisoning is to assume that all foods may cause foodborne illness. Infants, older persons, women who are pregnant and anyone with a compromised immune system are especially susceptible to foodborne illness. These people should never consume raw fish, raw seafood or raw meat-type products. You are the key to preventing foodborne illness. By observing the simple rules of good handling, food poisoning can be eliminated. Certain bacteria produce toxins that can cause severe food poisoning when ingested. Managing and monitoring these bacterial toxins is crucial for food safety.

Key benefits of monitoring bacterial toxins include:

- Early detection: Identifying the presence of bacterial toxins quickly to prevent foodborne illnesses.
- Hygiene control: Ensuring proper hygiene practices to reduce contamination risks.
- Consumer safety: Protecting public health by preventing severe food poisoning outbreaks.
- Regulatory compliance: Meeting food safety standards and regulations.

As a preventive measure to avoid food contamination and foodborne diseases, the World Health Organization proposes five keys for food safety (WHO, 2017):

- Keep clean: It refers to washing hands before and during food preparation, washing and sanitizing surfaces and equipment for food preparation and keeping them away from insects and animals.

- Separate raw and cooked food: Prepare raw and cooked food on different surfaces and use different equipment for each type of food.
- Cook thoroughly: Food cooked thoroughly allows the removal of bacteria and other pathogens; toxins produced by bacteria and pathogens can also be destroyed.
- Keep food at safe temperatures: Do not leave cooked food at room temperature for more than 2 h to avoid bacteria proliferation, and try not to store frozen food for long periods of time.
- Use safe water and raw materials: Safe treated water must be used when preparing food; use fresh food products and wash adequately. Pre-processed products such as pasteurized milk should be used as directed and not be used beyond their expiry dates.

4.11 Conclusion

Bacteria that produce toxins enter food products through adulterated raw foods and exposure to bacterial pathogens. Bacterial toxin production can either be endotoxins or exotoxins, depending on their mode of production. Both intrinsic and extrinsic factors contribute in one way or another to bacterial toxin production, which can eventually lead to food poisoning. Therefore, monitoring bacterial toxins in food is crucial to ensure consumer safety and prevent foodborne illnesses. Utilizing effective testing and control measures helps identify and alleviate the risks associated with toxin-producing bacteria like *Staphylococcus aureus* and enterohemorrhagic *Escherichia coli*. Implementing these measures are essential for maintaining high food safety standards and public health.

References

Adekoya, I., Obadina, A., Olorunfemi, M., Akande, O., Landschoot, S., De Saeger, S., et al. (2019). Occurrence of bacteria and endotoxins in fermented foods and beverages from Nigeria and South Africa. *International Journal of Food Microbiology*, 305.

Akhtar, S., Sarker, M. R., and Hossain, A. (2014). Microbiological food safety: A dilemma of developing societies. *Critical Reviews in Microbiology*, 40(4): 348–359. https://doi.org/10.3109/1040841X.2012.742036

Barbieri, J. T. (2009). Exotoxins. In: Schaechter, M., editor. *Encyclopedia of Microbiology*. 3rd ed. Academic Press; pp. 355–364.

Bertani, B., and Ruiz, N. (2018). Function and biogenesis of lipopolysaccharides – Review. *Cell Architecture and Growth*, 8: 1. https://doi.org/10.1128/ecosalplus.esp-0001-2018

Carrasco, E., Valero, A., Pérez-Rodríguez, F., García-Gimeno, R. M., and Zurera, G. (2011). Risk management in environment, production and economy. In: Savino, M., editor. *Food Safety Risk Management*. Croatia: Intech; pp. 77–102. https://doi.org/10.5772/17757.

Dashdorj, D., Amna, T., and Hwang, I. (2015). Influence of specific taste-active components on meat flavor as affected by intrinsic and extrinsic factors: An overview. *European Food Research and Technology*, 241(2): 157–171. https://doi.org/10.1007/s00217-015-2449-3

Dietrich, R., Moravek, M., Bürk, C., Granum, P. E., and Märtlbauer, E. (2005). Production and characterization of antibodies against each of the three subunits of the Bacillus cereus nonhemolytic enterotoxin complex. *Applied and Environmental Microbiology*, 71(12): 8214–8220.

Dolgun, H. T. Y., Kırkan, S., and Uğur Parın, U. (2020). Bacterial toxins. *Animal Health Production and Hygiene*, 9(2): 727–733.

Edae, M. C. K., and Wabalo, E. K. (2019). Bacterial toxins and their modes of action: A review article. *Cloning*, 55. DOI:10.7176/JMPB/55–03.

Farhana, A., and Khan, Y. S. (2023). *Biochemistry, Lipopolysaccharide*. Available from: https://www.ncbi.nlm.nih.gov/books/NBK554414/ [Accessed: August 15, 2024].

Fayyaz, K., Nawaz, A., Olaimat, A. N., Akram, K., Farooq, U., Fatima, M., Siddiqui, S. A., Rana, I. S., Mahnoor, M., and Shahbaz, H. M. (2022). Microbial toxins in fermented foods: Health implications and analytical techniques for detection. *Journal of Food and Drug Analysis*, 30(4): 523–537.

FDA (Food and Drug Administration). (2012). Clostridium perfringens. In: Lampel, K., Al-Khaldi, S., and Cahill, S., editors. *Bad Bug Book, Foodborne Pathogenic Microorganisms and Natural Toxins*. 2nd ed. Center for Food Safety and Applied Nutrition, of the Food and Drug Administration (FDA): The Food and Drug Administration (FDA), U.S. Department of Health and Human Services; pp. 83–86.

Ghazaei, C. (2022). Advances in the study of bacterial toxins, their roles and mechanisms in pathogenesis. *Malaysian Journal of Medical Sciences*, 29(1): 4–17. https://doi.org/10.21315/mjms2022.29.1.2

Gizaw, Z. (2019). Public health risks related to food safety issues in the food market: A systematic literature review. *Environmental Health and Preventive Medicine*, 24(68): 1–22. https://doi.org/10.1186/s12199-019-0825-5.

Hernández-Cortez, C., Palma-Martínez, I., Gonzalez-Avila, L. U., Guerrero-Mandujano, A., Solís, R. C., and Castro-Escarpulli, G. (2017). Food poisoining caused by bacteria. In: Malangu, N., editor. *Poisoning—From Specific Toxic Agents to Novel Rapid and Simplified Techniques for Analysis*. https://doi.org/10.5772/intechopen.69953

Keisam, S., Tuikhar, N., Ahmed, G., and Jeyaram, K. (2019). Toxigenic and pathogenic potential of enteric bacterial pathogens prevalent in the traditional fermented foods marketed in the Northeast region of India. *International Journal of Food Microbiology*, 296: 21e30. https://doi.org/10.1016/j.ijfoodmicro.2019.02.012.

Madigan, M. T., Martinko, J. M., Stahl, D., and Clark, D. P. (2010). *Brock Biology of Microorganisms.* 13th ed. U.K: Pearson Benjamin Cummings.
May, F. J., Polkinghorne B. J., and Fearnley, E. J. (2016). Epidemiology of bacterial toxin mediated foodborne gastroenteritis outbreaks in Australia, 2001 to 2013. *Communicable Diseases Intelligence,* 40(4).
Mi, E., Li, J., and McClane, B. A. (2018). NanR regulates sporulation and enterotoxin production by Clostridium perfringens type F strain F4969. *Infection and Immunity,* 86: e00416–18.
Michel, R. P. (2018). "Bacterial Toxins" section in the journal Toxins: A fantastic multidisciplinary interplay between bacterial pathogenicity mechanisms, physiological processes, genomic evolution, and subsequent development of identification methods, efficient treatment, and prevention of toxigenic bacteria. *Toxins,* 10(1): 44.
Peck, M. W., and Stringer, S. C. (2005). The safety of pasteurised in-pack chilled meat products with respect to the foodborne botulism hazard. *Meat Science,* 70(3): 461–475. https://doi.org/10.1016/j.meatsci.2004.07.019. PMID: 22063745
Peelman, N., Ragaert, P., Verguldt, E., Devlieghere, F., and Bruno Meulenaer, D. (2016). Applicability of biobased packaging materials for long shelf-life food products. *Packaging Research,* 1: 7–20.
Pimbley, D. W., and Patel, P. D. (1998). A review of analytical methods for the detection of bacterial toxins. *Journal of Applied Microbiology Symposium Supplement.* 84(S1): 98S–109S.
Popoff, M. R. (2024). Overview of bacterial protein toxins from pathogenic bacteria: Mode of action and insights into evolution. *Toxins,* 16(4): 182. https://doi.org/10.3390/toxins16040182
Putker, F., Bos, M. P., and Tommassen, J. (2015). Transport of lipopolysaccharide to the gram-negative bacterial cell surface. *FEMS Microbiology Reviews,* 39(6). https://doi.org/10.1093/femsre/fuv026
Rajkovic, A., (2014). Microbial toxins and low level of foodborne exposure. *Trends in Food Science & Technology,* 38(2): 149–157.
Rajkovic, A., Jovanovic, J., Monteiro, S., Decleer, M., Andjelkovic, M., Foubert, A., Beloglazova, N., Tsilla, V., Sas, B., Madder, A., Saeger, S., and Uyttendaele, M. (2020). Detection of toxins involved in foodborne diseases caused by Gram-positive bacteria. *Comprehensive Reviews in Food Science and Food Safety,* 19: 1605–1657. https://doi.org/10.1111/1541-4337.1257
Rivera-Chávez, F., and Mekalanos, J. J. (2019). Cholera toxin promotes pathogen acquisition of host-derived nutrients. *Nature,* 572: 244–248.
Rood, J. I., Adams, V., Lacey, J., Lyras, D., Mcclane, B. A., Melville, S. B., et al. (2018). Expansion of the Clostridium perfringens toxin-based typing scheme. *Anaerobe,* 53: 5–10.
Ross, T., and Nichols, D. S. (2014). Ecology of bacteria and fungi in foods | Influence of available water. In: Batt, C. A., and Tortorello, M. L., editors. *Encyclopedia of Food Microbiology.* 2nd ed. Amsterdam, The Netherlands: Academic Press. https://doi.org/10.1016/B978-0-12-384730-0.00086-0
Sampath, V. (2018). Bacterial endotoxin-lipopolysaccharide; structure, function and its role in immunity in vertebrates and invertebrates. *Agriculture and Natural Resources,* 52(2): 15–120.

Sengupta, M., and Austin, S. (2011). Prevalence and significance of plasmid maintenance functions in the virulence plasmids of pathogenic bacteria. *Infection and Immunity*, 79(7): 2502–2509.

Udebuani, A. C., and Abara, P. N. (2018). Introduction to food microbiology. In: Amadi, E. S., Ugbogu, O. C., and Ogugbue, C. J., editors. *Principles of General Microbiology*. 1st ed. Owerri, Nigeria: WEBSmedia Communications Ltd. ISBN: 978-978-53587-6-6

Wang, X., Meng, J. H., Zhang, N., Zhou, T., Zhang, Y. M., Yang, B. W., et al. (2012). Characterization of Staphylococcus aureus isolated from powdered infant formula milk and infant rice cereal in China. *International Journal of Food Microbiology*, 153(1–2): 142–147.

Wildman, R. E. (2016). *Handbook of Nutraceuticals and Functional Foods*. U.S.A: CRC Press; p. 543.

Willey, J. M., Sherwood, L. M., and Woolverton, C. J. (2008). *Prescott, Harley and Klein's Microbiology*. 7th ed. New York, NY: Mc Graw Hill.

World Health Organization. (2017). *WHO Estimates of the Global Burden of Foodborne Diseases: Foodborne Disease Burden Epidemiology Reference Group 2007–2015*. Available from: http://apps.who.Int/iris/bitstream/10665/199350/1/9789241565165_eng.pdf [Accessed: June 2024].

5

Mycotoxins and Global Food Safety

Isiaka Adedayo Adelere, David Oyeyemi Aboyeji, Helen Shnada Auta, Jayanthi Barasarathi, and Aziz Ahmed

5.1 Introduction

Mycotoxins are toxic secondary metabolites produced by certain species of fungi, primarily *Aspergillus*, *Penicillium*, and *Fusarium*. These toxic compounds can contaminate a wide range of food products, including grains, nuts, fruits, and animal feeds, posing significant risks to human and animal health (Ibrahim & Menkovska, 2018; Kępińska-Pacelik & Biel, 2021; Awuchi et al., 2021, 2022; El-Sayed et al., 2022; Yu & Pedroso, 2023). Mycotoxins are chemically diverse, with over 400 identified varieties, each with distinct biological effects and toxicity levels (Janik et al., 2020; Awuchi et al., 2021, Leslie et al., 2021; El-Sayed et al., 2022). The issue of mycotoxin contamination has been recognized for centuries. Historical records suggest ancient incidents of food-borne illness likely caused by mycotoxins. One of the earliest documented instances is the outbreak of ergotism in the middle ages, caused by the consumption of rye contaminated with ergot alkaloids produced by *Claviceps purpurea* (Agriopoulou, 2021; Grzybowski et al., 2021; Ashfaq et al., 2024).

In today's globalized food system, the importance of addressing mycotoxins in food safety cannot be overstated. These contaminants are not only a threat to public health but also a significant economic burden due to crop losses, reduced livestock productivity, and trade restrictions (Eshetu et al., 2016; Imran et al., 2020; Mamo et al., 2020). The World Health Organization (WHO) and the Food and Agriculture Organization (FAO) have identified mycotoxins as critical food safety concerns, urging countries to implement stringent monitoring and control measures (Ayelign & De Saeger, 2020; Mamo et al., 2020; Meneely et al., 2023).

This chapter aims to provide a comprehensive overview of mycotoxins and their impact on global food safety. It explores the various types of mycotoxins, their sources and occurrence, and the health implications associated with exposure. In addition, the methods used for detecting and analyzing mycotoxins, the regulatory frameworks established to control their presence in food, and the strategies employed to prevent and mitigate contamination are examined. The chapter also discusses the economic and social implications

DOI: 10.1201/9781003500605-6

of mycotoxin contamination and highlights global initiatives aimed at addressing this critical issue. Finally, future perspectives and research directions to improve the understanding and management of mycotoxins in the food supply are considered. By delving into these aspects, this chapter seeks to underscore the importance of mycotoxins in the broader context of global food safety and to highlight the need for continued vigilance and innovation in managing these insidious contaminants.

5.2 Types of Mycotoxins

Mycotoxins are a diverse group of toxic compounds produced by various fungi. Understanding the different types of mycotoxins, their sources, and their effects on the public health is crucial for developing effective food safety strategies. The diversity and complexity of mycotoxins necessitate the development of comprehensive monitoring and regulatory efforts to ensure food safety on a global scale (Marroquín-Cardona et al., 2014; Adeyeye et al., 2022; Chilaka et al., 2022; Zhang et al., 2024). The most significant mycotoxins in terms of their prevalence, toxicity, and impact on human and animal health are summarized in Table 5.1.

5.2.1 Aflatoxins

Aflatoxins are produced primarily by *Aspergillus flavus* and *Aspergillus parasiticus* (Ting et al., 2020; Nikolić et al., 2021; Lorán et al., 2022). They are highly toxic and carcinogenic, commonly found in crops such as corn, peanuts, cottonseed, and tree nuts (García & Heredia, 2014; Awuchi et al., 2020; Tumukunde et al., 2020; Smith, 2020). The various types of aflatoxins include aflatoxins B1, B2, G1, G2, and M1.

5.2.2 Ochratoxins

Ochratoxins are produced by *Aspergillus* and *Penicillium* species, with ochratoxin A being the most significant due to its prevalence and toxicity (Khoi et al., 2021; Więckowska et al., 2023). It is commonly found in cereals, coffee, dried fruits, wine, and grape juice.

5.2.3 Fusarium Toxins

Fusarium species produce several important mycotoxins that affect cereals such as wheat, maize, and barley (Gallo et al., 2022; Kościelecka et al., 2023). The various types of *Fusarium* toxins include deoxynivalenol (DON); zearalenone (ZEA); fumonisins; and fumonisin B1, T-2, and HT-2 toxins.

TABLE 5.1
Types of Mycotoxins and Their Effects on Human and Animal Health

Class of Mycotoxin	Sources	Crops Affected	Examples	Effects	References
Aflatoxin	*Aspergillus flavus* and *Aspergillus parasiticus*	Corn, peanuts, cottonseed, and tree nuts. It can also be found in dairy products.	Aflatoxin B1, B2, G1, G2, M1	It causes liver cancer. Chronic exposure can lead to liver cirrhosis and hepatocellular carcinoma.	Mungamuri & Benkerroum, 2020; Singh et al., 2021; Cao et al., 2022; Wang et al., 2023.
Ochratoxin	*Aspergillus* and *Penicillium* species	Cereals, coffee, dried fruits, wine, and grape juice.	Ochratoxin A (OTA)	It can cause kidney damage and has been linked to kidney and liver tumors. It can also impair immune function and has teratogenic effects.	Benkerroum, 2020; Khoi et al., 2021; Nour-bakhsh & Tajbakhsh, 2021; Longobardi et al., 2022; Stoev, 2022; Więckowska et al., 2023.
Fusarium Toxins	*Fusarium* species	Cereals such as wheat, maize, and barley.	Deoxynivalenol (DON); zearalenone (ZEA); fumonisins; and fumonisin B1, T-2, and HT-2 toxins	It causes nausea, vomiting, diarrhea, and immune suppression. It disrupts reproductive systems in animals, causing infertility, abortion, and other reproductive issues.	Pestka, 2007; Althouse et al., 2019; Rai et al., 2020; Zhou et al., 2020; Ekwomadu et al., 2021; Gallo et al., 2022; Kościelecka et al., 2023.
Patulin	*Penicillium*, *Aspergillus*, and *Byssochlamys* species	Rotting apples and apple products.	Patulin	Associated with gastrointestinal disturbances and immunotoxicity. It has shown potential carcinogenic properties in animal studies.	Ramalingam et al., 2019; Zhai et al., 2019; Wei et al., 2020; Zheng et al., 2021; Fan & Hu, 2024; Wang et al., 2024.
Ergot Alkaloids	*Claviceps* species	Rye and other cereals.	Ergotamine and ergometrine	It causes vasoconstriction, leading to severe health issues such as hallucinations, convulsions, and gangrene.	Al-Omari et al., 2018; Liu, 2018; Yonpiam, 2018; Ashfaq et al., 2024; Berraies et al., 2024.

TABLE 5.1 ***(Continued)***

Types of Mycotoxins and Their Effects on Human and Animal Health

Class of Mycotoxin	Sources	Crops Affected	Examples	Effects	References
Citrinin	*Penicillium* and *Aspergillus* species	Stored grains and cereals.	Citrinin	Known to cause kidney damage. It can also affect liver function and has been observed to cause cytotoxic effects in various cell lines.	Gupta et al., 2018, Silva et al., 2020; Gupta et al., 2022; de Menezes et al., 2023.
Alternaria Toxins	*Alternaria* species	Various fruits, vegetables, tomatoes, apples, and cereals.	Alternariol (AOH), alternariol monomethyl ether (AME)	It can disrupt endocrine function and has shown mutagenic properties in laboratory studies.	Crudo et al., 2019; Hohenbichler et al., 2020; Aichinger et al., 2021; Louro et al., 2024.
Sterigmato-cystin	*Aspergillus* species	Grains, cheese, and other foods.	Sterigmatocys-tin	It is a potent carcinogen and has been linked to liver and kidney cancers.	Nieto et al., 2018; Viegas et al., 2020; Zingales et al., 2020; Zhou et al., 2023.

5.2.4 Patulin

Patulin is produced by *Penicillium*, *Aspergillus*, and *Byssochlamys* species and is commonly found in rotting apples and apple products (Wei et al., 2020; Zheng et al., 2021; Fan & Hu, 2024).

5.2.5 Ergot Alkaloids

Ergot alkaloids produced by *Claviceps* species contaminate rye and other cereals, causing ergotism (Liu, 2018; Ashfaq et al., 2024). Ergotamine and ergometrine are the most significant.

5.2.6 Citrinin

Citrinin is produced by *Penicillium* and *Aspergillus* species, commonly found in stored grains and cereals (Gupta et al., 2022; de Menezes et al., 2023). It often occurs alongside ochratoxin A in contaminated foods.

5.2.7 Alternaria Toxins

Produced by *Alternaria* species, these mycotoxins are found in various fruits, vegetables, and grains (Aichinger et al., 2021; Louro et al., 2024). The main *Alternaria* toxins are alternariol (AOH) and alternariol monomethyl ether (AME).

5.2.8 Other Mycotoxins

Other mycotoxins include sterigmatocystin, produced by *Aspergillus* species (Zhou et al., 2023), and various emerging mycotoxins whose impacts are still being studied. They include enniatins, beauvericin, and moniliformin, which are gaining attention for their potential health impacts. Enniatins and beauvericin are ionophoric mycotoxins with antimicrobial and cytotoxic activities (Hasuda & Bracarense, 2023), while moniliformin affects cardiovascular health (Singh & Kumari, 2022).

5.3 Sources and Occurrence of Mycotoxins

Mycotoxins are ubiquitous in nature and can contaminate a wide range of agricultural products (Tola & Kebede, 2016; El-Sayed et al., 2022). Their presence in food and feed is influenced by various environmental, biological, and agricultural factors (Pleadin et al., 2019; Kępińska-Pacelik & Biel, 2021). Knowing the sources, occurrences, and conditions that favor mycotoxin production and proliferation is crucial for developing effective prevention and control strategies to ensure food safety.

5.3.1 Natural Occurrence in Crops

Mycotoxins are primarily produced by fungi during the growth, harvest, and storage of crops. The most common mycotoxin-producing fungi include species from the genera *Aspergillus, Penicillium, Fusarium,* and *Alternaria* (Sainz et al., 2018; Kaur & Verma, 2023). These fungi can infect crops both pre-harvest (in the field) and post-harvest (during storage and processing). In pre-harvest contamination, crops can be infected with mycotoxin-producing fungi while still in the field. Factors such as temperature, humidity, rainfall, and insect damage can influence fungal growth and mycotoxin production (Awuchi et al., 2021; Kos et al., 2023). For example, aflatoxins are commonly produced in hot, humid climates, while *Fusarium* toxins are more prevalent in cooler, temperate regions (Kos et al., 2023; Casu et al., 2024; Rangel-Muñoz et al., 2024). On the other hand, in post-harvest contamination, improper drying and storage conditions can lead to fungal growth and mycotoxin production. High moisture levels and warm temperatures in storage facilities create an ideal environment for fungal proliferation (Brambilla & Sangiorgio, 2020; Meno et al., 2021; Amobonye et al., 2023).

5.3.2 Factors Influencing Mycotoxin Production

Several factors can influence the production of mycotoxins in crops. They include

- **Climatic Conditions**: Temperature, humidity, and rainfall are critical factors. For instance, aflatoxin production is favored by high temperatures and high humidity, common in tropical and subtropical regions (Shekhar et al., 2018; Dövényi-Nagy et al., 2020). In contrast, cooler temperatures and wet conditions favor the production of *Fusarium* toxins like deoxynivalenol and zearalenone (Milani, 2013; Huang et al., 2023).
- **Agricultural Practices**: Farming practices such as crop rotation, irrigation, use of fertilizers, and pest control can affect fungal growth (Shah et al., 2021; Richard et al., 2022). For example, monoculture cropping systems can increase the risk of fungal infections.
- **Genetic Susceptibility**: Some crop varieties are more resistant to fungal infections and mycotoxin production. Breeding for resistance is an important strategy in managing mycotoxin risk (Buerstmayr & Lemmens, 2015; Rose, 2018)
- **Insect Damage**: Insects can create entry points for fungal infections and contribute to the spread of mycotoxin-producing fungi within crops (Biemond et al., 2021; Leslie et al., 2021).

5.3.3 Commonly Affected Foods

Mycotoxins can contaminate a wide range of food and feed products. The most commonly affected commodities include cereals and grains (corn, wheat, barley, oats, and rice are particularly susceptible to contamination by aflatoxins, ochratoxins, and *Fusarium* toxins) (El-Sayedet al., 2022; Gurikar et al., 2023), nuts and oilseeds (peanuts, almonds, pistachios, and cottonseed are prone to aflatoxin contamination) (Bhat & Reddy, 2017; El-Sayed et al., 2022), fruits and vegetables (apples, grapes, and other fruits can be contaminated by patulin and *Alternaria* toxins) (Nan et al., 2022; Bacha et al., 2023). Other foods affected include dairy products (aflatoxin M1 can be found in milk and dairy products via the ingestion of contaminated feeds by animals) (Min et al., 2021; Turna & Wu, 2021), spices and herbs (spices such as paprika, chili, and black pepper can be contaminated with aflatoxins and ochratoxins) (Syamilah et al., 2022; Demirhan & Demirhan, 2023) and animal feed(contaminated feed can lead to mycotoxin accumulation in animal tissues, milk, and eggs, posing indirect risks to human health) (Haque et al., 2020; Awuchi et al., 2022).

5.3.4 Geographical Distribution

The geographical distribution of mycotoxins varies based on climate, agricultural practices, and crop types. Aflatoxins are predominantly found in tropical and subtropical regions, affecting crops such as corn, peanuts, and tree nuts in countries like India, China, and Nigeria (Awuchi et al., 2020; Kaale et al., 2021; Meneely et al., 2023). Ochratoxins are found in a variety of climates, but especially in temperate regions, affecting cereals, coffee, dried fruits, and wine in Europe, North America, and parts of Asia (Li et al., 2021; Ganesan et al., 2022; González-Curbelo et al., 2023). *Fusarium* toxins are common in temperate regions, affecting wheat, barley, and maize in North America, Europe, and parts of Asia (El-Sayed et al., 2022; Kos et al., 2023). Patulins are found worldwide, particularly in apples and apple products, with significant occurrences reported in North America and Europe (Zhong et al., 2018; Vidal et al., 2019; Gomes et al., 2021).

5.3.5 Examples of Mycotoxin Outbreaks

Several notable mycotoxin outbreaks highlight the widespread impact of these contaminants. An outbreak of aflatoxicosis (turkey X disease)(1960s, UK) that killed over 100,000 turkey poults was traced back to peanut meal contaminated with aflatoxins (Ditta et al., 2018; Balan et al., 2024; Abdelhameed & Khalifa, 2024). High levels of fumonisins (fumonisin outbreak) (1989, USA) in corn were linked to cases of equine leukoencephalomalacia and porcine pulmonary edema (Smith, 2018; Wangia-Dixon & Nishimwe, 2020; Riet-Correa et al., 2024). High levels of Ochratoxin A (ochratoxin contamination) (2004, Europe) were found in baby food products, leading to recalls and heightened regulatory scrutiny (Kabak, 2012; Ozden et al., 2012; Hampikyan et al., 2015).

5.4 Health Impacts of Mycotoxins

Mycotoxins pose significant health risks to both humans and animals. Their effects can range from acute toxicity to chronic health problems, including cancer, immune suppression, and reproductive disorders. Understanding these health impacts is crucial for assessing the risks associated with mycotoxin exposure and implementing effective food safety measures to protect public health. Table 5.2 gives a summary of the health impacts of mycotoxins.

5.5 Detection and Analysis of Mycotoxins

Effective detection and analysis of mycotoxins are critical components to ensuring food safety and protecting public health (Adeyeye et al., 2022). Various analytical methods have been developed to detect and quantify

TABLE 5.2
Health Impacts of Mycotoxins

Health Impacts	Types of Mycotoxins Involved	Effects	References
Acute toxicity; acute mycotoxin toxicity often results from high doses consumed in a short period.	Aflatoxins, deoxynivalenol (DON), T-2 toxin, patulin	It can cause liver damage, jaundice, nausea, vomiting, diarrhea, abdominal pain, gastrointestinal distress, and even death.	Barac, 2019; Awuchi et al., 2021, 2022.
Chronic toxicity; chronic exposure to mycotoxins, even at low levels, can lead to long-term health issues that may not be immediately apparent.	Aflatoxins, ochratoxin A (OTA), fumonisins, zearalenone (ZEA), citrinin	It can cause immune suppression, stunted growth in children, and malnutrition. Chronic exposure can cause chronic kidney disease and disrupt endocrine function.	Tesfamariam et al., 2020; Kadan & Aral, 2021; Ráduly et al., 2021; Awuchi et al., 2022; Kościelecka et al., 2023.
Carcinogenicity; several mycotoxins are classified as carcinogens due to their ability to cause cancer in humans and animals.	Aflatoxin B1, ochratoxin A, fumonisin B1, sterigmatocystin	It is linked to liver and kidney cancers.	Ahmed-Adam et al., 2017; Chhonker et al., 2018; Omotayo et al., 2019; Awuchi et al., 2021, 2022; Yu & Pedroso, 2023; Gurikar et al., 2023.
Immunotoxicity; mycotoxins can impair the immune system, making individuals more susceptible to infections and diseases.	Aflatoxins, ochratoxin A, deoxynivalenol	Known to suppress the immune system, leading to increased susceptibility to infectious diseases and reduced vaccine efficacy. It can also cause chronic inflammatory diseases.	Pierron et al., 2016; Brown et al., 2021; Kraft et al., 2021; Awuchi et al., 2022; Saha Turna et al., 2023.
Reproductive and developmental toxicity; some mycotoxins can affect reproductive health and development, leading to birth defects and reproductive disorders.	Ochratoxin A, fumonisins, zearalenone	Mimics estrogen and can disrupt the reproductive system, leading to infertility, miscarriages, and developmental issues in offspring.	Malir et al., 2013; Eze et al., 2018; El. Khoury et al., 2019; Gönenç et al., 2020; Awuchi et al., 2022; Kościelecka et al., 2023.
Neurotoxicity; certain mycotoxins can affect the nervous system, leading to neurological disorders.	Fumonisins, T-2 toxin	Can cause severe neurological symptoms such as tremors, seizures, and brain damage in cases of high exposure.	Evans & Gupta, 2018; Barac, 2019; Janik et al., 2020; Richard et al., 2020; Nguyen et al., 2022.

mycotoxins in food and feed products. These methods range from traditional chromatographic techniques to modern biosensors.

5.5.1 Sampling and Preparation

The accuracy of mycotoxin analysis depends on proper sampling and sample preparation. Representative sampling is crucial due to the heterogeneous distribution of mycotoxins in bulk commodities (Rivas Casado et al., 2009; Wagner, 2015). Methods such as composite sampling (combining multiple samples) are used to ensure a more accurate representation of the contamination level (Ghosh et al., 2014). Samples must be prepared to isolate mycotoxins from the food matrix. This often involves grinding, homogenization, and extraction using solvents like methanol, acetonitrile, or water (Cigić & Prosen, 2009; Nakhjavan et al., 2020). Clean-up steps, such as solid-phase extraction (SPE), are used to remove interfering substances (Ötles & Kartal, 2016).

5.5.2 Chromatographic Techniques

Chromatographic methods are widely used for the detection and quantification of mycotoxins due to their accuracy and sensitivity. These include:

5.5.2.1 High-Performance Liquid Chromatography

High-performance liquid chromatography (HPLC) is a robust and widely used method for mycotoxin analysis. It often incorporates UV or fluorescence detection to identify and quantify mycotoxins (Turner et al., 2009; Singh & Mehta, 2020). For example, aflatoxins can be detected using HPLC with fluorescence detection after post-column derivatization (Shuib et al., 2017).

5.5.2.2 Liquid Chromatography-Mass Spectrometry

Liquid chromatography-mass spectrometry (LC-MS) combines the separation capabilities of liquid chromatography with the sensitivity and specificity of mass spectrometry. It is particularly useful for detecting multiple mycotoxins in a single run, making it a powerful tool for comprehensive mycotoxin screening (Malachová et al., 2018; Kunzet al., 2020).

5.5.2.3 Gas Chromatography-Mass Spectrometry

Gas chromatography-mass spectrometry (GC-MS) is used for volatile and semi-volatile mycotoxins, such as trichothecenes. Derivatization is often required to make the mycotoxins volatile for analysis (Köppen et al., 2010; Alsharif et al., 2015; Xu et al., 2021).

5.5.3 Immunochemical Methods

Immunochemical methods use antibodies to detect mycotoxins. These methods are often faster and more cost-effective than chromatographic techniques (Alsharif et al., 2015; Singh & Mehta, 2020; Raysyan et al., 2020; Alhazmi & Albratty, 2023).

5.5.3.1 Enzyme-Linked Immunosorbent Assay

Enzyme-linked immunosorbent assay (ELISA) is a widely used method for mycotoxin detection due to its simplicity, speed, and cost-effectiveness. It uses antibodies specific to the mycotoxin to capture and quantify the toxin based on colorimetric changes (Rahman et al., 2019; Majdinasab et al., 2020). ELISA kits are available for various mycotoxins, including aflatoxins, ochratoxins, and fumonisins.

5.5.3.2 Lateral Flow Devices

Lateral flow devices (LFDs), or rapid test strips, are userfriendly and provide quick results. They are commonly used for on-site testing of mycotoxins (Cvak et al., 2021; Wang et al., 2022). These devices work similarly to pregnancy tests, where a visible line indicates the presence of the mycotoxin.

5.5.4 Emerging Technologies

Advances in technology have led to the development of novel methods for mycotoxin detection.

5.5.4.1 Biosensors

Biosensors use biological molecules, such as enzymes or antibodies, to detect mycotoxins (Shrivastava & Sharma, 2022; Wang et al., 2022; Jubeen et al., 2024; Szelenberger et al., 2024). They offer high sensitivity and rapid detection. Examples include electrochemical biosensors, optical biosensors, and nanoparticle-based biosensors.

5.5.4.2 Molecular Techniques

Polymerase chain reaction (PCR) and quantitative PCR (qPCR) can detect the presence of mycotoxin-producing fungi by identifying specific DNA sequences (Rahman et al., 2019; Buslyk et al., 2022). These techniques are useful for predicting potential mycotoxin contamination.

5.5.4.3 Portable Devices

Portable devices, such as handheld spectrometers, are being developed for field testing of mycotoxins. These devices provide rapid and on-site analysis, which is particularly useful for farmers and food inspectors (Kademi et al., 2019; Jafari et al., 2021).

5.5.5 Challenges and Future Directions

Detecting and analyzing mycotoxins present several challenges, including the need for high sensitivity, specificity, and the ability to handle complex food matrices. Challenges such as matrix effects, the need for multi-mycotoxin detection, and the cost of analysis still exist (Agriopoulou et al., 2020; Iqbal, 2021). Complex food matrices can interfere with the detection of mycotoxins (Agriopoulou et al., 2020; Notardonato et al., 2021); hence, there is a need to develop effective sample clean-up and validation procedures. Standardization and rigorous validation of analytical techniques is required to ensuring consistent and reliable results across different laboratories (Peris-Vicente et al., 2015). In addition, developing methods capable of simultaneously detecting multiple mycotoxins is crucial due to the frequent co-occurrence of mycotoxins in food and feed. Reducing the cost and increasing the accessibility of mycotoxin detection methods, especially in developing countries, is essential for global food safety (Agriopoulou et al., 2020; Ndemera et al., 2020; Adeyeye et al., 2022).

5.6 Regulatory Standards and Guidelines of Mycotoxins

Regulatory standards and guidelines for mycotoxins are essential for ensuring food safety and protecting public health. International organizations, such as the Codex Alimentarius, together with national regulatory bodies, have established limits for mycotoxin levels in food and feed (Ibrahim & Menkovska, 2018; López-García, 2022). Effective monitoring, enforcement, and ongoing adaptation to emerging challenges are critical for managing mycotoxin risks and ensuring compliance with regulatory standards (López-García, 2022; Chilaka et al., 2022; Zhang et al., 2024). These regulations aim to minimize the risk of mycotoxin exposure and its associated health impacts.

5.6.1 International Standards

Several international organizations provide guidelines and standards for mycotoxin levels in food and feed (Duarte et al., 2010; Eskola et al., 2020; López-García, 2022). These standards help harmonize regulations across different countries and ensure global food safety.

5.6.1.1 Codex Alimentarius Commission

Codex Alimentarius Commission is jointly established by the Food and Agriculture Organization and the World Health Organization, the Codex

Alimentarius Commission develops international food standards, guidelines, and codes of practice (Halabi, 2015; Lee et al., 2021; Fink, 2023; Fortin, 2023). The Codex sets maximum levels for aflatoxins in various foods, such as 10 µg/kg for ready-to-eat peanuts and 0.5 µg/kg for aflatoxin M1 in milk (EFSA, 2018, 2020; Musawa, 2022; Schincaglia et al., 2023). The maximum level for ochratoxin A in cereals and cereal products is 5 µg/kg (Majeed et al., 2018; Celik & Kabak, 2022; Ben Miri et al., 2024). The Codex recommends a maximum level of 2 mg/kg for deoxynivalenol in cereal grains and 4 mg/kg for fumonisins (B1 + B2) in maize and maize products (Hanvi et al., 2019; Iqbal et al., 2020; Mahdjoubi et al., 2020).

5.6.2 European Union Regulations

The European Union (EU) has stringent regulations for mycotoxins in food and feed, enforced by the European Food Safety Authority (EFSA) and the European Commission (Cheli et al., 2014; Chilaka et al., 2022; Sorbo et al., 2022; Poroşnicu et al., 2023). Maximum levels are set for various foods, including 2 µg/kg for aflatoxin B1 in cereals and 4 µg/kg for total aflatoxins in groundnuts (EFSA, 2018, 2020). The maximum level for OTA is 3 µg/kg in cereals and 10 µg/kg in dried vine fruit and 1.75 mg/kg for DON in unprocessed wheat and 0.75 mg/kg in wheat-based products (Tantaoui-Elaraki et al., 2018; Agriopoulou et al., 2020). The maximum level is 4 mg/kg for fumonisins (B1 + B2) in maize intended for human consumption and 100 µg/kg for zearalenone (ZEA) in cereals and 50 µg/kg in cereal-based products (EFSA, 2014; Leite et al., 2021; Janić Hajnal et al., 2023).

5.6.3 National Regulations

Various countries have their own regulations and guidelines for the acceptable level of mycotoxins in food and feed that often align with international standards (Table 5.3). These limits align with international standards set by organizations such as Codex Alimentarius to ensure that food products meet global safety requirements

5.6.4 Monitoring and Enforcement

Effective monitoring and enforcement are critical for ensuring compliance with mycotoxin regulations. Regulatory agencies employ various strategies to monitor mycotoxin levels in food and feed, including regular sampling and analysis of food and feed products to detect mycotoxin contamination, evaluating the risk of mycotoxin exposure based on consumption patterns and contamination levels. They also conduct inspections of food production, storage, and distribution facilities to ensure adherence to regulations and also educate producers, processors, and consumers about mycotoxin risks and prevention measures (Omojokun, 2013; Fumagalli et al., 2021; Chatterjee et al., 2023).

TABLE 5.3

National Regulations for Mycotoxins in Food and Feed

Country	Regulatory Organization	Type of Mycotoxins/ Food or Feed	Maximum Allowable Limit	References
United States	Food and Drug Administration (FDA) and the Department of Agriculture (USDA)	Aflatoxin M1 in milk	0.5 µg/kg	Kos et al., 2014; Sangvikar, 2021.
		DON for finished wheat products	1 mg/kg	Chen et al., 2021; Mishra et al., 2022.
		DON for animal feed	5 mg/kg	Pack et al., 2021; Mishra et al., 2022.
		Fumonisins for maize products (human consumption)	2 mg/kg	Wu, 2004, 2006; Sabillón et al., 2023.
		Fumonisins for maize products (animal feed)	5 mg/kg	Wu, 2004, 2006; Sabillón et al., 2023
		ZEA in grains and animal feed	None, but the USDA monitors	Abdallah et al., 2015; Weaver et al., 2021.
Canada	Health Canada and the Canadian Food Inspection Agency (CFIA)	Aflatoxins in human food	15 µg/kg	Bhardwaj et al., 2023; Meneely et al., 2023.
		OTA in cereal grains and grains products	15 µg/kg	Shi et al., 2019; Yu & Pedroso, 2023
		DON for unprocessed wheat	2000 µg/kg	Chen et al., 2021; Gedion, 2022.
		DON in wheat (human consumption)	1000 µg/kg	Bosompem, 2020; Chen et al., 2021.
		Fumonisins for maize and maize products (human consumption)	2000 µg/kg	Donnelly et al., 2022; Gedion, 2022.
		ZEA in maize and maize products	100 µg/kg	Donnelly et al., 2022; Gedion, 2022; Stoev, 2024.
Japan	The Ministry of Health, Labour, and Welfare	Aflatoxin B1 in all foods	10 µg/kg	Benkerroum, 2020; Yoshinari et al., 2024.
		OTA in dried vine fruits	2 µg/kg	Özer, 2022; Fakhri et al., 2024.
		DON in wheat and wheat products	1100 µg/kg	Yoshinari et al., 2014; Nakamura et al., 2021.
		Fumonisins in corn and corn products	2000 µg/kg	Yoshinari et al., 2014; Kai et al., 2016.

TABLE 5.3 *(Continued)*

National Regulations for Mycotoxins in Food and Feed

Country	Regulatory Organization	Type of Mycotoxins/ Food or Feed	Maximum Allowable Limit	References
Australia and New Zealand	Food Standards Australia New Zealand (FSANZ)	Aflatoxins in peanuts	15 µg/kg	Bhardwaj et al., 2023; Meneely et al., 2023.
		DON in wheat and wheat products	2000 µg/kg	Baines & Borradale, 2020; Eskola et al., 2020.
		OTA in cereal grains and grains products	5 µg/kg	Carballo et al., 2019; Eskola et al., 2020.
		Fumonisins in maize and maize products	2000 µg/kg	Carballo et al., 2019; Eskola et al., 2020; Meneely et al., 2023.
Nigeria	National Agency for Food and Drug Administration and Control (NAFDAC) and Standards Organization of Nigeria (SON)	Aflatoxin B1	2 µg/kg	Onyeke, 2020; Nahunnaro et al., 2021.
		Total Aflatoxins (B1, B2, G1, and G2) in foods	4 µg/kg	Ubwa et al., 2014; Tor et al., 2020;
		OTA in cereal grains and grains products	5 µg/kg	Olotu, 2018; Onyeke, 2020; Awuchi et al., 2021.
		DON in wheat and wheat products	2000 µg/kg	Atanda et al., 2013; Onyeke, 2020; Awuchi et al., 2021.
		Fumonisins for maize and maize products	2000 µg/kg	Onyeke, 2020; Badmos, 2021.

5.6.5 Challenges and Future Directions

Despite the established regulations, there exist some challenges on how to effectively manage mycotoxin risks. The disparities in regulatory limits and guidelines among various countries can significantly hinder international trade. Efforts are ongoing to harmonize mycotoxin standards globally. New mycotoxins and masked mycotoxins (mycotoxins modified by plant metabolism) pose challenges for detection and regulation (Kovač et al., 2018; Ekwomadu et al., 2021; Iqbal, 2021). Also, changing climatic conditions can alter the prevalence and distribution of mycotoxin-producing fungi, requiring adaptive regulatory measures (Van der Fels-Klerx et al., 2016; Kos et al., 2023; Casu et al., 2024). Therefore, continued development and validation of advanced detection methods are necessary to improve monitoring and enforcement capabilities.

5.7 Prevention and Control Strategies for Mycotoxins

Prevention and control of mycotoxin contamination require a multi-faceted approach, crucial for ensuring food safety and protecting public health. Strategies to mitigate mycotoxin risks involve a combination of agricultural practices, effective post-harvest handling, biological and chemical control methods, regulatory measures, and technological innovations (Table 5.4). By integrating these strategies, it is possible to reduce the risk of mycotoxin contamination and ensure the safety of food and feed products. These strategies aim to reduce the occurrence of mycotoxins at all stages of the food production and supply chain.

5.8 Economic and Social Implications of Mycotoxins

The economic and social implications of mycotoxin contamination are profound and multifaceted, affecting not only public health but also agricultural economies, trade, and livelihoods. Economic losses due to reduced crop yields, trade restrictions, and healthcare costs are significant. Mycotoxin contamination also exacerbates food insecurity and public health issues, particularly in developing countries, where agriculture is a significant part of the economy and food security is a major concern (Gbashi et al., 2018; Kebede et al., 2020; Ajmal et al., 2022; Nji et al., 2022). Addressing these implications requires comprehensive strategies that integrate prevention, control, education, and support for affected populations to mitigate the adverse effects and promote sustainable development (Logrieco et al., 2018; Ndemara et al., 2020; Ortega-Beltran & Bandyopadhyay, 2021).

5.8.1 Economic Implications

5.8.1.1 Losses in Agriculture and Food Industry

Mycotoxin contamination can lead to significant economic losses at various stages of the food supply chain. Mycotoxin-producing fungi can infect crops in the field, leading to yield losses and reduced quality. Contaminated crops may be unsuitable for sale or consumption, resulting in direct financial losses for farmers. Improper storage and handling can exacerbate mycotoxin contamination, causing further losses during transportation, storage, and processing. Post-harvest losses due to mycotoxins can be substantial, especially in regions lacking proper storage facilities and technologies (Chilaka et al., 2017; Neme & Mohammed, 2017; Olorunfemi & Kayode, 2021). In addition, food manufacturers may face significant financial burdens due to the

TABLE 5.4

Prevention and Control Strategies for Mycotoxin Contamination

Control Strategies	Practices	Effects
	Crop rotation and diversity	Rotating crops and planting diverse species can reduce the build-up of mycotoxin-producing fungi in the soil.
Agricultural practices	Resistant varieties	Developing and planting crop varieties using genetic engineering and traditional breeding techniques that are resistant to fungal infections can significantly reduce mycotoxin contamination.
	Optimal planting and harvesting times	Planting and harvesting crops at optimal times can minimize exposure to conditions favorable for fungal growth, such as high humidity and warm temperatures.
	Proper irrigation and drainage	Ensuring adequate irrigation and drainage prevents water stress, which can make crops more susceptible to fungal infections.
	Integrated pest management (IPM)	Using biological control agents, chemical pesticides, and cultural practices to manage pests and diseases reduces the risk of fungal infections that can lead to mycotoxin production.
Post-harvest handling and storage	Clean and sanitary storage	Keeping storage facilities clean and free from previous crop residues minimizes fungal contamination.
	Controlled atmosphere storage	Low oxygen and high carbon dioxide levels can inhibit fungal growth and mycotoxin production.
	Temperature and humidity control	Maintaining low temperatures and humidity levels in storage facilities is crucial for preventing fungal growth.
	Drying	Rapid and thorough drying of crops to safe moisture levels (typically below 13–14%) immediately after harvest prevents fungal growth.
Biological control	Biocontrol agents	Beneficial microbes such as non-toxigenic strains of *Aspergillus flavus* can be applied to crops to reduce aflatoxin contamination.
	Plant extracts and natural compounds	Plant extracts and natural compounds such as neem oil, garlic extract, and thyme oil with antifungal properties can be used to control fungal growth and mycotoxin production.
Chemical control	Fungicides	Applying fungicides during crop growth can help control fungal infections.
	Detoxification agents	Chemical agents such as ozone treatment, ammoniation, and the use of binding agents can help detoxify or degrade mycotoxins.

(Continued)

TABLE 5.4 *(Continued)*

Prevention and Control Strategies for Mycotoxin Contamination

Control Strategies	Practices	Effects
Regulatory and policy measures	Regulatory standards Surveillance and monitoring Education and training	Establishing and enforcing maximum allowable levels of mycotoxins in food and feed ensures that contaminated products do not enter the market. Regular monitoring and surveillance programs help detect mycotoxin contamination early and prevent the distribution of contaminated products. Providing education and training to farmers, food processors, and consumers on mycotoxin risks and prevention methods is crucial for effective control.
	Support for research and development	Governments and organizations should support research and development of new technologies and methods for mycotoxin prevention and control.
Technological innovations	Biosensors and rapid detection kits	Developing rapid and cost-effective detection methods, such as biosensors and lateral flow devices, enables timely identification and management of mycotoxin contamination.
	Genetic engineering	Using genetic engineering to develop crops with enhanced resistance to mycotoxin-producing fungi can significantly reduce contamination levels.
	Blockchain and traceability systems	Implementing blockchain technology and traceability systems in the food supply chain help to ensure that mycotoxin levels are monitored and controlled at each stage.

need for mycotoxin testing, quality control measures, and potential recalls of contaminated products (Mitchell et al., 2016; Focker & van der Fels-Klerx, 2020; Chatterjee et al., 2023). These measures increase production costs and can impact profitability.

5.8.1.2 Trade Implications

Mycotoxin contamination can have severe implications for international trade, particularly for countries that rely on agricultural exports (Gbashi et al., 2018; Luo et al., 2021; López-García, 2022). Countries with strict mycotoxin regulations may reject contaminated imports, leading to trade restrictions and loss of export markets for affected countries. For example, the European Union has stringent limits on mycotoxins in imported food products, impacting exporters from regions with high contamination levels (Eskola et al., 2020; Luo et al., 2021; Chilaka et al., 2022; López-García, 2022). Mycotoxin contamination can also reduce the market value of agricultural commodities (Kebede et al., 2020; Luo et al., 2021). Contaminated products may be sold at lower prices or used for lower-value purposes, such as animal feed, resulting in reduced income for producers.

5.8.1.3 Healthcare Costs

The health impacts of mycotoxin exposure can lead to increased healthcare costs. Treating illnesses caused by mycotoxins, such as liver cancer, immune suppression, and acute poisoning, incurs significant healthcare costs (Mamo et al., 2020; Adeyeye et al., 2022). These costs can burden public health systems, especially in developing countries with limited healthcare infrastructure. Health issues related to mycotoxin exposure can reduce workforce productivity due to illness, absenteeism, and decreased capacity to work (Liew & Mohd-Redzwan, 2018; Sabino et al., 2019; Schlosser et al., 2020). This loss of productivity can have broader economic implications, affecting overall economic growth and development.

5.8.2 Social Implications

5.8.2.1 Food Security

Mycotoxin contamination directly impacts food security, particularly in regions where food availability and access are already limited (Moretti et al., 2017; Kebede et al., 2020; Nji et al., 2022). Contaminated crops and food products may be unsuitable for consumption, reducing the overall food supply. This can exacerbate food shortages and increase hunger and malnutrition, particularly among vulnerable populations. Economic losses due to mycotoxin contamination can reduce household income, limiting access to safe and nutritious food (Udomkun et al., 2017; Mamo et al., 2020; Adeyeye et al., 2022). This can have severe implications for food security and nutritional status, especially for low-income families.

5.8.2.2 Public Health

The public health implications of mycotoxin exposure are significant and multifaceted. Long-term exposure to mycotoxins, even at low levels, can lead to chronic health problems such as liver damage, cancer, immune suppression, and developmental issues in children (Kadan & Aral, 2021; Awuchi et al., 2022). These health impacts can reduce quality of life and increase morbidity and mortality rates. Acute mycotoxin poisoning, although less common, can cause severe and life-threatening symptoms (Awuchi et al., 2021, Navale et al., 2021). Outbreaks of acute aflatoxicosis, for example, have been reported in several countries, causing multiple fatalities (Kamala et al., 2018; Meijer et al., 2021).

5.8.2.3 Social Inequality

Mycotoxin contamination can exacerbate social inequalities, disproportionately affecting marginalized and vulnerable populations. Smallholder farmers, who often lack access to resources, technology, and education, are particularly vulnerable to mycotoxin contamination (Alberts et al., 2017; Chilaka et al., 2022; Nji et al., 2022). The economic losses they face can perpetuate poverty and limit opportunities for economic advancement. Women and children are often more affected by food insecurity and health issues related to mycotoxins. Women, as primary caregivers, bear the burden of caring for sick family members, while children are more susceptible to the health impacts of mycotoxins due to their developing bodies and higher consumption of staple foods (Tshalibe, 2019; Visser et al., 2020; Fredrick, 2021).

5.9 Global Initiatives and Collaboration

Global initiatives and collaboration are vital for effectively managing mycotoxin contamination and ensuring food safety. Various international organizations, regional bodies, research institutions, and governments work together to develop standards, conduct research, build capacity, and raise awareness to manage mycotoxin risks effectively (Logrieco et al., 2018; López-García, 2022; Zhang et al., 2024). Continued efforts in policy harmonization, technological innovation, and adaptation to emerging challenges are essential for mitigating the risks of mycotoxins and promoting sustainable agricultural practices worldwide (Logrieco et al., 2018; López-García, 2022; Chilaka et al., 2022). These initiatives aim to enhance food safety, improve public health, and support sustainable agricultural practices worldwide.

5.9.1 International Organizations

Several international organizations play pivotal roles in addressing mycotoxin contamination through research, policy development, and capacity-building initiatives. The Food and Agriculture Organizationworks to improve food security and safety by promoting good agricultural practices, providing technical assistance, and supporting research on mycotoxin management (Wagacha & Muthomi, 2008; Unnevehr & Grace, 2013; Grace et al., 2015; Xu et al., 2022). The FAO also collaborates with other organizations to develop guidelines and standards for mycotoxin levels in food and feed. The World Health Organization focuses on the public health aspects of mycotoxin contamination. It conducts risk assessments, provides health guidelines, and supports member countries in developing and implementing mycotoxin control measures (Dohlman, 2003; Wu, 2004; Sherif et al., 2009; López-García,

2022). Jointly established by the FAO and WHO, the Codex Alimentarius Commission develops international food standards, guidelines, and codes of practice to ensure food safety and facilitate international trade (Joint FAO/WHO, 2007; WHO, 2018; Godefroy, 2014; Fortin, 2023). The Codex sets maximum permissible levels for various mycotoxins in food and feed, providing a reference for national regulations.

5.9.2 Research and Development Collaborations

Research collaborations are crucial for advancing knowledge and developing innovative solutions for mycotoxin prevention and control. The International Maize and Wheat Improvement Center (CIMMYT) conducts research on improving maize and wheat production, including developing mycotoxin-resistant crop varieties (Ortiz et al., 2008; Mouton, 2014; Warburton & Williams, 2017). It collaborates with national and international partners to disseminate improved seeds and farming practices. The International Institute of Tropical Agriculture (IITA) works with local and international partners to develop and promote effective mycotoxin control strategies. Itfocuses on agricultural research in the tropics, including mycotoxin management in staple crops like maize and groundnuts (Ortiz et al., 2008; Bandyopadhyay et al., 2009; Grace et al., 2015; Xu et al., 2022).

5.9.3 Capacity Building and Education

Capacity building and education are essential for empowering stakeholders to implement effective mycotoxin control measures. International organizations and research institutions offer training programs for farmers, food processors, regulators, and health professionals on mycotoxin management (Alberts et al., 2017; Ndemara et al., 2020; Chilaka et al., 2022). These programs cover topics such as good agricultural practices, post-harvest handling, mycotoxin detection, and risk assessment. Organizations like the FAO and WHO provide technical assistance to countries in developing and implementing mycotoxin control strategies (Wagacha & Muthomi, 2008; Ndemara et al., 2020; Chilaka et al., 2022; López-García, 2022). This assistance includes support for laboratory infrastructure, regulatory frameworks, and surveillance programs. Raising awareness about the risks of mycotoxins and the importance of prevention measures is crucial for achieving widespread adoption of control strategies. Public awareness campaigns target various stakeholders, including farmers, consumers, and policymakers.

5.9.4 Policy and Regulatory Harmonization

Harmonizing mycotoxin regulations at the international level is vital for ensuring food safety and facilitating trade. The Codex Alimentarius Commission plays a key role in developing international standards for mycotoxin levels in food and feed (Duarte et al., 2010; Logrieco et al., 2018; López-García, 2022). These standards serve as benchmarks for national regulations and help ensure consistency and safety in the global food supply. International trade agreements often include provisions for food safety, including mycotoxin regulations. Harmonizing these regulations helps prevent trade barriers and ensures that food products meet safety standards across different countries (Hammoudi et al., 2009; Handford et al., 2015).

5.10 Future Perspectives and Research Directions on Mycotoxins

As the global food system faces increasing challenges from climate change, population growth, and evolving agricultural practices, addressing mycotoxin contamination remains a critical priority. Future perspectives and research directions must focus on innovative approaches, interdisciplinary collaborations, and proactive strategies to mitigate mycotoxin risks and enhance food safety. The development of rapid, accurate, and cost-effective detection methods for mycotoxins is essential for timely intervention and control. Advancements in biosensor technology, including nano-biosensors and lab-on-a-chip devices, offer promising solutions for real-time, on-site detection of mycotoxins in food and feed (Arora, 2018; Bhattacharya et al., 2022; Jafari, 2022). High-resolution mass spectrometry (HRMS) and tandem mass spectrometry (MS/MS) are becoming increasingly important for the precise quantification and identification of mycotoxins and their metabolites (Senyuva et al., 2015; Jensen et al., 2019; Arroyo-Manzanares et al., 2021). Developing portable and user-friendly diagnostic kits that can be used in the field by farmers and food processors can significantly improve early detection and reduce contamination levels.

Future perspectives and research directions in mycotoxin management should focus on advancing detection technologies, biological control methods, and genetic engineering to reduce contamination at the source. Climate change adaptation, innovations in storage and processing, and strengthened policy frameworks are essential for mitigating mycotoxin risks (Loi et al., 2023; Eruaga, 2024). Education and awareness initiatives, coupled with targeted research on health impacts and sustainable practices, will play a critical role in ensuring food safety and protecting public health in the face of evolving challenges. Through interdisciplinary collaborations and proactive strategies, the global community can effectively address mycotoxin contamination and promote a safer and more resilient food system (Fan et al., 2021; WHO, 2022; Eruaga, 2024).

Investigating the occurrence, toxicity, and health impacts of masked and emerging mycotoxins is crucial for comprehensive risk assessment. Also, conducting epidemiological studies to better understand the long-term health effects of mycotoxin exposure and identifying vulnerable populations can inform public health interventions (Wu et al., 2014; Alberts et al., 2017;

Phillips et al., 2022). Assessing the economic impacts of mycotoxin contamination on different sectors of the economy can help in prioritizing resources and policy measures. In addition, exploring sustainable agricultural practices, such as agroecology and organic farming, can provide holistic solutions for reducing mycotoxin risks while promoting environmental health (Bertola et al., 2021; Gomiero, 2018, 2021; Ratnadass et al., 2023).

5.11 Conclusion

Mycotoxins present a significant threat to global food safety, impacting public health, agriculture, and economies worldwide. Understanding the complexities of mycotoxin contamination and its wide-reaching effects is essential for developing effective prevention and control strategies. This chapter has explored the various facets of mycotoxin contamination, from types and sources to health impacts and economic implications, providing a comprehensive overview of the current state of knowledge and ongoing efforts to address this critical issue. Key strategies for mitigating mycotoxin risks include implementing good agricultural practices, improving post-harvest handling and storage, advancing detection and analysis technologies, and enforcing stringent regulatory standards. Looking ahead, future perspectives and research directions emphasize the need for innovative solutions, interdisciplinary approaches, and adaptive strategies to tackle the evolving challenges posed by mycotoxins. In conclusion, addressing mycotoxin contamination requires a coordinated global effort that integrates scientific research, policy development, and practical interventions. By leveraging the collective expertise of international organizations, researchers, policymakers, and industry stakeholders, we can mitigate the risks of mycotoxins, safeguard public health, and promote a more secure and resilient food system. Continued commitment to innovation, collaboration, and education will be essential in overcoming the challenges posed by mycotoxins and achieving sustainable food safety for future generations.

References

Abdallah, M. F., Girgin, G. Ö. Z. D. E., & Baydar, T. (2015). Occurrence, prevention and limitation of mycotoxins in feeds. *Animal Nutrition and Feed Technology, 15*(3), 471–490.

Abdelhameed, S. M., & Khalifa, B. A. (2024). Mycobiota contaminating some market cake samples with reference to their toxin and enzyme. *BMC Microbiology, 24*(1), 209.

Adeyeye, S. O., Ashaolu, T. J., & Idowu-Adebayo, F. (2022). Mycotoxins: Food safety, consumer health and Africa's food security. *Polycyclic Aromatic Compounds, 42*(8), 5779–5795.
Agriopoulou, S. (2021). Ergot alkaloids mycotoxins in cereals and cereal-derived food products: Characteristics, toxicity, prevalence, and control strategies. *Agronomy, 11*(5), 931.
Agriopoulou, S., Stamatelopoulou, E., & Varzakas, T. (2020). Advances in analysis and detection of major mycotoxins in foods. *Foods, 9*(4), 518.
Ahmed-Adam, M. A., Tabana, Y. M., Musa, K. B., & Sandai, D. A. (2017). Effects of different mycotoxins on humans, cell genome and their involvement in cancer. *Oncology Reports, 37*(3), 1321–1336.
Aichinger, G., Del Favero, G., Warth, B., & Marko, D. (2021). Alternaria toxins—Still emerging? *Comprehensive Reviews in Food Science and Food Safety, 20*(5), 4390–4406.
Ajmal, M., Bedale, W., Akram, A., & Yu, J. H. (2022). Comprehensive review of aflatoxin contamination, impact on health and food security, and management strategies in Pakistan. *Toxins, 14*(12), 845.
Alberts, J. F., Lilly, M., Rheeder, J. P., Burger, H. M., Shephard, G. S., & Gelderblom, W. C. A. (2017). Technological and community-based methods to reduce mycotoxin exposure. *Food Control, 73,* 101–109.
Alhazmi, H. A., & Albratty, M. (2023). Analytical techniques for the characterization and quantification of monoclonal antibodies. *Pharmaceuticals, 16*(2), 291.
Al-Omari, R., Al-Enazi, A., Ahmad, R., Ahmad, N., Naqvi, A. A., & Shehzad, A. (2018). Clinical uses and toxicity of Ergot, Claviceps purpurea An evidence-based comprehensive retrospective review. *Bioscience Biotechnology Research Communications, 1,* 356–362.
Alsharif, A. M., Tan, G. H., Choo, Y. M., & Lawal, A. (2015). Liquid phase microextraction for analysis of mycotoxins in food samples. *Research Journal of Chemistry Environmental Science, 3,* 5–21.
Althouse, G. C., Kauffold, J., & Rossow, S. (2019). Diseases of the reproductive system. *Diseases of Swine,* 373–392.
Amobonye, A., Aruwa, C., Aransiola, S. A., John, O., Alabi, T. D., & Lalung, J. (2023). Exploring the potential of fungi in the bioremediation of pharmaceutically active compounds. *Frontiers in Microbiology, 14,* 1207792, https://doi.10.3389/fmicb.2023.1207792
Arora, K. (2018). Advances in nano based biosensors for food and agriculture. *Nanotechnology, Food Security and Water Treatment,* 1–52.
Arroyo-Manzanares, N., Campillo, N., Lopez-Garcia, I., Hernandez-Cordoba, M., & Vinas, P. (2021). High-resolution mass spectrometry for the determination of mycotoxins in biological samples. A review. *Microchemical Journal, 166,* 106197.
Ashfaq, M., Mushtaq, I., Mehmood, M. A., Ahmad, F., & ur Rehman, S. (2024). Ergot alkaloids from Claviceps: Production and pharmacological properties. In *Fungal Secondary Metabolites* (pp. 241–257). Elsevier.
Atanda, O., Makun, H. A., Ogara, I. M., Edema, M., Idahor, K. O., Eshiett, M. E., & Oluwabamiwo, B. F. (2013). Fungal and mycotoxin contamination of Nigerian foods and feeds. *Mycotoxin and Food Safety in Developing Countries, 38.*
Awuchi, C. G., Amagwula, I. O., Priya, P., Kumar, R., Yezdani, U., & Khan, M. G. (2020). Aflatoxins in foods and feeds: A review on health implications, detection, and control. *Bulletin of Environment, Pharmacology and Life Sciences, 9,* 149–155.

Awuchi, C. G., Ondari, E. N., Eseoghene, I. J., Twinomuhwezi, H., Amagwula, I. O., & Morya, S. (2021). Fungal growth and mycotoxins production: Types, toxicities, control strategies, and detoxification. *Fungal Reproduction and Growth, 100207.*

Awuchi, C. G., Ondari, E. N., Nwozo, S., Odongo, G. A., Eseoghene, I. J., Twinomuhwezi, H., . . . Okpala, C. O. R. (2022). Mycotoxins' toxicological mechanisms involving humans, livestock and their associated health concerns: A review. *Toxins, 14*(3), 167.

Ayelign, A., & De Saeger, S. (2020). Mycotoxins in Ethiopia: Current status, implications to food safety and mitigation strategies. *Food Control, 113*, 107163.

Bacha, S. A. S., Li, Y., Nie, J., Xu, G., Han, L., & Farooq, S. (2023). Comprehensive review on patulin and Alternaria toxins in fruit and derived products. *Frontiers in Plant Science, 14*, 1139757.

Badmos, F. O. (2021). *Fusarium and Mycotoxins Profile of Maize (Zea mays) and Sorghum (Sorghum bicolor) Grown in Niger State, Nigeria* (Doctoral dissertation).

Baines, J., & Borradale, D. (2020). Food processing. In *Food and Nutrition* (pp. 74–99). Routledge.

Balan, B., Dhaulaniya, A. S., Kumar, M., Kumar, M., & Kumar, P. (2024). Aflatoxins in food: Prevalence, health effects, and emerging trends in its mitigation—An updated review. *Food Safety and Health*, 2(1), 39–71.

Bandyopadhyay, R., Hell, K., Menkir, A., & Kumar, P. L. (2009). *Annotated Bibliography of IITA Publications on Mycotoxins*. IITA.

Barac, A. (2019). Mycotoxins and human disease. *Clinically Relevant Mycoses: A Practical Approach*, 213–225.

Ben Miri, Y., Benabdallah, A., Chentir, I., Djenane, D., Luvisi, A., & De Bellis, L. (2024). Comprehensive insights into ochratoxin A: Accurrence, analysis, and control strategies. *Foods, 13*(8), 1184.

Benkerroum, N. (2020). Aflatoxins: Producing-molds, structure, health issues and incidence in Southeast Asian and Sub-Saharan African countries. *International Journal of Environmental Research and Public Health, 17*(4), 1215.

Berraies, S., Liu, M., Menzies, J. G., Tittlemier, S. A., Overy, D. P., & Walkowiak, S. (2024). Ergot of cereals: Toxins, pathogens and management. *Plant Pathology, 73*, 1301–1316.

Bertola, M., Ferrarini, A., & Visioli, G. (2021). Improvement of soil microbial diversity through sustainable agricultural practices and its evaluation by-omics approaches: A perspective for the environment, food quality and human safety. *Microorganisms, 9*(7), 1400.

Bhardwaj, K., Meneely, J. P., Haughey, S. A., Dean, M., Wall, P., Zhang, G.,. . . Elliott, C. T. (2023). Risk assessments for the dietary intake aflatoxins in food: A systematic review (2016–2022). *Food Control, 149*, 109687.

Bhat, R., & Reddy, K. R. N. (2017). Challenges and issues concerning mycotoxins contamination in oil seeds and their edible oils: Updates from last decade. *Food Chemistry, 215*, 425–437.

Bhattacharya, M., Paul, I. D., Jayachandran, L., Halder, S., & Banerjee, S. (2022). Nanobiosensors: Principles, techniques, and innovation in nanobiosensors. In *Biosensors in Food Safety and Quality* (pp. 85–110). CRC Press.

Biemond, P. C., Stomph, T. J., Kumar, P. L., & Struik, P. C. (2021). How maize seed systems can contribute to the control of mycotoxigenic fungal infection: A perspective. *Agronomy, 11*(11), 2168.

Bosompem, M. A. (2020). *Effect of Long-Term Feeding of Graded Levels of Deoxynivalenol to Grower-Finisher Pigs* (Doctoral dissertation, University of Saskatchewan).
Brambilla, A., & Sangiorgio, A. (2020). Mould growth in energy efficient buildings: Causes, health implications and strategies to mitigate the risk. *Renewable and Sustainable Energy Reviews, 132*, 110093.
Brown, R., Priest, E., Naglik, J. R., & Richardson, J. P. (2021). Fungal toxins and host immune responses. *Frontiers in Microbiology, 12*, 643639.
Buerstmayr, H., & Lemmens, M. (2015). Breeding healthy cereals: Genetic improvement of Fusarium resistance and consequences for mycotoxins. *World Mycotoxin Journal, 8*(5), 591–602.
Buslyk, T. V., Rosalovsky, V. P., & Salyha, Y. T. (2022). PCR-based detection and quantification of mycotoxin-producing fungi. *Cytology and Genetics, 56*(1), 16–30.
Cao, W., Yu, P., Yang, K., & Cao, D. (2022). Aflatoxin B1: Metabolism, toxicology, and its involvement in oxidative stress and cancer development. *Toxicology Mechanisms and Methods, 32*(6), 395–419.
Carballo, D., Tolosa, J., Ferrer, E., & Berrada, H. (2019). Dietary exposure assessment to mycotoxins through total diet studies. A review. *Food and Chemical Toxicology, 128*, 8–20.
Casu, A., Camardo Leggieri, M., Toscano, P., & Battilani, P. (2024). Changing climate, shifting mycotoxins: A comprehensive review of climate change impact on mycotoxin contamination. *Comprehensive Reviews in Food Science and Food Safety, 23*(2), e13323.
Celik, D., & Kabak, B. (2022). Assessment to propose a maximum permitted level for ochratoxin A in dried figs. *Journal of Food Composition and Analysis, 112*, 104705.
Chatterjee, S., Dhole, A., Krishnan, A. A., & Banerjee, K. (2023). Mycotoxin monitoring, regulation and analysis in India: A success story. *Foods, 12*(4), 705.
Cheli, F., Battaglia, D., Gallo, R., & Dell'Orto, V. (2014). EU legislation on cereal safety: An update with a focus on mycotoxins. *Food Control, 37*, 315–325.
Chen, C., Frank, K., Wang, T., & Wu, F. (2021). Global wheat trade and Codex Alimentarius guidelines for deoxynivalenol: A mycotoxin common in wheat. *Global Food Security, 29*, 100538.
Chhonker, S., Rawat, D., Naik, R. A., & Koiri, R. K. (2018). An overview of mycotoxins in human health with emphasis on development and progression of liver cancer. *Clinical Oncology, 3*, 1408.
Chilaka, C. A., De Boevre, M., Atanda, O. O., & De Saeger, S. (2017). The status of Fusarium mycotoxins in sub-Saharan Africa: A review of emerging trends and post-harvest mitigation strategies towards food control. *Toxins, 9*(1), 19.
Chilaka, C. A., Obidiegwu, J. E., Chilaka, A. C., Atanda, O. O., & Mally, A. (2022). Mycotoxin regulatory status in Africa: A decade of weak institutional efforts. *Toxins, 14*(7), 442.
Cigić, I. K., & Prosen, H. (2009). An overview of conventional and emerging analytical methods for the determination of mycotoxins. *International Journal of Molecular Sciences, 10*(1), 62–115.
Crudo, F., Varga, E., Aichinger, G., Galaverna, G., Marko, D., Dall'Asta, C., & Dellafiora, L. (2019). Co-occurrence and combinatory effects of Alternaria mycotoxins and other xenobiotics of food origin: Current scenario and future perspectives. *Toxins, 11*(11), 640.

Cvak, B., Warth, B., Atehnkeng, J., Parich, A., Moritz, A., Sulyok, M., & Krska, R. (2021). Evaluating the performance of lateral flow devices for total aflatoxins with special emphasis on their robustness under sub-Saharan conditions. *Toxins, 13*(11), 742.

de Menezes, A. A. P., Aguiar, R. P., Santos, J. V., Sarkar, C., Islam, M. T., Braga, A. L., . . . Sousa, J. M. (2023). Citrinin as a potential anti-cancer therapy: A comprehensive review. *Chemico-Biological Interactions, 381*, 110561.

Demirhan, B., & Demirhan, B. E. (2023). Analysis of multi-mycotoxins in commonly consumed spices using the LC-MS/MS method for assessing food safety risks. *Microorganisms, 11*(7), 1786.

Ditta, Y. A., Mahad, S., & Bacha, U. (2018). Aflatoxins: Their toxic effect on poultry and recent advances in their treatment. *Mycotoxins-Impact and Management Strategies, 2018*, 1–153.

Dohlman, E. (2003). Mycotoxin hazards and regulations. *International Trade and Food Safety, 97.*

Donnelly, R., Elliott, C., Zhang, G., Baker, B., & Meneely, J. (2022). Understanding current methods for sampling of aflatoxins in corn and to generate a best practice framework. *Toxins, 14*(12), 819.

Dövényi-Nagy, T., Rácz, C., Molnár, K., Bakó, K., Szláma, Z., Jóźwiak, Á.,. . . Dobos, A. C. (2020). Pre-harvest modelling and mitigation of aflatoxins in maize in a changing climatic environment—A review. *Toxins, 12*(12), 768.

Duarte, S. C., Lino, C. M., & Pena, A. (2010). Mycotoxin food and feed regulation and the specific case of ochratoxin A: A review of the worldwide status. *Food Additives and Contaminants, 27*(10), 1440–1450.

EFSA Panel on Contaminants in the Food Chain (CONTAM), Knutsen, H. K., Alexander, J., Barregård, L., Bignami, M., Brüschweiler, B.,. . . Petersen, A. (2018). Effect on public health of a possible increase of the maximum level for 'aflatoxin total' from 4 to 10 μg/kg in peanuts and processed products thereof, intended for direct human consumption or use as an ingredient in foodstuffs. *EFSA Journal, 16*(2), e05175.

EFSA Panel on Contaminants in the Food Chain (CONTAM), Schrenk, D., Bignami, M., Bodin, L., Chipman, J. K., del Mazo, J.,. . .Wallace, H. (2020). Risk assessment of aflatoxins in food. *EFSA Journal, 18*(3), e06040.

Ekwomadu, T. I., Akinola, S. A., & Mwanza, M. (2021). Fusarium mycotoxins, their metabolites (free, emerging, and masked), food safety concerns, and health impacts. *International Journal of Environmental Research and Public Health, 18*(22), 11741.

El. Khoury, D., Fayjaloun, S., Nassar, M., Sahakian, J., & Aad, P. Y. (2019). Updates on the effect of mycotoxins on male reproductive efficiency in mammals. *Toxins, 11*(9), 515.

El-Sayed, R. A., Jebur, A. B., Kang, W., & El-Demerdash, F. M. (2022). An overview on the major mycotoxins in food products: Characteristics, toxicity, and analysis. *Journal of Future Foods, 2*(2), 91–102.

Eruaga, M. A. (2024). Policy strategies for managing food safety risks associated with climate change and agriculture. *International Journal of Scholarly Research and Reviews, 4*(1), 21–32.

Eshetu, E., Habtamu, A., & Gebretensa, A. (2016). An overview on major mycotoxin in animal: Its public health implication, economic impact and control strategies. *Journal of Health, Medicine and Nursing, 25*, 64–73.

Eskola, M., Kos, G., Elliott, C. T., Hajšlová, J., Mayar, S., & Krska, R. (2020). Worldwide contamination of food-crops with mycotoxins: Validity of the widely cited 'FAO estimate' of 25%. *Critical Reviews in Food Science and Nutrition*, *60*(16), 2773–2789.

European Food Safety Authority. (2014). Evaluation of the increase of risk for public health related to a possible temporary derogation from the maximum level of deoxynivalenol, zearalenone and fumonisins for maize and maize products. *EFSA Journal*, *12*(5), 3699.

Evans, T. J., & Gupta, R. C. (2018). Tremorgenic mycotoxins. In *Veterinary Toxicology* (pp. 1033–1041). Academic Press.

Eze, U. A., Routledge, M. N., Okonofua, F. E., Huntriss, J., & Gong, Y. Y. (2018). Mycotoxin exposure and adverse reproductive health outcomes in Africa: A review. *World Mycotoxin Journal*, *11*(3), 321–339.

Fakhri, Y., Mahdavi, V., Ranaei, V., Pilevar, Z., Sarafraz, M., Mahmudiono, T., & Khaneghah, A. M. (2024). Ochratoxin A in coffee and coffee-based products: A global systematic review, meta-analysis, and probabilistic risk assessment. *Reviews on Environmental Health*, *39*(2), 211–220.

Fan, L., & Hu, H. (2024). Involvement of multiple forms of cell death in patulin-induced toxicities. *Toxicon*, 107768.

Fan, S., Cho, E. E., Meng, T., & Rue, C. (2021). How to prevent and cope with coincidence of risks to the global food system. *Annual Review of Environment and Resources*, *46*(1), 601–623.

Fink, B. A. (2023). Codex Alimentarius at home and abroad: The regulatory costs of developing and implementing international and national food-safety standards. In *Research Handbook on International Food Law* (pp. 347–367). Edward Elgar Publishing.

Focker, M., & van der Fels-Klerx, H. J. (2020). Economics applied to food safety. *Current Opinion in Food Science*, *36*, 18–23.

Fortin, N. D. (2023). Global governance of food safety: The role of the FAO, WHO, and Codex Alimentarius in regulatory harmonization. In *Research Handbook on International Food Law* (pp. 227–242). Edward Elgar Publishing.

Fredrick, R. (2021). *Assessment of Nutritional Status and Dietary Aflatoxins Exposure in Children in Singida District Council* (Doctoral dissertation, NM-AIST).

Fumagalli, F., Ottoboni, M., Pinotti, L., & Cheli, F. (2021). Integrated mycotoxin management system in the feed supply chain: Innovative approaches. *Toxins*, *13*(8), 572.

Gallo, A., Mosconi, M., Trevisi, E., & Santos, R. R. (2022). Adverse effects of Fusarium toxins in ruminants: A review of in vivo and in vitro studies. *Dairy*, *3*(3), 474–499.

Ganesan, A. R., Mohan, K., Rajan, D. K., Pillay, A. A., Palanisami, T., Sathishkumar, P., & Conterno, L. (2022). Distribution, toxicity, interactive effects, and detection of ochratoxin and deoxynivalenol in food: A review. *Food Chemistry*, *378*, 131978.

García, S., & Heredia, N. L. (2014). Aflatoxins: An overview. In J. B. Dixon, A. L. Barrientos Velázquez, & Y. Deng, (Eds.) *Aflatoxin Control: Safeguarding Animal Feed with Calcium Smectite* (pp. 1–10). John Wiley & Sons.

Gbashi, S., Madala, N. E., De Saeger, S., De Boevre, M., Adekoya, I., Adebo, O. A., & Njobeh, P. B. (2018). The socio-economic impact of mycotoxin contamination in Africa. In *Mycotoxins-Impact and Management Strategies*. IntechOpen. https://doi.10.5772/intechopen.79328

Gedion, B. W. (2022). *Improved Sampling and Detection of Mycotoxins in Maize (Zea mays L.)* (Doctoral dissertation, University of Guelph).

Ghosh, U., Kane Driscoll, S., Burgess, R. M., Jonker, M. T., Reible, D., Gobas, F.,. . . Beegan, C. (2014). Passive sampling methods for contaminated sediments: Practical guidance for selection, calibration, and implementation. *Integrated Environmental Assessment and Management*, *10*(2), 210–223.
Godefroy, S. B. (2014). Codex Alimentarius Commission at 50: Major achievements and challenges ahead. *International Food Risk Analysis Journal*, *4*.
Gomes, I. A., Marková, E., da Silva, J. P. L., Venâncio, A., & Freitas-Silva, O. (2021). Global trends for patulin adsorption: A review. *Research, Society and Development*, *10*(6), e58310616162–e58310616162.
Gomiero, T. (2018). Food quality assessment in organic vs. conventional agricultural produce: Findings and issues. *Applied Soil Ecology*, *123*, 714–728.
Gomiero, T. (2021). Organic agriculture: Impact on the environment and food quality. In *Environmental Impact of Agro-food Industry and Food Consumption* (pp. 31–58). Academic Press.
Gönenç, İ. M., Yilmaz Sezer, N., & Yilmaz, S. (2020). Mycotoxin exposure and pregnancy. *Critical Reviews in Toxicology*, *50*(7), 594–604.
González-Curbelo, M. Á., & Kabak, B. (2023). Occurrence of mycotoxins in dried fruits worldwide, with a focus on aflatoxins and ochratoxin A: A review. *Toxins*, *15*(9), 576.
Grace, D., Mahuku, G., Hoffmann, V., Atherstone, C., Upadhyaya, H. D., & Bandyopadhyay, R. (2015). International agricultural research to reduce food risks: Case studies on aflatoxins. *Food Security*, *7*, 569–582.
Grzybowski, A., Pawlikowska-Łagód, K., & Polak, A. (2021). Ergotism and Saint Anthony's fire. *Clinics in Dermatology*, *39*(6), 1088–1094.
Gupta, R. C., Doss, R. B., Lall, R., Srivastava, A., & Sinha, A. (2022). Aflatoxins, ochratoxins, and citrinin. In *Reproductive and Developmental Toxicology* (pp. 983–1002). Academic press.
Gupta, R. C., Srivastava, A., & Lall, R. (2018). Ochratoxins and citrinin. In *Veterinary Toxicology* (pp. 1019–1027). Academic Press.
Gurikar, C., Shivaprasad, D. P., Sabillón, L., Gowda, N. N., & Siliveru, K. (2023). Impact of mycotoxins and their metabolites associated with food grains. *Grain & Oil Science and Technology*, *6*(1), 1–9.
Halabi, S. (2015). The Codex Alimentarius Commission, corporate influence, and international trade. *American Journal of Law and Medicine*, *41*(2).
Hammoudi, A., Hoffmann, R., & Surry, Y. (2009). Food safety standards and agri-food supply chains: An introductory overview. *European Review of Agricultural Economics*, *36*(4), 469–478.
Hampikyan, H., Bingol, E. B., Colak, H., Cetin, O., & Bingol, B. (2015). Determination of ochratoxin a in baby foods by ELISA and HPLC. *Acta Alimentaria*, *44*(4), 578–584.
Handford, C. E., Elliott, C. T., & Campbell, K. (2015). A review of the global pesticide legislation and the scale of challenge in reaching the global harmonization of food safety standards. *Integrated Environmental Assessment and Management*, *11*(4), 525–536.
Hanvi, D. M., Lawson-Evi, P., De Boevre, M., Goto, C. E., De Saeger, S., & Eklu-Gadegbeku, K. (2019). Natural occurrence of mycotoxins in maize and sorghum in Togo. *Mycotoxin Research*, *35*(4), 321–327.
Haque, M. A., Wang, Y., Shen, Z., Li, X., Saleemi, M. K., & He, C. (2020). Mycotoxin contamination and control strategy in human, domestic animal and poultry: A review. *Microbial Pathogenesis*, *142*, 104095.

Hasuda, A. L., & Bracarense, A. P. F. (2023). Toxicity of the emerging mycotoxins beauvericin and enniatins: A mini-review. *Toxicon*, 107534.

Hohenbichler, J., Aichinger, G., Rychlik, M., Del Favero, G., & Marko, D. (2020). Alternaria alternata toxins synergistically activate the aryl hydrocarbon receptor pathway in vitro. *Biomolecules, 10*(7), 1018.

Huang, W., Zhou, P., Shen, G., Gao, T., Liu, X., Shi, J.,. . . Qiu, J. (2023). Relationship Between Mycotoxin Production and Gene Expression in Fusarium graminearum Species Complex Strains Under Various Environmental Conditions. *Journal of Microbiology, 61*(5), 525–542.

Ibrahim, O. O., & Menkovska, M. (2018). The nature, sources, detections and regulations of mycotoxins that contaminate foods and feeds causing health hazards for both human and animals. *Journal of Agricultural Chemistry and Environment, 8*(1), 33–57.

Imran, M., Cao, S., Wan, S. F., Chen, Z., Saleemi, M. K., Wang, N.,. . . Munawar, J. (2020). Mycotoxins–a global one health concern: A review. *Agrobiological Records*, 2, 1–16.

Iqbal, S. Z. (2021). Mycotoxins in food, recent development in food analysis and future challenges; a review. *Current Opinion in Food Science, 42*, 237–247.

Iqbal, S. Z., Usman, S., Razis, A. F. A., Basheir Ali, N., Saif, T., & Asi, M. R. (2020). Assessment of deoxynivalenol in wheat, corn and its products and estimation of dietary intake. *International Journal of Environmental Research and Public Health, 17*(15), 5602.

Jafari, S. (2022). *Development of Smartphone-based Electrochemical Biosensors for Point-of-need Food Safety Testing* (Doctoral dissertation, ETH Zurich).

Jafari, S., Guercetti, J., Geballa-Koukoula, A., Tsagkaris, A. S., Nelis, J. L., Marco, M. P.,. . . Sturla, S. J. (2021). ASSURED point-of-need food safety screening: A critical assessment of portable food analyzers. *Foods, 10*(6), 1399.

Janić Hajnal, E., Kos, J., Radić, B., Anić, M., Radović, R., Kudumija, N.,. . . Pleadin, J. (2023). Impact of climate changes on the natural prevalence of Fusarium mycotoxins in maize harvested in Serbia and Croatia. *Foods, 12*(5), 1002.

Janik, E., Niemcewicz, M., Ceremuga, M., Stela, M., Saluk-Bijak, J., Siadkowski, A., & Bijak, M. (2020). Molecular aspects of mycotoxins—A serious problem for human health. *International Journal of Molecular Sciences, 21*(21), 8187.

Jensen, T., De Boevre, M., Preußke, N., De Saeger, S., Birr, T., Verreet, J. A., & Sönnichsen, F. D. (2019). Evaluation of high-resolution mass spectrometry for the quantitative analysis of mycotoxins in complex feed matrices. *Toxins, 11*(9), 531.

Joint FAO/WHO Codex Alimentarius Commission, World Health Organization, & Joint FAO/WHO Food Standards Programme. (2007). *Codex Alimentarius: Food Import and Export Inspection and Certification Systems*. Food & Agriculture Org.

Jubeen, F., Batool, A., Naz, I., Sehar, S., Sadia, H., Hayat, A., & Kazi, M. (2024). Mycotoxins detection in food using advanced, sensitive and robust electrochemical platform of sensors: A review. *Sensors and Actuators A: Physical*, 115045.

Kaale, L. D., Kimanya, M. E., Macha, I. J., & Mlalila, N. (2021). Aflatoxin contamination and recommendations to improve its control: A review. *World Mycotoxin Journal, 14*(1), 27–40.

Kabak, B. (2012). Aflatoxin M1 and ochratoxin A in baby formulae in Turkey: Occurrence and safety evaluation. *Food Control, 26*(1), 182–187.

Kadan, G., & Aral, N. (2021). Effects of mycotoxins on child development. *Current Molecular Pharmacology, 14*(5), 770–781.

Kademi, H. I., Ulusoy, B. H., & Hecer, C. (2019). Applications of miniaturized and portable near infrared spectroscopy (NIRS) for inspection and control of meat and meat products. *Food Reviews International, 35*(3), 201–220.
Kai, S., Kosuge, N., Waki, M., Miyazawa, M., & Kanazawa, H. (2016). Analysis of Fusarium toxins in processed grain products using high-performance liquid chromatography/tandem mass spectrometry. *Chromatography, 37*(2), 79–85.
Kamala, A., Shirima, C., Jani, B., Bakari, M., Sillo, H., Rusibamayila, N., . . . Investigation Team. (2018). Outbreak of an acute aflatoxicosis in Tanzania during 2016. *World Mycotoxin Journal, 11*(3), 311–320.
Kaur, Y., & Verma, R. K. (2023). Mycotoxins produced in plant-pathogen interactions. In *Plant-Microbe Interaction-Recent Advances in Molecular and Biochemical Approaches* (pp. 257–279). Academic Press.
Kebede, H., Liu, X., Jin, J., & Xing, F. (2020). Current status of major mycotoxins contamination in food and feed in Africa. *Food Control, 110*, 106975.
Kępińska-Pacelik, J., & Biel, W. (2021). Mycotoxins—prevention, detection, impact on animal health. *Processes, 9*(11), 2035.
Khoi, C. S., Chen, J. H., Lin, T. Y., Chiang, C. K., & Hung, K. Y. (2021). Ochratoxin A-induced nephrotoxicity: Up-to-date evidence. *International Journal of Molecular Sciences, 22*(20), 11237.
Köppen, R., Koch, M., Siegel, D., Merkel, S., Maul, R., & Nehls, I. (2010). Determination of mycotoxins in foods: Current state of analytical methods and limitations. *Applied Microbiology and Biotechnology, 86*, 1595–1612.
Kos, J., Anić, M., Radić, B., Zadravec, M., Janić Hajnal, E., & Pleadin, J. (2023). Climate change—A global threat resulting in increasing mycotoxin occurrence. *Foods, 12*(14), 2704.
Kos, J., Lević, J., Đuragić, O., Kokić, B., & Miladinović, I. (2014). Occurrence and estimation of aflatoxin M1 exposure in milk in Serbia. *Food Control, 38*, 41–46.
Kościelecka, K., Kuć, A., Kubik-Machura, D., Męcik-Kronenberg, T., Włodarek, J., & Radko, L. (2023). Endocrine effect of some mycotoxins on humans: A clinical review of the ways to mitigate the action of mycotoxins. *Toxins, 15*(9), 515.
Kovač, M., Šubarić, D., Bulaić, M., Kovač, T., & Šarkanj, B. (2018). Yesterday masked, today modified; what do mycotoxins bring next? *Archives of Industrial Hygiene and Toxicology, 69*(3), 196–214.
Kraft, S., Buchenauer, L., & Polte, T. (2021). Mold, mycotoxins and a dysregulated immune system: A combination of concern?. *International Journal of Molecular Sciences, 22*(22), 12269.
Kunz, B. M., Wanko, F., Kemmlein, S., Bahlmann, A., Rohn, S., & Maul, R. (2020). Development of a rapid multi-mycotoxin LC-MS/MS stable isotope dilution analysis for grain legumes and its application on 66 market samples. *Food Control, 109*, 106949.
Lee, J. G., Lee, Y., Kim, C. S., & Han, S. B. (2021). Codex Alimentarius commission on ensuring food safety and promoting fair trade: Harmonization of standards between Korea and codex. *Food Science and Biotechnology, 30*(9), 1151–1170.
Leite, M., Freitas, A., Silva, A. S., Barbosa, J., & Ramos, F. (2021). Maize food chain and mycotoxins: A review on occurrence studies. *Trends in Food Science & Technology, 115*, 307–331.
Leslie, J. F., Moretti, A., Mesterházy, Á., Ameye, M., Audenaert, K., Singh, P. K.,. . . Logrieco, A. F. (2021). Key global actions for mycotoxin management in wheat and other small grains. *Toxins, 13*(10), 725.

Li, X., Ma, W., Ma, Z., Zhang, Q., & Li, H. (2021). The occurrence and contamination level of ochratoxin A in plant and animal-derived food commodities. *Molecules, 26*(22), 6928.

Liew, W. P. P., & Mohd-Redzwan, S. (2018). Mycotoxin: Its impact on gut health and microbiota. *Frontiers in Cellular and Infection Microbiology, 8*, 60.

Liu, D. (2018). Ergot alkaloids. In *Handbook of Foodborne Diseases* (pp. 925–931). Taylor & Francis Group, CRC Press.

Logrieco, A. F., Miller, J. D., Eskola, M., Krska, R., Ayalew, A., Bandyopadhyay, R., . . Leslie, J. F. (2018). The mycotox charter: Increasing awareness of, and concerted action for, minimizing mycotoxin exposure worldwide. *Toxins, 10*(4), 149.

Loi, M., Logrieco, A. F., Pusztahelyi, T., Leiter, É., Hornok, L., & Pócsi, I. (2023). Advanced mycotoxin control and decontamination techniques in view of an increased aflatoxin risk in Europe due to climate change. *Frontiers in Microbiology, 13*, 1085891.

Longobardi, C., Ferrara, G., Andretta, E., Montagnaro, S., Damiano, S., & Ciarcia, R. (2022). Ochratoxin A and kidney oxidative stress: The role of nutraceuticals in veterinary medicine—a review. *Toxins, 14*(6), 398.

López-García, R. (2022). Mycotoxin management: An international challenge. In *Ensuring Global Food Safety* (pp. 213–219). Academic Press.

Lorán, S., Carramiñana, J. J., Juan, T., Ariño, A., & Herrera, M. (2022). Inhibition of Aspergillus parasiticus growth and aflatoxins production by natural essential oils and phenolic acids. *Toxins, 14*(6), 384.

Louro, H., Vettorazzi, A., López de Cerain, A., Spyropoulou, A., Solhaug, A., Straumfors, A.,. . . Marko, D. (2024). Hazard characterization of Alternaria toxins to identify data gaps and improve risk assessment for human health. *Archives of Toxicology, 98*(2), 425–469.

Luo, S., Du, H., Kebede, H., Liu, Y., & Xing, F. (2021). Contamination status of major mycotoxins in agricultural product and food stuff in Europe. *Food Control, 127*, 108120.

Mahdjoubi, C. K., Arroyo-Manzanares, N., Hamini-Kadar, N., García-Campaña, A. M., Mebrouk, K., & Gámiz-Gracia, L. (2020). Multi-mycotoxin occurrence and exposure assessment approach in foodstuffs from Algeria. *Toxins, 12*(3), 194.

Majdinasab, M., Ben Aissa, S., & Marty, J. L. (2020). Advances in colorimetric strategies for mycotoxins detection: Toward rapid industrial monitoring. *Toxins, 13*(1), 13.

Majeed, M., Khaneghah, A. M., Kadmi, Y., Khan, M. U., & Shariati, M. A. (2018). Assessment of ochratoxin A in commercial corn and wheat products. *Current Nutrition & Food Science, 14*(2), 116–120.

Malachová, A., Stránská, M., Václavíková, M., Elliott, C. T., Black, C., Meneely, J.,. . . Krska, R. (2018). Advanced LC–MS-based methods to study the co-occurrence and metabolization of multiple mycotoxins in cereals and cereal-based food. *Analytical and Bioanalytical Chemistry, 410*, 801–825.

Malir, F., Ostry, V., Pfohl-Leszkowicz, A., & Novotna, E. (2013). Ochratoxin A: Developmental and reproductive toxicity—An overview. *Birth Defects Research Part B: Developmental and Reproductive Toxicology, 98*(6), 493–502.

Mamo, F. T., Abate, B. A., Tesfaye, K., Nie, C., Wang, G., & Liu, Y. (2020). Mycotoxins in Ethiopia: A review on prevalence, economic and health impacts. *Toxins, 12*(10), 648.

Marroquín-Cardona, A. G., Johnson, N. M., Phillips, T. D., & Hayes, A. W. (2014). Mycotoxins in a changing global environment–a review. *Food and Chemical Toxicology, 69*, 220–230.

Meijer, N., Kleter, G., de Nijs, M., Rau, M. L., Derkx, R., & van der Fels-Klerx, H. J. (2021). The aflatoxin situation in Africa: Systematic literature review. *Comprehensive Reviews in Food Science and Food Safety, 20*(3), 2286–2304.
Meneely, J. P., Kolawole, O., Haughey, S. A., Miller, S. J., Krska, R., & Elliott, C. T. (2023). The challenge of global aflatoxins legislation with a focus on peanuts and peanut products: A systematic review. *Exposure and Health, 15*(2), 467–487.
Meno, L., Escuredo, O., Rodríguez-Flores, M. S., & Seijo, M. C. (2021). Prevalence of airborne fungal spores in two potato warehouses with different storage conditions. *Aerobiologia, 37*, 309–320.
Milani, J. M. (2013). Ecological conditions affecting mycotoxin production in cereals: A review. *Veterinarni Medicina, 58*(8).
Min, L., Fink-Gremmels, J., Li, D., Tong, X., Tang, J., Nan, X.,. . . Wang, G. (2021). An overview of aflatoxin B1 biotransformation and aflatoxin M1 secretion in lactating dairy cows. *Animal Nutrition, 7*(1), 42–48.
Mishra, S., Srivastava, S., Dewangan, J., Divakar, A., & Kumar Rath, S. (2022). Global occurrence of deoxynivalenol in food commodities and exposure risk assessment in humans in the last decade: A survey. *Critical Reviews in Food Science and Nutrition, 60*(8), 1346–1374.
Mitchell, N. J., Bowers, E., Hurburgh, C., & Wu, F. (2016). Potential economic losses to the US corn industry from aflatoxin contamination. *Food Additives & Contaminants: Part A, 33*(3), 540–550.
Moretti, A., Logrieco, A. F., & Susca, A. (2017). Mycotoxins: An underhand food problem. *Mycotoxigenic Fungi: Methods and Protocols*, 3–12.
Mouton, M. (2014). *Resistance in South African Maize Inbred Lines to the Major Ear Rot Diseases and Associated Mycotoxin Contamination* (Doctoral dissertation, Stellenbosch: Stellenbosch University).
Mungamuri, S. K., & Mavuduru, V. A. (2020). Role of epigenetic alterations in aflatoxin-induced hepatocellular carcinoma. *Liver Cancer International, 1*(2), 41–50.
Musawa, G. (2022). *Exposure Risk Assessment to Aflatoxins through the Consumption of Peanut among Children Aged 6–59 Months in Lusaka District* (Doctoral dissertation, The University of Zambia).
Nahunnaro, H., Channya, F. K., Chimbekwuju, I. B., & Bayaso, I. (2021). Surveillance and determination of levels of aflatoxin B1 (Afb1) in imported and locally milled rice in Adamawa State, Nigeria. *FUW Journal of Agriculture & Life Sciences, 4*(1), 247–266.
Nakamura, A., Aoyagi, M., Fukuyama, M., Maeki, M., Ishida, A., Tani, H.,. . . Tokeshi, M. (2021). Determination of deoxynivalenol in wheat, barley, corn meal, and wheat-based products by simultaneous multisample fluorescence polarization immunoassay using a portable analyzer. *ACS Food Science & Technology, 1*(9), 1623–1628.
Nakhjavan, B., Ahmed, N. S., & Khosravifard, M. (2020). Development of an improved method of sample extraction and quantitation of multi-mycotoxin in feed by LC-MS/MS. *Toxins, 12*(7), 462.
Nan, M., Xue, H., & Bi, Y. (2022). Contamination, detection and control of mycotoxins in fruits and vegetables. *Toxins, 14*(5), 309.
Navale, V., Vamkudoth, K. R., Ajmera, S., & Dhuri, V. (2021). Aspergillus derived mycotoxins in food and the environment: Prevalence, detection, and toxicity. *Toxicology Reports, 8*, 1008–1030.

Ndemera, M., De Boevre, M., & De Saeger, S. (2020). Mycotoxin management in a developing country context: A critical review of strategies aimed at decreasing dietary exposure to mycotoxins in Zimbabwe. *Critical Reviews in Food Science and Nutrition, 60*(4), 529–540.

Neme, K., & Mohammed, A. (2017). Mycotoxin occurrence in grains and the role of postharvest management as a mitigation strategies. A review. *Food Control, 78,* 412–425.

Nguyen, V. T. T., König, S., Eggert, S., Endres, K., & Kins, S. (2022). The role of mycotoxins in neurodegenerative diseases: Current state of the art and future perspectives of research. *Biological Chemistry, 403*(1), 3–26.

Nieto, C. H. D., Granero, A. M., Zon, M. A., & Fernández, H. (2018). Sterigmatocystin: A mycotoxin to be seriously considered. *Food and Chemical Toxicology, 118,* 460–470.

Nikolić, M., Savić, I., Nikolić, A., Jauković, M., Kandić, V., Stevanović, M., & Stanković, S. (2021). Toxigenic species Aspergillus parasiticus originating from Maize Kernels grown in Serbia. *Toxins, 13*(12), 847.

Nji, Q. N., Babalola, O. O., Ekwomadu, T. I., Nleya, N., & Mwanza, M. (2022). Six main contributing factors to high levels of mycotoxin contamination in African foods. *Toxins, 14*(5), 318.

Notardonato, I., Gianfagna, S., Castoria, R., Ianiri, G., De Curtis, F., Russo, M. V., & Avino, P. (2021). Critical review of the analytical methods for determining the mycotoxin patulin in food matrices. *Reviews in Analytical Chemistry, 40*(1), 144–160.

Nourbakhsh, F., & Tajbakhsh, E. (2021). Neurotoxicity mechanism of Ochratoxin A. *Quality Assurance and Safety of Crops & Foods, 13*(2), 34–45.

Olorunfemi, B. J., & Kayode, S. E. (2021). Post-harvest loss and grain storage technology-a review. *Turkish Journal of Agriculture-Food Science and Technology, 9*(1), 75–83.

Olotu, I. O. (2018). *Safety Assessment of Some Traditionally Fermented Foods Produced in Nigeria and South Africa* (Doctoral dissertation, University of Johannesburg (South Africa)).

Omojokun, J. (2013). Regulation and enforcement of legislation on food safety in Nigeria. *Mycotoxin and Food Safety in Developing Countries, 10,* 251–268.

Omotayo, O. P., Omotayo, A. O., Mwanza, M., & Babalola, O. O. (2019). Prevalence of mycotoxins and their consequences on human health. *Toxicological Research, 35,* 1–7.

Onyeke, C. C. (2020). Review of mycotoxins in foods in Nigeria. *Food Control, 118,* 107376.

Ortega-Beltran, A., & Bandyopadhyay, R. (2021). Contributions of integrated aflatoxin management strategies to achieve the sustainable development goals in various African countries. *Global Food Security, 30,* 100559.

Ortiz, R., Ban, T., Ranajit Bandyopadhyay, R. B., Banziger, M., Bergvinson, D., Hell, K.,. . . Waliyar, F. (2008). CGIAR research-for-development program on mycotoxins. In *Mycotoxins: Detection Methods, Management, Public Health and Agricultural Trade* (pp. 413–422). CABI.

Ötles, S., & Kartal, C. (2016). Solid-Phase Extraction (SPE): Principles and applications in food samples. *Acta Scientiarum Polonorum Technologia Alimentaria, 15*(1), 5–15.

Ozden, S., Akdeniz, A. S., & Alpertunga, B. (2012). Occurrence of ochratoxin A in cereal-derived food products commonly consumed in Turkey. *Food Control, 25*(1), 69–74.

Özer, K. B. (2022). Mycotoxins in figure. In *Advances in Fig Research and Sustainable Production* (pp. 318–340). CABI.

Pack, E. D., Weiland, S., Musser, R., & Schmale, D. G. (2021). Survey of zearalenone and type-B trichothecene mycotoxins in swine feed in the USA. *Mycotoxin Research, 37*(4), 297–313.

Peris-Vicente, J., Esteve-Romero, J., & Carda-Broch, S. (2015). Validation of analytical methods based on chromatographic techniques: An overview. *Analytical Separation Science*, 1757–1808.

Pestka, J. J. (2007). Deoxynivalenol: Toxicity, mechanisms and animal health risks. *Animal Feed Science and Technology, 137*(3–4), 283–298.

Phillips, E., Turner, P. C., Ngure, F. M., Kassim, N., Makule, E., Smith, L. E.,. . . Stoltzfus, R. J. (2022). Ethical considerations in the design and conduct of a cluster-randomised mycotoxin mitigation trial in Tanzania. *World Mycotoxin Journal, 15*(3), 213–222.

Pierron, A., Alassane-Kpembi, I., & Oswald, I. P. (2016). Impact of mycotoxin on immune response and consequences for pig health. *Animal Nutrition, 2*(2), 63–68.

Pleadin, J., Frece, J., & Markov, K. (2019). Mycotoxins in food and feed. *Advances in Food and Nutrition Research, 89*, 297–345.

Poroşnicu, I., Ailincăi, L. I., Neculai-Văleanu, A. S., Ariton, M. A., & Mareş, M. (2023). Legislative Aspects Regarding the Control of Mycotoxins. *Scientific Papers Animal Science and Biotechnologies, 56*(2), 153–153.

Ráduly, Z., Price, R. G., Dockrell, M. E., Csernoch, L., & Pócsi, I. (2021). Urinary biomarkers of mycotoxin induced nephrotoxicity—Current status and expected future trends. *Toxins, 13*(12), 848.

Rahman, H. U., Yue, X., Yu, Q., Xie, H., Zhang, W., Zhang, Q., & Li, P. (2019). Specific antigen-based and emerging detection technologies of mycotoxins. *Journal of the Science of Food and Agriculture, 99*(11), 4869–4877.

Rai, A., Das, M., & Tripathi, A. (2020). Occurrence and toxicity of a fusarium mycotoxin, zearalenone. *Critical Reviews in Food Science and Nutrition, 60*(16), 2710–2729.

Ramalingam, S., Bahuguna, A., & Kim, M. (2019). The effects of mycotoxin patulin on cells and cellular components. *Trends in Food Science & Technology, 83*, 99–113.

Rangel-Muñoz, E. J., Valdivia-Flores, A. G., Cruz-Vázquez, C., de-Luna-López, M. C., Hernández-Valdivia, E., Vitela-Mendoza, I., . . . Quezada-Tristán, T. (2024). Increased dissemination of aflatoxin-and zearalenone-producing Aspergillus spp. and Fusarium spp. during wet season via houseflies on dairy farms in Aguascalientes, Mexico. *Toxins, 16*(7), 302.

Ratnadass, A., Deberdt, P., Martin, T., Sester, M., & Deguine, J. P. (2023). Impacts of crop protection practices on human infectious diseases: Agroecology as the preferred strategy to integrate crop plant health within the extended "One Health" framework. *One Health: Human, Animal, and Environment Triad*, 287–308.

Raysyan, A., Eremin, S. A., Beloglazova, N. V., De Saeger, S., & Gravel, I. V. (2020). Immunochemical approaches for detection of aflatoxin B1 in herbal medicines. *Phytochemical Analysis, 31*(5), 662–669.

Richard, B., Qi, A., & Fitt, B. D. (2022). Control of crop diseases through Integrated Crop Management to deliver climate-smart farming systems for low-and high-input crop production. *Plant Pathology, 71*(1), 187–206.

Richard, S. A., Manaphraim, N. Y., & Kortei, N. K. (2020). The novel neurotoxic and neuroimmunotoxic capabilities of aflatoxin B1 on the nervous system: A review. *Advances in Bioscience and Clinical Medicine, 8*(3), 1–8.

Riet-Correa, F., Cook, D., Micheloud, J. F., Machado, M., Mendonça, F. S., Schild, A. L., & Lemos, R. A. (2024). A review on mycotoxins and mycotoxicoses in ruminants and Equidae in South America. *Toxicon*, 107827.

Rivas Casado, M., Parsons, D. J., Weightman, R. M., Magan, N., & Origgi, S. (2009). Modelling a two-dimensional spatial distribution of mycotoxin concentration in bulk commodities to design effective and efficient sample selection strategies. *Food Additives and Contaminants, 26*(9), 1298–1305.

Rose, L. J., Okoth, S., Flett, B. C., Van Rensburg, B. J., & Viljoen, A. (2018). Preharvest management strategies and their impact on mycotoxigenic fungi and associated mycotoxins. *Mycotoxins–Impact and Management Strategies*, 41–57.

Sabillón, L., Alvarado, J., Leiva, A., Mendoza, R., Espinal, R., Leslie, J. F., & Bianchini, A. (2023). Presence, co-occurrence, and daily intake estimates of aflatoxins and fumonisins in maize consumed in food-insecure regions of Western Honduras. *Toxins, 15*(9), 559.

Sabino, R., Veríssimo, C., Viegas, C., Viegas, S., Brandão, J., Alves-Correia, M., . . . Richardson, M. (2019). The role of occupational Aspergillus exposure in the development of diseases. *Medical Mycology, 57*(Supplement_2), S196–S205.

Saha Turna, N., Comstock, S. S., Gangur, V., & Wu, F. (2023). Effects of aflatoxin on the immune system: Evidence from human and mammalian animal research. *Critical Reviews in Food Science and Nutrition*, 1–19.

Sainz, M. J., González-Jartín, J. M., Aguín, O., Mansilla, J. P., & Botana, L. M. (2018). Isolation, characterization, and identification of mycotoxin-producing fungi. In *Environmental Toxicology* (pp. 202–245). De Gruyter.

Sangvikar, R. V. (2021). Food safety concern related to aflatoxins and control. In *Fungi Bio-Prospects in Sustainable Agriculture, Environment and Nano-technology* (pp. 347–380). Academic Press.

Schincaglia, A., Aspromonte, J., Franchina, F. A., Chenet, T., Pasti, L., Cavazzini, A., . . . Beccaria, M. (2023). Current developments of analytical methodologies for aflatoxins' determination in food during the last decade (2013–2022), with a particular focus on nuts and nut products. *Foods, 12*(3), 527.

Schlosser, O., Robert, S., & Noyon, N. (2020). Airborne mycotoxins in waste recycling and recovery facilities: Occupational exposure and health risk assessment. *Waste Management, 105*, 395–404.

Senyuva, H. Z., Gökmen, V., & Sarikaya, E. A. (2015). Future perspectives in Orbitrap™-high-resolution mass spectrometry in food analysis: A review. *Food Additives & Contaminants: Part A, 32*(10), 1568–1606.

Shah, K. K., Modi, B., Pandey, H. P., Subedi, A., Aryal, G., Pandey, M., & Shrestha, J. (2021). Diversified crop rotation: An approach for sustainable agriculture production. *Advances in Agriculture, 2021*(1), 8924087.

Shekhar, M., Singh, N., Bisht, S., Singh, V., & Kumar, A. (2018). Effects of climate change on occurrence of aflatoxin and its impacts on maize in India. *International Journal of Current Microbiology and Applied Science, 7*(6), 109–116.

Sherif, S. O., Salama, E. E., & Abdel-Wahhab, M. A. (2009). Mycotoxins and child health: The need for health risk assessment. *International Journal of Hygiene and Environmental Health, 212*(4), 347–368.

Shi, H., Schwab, W., & Yu, P. (2019). Natural occurrence and co-contamination of twelve mycotoxins in industry-submitted cool-season cereal grains grown under a low heat unit climate condition. *Toxins, 11*(3), 160.

Shrivastava, A., & Sharma, R. K. (2022). Biosensors for the detection of mycotoxins. *Toxin Reviews, 41*(2), 618–638.
Shuib, N. S., Makahleh, A., Salhimi, S. M., & Saad, B. (2017). Determination of aflatoxin M1 in milk and dairy products using high performance liquid chromatography-fluorescence with post column photochemical derivatization. *Journal of Chromatography A, 1510*, 51–56.
Silva, L. J., Pereira, A. M., Pena, A., & Lino, C. M. (2020). Citrinin in foods and supplements: A review of occurrence and analytical methodologies. *Foods, 10*(1), 14.
Singh, J., & Mehta, A. (2020). Rapid and sensitive detection of mycotoxins by advanced and emerging analytical methods: A review. *Food Science & Nutrition, 8*(5), 2183–2204.
Singh, K., & Kumari, A. (2022). Emerging Mycotoxins and their Clinicopathological effects. In *Mycotoxins and Mycotoxicoses* (pp. 65–104). Singapore: Springer Nature Singapore.
Singh, U., Gupta, S., & Gupta, M. (2021). A review study on biological ill effects and health hazards of aflatoxins. *Asian Journal of Advances in Medical Science*, 1–8.
Smith, G. W. (2018). Fumonisins. In *Veterinary Toxicology* (pp. 1003–1018). Academic Press.
Smith, J. E. (2020). Aflatoxins. In *Handbook of Plant and Fungal Toxicants* (pp. 269–285). CRC Press.
Sorbo, A., Pucci, E., Nobili, C., Taglieri, I., Passeri, D., & Zoani, C. (2022). Food safety assessment: Overview of metrological issues and regulatory aspects in the European Union. *Separations, 9*(2), 53.
Stoev, S. D. (2022). New evidences about the carcinogenic effects of ochratoxin A and possible prevention by target feed additives. *Toxins, 14*(6), 380.
Stoev, S. D. (2024). Food security and foodborne mycotoxicoses—What should be the adequate risk assessment and regulation? *Microorganisms, 12*(3), 580.
Syamilah, N., Nurul Afifah, S., Effarizah, M. E., & Norlia, M. (2022). Mycotoxins and mycotoxigenic fungi in spices and mixed spices: A review. *Food Research, 6*, 30–46.
Szelenberger, R., Cichoń, N., Zajaczkowski, W., & Bijak, M. (2024). Application of biosensors for the detection of mycotoxins for the improvement of food safety. *Toxins, 16*(6), 249.
Tantaoui-Elaraki, A., Riba, A., Oueslati, S., & Zinedine, A. (2018). Toxigenic fungi and mycotoxin occurrence and prevention in food and feed in northern Africa–a review. *World Mycotoxin Journal, 11*(3), 385–400.
Tesfamariam, K., De Boevre, M., Kolsteren, P., Belachew, T., Mesfin, A., De Saeger, S., & Lachat, C. (2020). Dietary mycotoxins exposure and child growth, immune system, morbidity, and mortality: A systematic literature review. *Critical Reviews in Food Science and Nutrition, 60*(19), 3321–3341.
Ting, W. E., Chang, C. H., Szonyi, B., & Gizachew, D. (2020). Growth and aflatoxin B1, B2, G1, and G2 production by Aspergillus flavus and Aspergillus parasiticus on ground flax seeds (Linum usitatissimum). *Journal of Food Protection, 83*(6), 975–983.
Tola, M., & Kebede, B. (2016). Occurrence, importance and control of mycotoxins: A review. *Cogent Food & Agriculture, 2*(1), 1191103.
Tor, P. N., Yande, J. T., Ijuo, G. A., & Oloruntoba, S. O. (2020). Assessment of total aflatoxins level of two major nuts consumed in Gboko Benue State, Nigeria. *World Scientific News*, (143), 170–180.

Tshalibe, R. S. (2019). *The Effect of Mycotoxin Exposure on the Growth of Infants and Young Children in Deep Rural Areas of the Eastern Cape Province, South Africa* (Doctoral dissertation, North-West University (South-Africa). Potchefstroom Campus).

Tumukunde, E., Ma, G., Li, D., Yuan, J., Qin, L., & Wang, S. (2020). Current research and prevention of aflatoxins in China. *World Mycotoxin Journal, 13*(2), 121–138.

Turna, N. S., & Wu, F. (2021). Aflatoxin M1 in milk: A global occurrence, intake, & exposure assessment. *Trends in Food Science & Technology, 110*, 183–192.

Turner, N. W., Subrahmanyam, S., & Piletsky, S. A. (2009). Analytical methods for determination of mycotoxins: A review. *Analytica chimica acta, 632*(2), 168–180.

Ubwa, S. T., Abah, J., Atu, B. O., Tyohemba, R. L., & Yande, J. T. (2014). Assessment of total aflatoxins level of two major nuts consumed in Makurdi Benue State, Nigeria. *International Journal of Nutrition and Food Sciences, 3*(5), 397–403.

Udomkun, P., Wiredu, A. N., Nagle, M., Bandyopadhyay, R., Müller, J., & Vanlauwe, B. (2017). Mycotoxins in Sub-Saharan Africa: Present situation, socio-economic impact, awareness, and outlook. *Food Control, 72*, 110–122.

Unnevehr, L., & Grace, D. (Eds.). (2013). *Aflatoxins: Finding Solutions for Improved Food Safety* (Vol. 20). International Food Policy Research Institute.

Van der Fels-Klerx, H. J., Liu, C., & Battilani, P. (2016). Modelling climate change impacts on mycotoxin contamination. *World Mycotoxin Journal, 9*(5), 717–726.

Vidal, A., Ouhibi, S., Ghali, R., Hedhili, A., De Saeger, S., & De Boevre, M. (2019). The mycotoxin patulin: An updated short review on occurrence, toxicity and analytical challenges. *Food and Chemical Toxicology, 129*, 249–256.

Viegas, C., Nurme, J., Piecková, E., & Viegas, S. (2020). Sterigmatocystin in foodstuffs and feed: Aspects to consider. *Mycology, 11*(2), 91–104.

Visser, M. E., Schoonees, A., Ezekiel, C. N., Randall, N. P., & Naude, C. E. (2020). Agricultural and nutritional education interventions for reducing aflatoxin exposure to improve infant and child growth in low-and middle-income countries. *Cochrane Database of Systematic Reviews*, (4).

Wagacha, J. M., & Muthomi, J. W. (2008). Mycotoxin problem in Africa: Current status, implications to food safety and health and possible management strategies. *International Journal of Food Microbiology, 124*(1), 1–12.

Wagner, C. (2015). Critical practicalities in sampling for mycotoxins in feed. *Journal of AOAC International, 98*(2), 301–308.

Wang, F., Ma, L., Wang, Q., Hammock, B. D., Xiao, G., & Liu, R. (2024). Evaluation of the immune response of patulin by proteomics. *Biosensors, 14*(7), 322.

Wang, Y., Wang, X., & Li, Q. (2023). Aflatoxin B1 in poultry liver: Toxic mechanism. *Toxicon*, 107262.

Wang, Y., Zhang, C., Wang, J., & Knopp, D. (2022). Recent progress in rapid determination of mycotoxins based on emerging biorecognition molecules: A review. *Toxins, 14*(2), 73.

Wangia-Dixon, R. N., & Nishimwe, K. (2020). Molecular toxicology and carcinogenesis of fumonisins: A review. *Journal of Environmental Science and Health, Part C, 39*(1), 44–67.

Warburton, M. L., & Williams, W. P. (2017). Advances in mycotoxin-resistant maize varieties Resistance Unit, USA. In *Achieving Sustainable Cultivation of Maize Volume 1* (pp. 147–160). Burleigh Dodds Science Publishing.

Weaver, A. C., Weaver, D. M., Adams, N., & Yiannikouris, A. (2021). Co-occurrence of 35 mycotoxins: A seven-year survey of corn grain and corn silage in the United States. *Toxins, 13*(8), 516.

Wei, C., Yu, L., Qiao, N., Zhao, J., Zhang, H., Zhai, Q.,. . . Chen, W. (2020). Progress in the distribution, toxicity, control, and detoxification of patulin: A review. *Toxicon, 184,* 83–93.

Więckowska, M., Szelenberger, R., Niemcewicz, M., Harmata, P., Poplawski, T., & Bijak, M. (2023). Ochratoxin A—the current knowledge concerning hepatotoxicity, mode of action and possible prevention. *Molecules, 28*(18), 6617.

World Health Organization. (2018). *Understanding the Codex Alimentarius.* Food & Agriculture Organization.

World Health Organization. (2022). *WHO Global Strategy for Food Safety 2022–2030: Towards Stronger Food Safety Systems and Global Cooperation.* World Health Organization.

Wu, F. (2004). Mycotoxin risk assessment for the purpose of setting international regulatory standards. *Environmental Science & Technology, 38*(15), 4049–4055.

Wu, F. (2006). Economic impact of fumonisin and aflatoxin regulations on global corn and peanut markets. In *The Mycotoxin Factbook* (pp. 83–93). Wageningen Academic.

Wu, F., Groopman, J. D., & Pestka, J. J. (2014). Public health impacts of foodborne mycotoxins. *Annual Review of Food Science and Technology, 5*(1), 351–372.

Xu, F., Baker, R. C., Whitaker, T. B., Luo, H., Zhao, Y., Stevenson, A.,. . . Zhang, G. (2022). Review of good agricultural practices for smallholder maize farmers to minimise aflatoxin contamination. *World Mycotoxin Journal, 15*(2), 171–186.

Xu, M. L., Gao, Y., Wang, X., Han, X. X., & Zhao, B. (2021). Comprehensive strategy for sample preparation for the analysis of food contaminants and residues by GC–MS/MS: A review of recent research trends. *Foods, 10*(10), 2473.

Yonpiam, R. (2018). *Vasoactive Effects of Ergot Alkaloid Exposure on Ovine Pedal Artery and Umbilical Blood Vessels* (Doctoral dissertation, University of Saskatchewan).

Yoshinari, T., Sugita-Konishi, Y., Sato, E., Takeuchi, H., Taniguchi, M., Fukumitsu, T.,. . . Hara-Kudo, Y. (2024). Survey and risk assessment of aflatoxins and sterigmatocystin in Japanese staple food items and the evaluation of an in-house ELISA technique for rapid screening. *Food Control, 157,* 110154.

Yoshinari, T., Takeuchi, H., Aoyama, K., Taniguchi, M., Hashiguchi, S., Kai, S.,. . . Sugita-Konishi, Y. (2014). Occurrence of four Fusarium mycotoxins, deoxynivalenol, zearalenone, T-2 toxin, and HT-2 toxin, in wheat, barley, and Japanese retail food. *Journal of Food Protection, 77*(11), 1940–1946.

Yu, J., & Pedroso, I. R. (2023). Mycotoxins in cereal-based products and their impacts on the health of humans, livestock animals and pets. *Toxins, 15*(8), 480.

Zhai, Q., Gong, X., Wang, C., Zhao, J., Zhang, H., Tian, F., & Chen, W. (2019). Foodborne patulin toxicity is related to gut barrier disruption and can be prevented by docosahexaenoic acid and probiotic supplementation. *Food & Function, 10*(3), 1330–1339.

Zhang, K., Flannery, B., & Zhang, L. (2024). Challenges and future state for mycotoxin analysis: A review from a regulatory perspective. *Journal of Agricultural and Food Chemistry, 72*(15), 8380–8388.

Zheng, X., Wei, W., Zhou, W., Li, H., Rao, S., Gao, L., & Yang, Z. (2021). Prevention and detoxification of patulin in apple and its products: A review. *Food Research International, 140,* 110034.

Zhong, L., Carere, J., Lu, Z., Lu, F., & Zhou, T. (2018). Patulin in apples and apple-based food products: The burdens and the mitigation strategies. *Toxins, 10*(11), 475.

Zhou, H., Guog, T., Dai, H., Yu, Y., Zhang, Y., & Ma, L. (2020). Deoxynivalenol: Toxicological profiles and perspective views for future research. *World Mycotoxin Journal, 13*(2), 179–188.
Zhou, Y., Hu, L., Zhou, G., Luo, Y., & Liu, R. (2023). Sterigmatocystin induced cytotoxicity and disturbed lipid metabolism. *Journal of Agriculture and Food Research, 14*, 100673.
Zingales, V., Fernández-Franzón, M., & Ruiz, M. J. (2020). Sterigmatocystin: Occurrence, toxicity and molecular mechanisms of action–A review. *Food and Chemical Toxicology, 146*, 111802.

6

Challenges and Prevention of Marine Biotoxins in Seafoods

Olutayo, I. Falodun, Blessing I. Nwadike, Abolade A. Oyelade, and Adeniyi A. Ogunjobi

6.1 Overview of Seafoods

Fish and shellfish are nutritious foods that constitute desirable components of a healthy diet. Some seafood available to the markets are wholesome and unlikely to cause illness in the consumer. Nevertheless, there are areas of risk where the water bodies in which the seafood is obtained are contaminated. The major risk of acute disease is associated with consuming raw shellfish or inadequately processed seafood. For persons living in areas in which reef fish are consumed (Hawaii, Puerto Rico, the Virgin Islands), there is a risk of ciguatera; other natural toxins (paralytic shellfish poisoning, neurotoxic shellfish poisoning, etc.) have been associated with shellfish from endemic areas.

Furthermore, there are less well-defined risks of acute and chronic diseases related to environmental contamination of aquatic food animals. Dealing with such dangers on a short-term basis requires improvements in regulatory control systems. In the long term, amelioration and eventual elimination of some hazards require strengthening and more effective application of control measures to prevent the disposal of human and industrial waste into offshore marine and fresh waters. A variety of seafood products are available in the marketplace from many different sources. In Nigeria, for example, wild fish and shellfish are harvested by commercial fishermen in both near-shore and open ocean waters and freshwater lakes or rivers. Farm-raised (aquacultured) seafood products are raised both in ponds (catfish) and re-circulating tanks (tilapia and hybrid bass) and in near-shore coastal waters (salmon and shellfish). These same methods are used to farm a wide variety of fish and shellfish in other countries around the world.

Once seafood products are harvested, they are generally processed or packaged for distribution to retail stores and restaurants. Wild fish and shellfish are unloaded from harvest vessels, and farmed products are harvested

DOI: 10.1201/9781003500605-7

from facilities and then transported and packed for distribution to processing plants or wholesalers. Processors convert whole fish or shellfish to various other product forms such as fresh fish fillets or steaks or other items such as frozen products, breaded fish portions, and canned or smoked products.

Some of these products may be further converted by secondary processors to heat and serve or ready-to-eat products like seafood salads, entrees, or other items. Wholesalers and food service distributors receive both raw and processed products from many different domestic and foreign sources and distribute them to retail stores and restaurants. Consumers purchase these products from retail stores for home consumption or at restaurants and other food service establishments.

Seafood is also a unique food in that a large number of fish and shellfish are harvested from the wild by individuals for recreational purposes, and some of that harvest is also consumed. Because of the strong public interest in seafood safety, there is a need to introduce innovative methodologies for control that address important health issues associated with seafood consumption. This overview reviews the nature and extent of public health risks associated with seafood and examines the scope and adequacy of current seafood safety programs.

Most current health risks associated with seafood safety originate in the environment and should be dealt with by control of harvest or at the point of capture. With minor exceptions, risks cannot be identified by an organoleptic inspection system. Inspection at the processing level is important to maintain the safety of seafood, but there is little evidence that increased inspection activities at this level would effectively reduce the incidence of seafood-borne disease. With currently available data, it is possible to identify the source of much of the acute illness associated with seafood consumption, though the dimensions of the problems are not always known; these data, in turn, can form the basis for national control programs.

Chronic illness resulting from seafood consumption is associated primarily with environmental contamination; thus, control depends on an improved understanding of the occurrence and distribution of the chemical agents involved, the exclusion of contaminated seafood from the market, and increased action to prevent additional pollution of the waters. Because well over half some nation's seafood supply is imported and environmental contamination is globally pervasive, the safety of imported seafood must be ensured through equivalent control measures in exporting countries.

One-fifth of the fish and shellfish eaten in the United States is derived from recreational or subsistence fishing, and these products are not subject to health-based control; there is a need to improve protection for consumers of these products by regulation of harvest and by education concerning risks associated with their consumption. Since the problems are largely regional, the primary effective control—except for imports—is at the state level, and this effort should be strengthened and supported to ensure the effectiveness of state-based programs and to provide expert assistance and specialized facilities.

There is a lack of understanding of the nature of seafood hazards in the food service sectors and by the consuming public and health professionals; a vigorous campaign for information dissemination and education in these matters is needed, particularly for high-risk consumers and high-risk products such as raw shellfish. An improved national surveillance system should be developed to provide more reliable and comprehensive information on seafood-borne disease incidence. Data will then permit meaningful risk identification and risk assessment as a basis for effective regulation of seafood (current data on disease occurrence in seafood consumption are too fragmentary to allow reliable risk assessment of microbiological and natural toxin hazards).

Foods derived from salt water are considered "seafood," whereas all food derived from water environments, be they fresh or salt, are considered marine foods. The principal marine foods are saltwater fish, crustaceans, and shellfish such as shrimp, lobster, crab, clams, and oysters and certain freshwater fish and crustaceans. Seafood also includes other sea animals and plants such as seaweed and sea cucumber. Seafoods are also converted into large quantities of manufactured or processed foods, most of which are frozen or canned. Examples include precooked, battered, breaded, and frozen fillets, fish sticks, and shrimp, as well as canned tuna, salmon, and sardines.

In addition, fish are salted, smoked, pickled, or dried. Currently, Americans consume about 16 lb of seafood per capita per year, compared to 112 lb of red meats and 64 lb of chicken. In other parts of the world, seafood makes up the major source of protein in the diet. Although the United States is a major exporter of fish, over 60% of the seafood consumed in this country is from imports, reflecting market demand for selected species.

6.2 Biotoxin-Producing Organisms in Seafoods

Biotoxins are chemical substances produced by microorganisms. In the marine environment, they accumulate in fish or bivalve molluscs such as oysters and mussels. They are produced mainly by naturally occurring marine algae known as phytoplanktons. When there is algal bloom, that is, excessive proliferation of algae, they produce toxins which accumulate in fish and other sea foods (Grattan et al., 2016; Nicolas et al., 2017; Lee et al., 2024). Marine biotoxins are poisonous substances, which can accumulate in seafoods mainly as a result of feeding on plankton containing toxins. According to Smith et al. (2010) seafood can be defined as fish and shellfish collected from capture fisheries and aquaculture production in marine and freshwater environments.

Among the species of microalgae, only a few are known to produce persistent natural toxins that can cause intoxication and even deaths in humans

TABLE 6.1

Some Biotoxins and their producing microorganisms

Biotoxin	Producing Organism
Palytoxin	*Palythoa* species
Palytoxin derivatives	*Ostreopsis* species
Gymnodimine A, B, C (GYMS)	*Karenia selliformis*
Spirolides	*Alexandrium ostenfeldii, A. peruvianum*
Pinnatoxins	*Vulcanodinium rugosum*
Ciguatoxins	*Gambierdiscus toxicus*
Brevetoxins	*Karenia brevis*
Saxitoxin and its analogue paralytic shellfish toxins	*Alexandrium* spp., *Pyrodinium bahamense,* and *Gymnodinium catenatum*
Domoic acid (amnestic shellfish Poisoning toxin)	*Pseudo-nitzschia* species
Yessotoxins	*Protoceratium reticulatum, Patinopecten yessoensis, Lingulodinium polyedrum,* and *Gonyaulax spinifera*
Okadaic acid and dinophysistoxins	*Dinophysis* and *Prorocentrum* species
Pectenotoxins	*Dinophysis* species
Azaspiracids	*Azadinium spinosum* and *Amphidoma* species

and animals. Some of the different organisms that produce marine toxins and the toxins they produce are listed in Table 6.1.

6.3 Aquatic Biotoxin Production

Biotoxins are hazards produced naturally by certain species of algae or bacteria that can accumulate in shellfish grown in coastal waters, and that may cause illnesses including paralytic shellfish poisoning (PSP), amnesic shellfish poisoning (ASP), diarrhetic shellfish poisoning (DSP), or azaspiracid shellfish poisoning. These toxins have been responsible for incidents of wide-scale death of sea life and are increasingly responsible for human intoxication. There are several different seafood poisoning syndromes associated with toxic marine algae, and these include paralytic shellfish poisoning, amnesic shellfish poisoning, diarrhetic shellfish poisoning, neurotoxic shellfish poisoning (NSP), and azaspiracid shellfish poisoning (AZP). There are also different types of food poisoning associated with finfish, and these include ciguatera poisoning and pufferfish poisoning. Consumption of raw molluscan shellfish poses well-known risks of food poisoning; however, intoxication from finfish is not so well known. Most of the algal toxins associated with seafood poisoning are heat stable and are not inactivated by cooking. It is also not possible to visually distinguish toxic from non-toxic fish and shellfish. Many countries rely on biotoxin monitoring programs to protect public health and close harvesting areas when toxic algal blooms or shellfish are detected. In non-industrialized countries, particularly in rural areas, monitoring for harmful algal blooms does not routinely occur, and death due to "red tide toxins" commonly occurs.

Harmful algal blooms are natural phenomena caused by the massive growth of phytoplankton that may contain highly toxic chemicals, the so-called marine biotoxins causing illness and even death to both aquatic organisms and humans. Their occurrence has increased in frequency and severity, suggesting a worldwide public health risk. Marine biotoxins can accumulate in bivalve molluscs, and regulatory limits have been set for some classes according to European Union legislation. These compounds can be distinguished into water- and fat-soluble molecules. The first group involves those of PSP and ASP, whereas the toxins soluble in fat can cause DSP and NSP. Due to the lack of long-term toxicity studies, establishing tolerable daily intakes for any of these marine biotoxins has not been possible, but an acute reference dose can be considered more appropriate because these molecules show acute toxicity. Dietary exposure assessment is linked both to the levels of marine biotoxins present in bivalve molluscs and the portion that could be eaten by consumers. Symptoms may vary from severe gastrointestinal intoxication with diarrhoea, nausea, vomiting, and abdominal cramps to neurological disorders such as ataxia, dizziness, partial paralysis, and respiratory distress. The official method for the detection of marine biotoxins is the mouse bioassay (MBA) showing some limits due to ethical restrictions and insufficient specificity. For this reason, the liquid chromatography-mass spectrometry method has replaced MBA as the reference technique. However, the monitoring of algal blooms producing marine biotoxins should be regularly assessed to obtain more reliable, accurate estimates of bloom toxicity and their potential impacts.

6.4 Marine Biotoxins

Harmful algal blooms (HABs) periodically kill fish or disrupt food sources for fish and shellfish. When HABs are not detected, seafood taken from such waters may be harmful to human health. HABs can cover huge areas, often stimulated by the right combination of temperature, salinity, nutrients, sunlight, and tidal conditions. When they discolor the water, they are typically called "red tides." Sometimes HABs can be highly localized, as in the case of coral reefs where reef damage due to storms or construction can disrupt the marine ecology. Human intoxications by planktonic biotoxins result from the consumption of contaminated seafood, such as shellfish and fish. Marine biotoxins are produced by various species of dinoflagellates under certain conditions. Shellfish, which are filter feeders, accumulate the biotoxins without adverse effects and any apparent organoleptic changes.

Warming of the world's oceans has been reported to alter the distribution and range of dinoflagellates that make these toxins, introducing the problem to previously unaffected areas (Moy and Todd, 2014; Aransiola et al., 2024).

Ciguatoxin is another type of marine biotoxin, which causes ciguatera fish poisoning. Ciguatoxin is a neurotoxin which can produce symptoms lasting for several weeks, months, or years. It is a serious disease with a case/fatality rate that may range up to 4.5%. Ciguatera has been associated with the consumption of a variety of tropical and subtropical fish, mainly coral fish, feeding on toxin-producing dinoflagellates, or predatory fish consuming such coral fish.

It should also be noted that certain fish species use biotoxins for their protection and can present risks to the consumer if consumed inadvertently or intentionally without proper handling (Moy and Todd, 2014).

A lesser-known group of biotoxins are derived from certain cyanobacteria (blue-green algae) in brackish or freshwater. These bacteria produce cyanotoxins, which are some of the most powerful natural poisons known. Although not normally affecting commercial fisheries, exposure to these toxins has occurred through drinking water and occupational and recreational contact. The toxins are accumulated in the digestive gland of the shellfish (hepatopancreas) and do not affect the shellfish themselves. The shellfish may reduce toxicity in clean water, but depuration times vary greatly according to the bivalve species involved, the pumping activity of the bivalve, and the hygrographic conditions. Fish may also consume toxic algae and cause disease in humans (ciguatera). Also, there are toxins in some fish species that do not involve marine algae (pufferfish poisoning); see Table 6.2.

TABLE 6.2

Aquatic Biotoxins and the Associated Poisonings

The Disease	Toxins	Occurrence
Paralytic shellfish poisoning	Saxitoxin	Worldwide
Diarrheic shellfish poisoning	Okadaic acid diaphysis toxin	Worldwide
Neurotoxic shellfish poisoning	Brevetoxins	USA, Caribbean, New Zealand
Amnesic shellfish poisoning	Domoic acid	North America
Ciguatera fish poisoning	Ciguatoxin (CTX)	Tropical, subtropical
Pufferfish (tetrodotoxin) poisoning	Tetrodotoxin (TTX)	Japan, South Pacific

Source: Moy and Toddy, 2014

6.4.1 Marine Biotoxin Production in Seafoods

Biotoxins are naturally present in the marine environment all year round, normally at very low concentrations, and could be of no concern for most people that are immunocompetent and eat fair amounts of seafood. Nevertheless, an increase in the population of algae in the marine environment could trigger an increase in the quantities of biotoxin-producing species. These biotoxins are considered secondary metabolites that are used for survival when competing for space due to overgrowth of other species or a defence mechanism against predators (Botana et al., 1996). The more of these algae the marine filter feeders consume, the more biotoxin they accumulate. Biotoxins could be a public health issue when humans are exposed to it through consumption of seafoods that are contaminated with toxins (Visciano et al., 2016). Certain phytoplankton, also known as microscopic algae, are responsible for the production of biotoxins in the marine environment. An increase in the population (algal bloom) of algae in a marine environment could be influenced by changes in the climatic and hydrographic conditions (Van Egmond and Speijers, 1999) or nutrient availability, salinity, and winds (Bower et al., 1981).

There has been an increase in the global distribution of toxin-producing algae which has led to the increase in reports of biotoxins found in seafood due to a rise in water transportation and increased aquaculture, which has helped in the spreading of algae in the marine ecosystem (Maso and Garces, 2006; Smayda, 2007). Other causes attributed to the proliferation of harmful algal blooms are increased scientific research on toxin-producing algae, eutrophication, untreated agricultural and industrial wastes that find their way into the marine environment, and an increase in the practice of transferring shellfish stock from one growing area to another (Hallegraeff et al., 1995; McMinn et al., 1997). It is important to note that biotoxins are not inactivated or destroyed by processes such as freezing, smoking, canning, cooking, or frying of seafoods. As a result, effective seafood safety programs that focus on the sources, fate, and control and management plans of marine biotoxins are highly important in ensuring the safety of seafood before it gets to consumers (Wiggins and Anderson, 2022)

Marine biotoxins can be classified as either hydrophilic of lipophilic; also, they can be classified based on the clinical presentations (symptoms) or the kind of toxic syndrome produced. On the basis of types of toxic syndrome, they can be classified as:

1. Paralytic shellfish poisoning
2. Amnesic shellfish poisoning
3. Neurotoxic shellfish poisoning
4. Diarrhetic shellfish poisoning
5. Azaspiracid shellfish poisoning
6. Ciguatera fish poisoning

Understanding the sources and distribution (locally and globally) of the toxins responsible for each syndrome is critical in the implementation of control and management plans targeted at preventing harvesting and sales of contaminated seafoods to the public (Wiggins and Anderson, 2022). Accordingly, marine biotoxins can be classified on the basis of their chemical structure as: azaspiracid (AZA), brevetoxin (BTX), cyclic imine (CI), domoic acid (DA), okadaic acid (OA), pectenotoxin (PTX), saxitoxin (STX), and yessotoxin (YTX) palytoxin (PlTX), and ciguatoxin (CTX) (EFSA, 2009).

6.4.1.1 Paralytic Shellfish Poisoning

Paralytic shellfish poisoning toxins, otherwise known as saxitoxins, are hydrophilic tetrahydropurine toxins primarily produced by dinoflagellates, which belong to the genus *Alexandrium*. Other PSP-producing dinoflagellates are *Pyrodinium bahamense* and *Gymnodinium catenatum*. Saxitoxin is one of many toxins that are grouped together in the PSP toxin family, which include several variants and are subject to frequent conversions depending on pH (Wiggins and Anderson, 2022).

6.4.1.2 Amnesic Shellfish Poisoning

Amnesic shellfish poisoning toxin, also known as domoic acid, is produced by certain microalgae, referred to as diatoms of the genus *Pseudo-nitzschia*. It is usually difficult to differentiate toxic species from non-toxic ones through light microscopy; however, the use of molecular methods or a specialized microscope can be used to effectively differentiate toxic species from non-toxic ones. The ASP-producing algae has been documented to occur off the US northeast and west coasts and the coast of Florida (US National office of HABs, 2019). It has been documented to produce a toxic effect on marine wildlife such as birds and mammals.

6.4.1.3 Neurotoxic Shellfish Poisoning

Neurotoxic shellfish poisoning toxins, also known as brevetoxins, are metabolites of the dinoflagellate *Karenia brevis*. Many toxins capable of being transformed into different forms through metabolic processes in shellfish have been reported to make up the NSP family. The western hemisphere is mostly affected by illness through consumption of contaminated shellfish or inhalation of aerosolized toxin from the sea spray of red tides. The affected regions include the Gulf of Mexico and the southeastern coast of the US, as well as the eastern coast of the USA and New Zealand (Cassell et al., 2015; EFSA, 2010; Ansdell, 2023) (Figure 6.1).

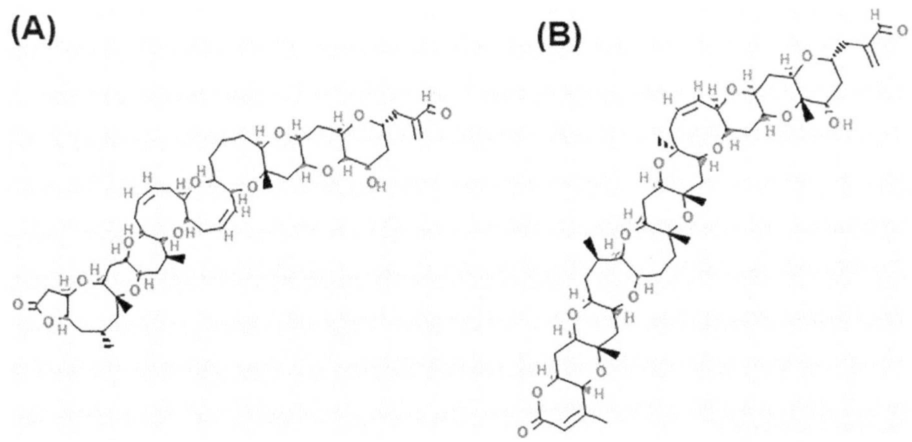

FIGURE 6.1
Chemical structures of brevetoxin A (A) and B (B). Source: PubChem https://pubchem.ncbi.nlm.nih.gov/compound/Brevetoxin-A and https://pubchem.ncbi.nlm.nih.gov/compound/Brevetoxin-B#section=2D-Structure.

6.4.1.4 Diarrhetic Shellfish Poisoning

Diarrhetic shellfish poisoning biotoxins comprise okadaic acid and dinophysistoxins. These toxins are produced by dinoflagellates, *Dinophysis* and *Prorocentrum.* Diarrheic shellfish poisoning results from the consumption of okadaic acid–contaminated shellfish and is known to be a global phenomenon; outbreaks have been reported in the Americas, Asia, Europe, and Africa (Zendong et al., 2016). Multiple toxins have been identified in this family of toxins with the ability of shellfish to add fatty acid esters to the toxins upon ingestion. They can be grouped into four chemical structures: okadaic acid and its derivatives (dinophysistoxin), pectenotoxin, yessotoxin and its derivatives, and azaspiracid (Trainer et al., 2013; Ansdell, 2023).

6.4.1.5 Azaspiracid Shellfish Poisoning

Azaspiracid shellfish poisoning is caused by azaspiracids produced by the genus *Azadinium*, a very small dinoflagellate. Their small size makes it very difficult to identify toxic species from non-toxic ones through standard microscope. Azaspiracids are nitrogen-containing polyether toxins comprising a unique spiral ring assembly with a heterocyclic amine and an aliphatic carboxylic acid component. Although 21 different analogues of azaspiracids have been identified, AZA1, AZA2, and AZA3 are the most critical ones based on occurrence and toxicity (EFSA, 2008).

6.4.1.6 Ciguatera Fish Poisoning

Ciguatera fish poisoning results from consumption of contaminated reef fish with biotoxins such as ciguatoxin or maitotoxin. These toxins are potent and originate from a minute marine dinoflagellate named *Gambierdiscus toxicus* that is commonly found around coral reefs. This dinoflagellate is consumed by herbivorous fish which are capable of modifying and concentrating the toxins produced by *G. toxicus* as they go through the marine trophic levels to carnivorous fish and finally to humans. Ciguatoxins have been reported to be concentrated mainly in fish liver, intestines, roe, and heads (Ansdell, 2023)

6.5 Challenges of Marine Biotoxins in Seafoods

It is an undeniable fact that seafoods are very important to the Indigenous population in coastal areas, yet harvesting and consuming seafoods is attributed to significant risk to the health of the consumers, and the risk is that they can be exposed to marine biotoxins (McIntyre et al., 2021). Different organisms produce marine biotoxins, especially when the environmental conditions favour their growth and proliferation. Such favourable conditions include nutrient content elevation; for example, the proliferation of algae occurs in such conditions and could lead to the event referred to as harmful algal blooms (Grattan et al., 2016). When HAB events occur, biotoxins will be produced, and when ingested by different species of shellfish, fish, and other marine animals, the toxins could accumulate in them. Shellfish toxins are greatly important to shellfish consumers, producers, and those involved in food safety regulations.

Microalgae are fond of producing toxins which have dangerous effects on the health of humans, aquatic ecosystems, and the resources of coastal systems. The accumulation of these algal blooms has been on the increase for some time with regard to rate of occurrence, severity, and biogeographical level, constituting serious health risks which result from consuming contaminated seafood. Microalgae-produced toxins lead to many clinical syndromes which are associated with a number of symptoms such as amnesic, diarrhoetic, azaspirazid, neurotoxic, paralytic shellfish, and ciguatera fish poisoning (Morabito et al., 2018).

The consumption of toxin-contaminated seafoods is the main source by which human beings are exposed to these toxins (Visciano et al., 2016). Those at higher risk of marine biotoxin exposure are the Indigenous populations of coastal regions because of the general practice of increased rates of harvesting and consuming seafoods compared to the non-Indigenous populace. For example, it was estimated that the rate at which seafoods were consumed was more than 1,900 per capita among the Indigenous populace in about 87 countries, on average 15 times higher than that of non-Indigenous populations (Cisneros-Montemayor et al., 2016). Evidence exists on concerns about the risk to health with just exposure to a single marine biotoxin at a single point in time; although the exposure is a short term, it can result in the manifestation of many symptoms, which could range from diarrhoea, vomiting, and nausea to paralysis, loss of memory, and even death.

The ingestion of seafood contaminated by phycotoxins has resulted in human poisoning in the past, and the previous records on the normal habits of people who reside in coastal areas and the tropics have shown that HABs are events that occur naturally. For over three decades, the attention of the scientific community as well as society has been attracted to the problems associated with HABs. The reported cases of the occurrences of human poisoning due to consumption of seafood contaminated with toxins that affected many people in different parts of the world and the eventual consequences on the health of humans have brought more attention to HABs. This attention has led to an increase in the record of toxic algae and HABs in coastal waters in different parts of the world. In addition, there are other factors that have been recognized to have contributed to the increase in the rate of occurrence of the outbreaks of HABs. Some of the factors that are proposed to have contributed to the overall rise in HABs include eutrophication of coastal waters, which has resulted from the effect of aquaculture practices; the use of fertilizers and agricultural runoff; economic activities, which have a link with urbanization; climatic change conditions; and the transportation of toxic algae as well as their cysts from one coastal area to another, which could be a result of their presence in the ballast water of ships or when shellfish stocks are moved from one place to another (Hallegraeff, 2004). This therefore suggests that HABs and seafood contamination constitute a significant issue with regard to social issues because of the challenges to human health and economic activities and the impact on recreational activities and tourism.

Seafood biotoxins can accumulate in humans through the consumption of fish products, which can eventually result in various kinds of ailments, referred to as biointoxication. It has been observed that biotoxin synthesis can arise through phytoplankton and phytobenthos. The resultant effect can be through changes in metabolic processes, which may happen at different food chain steps. Some of the most important biotoxins are those produced by algae when the environmental conditions they are subjected to are favourable. In such situations, multiplication of cellular algae occurs, thereby leading to aggregation of cells that are referred to as algal blooms, the development of which has been defined as toxic or harmful. The algal bloom increase has been linked to the consequences of different anthropogenic activities as well as climate change, which has had an influence on marine planktonic systems (Grattan et al., 2016).

6.6 Poisoning Caused by Marine Biotoxins and Effects on Human Health

Toxins can produce a wide range of symptoms and therefore have been associated with several clinically described syndromes. The main HAB-related syndromes are amnesic, diarrhoetic, azaspirazid, paralytic, and neurotoxic shellfish poisoning and ciguatera fish poisoning.

Paralytic shellfish poisoning: This is one of the most common disorders that affect humans who consume seafood and seafood products contaminated with biotoxins. This type of biointoxication occurs when toxic shellfish such as clams, oysters, mussels, or various other molluscs that feed on toxic dinoflagellates are consumed. This type of poisoning is produced by the microalgae belonging to the taxon Dinoficee. The consequence of this poisoning is neurological symptoms, while in some cases it could lead to paralysis of the respiratory system that could thereafter lead to death. The toxin that is implicated in this symptom is called saxitoxin and is derived from *Saxidomus giganteus,* the algae that produce it. The saxitoxin toxic effect in humans is entirely acute and acts on the voltage-dependent sodium ion channel, thereby preventing channel conductance and resulting in blocking neuronal activity. The primary site by which saxitoxin exerts its action is the peripheral nervous system of humans, where it causes a quick onset of symptoms: numbness or tingling sensation around lips; these feelings can eventually spread to the face and neck. Other frequent symptoms that are associated with this toxin include pain in toes and fingertips, nausea, vomiting, diarrhoea, dizziness, and headaches, and, in rare cases, transitory blindness may be seen. Most of the time, the occurrence of the symptoms is rapid, and they may also continue for some days. Severe forms may be characterized by paraesthesia progressing to the legs and arms; motor weakness; giddiness; incoherent speech; and cerebellar manifestations such as ataxia, motor incoordination, and dysmetria. This can also lead to respiratory challenges appearing as constriction around the throat. More severe poisoning may manifest as muscular paralysis or serious respiratory problems and may also lead to death within 24 hours of ingestion (Deeds et al., 2008, Morabito et al., 2018).

Amnesic shellfish poisoning: This is also called domoic acid poisoning and was first discovered to have been produced by *Pseudo-nitzschia pungens* f. multiseries, a species of diatom. The action of domoic acid is on the excitatory amino acid receptors and on synaptic transmission; thus, it is regarded as excitatory amino acid, a neurotransmitter, and a neurotoxin to the central nervous system. The hippocampus areas (CA1 and CA3) which are responsible for the processing of learning and memory are the susceptible parts, which is the reason memory deficits in both animals and humans occur in cases of poisoning. Other toxic effects of domoic acid poisoning include neurotoxic activity and gastrotoxic or enterotoxic action. In humans, the symptoms associated with this poisoning could range from gastrointestinal effects such as nausea, vomiting, diarrhoea, and abdominal cramps to neurological signs, including confusion, lethargy, disorientation, paresthesia, and short-term memory loss. However, it could also lead to death in some rare cases (Ramsdell and Gulland, 2014; Morabito et al., 2018).

Diarrhoeic shellfish poisoning: This seafood intoxication consists of the rapid onset of gastrointestinal symptoms, usually within three hours, such as vomiting and diarrhoea, which generally resolve in about two to three days. The cause of this toxicity is accumulation of toxic Dinoficee in bivalves, and it is an important health challenge to humans globally. The main producer of this toxin is the dinoflagellate that belongs to the genus *Dinophysis*. The DSP toxin is usually grouped into acidic toxins (such as okadaic acid and its derivatives) and neutral toxins (including pectenotoxins and sulphated polyether compounds). Poisoning by kadaic acid and its derivatives mainly cause diarrhoea in humans, attributable to a swift increase in phosphorylated proteins that control sodium ion secretion in the cells of the intestine. Pectenotoxins are among the group of toxins that are generally associated with DSP, but the mode of its action is not yet fully understood, although some have shown *in vitro* toxicity and exert effects on the cytoskeleton that involve microtubules and actin (Morabito et al., 2018).

Azaspiracid shellfish poisoning: This toxin was formerly included in the DSP toxin group because of the relatedness in the production of severe acute symptoms, including nausea, diarrhoea, vomiting, and stomach cramps, when ingested with contaminated seafoods. It was initially hypothesized that AZA had similarity of action with okadaic acid in protein phosphatase inhibition, but successive studies revealed that purified AZA had no enzyme activity but could be possibly involved in the inhibition of other types of serine/threonine protein phosphatase. It can also exert toxicity effects using human bladder carcinoma cells (ECV-304) and HepG2 hepatoblastoma cells exposed to crude mussel extracts (Román et al., 2004).

Neurotoxic shellfish poisoning: Brevetoxin is produced by the dinoflagellate *Karenia brevis* and is implicated in massive mortality of fish and marine mammals in the Gulf of Mexico, the east coast of the United States, and New Zealand. Brevetoxins cause NSP and asthma-like symptoms in humans through inhalation and are associated with both neurological and gastrointestinal abnormalities such as nausea, vomiting, diarrhoea, paraesthesia, cramps, bronchoconstriction, paralysis, seizures, and coma and could also lead to death in some rare cases. Likewise, respiratory effects that are related to aerosolized red tide, including sneezing, throat irritation, burning, and itching, have been observed, while in asthmatic individuals, a considerable increase in these symptoms has been noted (Sun et al., 2016; Visciano et al., 2016).

Ciguatera fish poisoning: This type of poison is due to ciguatoxins produced by a benthic dinoflagellate that belongs to the genus *Gambierdiscus toxicus.* The site ciguatoxins affect is the 5-alpha subunit of the sodium channel, thereby inducing extended opening of sodium channels. The aftermath of the effect on the 5-alpha subunit of the sodium channel is the inability of the cell to maintain its internal ion balance, which could therefore alter the bioenergetic mechanisms, swelling of cell, and mitochondrial formation of blebs on the cell surfaces. The occurrence of ciguatoxin-induced intracellular transport of calcium is in the intestinal epithelia cells, which leads to fluids being secreted, resulting in diarrhoea. The signs associated with CFP include gastrointestinal, cardiovascular, neurological, and neuropsychiatric symptoms. The gastrointestinal symptoms are vomiting, diarrhoea, abdominal pain, and nausea. The development of these is between 6 and 24 hours from the time the contaminated fish is consumed but is resolved spontaneously within a time range of one to four days (Robertson et al., 2014; Reverté et al., 2014). The neurologic symptoms are associated with temperature sensation reversal, paraesthesia in the extremities, headache, myalgia, arthralgia, generalised pruritis, muscle and joint aches, and fatigue. Moreover, neuropsychiatric symptoms include anxiety, depression, and memory loss. The outcome of this intoxication is rarely fatal, but acute intoxication can lead to a chronic stage continuing for several weeks and years (Morabito et al., 2018).

Tridacna clam poisoning: This kind of biointoxication is produced by giant clams that belong to the species *Tridacna maxima,* the ingestion of which leads to disorders of the digestive system and severe nervous system disturbances, including paraesthesia, lack of motor co-ordination, ataxia, and tremor. Sometimes it can lead to fatal outcomes in both humans and animals that consume the remnants of the toxic products.

Palytoxin: This type of toxin is a potent non-protein marine compound that is produced by corals in the genus *Palythoa* and dinoflagellate in the genus *Ostreopsis.* Some of the symptoms that have been reported to be associated with the consumption of contaminated shellfish are metallic taste, gastrointestinal malaise, diarrhoea, nausea, vomiting, ataxias, dizziness, myalgia, dyspnoea, convulsion, and bradycardia. In addition, exposure to marine aerosols that contain palytoxin has resulted in cutaneous and respiratory challenges; also, in some cases, the outcome of ingestion could be fatal (Visciano et al., 2016).

Venerupin shellfish poisoning: This form of poisoning occurs when toxic bivalve shellfish recovered from certain regions of Japan are consumed. The contamination of shellfish occurs when they feed on the toxic dinoflagellate *Exuviaella mariae-lebouriae*. The two species of shellfish that have been implicated in biointoxication are *Crassostrea gigas* and *Venerupis semidecussata*. The symptoms that arise from the consumption of this toxin develop within 48 hours and include but are not limited to upset of the gastrointestinal tract, headache, gum bleeding, jaundice, anaemia, blood-clotting retardation time, and liver function disturbances and enlargement. In some cases, it could also result in death.

Cephalopod poisoning: This form of intoxication results when squid or octopus contaminated with toxins is ingested. The development of symptoms usually occurs within a period of 10–20 hours, and they manifest as gastrointestinal upset, abdominal pain, headache, weakness, paralysis, and convulsions. In most cases, recovery of the victims happens within a 48-hour period. The toxin is heat stable; hence destruction of the toxin cannot be done with ordinary cooking.

Whelk poisoning: This is from the ingestion of whole whelks or ivory shells; the mollusc that belongs to the genus *Neptunea* leads to this form of poisoning, and the toxin is present in the salivary glands of the mollusc. Although ordinary cooking cannot be employed to destroy the toxins, it has not been associated with any deaths. The symptoms associated with this poison include intense headaches, dizziness, nausea, vomiting, visual impairment, and mouth dryness.

Abalone poisoning: The occurrence of this form of poisoning is a result of consuming the viscera of abalone, which is also referred to as ormers and has long been identified, with two species, *Haliotis discus* and *Haliotis sieboldin*, implicated. The symptoms that manifest include serious local reactions with urticaria, erythema, pruritus, subcutaneous infiltration, and occasionally skin ulceration. The lesions in the skin are usually restricted to body parts that are exposed to the sun. This form of poisoning is a rare condition leading to photosensitization because of animal product consumption.

Crab and lobster poisoning: The consumption of crabs and lobsters with lethal biointoxication nearly identical to saxitoxin has been reported in the tropical Pacific islands but with little research carried out on it. The clinical manifestation of the biotoxin includes gastrointestinal upset, mouth anaesthesia, limb numbness, loss of motor co-ordination, unconsciousness, aphasia, muscular paralysis, and death within a period of several hours. It can, however, not be destroyed with ordinary cooking procedures.

6.7 Detoxification and Prevention of Marine Biotoxins

The prevention of marine biotoxins involves detoxification with the aim of reducing the off-market time duration. In PSP, one of the methods employed in detoxification is transferring contaminated shellfish to water that is free of toxic microorganisms, thereby allowing them to self-depurate. The disadvantages associated with transferring a large number of shellfish are that it is costly and labour intensive. The rate at which detoxification also occurs differs from species to species, since some, such as Crassostrea, Plactopecten, and Spisula, may remain toxic for many months. In addition, there is also variation in the required time to eliminate toxins in mussel tissues of shellfish; for instance, if the dinoflagellates that contaminated the water have disappeared, there will be a gradual reduction in the amount of toxins. For example, in dinoflagellate-free salt water with a temperature between 15 to 20°C, mussel *Mytilus edulis* toxin can be reduced by 50% within a period of 12 days. However, in the case of the clam *Saxidomus giganteus*, the time required for PSP toxins to be eliminated could take up to a year from the time it was exposed to toxic dinoflagellates.

Other factors that affect the variation rate of detoxification include seasons, low water temperature that cause retardation in the loss of toxins, and the site of storage within the shellfish. Elimination of toxins stored in the gastrointestinal tract occurs readily compared to those stored in tissues. The rate of toxin accumulation is also another factor that influences detoxification; for example, the rate at which mussels accumulate toxins is faster, and the rate at which they eliminate the poison is also fast, but for oysters, the rate of toxin accumulation is slow, and detoxification takes a longer time (Mons et al., 1998). Paralytic Shellfish Poisoning (PSP) toxin detoxification can also be carried out with the use of temperature or salinity stress, but with little success. Moreover, shellfish contaminated with PSP toxins can also be detoxified with cooking. The challenge with cooking is that though the level of toxins may be reduced, the danger associated with toxins cannot be eliminated. Cooking may be very effective in reducing toxicity to a safe level, but pan frying is more effective, while boiling is not sufficient for the detoxification of highly toxic shellfish (FAO, 2004).

In addition, seasons affect the rate at which DSP toxin is lost, and retardation of toxin loss also occurs at low water temperatures, while the rate at which toxins are detoxified depends largely on the site where the toxins are stored. Elimination of toxins in the gastrointestinal tract of *Mytilus* occurs much more readily than in tissues. The quality of food that is made available to shellfish during the period of detoxification could influence the rate of toxin elimination. The depuration rate, the rate of toxin removal from shellfish, has a dependence on the species, coupled with feeding, pumping, temperature, salinity, and the level of non-toxic algae and particulate matter present.

Generally, detoxifying PSP-contaminated shellfish at a large scale in artificial systems, especially in areas predisposed to regular toxic algae outbreaks, is not feasible; hence putting preventive measures in place is more appropriate. Such preventive measures include inspecting seawater bodies where shellfish are grown regularly for the appearance of toxic dinoflagellates, especially during the occurrences of algal blooms. This is in addition to the exploration of dinoflagellate cysts and routine inspection of shellfish. Other preventive measures include organization of training for diverse groups and disseminating key information on the effects of harmful algal blooms as a means of providing orientation for the public, and, in the case of shellfish contamination, measures that will prevent consumption should be put in place in addition to prompt reporting of cases of human intoxication (FAO, 2004).

The preventive measures required for DSP shellfish-borne diseases involve the marine environment and shellfish flesh monitoring. This is in addition to frequently carrying out monitoring of the seawater around shellfish farms in other to discover whether toxin-producing phytoplankton are present. Such monitoring processes might provide information on the type and concentration of toxic alga species present, which is an indication of expected toxins during a particular period of bloom and seafood products for analytical monitoring consideration. However, some species that have not been encountered in certain areas may appear unexpectedly, causing problems. In general, effective monitoring is the main preventive means for DSP toxins so that toxin-contaminated products will not get to the market for consumers. In endemic areas, weekly sampling is insufficient to provide human health protection; hence, a more reliable plan in addition to detection means is needed. Nevertheless, there are some factors that make monitoring complicated, and these include variation in the cell numbers of toxin-producing algae that will be required for the production of toxic mussels; variation in the time period of toxicity with region and episode in different regions; implicated toxins and algae may be different; and the presence of different types of toxins at the same time.

In all the methods that have been used to reduce ASP toxin-contaminated shellfish, none has proved useful for reduction. Tested methods have either not been safe, they have been too slow or costly, or they have led to the generation of a product that is not acceptable in appearance and taste. The rate at which mussels take up ASP toxin is rapid, and at the same time, elimination of the toxin is also rapid compared to the longer period of retention in other bivalves. At freezing temperatures, DA are transferred from hepatopancreas into the other body parts, and the elimination of the DA is lost, but toxin loss might take considerable time. In this case, providing preventive measures may be difficult because the effect of the toxic bloom in commercial harvest areas and aquaculture facilities may be adversely affected and unpredictable. This is due to the fact that some algal species that have never been encountered may just appear, causing problem at facilities. Hence, it may be practically impossible to put effective preventive measures in place. Therefore, strict, extensive marine environment regulation will be needed for prevention to be achieved. In addition, the step of stopping product harvest may be taken if the level of observed toxin exceeds the limit and a waiting period observed until the toxin level drops to a limit that is acceptable. This is in addition to destroying the harvested fishery products with a very high toxin content (FAO, 2004).

The rate at which NSP toxins are lost from bivalves is dependent on the site of toxin accumulation, which may be different between phycotoxins. There are two phases through which toxins are eliminated from scallops: initial rapid loss, which is also similar to the rate of accumulation, followed by a slower phase. During this period, there may be changes in the toxin profile between tissues, with the transfer of toxins between the compartment of the tissues or organs before they are finally excreted or secreted into the surrounding environment. The common way of depurating bivalves is by self-depuration, which is usually accomplished by transferring shellfish stock to clear water. While it has been observed that ozone has proven to assist in depuration, cooking and freezing are not effective in eliminating NSP from tissues (Van Apeldoorn, 2001; FAO, 2004). Detection of toxic blooms is usually through visual observation, which involves water discolouration and fish kills, illness for shellfish consumers, and human respiratory irritation. Verification of actual toxicity is by chemical analyses for brevetoxins within shellfish samples and by mouse bioassays; however, this is time consuming. Prediction of the occurrence and bloom magnitude is very difficult because the actual environmental conditions that are responsible for algal blooms are poorly known. This is the reason management strategy can only be based on the accuracy of water quality evaluation. Hence, reliance on monitoring programmes is on identifying and enumerating harmful taxa microscopically to prevent human intoxication, which, however, is time consuming and could vary with individuals.

Furthermore, information on AZP intoxication is sparse. This could be as a result of its similarity with DSP that might have been responsible for the underreporting of cases. The duration of AZP intoxication is usually about six months, and the toxin is stored in the digestive glands and can migrate to other tissues, making intoxication persistent, and could also lead to slow natural depuration. In other to protect human health, it is recommended that analysis be carried out for the detection of AZA in aquatic environments (Ettoubi et al., 2020)

Identification of CFP toxin cannot be done using odour and taste. It is not susceptible to temperature; hence it cannot be destroyed either by cooking, freezing, salting, drying, smoking, or marinating; fish that has been contaminated could remain toxic for years. Preventive measures include the use of animal screening tests, avoiding the consumption of large predatory fish, and public education on the dangers of consuming contaminated fish.

6.8 Benefits of Marine Biotoxins in Seafoods

Seafood plays a vital role in meeting the diet needs of many coastal Indigenous populations, as it has been shown that over 90% of the required protein in the diet of some people living in coastal areas is obtained from marine sources, thereby putting more emphasis on the traditional value of marine foods (Batal et al., 2021; Lee et al., 2024). Furthermore, along with the cultural significance of seafood being substantially retained, Indigenous communities are also provided with livelihoods: it contributes to the general well-being and welfare of the Indigenous population and gives strong support to food security and sovereignty, as well as serving as a significant source of nutrients in the diet (Batal et al., 2021; Marushka et al., 2021). There are reports that has shown Indigenous groups that eat more traditional foods such as seafoods have better intake of nutrients, lower obesity levels, and a reduction in other metabolic disorders like type 2 diabetes (Vogliano et al., 2020).

6.9 Conclusion

Fish and shellfish constitute nutritious foods with desirable components of a healthy diet. Some seafoods are wholesome, but some could be responsible for infection, leading to illnesses in the consumer. Biotoxins are substances produced by microbes, and in the marine environment, they accumulate in fish or bivalve molluscs such as oysters and mussels. Harmful algal blooms are periodically responsible for the death of fish, thereby disrupting food sources for fish and shellfish. In situations where HABs are not detected, seafood harvested from such waters may constitute a risk to human health. The knowledge of the sources and distribution of toxins in seafoods is very important to putting in place effective control and management plans that will be targeted at preventing harvesting and sales of contaminated seafoods to the public. Some of the preventive measures that can be utilized include detoxification with the aim of reducing the off-market time duration. However, there may be variation in the rate of detoxification, which is dependent on the seasons, low water temperature, and site of storage within the shellfish. Generally, elimination of toxins in the gastrointestinal tract occurs at a faster rate readily compared to those stored in tissues

References

Ahmed, F.E. 1991. *Seafood Safety*. Washington, DC: National Academy Press.

Aitken, A. et al. 1982. *Fish Handling & Processing*. 2nd ed. Edinburgh: Aberdeen Ministry of Agriculture.

Ansdell, V. 2023. *Food Poisoning from Marine Toxins*. CDC Yellow Book 2024. https://wwwnc.cdc.gov/travel/yellowbook/2024/environmental-hazards-risks/food-poisoning-from-marine-toxins.

Aransiola, S.A. et al., eds. 2024. *Marine Greens: Environmental, Agricultural, Industrial and Biomedical Applications*. 1st ed. Boca Raton, FL: CRC Press, Taylor and Francis Group. https://doi.org/10.1201/9781003369738

Batal, M. et al. 2021. Importance of the traditional food systems for First Nations adults living on reserves in Canada. *Canadian Journal of Public Health*, 112, 20–28.

Botana, L.M., Rodriguez-Vieytes, M., Alfonso, A., and Louzao, M.C. 1996. Phycotoxins: Paralytic shellfish poisoning and diarrhetic shellfish poisoning. In L.M.L. Nollet, ed. *Handbook of Food Analysis—Residues and Other Food Component Analysis*, Vol. 2, pp. 1147–1169. Taylor & Francis.

Bower, D.J., Hart, R.J., Matthews, P.A., and Howden, M.E.H. 1981. Nonprotein neurotoxins. *Clinical Toxicology*, 18, 813–843.

Cassell, R.T., Chen, W., Thomas, S., Liu, L., and Rein, K.S. 2015. Brevetoxin, the dinoflagellate neurotoxin, localizes to thylakoid membranes and interacts with the light harvesting complex II (LHCII) of photosystem II. *ChemBioChem*, 16, 1060–1067. https://doi.org/10.1002/cbic.201402669

Cisneros-Montemayor, A.M., Pauly, D., Weatherdon, L.V., and Ota, Y. 2016. A global estimate of seafood consumption by coastal Indigenous peoples. *PLoS One*, 11(12), e0166681

Connell, J.J. 1990. *Control of Fish Quality*. 3rd ed. Oxford: Fishing News Books.

Deeds, J.R., Landsberg, J.H., Etheridge, S.M., Pitcher, G.C., and Longman, S.W. 2008. Non-traditional vectors for paralytic shellfish poisoning. *Marine Drugs*, 6, 308–348.

EFSA. 2008. Scientific opinion of the panel on contaminants in the food chain on a request from the European Commission on marine biotoxins in shellfish—azaspiracids. *EFSA Journal*, 723, 1–52.

EFSA. 2009. Scientific opinion of the panel on contaminants in the food chain on a request from the European Commission on marine biotoxins in shellfish—pectenotoxin group. *EFSA Journal*, 1109, 1–47.

EFSA. 2010. Scientific opinion on marine biotoxins in shellfish—emerging toxins: Brevetoxin group. *EFSA Journal*, 1677, 1–29.

Ettoubi, E., Akif, F., Genten, F., and Blaghen, M. 2020. Marine biotoxins: Origins, effects, distribution, prevention and treatment. *International Journal of Innovative Science and Research Technology*, 5(11), 928–941.

FAO. 2004. *Food and Agriculture Organization of the United Nations Rome*. file:///C:/Users/HomePC/Desktop/chp%205/Prevention

Grattan, L.M., Holobaugh, S., and Morris, J.G. 2016. Harmful algal blooms and public health. *Harmful Algae*, 57, 2–8.

Hallegraeff, G.M. 2004. Harmful algal blooms: A global overview. In G.M. Hallegraeff, D.M. Anderson, and A.D. Cembella, eds. *Manual on Harmful Marine Microalgae*, 2nd ed., pp. 25–49. Paris: UNESCO.

Lee, M.J., Hendersona, S.B., Clermontb, H., Turna, N.S., and McIntyre, L. 2024. The health risks of marine biotoxins associated with high seafood consumption: Looking beyond the single dose, single outcome paradigm with a view towards addressing the needs of coastal Indigenous populations in British Columbia. *Heliyon*, 10, e27146. https://doi.org/10.1016%2Fj.heliyon.2024.e27146

Marushka, L. et al. 2021. Importance of fish for food and nutrition security among First Nations in Canada. *Canadian Journal of Public Health*, 112, 64–80.

Maso, M., and Garcés, E. 2006. Harmful microalgae blooms (HAB); problematic and conditions that induce them. *Marine Pollution Bulletin*, 53, 620–630. https://doi.org/10.1016/j.marpolbul.2006.08.006

McIntyre, L., Miller, A., and Kosatsky, T. 2021. Changing trends in paralytic shellfish poisonings reflect increasing sea surface temperatures and practices of Indigenous and recreational harvesters in British Columbia, Canada. *Marine Drugs*, 19(10), 568.

McVey, J.P. 1983. *Handbook of Mariculture*. Vol. 1. Boca Raton, FL: CRC Press.

Mons, M.N., Van Egmond, H.P., and Speijers, G.J.A. 1998. Paralytic shellfish poisoning: A review. *RIVM Report*, 388802 005. June.

Morabito, S., Silvestro, S., and Faggio, C. 2018. How the marine biotoxins affect human health. *Natural Product Research*, 32(6), 621–631. https://doi.org/10.1080/14786419.2017.1329734

Motarjemi, Y., Moy, G.G., and Todd, E.C.D. 2014. *Encyclopedia of Food Safety*. Elsevier.

Negedly, R. 1990. *Elsevier's Dictionary of Fishery, Processing, Fish, and Shellfish Names of the World in Five Languages, English, French, Spanish, German, and Latin*. New York: Elsevier.

Nicolas, J. et al. 2017. Marine biotoxins and associated outbreaks following seafood consumption: Prevention and surveillance in the 21st century. *Global Food Security*, 15, 11–21.

Quilliam, M.A. et al. 2001. Recent developments in the analysis of phycotoxins by liquid chromatography — mass spectrometry. In W.J.de Koe et al., eds. *Mycotoxins and Phycotoxins in Perspective at the Turn of the Millennium*, pp. 383–391. Netherlands: W.J. deKoe.

Ramsdell, J.S., and Gulland, F.M. 2014. Domoic acid epileptic disease. *Marine Drugs*, 12, 1185–1207, March 6. Epub.

Regenstein, J.M., and Regenstein, C. 1991. *An Introduction to Fish Technology*. London and New York: Chapman & Hall.

Reverté, L., Soliño, L., Carnicer, O., Diogène, J., and Campàs, M. 2014. Alternative methods for the detection of emerging marine toxins: Biosensors, biochemical assays and cell-based assays. *Marine Drugs*, 12, 5719–5763.

Robertson, A., Garcia, A.C., Quintana, H.A.F., Smith, T.B., Castillo, B.F., Reale-Munroe, K., Gulli, J.A., Olsen, D.A., Hooe-Rollman, J.I., Jester, E.L.E., Klimek, B.J., and Plakas, S.M. 2014. Invasive lionfish (Pterois volitans): A potential human health threat for ciguatera fish poisoning in tropical waters. *Marine Drugs*, 12(1), 88–97.

Román, Y., Alfonso, A., Vieytes, M.R., Ofuji, K., Satake, M., Yasumoto, T., and Botana, L.M. 2004. Effects of azaspiracids 2 and 3 on intracellular cAMP, [Ca 2+], and pH. *Chemical Research in Toxicology*, 17, 1338–1349, October.

Sikorski, Z.E., Pan, B.S., and Shahidi, F., eds. 1994. *Seafood Proteins*. London and New York: Chapman & Hall.

Smayda, T.J. 2007. Reflections on the ballast water dispersal-harmful algal bloom paradigm. *Harmful Algae*, 6, 601–622. https://doi.org/10.1016/j.hal.2007.02.003

Smith, M.D. et al. 2010. Sustainability and global seafood. *Science*, 327, 784–778.

Straus, K. 1991. *The Seafood Handbook: Seafood Standards: Establishing Guidelines for Quality*. Rockland, ME: Seafood Business.

Trainer, V.L. et al. 2013. Diarrhetic shellfish toxins and other lipophilic toxins of human health concern in Washington State. *Marine Drugs*, 11, 1815–1835. https://doi.org/10.3390/md11061815

U.S. National Office for Harmful Algal Blooms. 2019. *Distribution of HABs in the U.S. Wood Hole Oceanographic Institute*. https://hab.whoi.edu/maps/regions-us-distribution/.

Van Apeldoorn, M.E. 2001. Neurotoxic shellfish poisoning: A review. *RIVM Report*, 388802023. September 2001.

Van Egmond, H.P., and Speijers, G.J.A. 1999. Natural toxins II. Phycotoxins. In K. Van der Heijden et al., eds. *International Food Safety Handbook. Science, International Regulation and Control*, pp. 357–368. New York: Marcel Dekker Inc.

Visciano, P., Schirone, M., Berti, M., Milandri, A., Tofalo, R., and Suzzi, G. 2016. Marine biotoxins: Occurrence, toxicity, regulatory limits and reference methods. *Frontiers in Microbiology*, 7, 1051. https://doi.org/10.3389/fmicb.2016.01051

Vogliano, C., Raneri, J.E., Maelaua, J., Coad, J., Wham, C., and Burlingame, B. 2020. Assessing diet quality of Indigenous food systems in three geographically distinct Solomon Islands sites (Melanesia, Pacific Islands). *Nutrients*, 13(1), 30.

Wiggins, S., and Anderson, E. 2022. Marine biotoxin control for molluscan shellfish. *Food Safety Magazine*. https://www.food-safety.com/articles/7557-marine-biotoxin-control-for-molluscan-shellfish

Zendong, Z., Kadiri, M., Herrenknecht, C., Nézan, E., Mazzeo, A., and Hess, P. 2016. Algal toxin profiles in Nigerian coastal waters (Gulf of Guinea) using passive sampling and liquid chromatography coupled to mass spectrometry. *Toxicon*, 114, 16–27. https://doi.org/10.1016/j.toxicon.2016.02.011

Section 2

Applications of Biotoxins

7

Plant-Based Biotoxins: Applications and Controls

Maria M. Adeyemi, Ifeoluwa O. Olayemi, Adedola Adeboye, and Susan N. Thera-Sekgweng

7.1 Introduction

Toxins are small molecules, peptides, or proteins capable of causing disease on contact with or absorption by body tissues by interacting with biological macromolecules such as enzymes or cellular receptors. Plant toxins are secondary metabolites in plants to defend themselves against threats like insects, predators, and microorganisms. Some common examples include lectins in beans, cyanogenic glycosides in cassava, and glycoalkaloids in potatoes (Kocyigit et al., 2023). Plant-based biotoxins, also known as phytotoxins, are poisonous substances synthesized by plants or plant pathogens through naturally occurring biochemical reactions (Chen et al., 2020; Tampakaki et al., 2009; Xu et al., 2021). Plant-based toxins can have both beneficial and harmful effects. The symptoms of plant biotoxin poisoning may include cardiovascular, hematologic, neurologic, respiratory, renal, and gastrointestinal symptoms. These plant-based toxins can be harmful to humans if consumed in large quantities, causing issues like vomiting, diarrhea, and even death in severe cases (Ogori, 2019). Despite the obvious health concerns of being exposed to toxins, scientific interest in plant-based biotoxins has grown significantly due to their potential applications in medicine, agriculture, and other industries (Assuncao et al., 2017; Clark et al., 2019; Suresh et al., 2014; Xu et al., 2021). They are having substantial positive impacts in industrial sectors, which include clinical, veterinary, and agrochemical uses. These toxic substances have evolved over millions of years, resulting in a diverse array of compounds with potent biological activities (Wink, 2010). These compounds can be classified based on their chemical structure, mode of action, or the plant families that produce them. Common classifications include:

1. Alkaloids (e.g., nicotine, atropine, morphine)
2. Glycosides (e.g., digitoxin, amygdalin)

DOI: 10.1201/9781003500605-9

3. Terpenoids (e.g., paclitaxel, artemisinin)
4. Peptides and proteins (e.g., ricin, abrin)

The diversity of these compounds reflects the wide range of ecological roles they play in plant defense and survival (Mithofer & Boland, 2012). Plant-based biotoxins can affect various biological processes in target organisms, altering biological mechanisms such as:

1. Disruption of cell membranes
2. Inhibition of enzyme activity
3. Interference with neurotransmission
4. Alteration of DNA or RNA synthesis
5. Induction of apoptosis (programmed cell death)

7.2 Applications of Plant-Based Biotoxins

Plant-based biotoxins are used in various applications ranging from medicinal to agricultural to biotechnological and research purposes.

1. **Medicinal Applications:**

   Plant-based biotoxins play a significant role in drug discovery and the field of medicine, especially in forensic medicine, clinical toxicology, pharmacology, and veterinary medicine (Thakur et al., 2018). They are a valuable source of novel therapeutic agents, such as:

   a. **Cancer treatment**: Paclitaxel (Taxol), derived from the Pacific yew tree (*Taxus brevifolia*), is widely used in the treatment of various cancers, including ovarian, breast, and lung cancer (Weaver, 2014).

   b. **Pain management**: Capsaicin, found in chili peppers (*Capsicum* species), is used in topical creams for pain relief in conditions such as arthritis and neuropathic pain (Anand & Bley, 2011).

   c. **Cardiovascular medicine:** Digoxin, derived from foxglove plants (*Digitalis* species), is used to treat heart failure and atrial fibrillation (Gheorghiade et al., 2006).

   d. **Neurodegenerative diseases:** Botulinum toxin produced by *Clostridium botulinum* is used in facial remodeling and for the treatment of migraines, excessive perspiration, brain and spinal cord disorders, prostate enlargement, and bladder function (Thakur et al., 2018).

   e. **Antimalaria:** Artemisinin, isolated from sweet wormwood (*Artemisia annua*), is a potent antimalarial compound that has revolutionized malaria treatment (Tu, 2011).

2. **Agricultural Applications:**

   Plant-based biotoxins have applications in agriculture, particularly in pest management and crop protection.

   a. **Biopesticides:** Natural plant toxins like pyrethrin (from *Chrysanthemum cinerariaefolium*) and rotenone (from tropical legumes) are used as alternatives to synthetic pesticides (Isman, 2006).

   b. **Insect repellents:** Essential oils containing various plant-based compounds are used as natural insect repellents (Nerio et al., 2010). Biotoxins such as pyrethrins and neem oil play a vital role in pest management. These natural insecticides offer an eco-friendly alternative to synthetic chemicals, reducing negative environmental impacts and promoting sustainable farming practices. Their effectiveness in pest control underscores their importance in agriculture (Evidente et al., 2019)

   c. **Herbicides:** Some plant-derived compounds show potential as natural herbicides, offering environmentally friendly alternatives to synthetic weed killers (Duke et al., 2000).

3. **Biotechnological Applications:**

   The use of biotoxins like ricin in biotechnology for targeted cancer therapy exemplifies the innovative applications of these substances. By leveraging the specificity of antibodies, ricin can be directed to cancer cells, minimizing damage to healthy tissues and enhancing treatment efficacy.

4. **Scientific Research:**

   Plant-based biotoxins serve as valuable tools in scientific research:

   a. **Molecular probes:** Toxins with specific cellular targets are used to study biological processes and signaling pathways (Strebhardt & Ullrich, 2008).

   b. **Drug development**: Plant-based toxins serve as lead compounds for new drugs with improved efficacy and reduced side effects (Newman & Cragg, 2016).

7.3 Control Measures for Plant-Based Biotoxins

1. **Regulatory Frameworks**

   Regulatory frameworks are essential for managing the use and distribution of plant-based biotoxins. Governments and international bodies have established regulations to ensure the safe and effective use of these substances.

a. International Regulations
   i. **U.S. Environmental Protection Agency (EPA):** Regulates biopesticides under the Federal Insecticide, Fungicide, and Rodenticide Act (FIFRA), assessing their safety and efficacy before market approval.
   ii. **Chemical Weapons Convention (CWC):** This international treaty prohibits the development, production, acquisition, stockpiling, retention, transfer, or use of chemical weapons, including plant-based toxins like ricin (OPCW, 2005).
   iii. **The Biological Weapons Convention (BWC):** This treaty bans the development, production, and stockpiling of biological and toxin weapons, including plant-based toxins (United Nations, 1972).
   iv. **National Regulations:** Many countries have specific regulations governing the use, possession, and transport of plant-based biotoxins, such as the United States, European Union, and so on.

2. **Detection and Monitoring**

   Advanced analytical techniques are employed to detect and monitor biotoxins in various environments. Techniques such as chromatography, mass spectrometry, and immunoassays enable rapid and accurate detection, which is crucial for managing contamination events and ensuring food and water safety. Enzyme-linked immunosorbent assays (ELISA) and high-performance liquid chromatography (HPLC) are used to monitor aflatoxins in crops, preventing exposure to these carcinogenic compounds.

3. **Mitigation Strategies**

   Mitigation strategies involve preventive and corrective actions to manage the risks associated with biotoxins. Integrated pest management (IPM) combines biological, cultural, and chemical controls to minimize the impact of biotoxins by reducing reliance on synthetic pesticides. Biological control using pathogens, parasites, or natural predators offers an effective and eco-friendly approach to pest management. For example, *Bacillus thuringiensis* (Bt) formulations are used in organic farming and genetically engineered crops to provide built-in pest resistance.

7.4 Conclusion

Plant-based biotoxins represent a vast and diverse group of compounds with significant potential across various fields, from medicine to agriculture.

Ensuring a sustainable and stable supply of plant-based biotoxins can be very difficult, especially for rare or slow-growing species, and most times, navigating the complex regulatory landscape for the development and use of plant-based biotoxins can be time consuming and costly. Their unique properties and mechanisms of action make them valuable tools in drug discovery, pest management, and scientific research. However, the potent nature of these compounds necessitates careful regulation and control to ensure safe and responsible use. New applications emerge, along with improved methods for harnessing the power of these natural compounds while mitigating their risks. The future of plant-based biotoxins lies in striking a balance between exploiting their unique properties and ensuring the safety of humans and the environment. By implementing the recommended strategies for sustainable production and increased bioprospecting efforts, we can maximize the potential benefits of plant-based biotoxins.

References

Anand, P., & Bley, K. (2011). Topical capsaicin for pain management: Therapeutic potential and mechanisms of action of the new high-concentration capsaicin 8% patch. *British Journal of Anaesthesia, 107*(4), 490–502. https://doi.org/10.1093/bja/aer260

Assuncao, J., Guedes, A. C., & Malcata, F. X. (2017). Biotechnological and pharmacological applications of biotoxins and other bioactive molecules from dinoflagellates. *Marine Drugs, 15*(12), 393.

Chen, H., Singh, H., Bhardwaj, N., Bhardwaj, S. K., Khatri, M., Kim, K.-H., & Peng, W. (2020). An exploration of the toxicity mechanisms of phytotoxins and their potential utilities. *Critical Reviews in Environmental Science and Technology, 52*(3), 395–435. https://doi.org/10.1080/10643389.2020.1823172

Clark, G. C., Casewell, N. R., Elliot, C. T., Harvey, A. L., Jamison, A. G., Strong, P. N., & Turner, A. D. (2019). Friends or foes? Emerging impacts of biological toxins. *Trends in Biochemical Sciences, 44*(4), 365–379.

Duke, S. O., Dayan, F. E., Romagni, J. G., & Rimando, A. M. (2000). Natural products as sources of herbicides: Current status and future trends. *Weed Research, 40*(1), 99–111. https://doi.org/10.1046/j.1365-3180.2000.00161.x

Evidente, A., Cimmino, A., & Masi, M. (2019). Phytotoxins produced by pathogenic fungi of agrarian plants. *Phytochemistry Reviews, 18*, 843–870. https://doi.org/10.1007/s11101-019-09624-0

Gheorghiade, M., Van Veldhuisen, D. J., & Colucci, W. S. (2006). Contemporary use of digoxin in the management of cardiovascular disorders. *Circulation, 113*(21), 2556–2564. https://doi.org/10.1161/CIRCULATIONHA.105.560110

Isman, M. B. (2006). Botanical insecticides, deterrents, and repellents in modern agriculture and an increasingly regulated world. *Annual Review of Entomology.* (51), 45–66. https://doi.org/10.1146/annurev.ento.51.1101014.151146

Kocyigit, E., Kocaadam-Bozkurt, B., Bozkurt, O., Ağagündüz, D., & Capasso, R. (2023). Plant Toxic proteins: Their biological activities. *Mechanism of Action and Removal Strategies, 15*(6), 356. http://doi.org/10.3390/toxins15060356

Mithofer, A., & Boland, W. (2012). Plant defense against herbivores: Chemical aspects. *Annual Review of Plant Biology, 63,* 431–450. https://doi.org/10.1146/annurev-arplant-042110-103854

Nerio, L. S., Olivero-Verbel, J., & Stashenko, E. (2010). Repellent activity of essential oils: A review. *Biosource Technology, 101*(1), 372–378. https://doi.org/10.1016/j.biotech.2009.07.048

Newman, D. J., & Cragg, G. M. (2016). Natural products as sources of new drugs from 1981 to 2014. *Journal of Natural Products, 79*(3), 629–661. https://doi.org/10.1021/acs.jnatprod.5b01055

Ogori, A. (2019). Plant toxins. *American Journal of Biomedical Science & Research, 4*(3), 2642–1747. https://doi.org/10.34297/AJBSR.2019.04.000793

Organization for the Prohibition of Chemical Weapons (OPCW). (2005). *Convention on the Prohibition of the Development, Production, Stockpiling and Use of Chemical Weapons and on their Destruction.* Retrieved from https://www.opcw.org/chemical-weapons-convention

Strebhardt, K., & Ullrich, A. (2008). Paul Ehrlich's magic bullet concept: 100 years of progress. Nature reviews. *Cancer, 8*(6), 473–480. https://doi.org/10.1038/nrc2394

Suresh, S. P., Gauri, S., Desai, S., Kartha, M., & Padmavathy, P. (2014). Marine biotoxins and its detection. *African Journal of Environmental Science and Technology, 896,* 350–365.

Tampakaki, A. P., Hatziloukas, E., & Panopoulos, N. J. (2009). Plant pathogens, bacterial. *Encyclopedia of Microbiology,* 655–677. https://doi.org/10.1016/b978-012373944-5.00346-1

Thakur, A., Sharma, V., & Thakuar, A. (2018). Phytotoxins—A mini review. *Journal of Pharmacognosy and Phytochemistry, 7*(6), 2705–2708.

Tu, Y. (2011). The discovery of artemisinin (qinghaosu) and gifts from Chinese medicine. *Nature Medicine, 17*(10), 1217–1220. https://doi.org/10.1038/nm.2471

United Nations. (1972). *Convention on the Prohibition of the Development, Production, and Stockpiling of Bacteriological (Biological) and Toxin Weapons and on their Destruction. United Nations Office for Disarmament Affairs.* Retrieved from https://www.un.org/disarmament/biological-weapons/

Weaver, B. A. (2014). How taxol/paclitaxel kills cancer cells. *Molecular Biology of the Cell, 25*(18), 2677–2681. https://doi.org/10.1091/mbc.E14-04-0916

Wink, M. (2010). Introduction: Biochemistry, physiology and ecological functions of secondary metabolites. *Annual Plant Reviews, 40,* 1–19. https://doi.org/10.1002/9781444320503.ch1

Xu, D., Xue, M., Shen, Z., Jia, X., Hou, X., Lai, D., & Zhou, L. (2021). Phytotoxic secondary metabolites from fungi. *Toxins, 13*(4), 261. https://doi.org/10.3390/toxins13040261

8

Industrial Applications of Biotoxins

Folorunso, O.A., Adeleke, A.J., Egbeagu, U.U., and Adebayo-Olajide, T.C.

8.1 Overview/History and Traditional Applications of Biotoxins

Biotoxins are toxic substances from natural sources such as microorganisms, plants and animals. These toxins are produced by living organisms in response to threats such as predators and harsh environmental conditions including unfavourable humidity, temperature, drought, pH and salt (Kocyigit et al., 2023). The toxicity of these substances means they are viewed in a negative light. However, studies have shown their use in cancer therapy. As early as the 1910s, botulinum toxin (produced by the bacterium *Clostridium botulinum*) was used for warfare during the Mexican Revolution. Also, ricin (produced by the castor plant, *Ricinus communis*) was used in the umbrella assassination in 1978, as alleged by the United States of America (Alexa et al., 2020).

8.2 Classifications of Biotoxins

Biotoxins can classified based on their origin, chemical structure and mode of action (Zhu et al., 2024). Based on chemical structure, a biotoxin can be a polyether, peptide or alkaloid toxin Based on their origin, biotoxins may be of bacterial, algal, fungal, animal or plant origin as well as from marine organisms. Based on their mode of action, we have necrotoxins (toxins that destroy tissues in the bloodstream through cell death), neurotoxins (biotoxins that affect the nervous system) and hemotoxins (biotoxins that target red blood cells) (Alvarez et al., 2021).

DOI: 10.1201/9781003500605-10

8.3 Production of Biotoxins

The production of biotoxins involves cultivating specific organisms under controlled conditions to maximize the yield of the desired toxin. The production process involves selection of the source organism, cultivation of the selected source organism, harvesting of biotoxins and purification (Ochieng et al., 2022).

8.3.1 Selection of Source Organism

Choose the microorganism or plant known to produce the desired biotoxin. This can include bacteria, fungi, algae or plants. Pure culture of microorganisms can be obtained and the inoculum prepared using the appropriate media. For instance, inoculum of bacteria like *Clostridium botulinum* can be prepared in a suitable medium, such as trypticase-peptone-glucose-yeast extract (TPGY) broth, under anaerobic conditions (Hamad et al., 2023), while inoculum of fungi like *Aspergillus flavus* can be prepared using potato dextrose agar (Ochieng et al., 2022).

8.3.2 Cultivation

Cultivation is the growth of the selected organisms under optimal conditions to enhance toxin production. Optimal conditions can involve specific nutrient media, temperature, pH and aeration conditions. Spores or mycelial fragments of fungi can be used for cultivation in a liquid medium such as Czapek-Dox medium, in flasks or bioreactors and incubated under optimal conditions (e.g., 28–30°C, shaking or static) for several days to allow aflatoxin production. Bacteria prefer 37°C incubation temperature. Some biotoxins require specific induction conditions such as stress or the presence of certain substrates to initiate or enhance production (Ochieng et al., 2022).

8.3.3 Harvesting

After the appropriate growth period, the culture is then harvested. This can involve centrifugation to collect cells or filtration for liquid cultures. For bacterial toxins, centrifuge the culture to separate the bacterial cells from the supernatant containing the toxin. For fungi, filter the culture to remove fungal biomass and collect the filtrate containing aflatoxin. Thereafter, the filtrate is subjected to various procedures which may include cell lysis and chromatographic techniques to obtain a pure form of the toxin (Ochieng et al., 2022).

8.4 Industrial Application of Bacterial Toxins

Bacterial toxins have several industrial applications across various fields, including medicine, agriculture and biotechnology.

8.4.1 Medical Applications

Botulinum toxin (Botox) is used in small, controlled doses to treat conditions like chronic migraines (Ilgaz Aydinlar et al., 2013) and muscle spasticity and in cosmetic applications (Kattimani et al., 2019) to reduce wrinkles. Botulinum toxin A is a neurotoxin produced by the anaerobic bacterium *Clostridium botulinum*. When used to treat hyperhidrosis, botulinum toxin is injected intradermally and acts to inhibit the release of acetylcholine at the neuromuscular junction and from sympathetic nerves that innervate eccrine sweat glands, which results in improvement in sweating (Wolosker et al., 2016).

Diphtheria toxin is engineered to create immunotoxins for cancer therapy, targeting and killing cancer cells while sparing healthy cells (Shafiee et al., 2019). Clostridial collagenase is used in wound debridement and treatment of conditions like Dupuytren's contracture, where collagen buildup restricts movement (Brazzelli et al., 2015). Tetanus and diphtheria toxoids are inactivated forms of toxins used in vaccines to prevent tetanus and diphtheria. Cholera toxin is utilized as a model for developing oral vaccines and adjuvants to enhance immune responses (Harris, 2018).

8.4.2 Agricultural Applications

Bacillus thuringiensis (Bt) Toxin is widely used as a biopesticide in agriculture to control insect pests. Bt toxins are specific to certain insect larvae and are safe for humans, animals, and nontarget insects (Ibrahim et al., 2010). *Photorhabdus luminescens* toxin complexes are used in biological control of pests, particularly in combination with nematodes (Abd-Elgawad, 2021). Antimicrobial peptides (AMPs) are produced by bacteria and used to protect crops from bacterial and fungal infections. Examples include nisin and subtilin. Listeriolysin O is used in diagnostic tests to detect *Listeria monocytogenes* contamination in food products (Huan et al., 2020).

8.4.3 Biotechnology Applications

Cholera and pertussis toxins are used as tools in cell biology research to study cell signalling pathways and membrane trafficking (Kenworthy et al., 2021). Shiga toxin is utilized in research to understand mechanisms of disease and host-pathogen interactions (Paton & Paton, 1998). Toxins can be used as delivery systems. Modified bacterial toxins are used to deliver therapeutic agents, such as drugs or genetic material, into cells. Affinity tags derived from bacterial toxins are also used in the purification of recombinant proteins (Pandey et al., 2022; Kimple et al., 2013; Aransiola et al., 2021)

8.4.4 Industrial Processes

Enzymes from Clostridia are used in industrial processes, such as the production of biofuels and bioplastics, due to their ability to break down complex carbohydrates and produce solvents like butanol (Bala et al., 2022; Fu & Yang, 2022). Certain bacterial toxins can degrade environmental pollutants, helping in the cleanup of contaminated sites (Bala et al., 2022; Fu & Yang, 2022).

8.4.5 Veterinary Applications

Botulinum toxin is used in veterinary medicine to treat muscle disorders in animals (McGeachan et al., 2020)

8.5 Industrial Applications of Algal Toxins

Algal toxins, which are produced by a number of different species of microalgae, have important industrial applications due to their strong biological activities. Although produced by harmful algal blooms (HABs), these microorganisms have the potential for various industrial and therapeutic applications despite the harmful effects that HABs can have on human health and aquatic ecosystems. The comprehension and manipulation of these toxins may facilitate the development of groundbreaking solutions across a spectrum of disciplines, including medicine, agricultural science, food security, biotechnology and environmental management (Hudnell, 2008). It is important to note the main points as regards the industrial implementation of algal biotoxins, such as drug delivery and development, understanding the mode of action of algal toxins, which guides research geared towards the development of medicines for the treatment of certain illnesses. For example, some toxins, such as dinoflagellate phycotoxins, could be used to develop antiarrhythmia medicines, anticholinergics and medicines for stroke recovery (Cho et al., 2020). Additionally, saxitoxin may also be a potent neurotoxin with potential application in pain management (Cho et al., 2020; Llewellyn, 2006), while brevetoxins, ciguatoxins and maitotoxins could be exploited for the development of new neurological therapeutics or probes for the study of neurological disorders (Carmichael, 1992; Aransiola et al., 2024). Brevetoxins, which act on ion channels in cell membranes, are also being studied for their potential to treat cystic fibrosis (Assunção et al., 2017). Also, amphidinols (antibacterial) and karlotoxins (antifungal) (Pradhan et al., 2022). Some applications of algal toxins include:

1. *Anticancer Properties*: Some algal toxins (e.g. azaspiracids, okadaic acid and yessotoxins) (Wang, 2008) have demonstrated anticancer properties by inducing apoptosis (programmed cell death) in cancer cells (Pradhan et al., 2022). This suggests that they are promising candidates for the development of new anticancer drugs.
2. *Obesity and Metabolic Disorders*: Algae-derived compounds such as okadaic acid and caliculin A have been shown to be capable of modulating lipid metabolism, which suggests their use in the treatment of obesity, lipid disorders and related metabolic disorders (Pradhan et al., 2022).
3. *Cosmetic and Pharmaceutical Industry*: The use of biotoxins such as okadaic acid and calyculin A is permissible in the cosmetic and pharmaceutical industries, as these substances possess the capacity to impede protein phosphatases, which are implicated in numerous cellular functions (Cho et al., 2020).
4. *Agriculture*: Agricultural use of algal toxins must be carefully managed to avoid unintended harm to non-targeted species and ecosystems. These toxins are particularly used for pest and weed control. For example, microcystins can reduce the need for broad-spectrum chemical pesticides by targeting pest populations (Hudnell, 2008), while some of the algal toxins have herbicidal properties that can be used to control the growth of weeds without the adverse effects on the environment associated with synthetic herbicides. Also, gymnodimine has the potential to be developed as a biopesticide, having been shown to have insecticidal activity against fruit flies (Cho et al., 2020). In addition, brevetoxins and ciguatoxins have been shown to have insecticidal and molluscicidal activities, suggesting the potential development of these toxins as crop protection products (Assunçao et al., 2017; Cho et al., 2020).
5. *Food Industry*: In order to ensure consumer safety, the food industry must comply with regulations on the permissible level of algal toxins in food. The monitoring and management of algal toxin levels in seafood are crucial to the prevention of foodborne diseases such as paralytic shellfish poisoning, diarrhoea and amnesic shellfish poisoning. In order to guarantee that food products comply with safety standards, advanced detection methods, including biosensors and immunoassays, are used (Sellner et al., 2003).
6. *Biotechnology and Industrial Processes*: In a variety of biotechnological applications, algal toxins could also be valuable as: (a) research

tool: saxitoxin has been employed in neurobiological research with a view to investigating ion channels as well as the functional properties of nerve cells (Llewellyn, 2006); (b) diagnostic tools: microcystins are utilized as a detection method in environmental biosensors (Meriluoto & Spoof, 2008); (c) biofuel production: research is investigating the potential use of certain algae, which can produce toxins in response to stress, as a source of biofuel, taking advantage of their high lipid content (Anderson et al., 2002); and (d) bioremediation: the potential of algal toxins for bioremediation has been the subject of investigation, with a particular focus on their capacity to degrade environmental pollutants (Sellner et al., 2003).

7. *Environmental Management*: The management of algal blooms and the toxins associated with them is of paramount importance for the protection of the environment in the following ways: (a) water quality monitoring: the presence of algal toxins represents a vital aspect in the administration of monitoring programs designed to assess water quality and detect the occurrence of harmful algal blooms (Hudnell, 2008); (b) HAB control: the control of harmful algal blooms is achieved through the implementation of various strategies. These include the utilization of algicides, the modification of nutrient inputs and the employment of biological control agents, all with the goal of reducing the population of algae (Anderson et al., 2002); and (c) environmental monitoring: the continuous monitoring of algal toxin levels is of great benefit both in terms of the protection of aquatic ecosystems and public health (Sellner et al., 2003).
8. *Economic and Regulatory Aspects:* The economic impact of dealing with algal toxins spans several industries: (a) economic impact: the costs of the management of algal blooms and their toxins can be significant and have an impact on tourism, fisheries and public health (Hudnell, 2008); (b) regulatory framework: the regulation of algal toxins in food and water is governed by national and international legislation, with the intention of ensuring public safety; and (c) compliance and best practices: in order to minimize the risks associated with the presence of algal toxins, it is imperative that industries adhere to best practices and regulatory guidelines (Hallegraeff, 1993).

8.6 Industrial Applications of Fungal Toxins

Mycotoxins, also referred to as fungal toxins, are a class of secondary metabolites which are produced by fungi. These fungal toxins are used in various industrial applications due to the contingent properties of their biotoxins.

These toxins, which are produced by a variety of fungal species, are mainly known for their detrimental effects on both plant and animal kingdoms. The severity of the toxin's effects is contingent upon the toxin's specific type and the extent of the individual's exposure. Nevertheless, the bioactivity of these compounds has been exploited in a number of industrial sectors, including biotechnology, pharmaceuticals, agriculture and food safety.

Agriculture and Pest Control: Fungal toxins have been the subject of extensive study in order to assess their suitability for use in pest control and have the potential to serve as biopesticides, offering an environmentally friendly alternative to conventional chemical pesticides. For example, fumonisin, which is produced by *Fusarium* spp., has been subjected to research with a view to determining its potential for use in the control of insect pests and plant pathogens. Its use can promote sustainable agricultural practices by reducing reliance on synthetic chemicals (Vinale et al., 2017).

Pharmaceutical Industry: In the field of pharmaceutical science, fungal toxins represent a promising avenue for the discovery of new drug candidates. It has been demonstrated that these toxins possess potent biological activity, which can be leveraged in order to develop new medications. For example, cyclosporine, which is a derivative of *Tolypocladium inflatum*, is an immunosuppressant that has transformed the field of organ transplantation, offering a new approach to preventing rejection (Kovacs et al., 2021). Furthermore, ergot alkaloids, which are produced by certain species of the fungus *Claviceps* because of their vasoconstriction properties, are employed in the treatment of migraines and induction of labour (Flieger et al., 2019).

Food Safety and Quality Control: It is of paramount importance to detect and manage mycotoxins in the food industry in order to guarantee the safety of the food produced. Some advanced analytic techniques are now available to enable the monitoring of the presence of toxins in food products. The efficacy of these detection methods is of great importance in order to ensure the quality of food products and to protect public health. For instance, liquid chromatography-mass spectrometry (LC-MS) and enzyme-linked immunosorbent assay (ELISA) are employed in the routine detection of aflatoxins, which are a group of highly toxic secondary metabolites synthesized by *Aspergillus* species (Marin et al., 2018).

Biotechnology and Biotransformation: The utilization of fungal toxins in the field of biotechnology encompasses their application within the context of biotransformation processes. It has been demonstrated that certain mycotoxins possess the ability to catalyse the biological conversion of organic substances to very useful products. An example is *Mycotoxin patulin*, which is produced by *Penicillium* spp. and has been studied in relation to its role in converting steroids into more bioactive forms well utilized in pharmaceutical formulations (Moss, 2018).

Industrial Enzyme Production: Furthermore, fungal toxins have been identified as a potential factor in the industrial production of enzymes. The production of mycotoxins by fungi often results in the secretion of a range of enzymes, which can be exploited for the purposes of industrial processes. As an illustrative example, *Aspergillus* spp. is known for its capacity to produce aflatoxins. Nevertheless, these fungi have the ability to secrete other essential enzymes, such as cellulases and proteases. Such enzymes are of significant value in a variety of industrial applications, which include the production of biofuels, the processing of food and manufacturing textiles (Hölker et al., 2004).

8.7 Industrial Applications of Plant Toxins

Plant toxins are secondary metabolites produced by plants to protect themselves, and they are also called phytotoxins (Matel et al., 2013). Plant toxins have been known to have both beneficial and harmful uses. Industrially, they have been harnessed in the manufacture of cosmetics and medications used in the treatment of ulcers, cancer, menstrual cramps and other human diseases (Chandrar et al., 2012).

A common one is ricin, which causes apoptosis of cancer cells. It is a ribosome-inactivating plant protein that is cytotoxic and obtained from the castor bean seed. Ricin acts by inhibiting the synthesis of protein and, by so doing, destroying cells. The discovery of nanotechnology has improved its use, as nanoparticles are used in drug delivery (Tyagi et al., 2015). Other phytotoxins with antitumour activity include chamaejasmenin B, neochamaejasmin C and gnidimacrin obtained from *Stellera chamaejasme* L, with activity against leukaemia L-1210 and P-388 in vivo (Liu et al., 2014). Persin obtained from avocado has been found to induce apoptosis in breast cancer cells (Butt et al., 2006). Table 8.1 shows the health benefits of phytotoxins.

TABLE 8.1

Phytotoxins with Health Benefits

Plant Source	Chemical Composition	Benefits
Banberry (*Actaea rubra*)	Cardiogenic toxins, beta-sitosterol glycoside	Menstrual cramp
Apricot (*Prunus americana*)	Cyanogenic glycosides	Constipation, detoxification, ulcers, cancer
Bindweed (*Convolvulus arvensis*)	Convolamine, conolidine, convosine, confoline	Insomnia, diuretic brain tonic
Bleeding heart (*Dicentra eximia*)	Alkaloids	Treatment of toothache
Black walnut (*Juglans nigra*)	—	Anti-inflammatory, laxative, treatment of leprosy and blood purifier

Source: (Chandrar et al., 2012)

8.8 Industrial Applications of Marine Toxins

The high nutritional content of marine environments often encourages the growth of aquatic organisms such as phytoplanktons. These, in turn, are capable of producing various toxins that are mostly known to be damaging. Marine toxins have been widely studied and given attention in recent times, particularly those produced by dinoflagellates. Regardless of the poisonous nature of these toxins, a number of them have been studied and found to have the potential to treat ailments such as Alzheimer's disease, diabetes, cancer and AIDS (Pradhan & Ki, 2022).

Saxitoxin (STX) produced by marine dinoflagellates has shown the potential to be used as an anaesthetic as well as having antibacterial, antiprotozoal, antifungal and antialgal activities in vitro. (Pradhan et al., 2022). It has also been found to have neuroprotective ability in Alzheimer's disease (Alonso et al., 2011). Yessotoxins (YTXs) are capable of treating and preventing issues related to glucose and lipid metabolism in glioma cells and liver and pancreatic abnormalities associated with transcription (Rubiolo et al., 2014). An invention based on derivatives from brevetoxin (BTX) has been used to treat mucus transport amplification and cystic fibrosis (Baden et al., 2008). Palytoxin (PLTX) obtained from *Palythoa clavate* polyps has shown the potential to treat myelogenous or lymphoblastic leukaemia (Patocka et al., 2015).

8.9 Future Directions and Innovation in Biotoxin Research and Development

The presence of biotoxins, which are toxins produced by living organisms, has the potential to have a significant impact on a number of different areas, which include biomedicine, public health and agriculture. It is of great importance to undertake further research and development of biotoxins in order to advance our understanding of their underlying mechanisms, plausible therapeutic applications and development of effective mitigation strategies (Chen et al., 2017). For example:

1. Advancements in Detection Technologies: It is of the utmost importance to develop sensitive, quick and precise detection techniques for biotoxins. The incorporation of nanomaterials into biosensor technology has markedly enhanced the sensitivity and precision of biotoxin detection, thereby significantly advancing the field. Such advancements facilitate the real-time monitoring and timely detection of outbreaks and contamination events, thereby reducing their potential to become large scale (Chen et al., 2017).

2. Genomic and Proteomic Approaches: The application of modern genomic and proteomic techniques has enabled researchers to gain a more profound understanding of the underlying molecular mechanisms, production and action of biotoxins. The identification of toxin genes and their regulatory pathways is currently being achieved through the application of high-throughput sequencing and mass spectrometry. The acquisition of such knowledge allows the design of specific interventions and the engineering of microbial organisms for the creation of biopharmaceuticals and other beneficial products and substances (Jiang et al., 2018).
3. Therapeutic Applications: Biotoxins present significant potential for use as therapeutic agents, given their notable biological activity. Research is being conducted with the aim of utilizing these properties for the development of new pharmaceutical agents, particularly in the fields of oncology and neurology. For example, certain venom components from snakes are currently under investigation with a view to determining their efficacy in the inhibition of the growth of tumours and metastasis (Kang et al., 2011). Furthermore, the ongoing advancements in peptide synthesis and modification have the potential to facilitate the development of biotoxin-based therapeutics with enhanced efficacy and a reduction in side effects.
4. Bioremediation and Environmental Management: The presence of biotoxins in the environment can have severe consequences, particularly in aquatic ecosystems. New and innovative bioremediation techniques are being devised in order to mitigate the adverse effects that have been observed. The use of microorganisms and plants that are genetically modified to degrade or neutralize biotoxins represents a viable and sustainable strategy for the management of a contaminated environment (Singh et al., 2018). The integration of these methods with ecological engineering practices has been observed to facilitate ecosystem restoration in affected ecosystems.
5. Synthetic Biology and Bioengineering: The use of synthetic biology in the field of biotoxin research is paving the way for the generation of novel biotoxins with specific properties that can be tailored to meet specific needs. By means of genetic engineering, researchers are able to create microbes that produce biotoxins with particular characteristics, which may include enhancing stability or target specificity. This approach not only facilitates an in-depth understanding of the basic biology of toxins but can also enable the development of new tools and products for biotechnology (Nielsen et al., 2016).
6. Regulatory and Safety Innovations: As research into biotoxins continues to progress, it becomes increasingly apparent that there is a pressing need for the implementation of robust regulatory

frameworks alongside comprehensive safety protocols. The development of novel approaches to the assessment of risk and the conduct of safety testing is of the utmost importance in ensuring the secure deployment of biotoxins across a range of applications. It is of paramount importance that collaborative initiatives be undertaken between researchers, regulatory authorities and industry stakeholders in order to facilitate the development of regulatory frameworks which can adapt to the pace of technological advancement (Wu et al., 2019).

7. Interdisciplinary Collaboration: In order to advance the field of biotoxin research, it is imperative to foster interdisciplinary collaboration. By integrating knowledge from diverse fields, including biochemistry, computational biology, microbiology and environmental science, we can gain a comprehensive understanding of biological toxins and their potential usage. The advancement of comprehensive strategies to address biotoxin-related challenges is being propelled by collaborative research initiatives and international consortia (Zhou et al., 2017).

8.10 Conclusion

In conclusion to this examination of biotoxins, it becomes evident that a compelling image emerges. The potential applications of biotoxins across a wide range of industries are extensive, with considerable scope for innovation and exploitation in a multitude of ways. In the pharmaceutical and medical fields for drug development and therapeutics, pain management and cancer treatment; in agriculture, a novel approach to pest management involves harnessing naturally occurring biotoxins to provide an alternative to the use of synthetic chemicals; in the cosmetic industry, which confers particular advantages in the field of anti-ageing and skincare products; in industrial applications for prevention of biofouling, disruption of biofilms and bioremediation.

As research progresses, it is likely that the scope of applications for biotoxins will be extended. Their exceptional qualities, derived from the natural world, present novel solutions to some of humanity's most urgent concerns across a diverse range of fields. The utilization of biotoxins by industry enables greater efficiency and effectiveness while also contributing to the sustainability of the planet. This, in turn, facilitates a future where bio-solutions will play a pivotal role in the advancement of industries and technology. Nevertheless, the advancement and implementation of biotoxins must be undertaken with a resolute commitment to the observance of safety regulations and the upholding of ethical standards. The concept of responsible development is contingent upon rigorous testing and compliance with safety regulations and ethical considerations. By prioritizing the principles of safety and ethical responsibility, industries can responsibly exploit the potential benefits of biotoxins, ensuring that these benefits are not compromised by any ethical lapses or breaches of public safety standards. As society increasingly values sustainability and natural solutions, the role of biotoxins in driving innovation and addressing global challenges will become ever more significant.

Overall, while there are inherent risks associated with biotoxins, their potential applications across numerous fields are significant. By giving priority to the principles of safety, ethics and responsibility, research into biotoxins can make a significant contribution to scientific development and societal well-being. The field has considerable promise in addressing some of the most pressing challenges humanity currently faces, including those related to agriculture, health and environmental management.

References

Abd-Elgawad, M. M. M. (2021). Photorhabdus spp.: An overview of the beneficial aspects of mutualistic bacteria of insecticidal nematodes. *Plants (Basel, Switzerland), 10*(8), 1660. https://doi.org/10.3390/plants10081660

Alexa, M., Kaufer, A. C., Theis, T., Lau, K. A., Gray, J. L., & Rawlinson, W. D. (2020). Biological warfare: The history of microbial pathogens, biotoxins and emerging threats. *Microbiology Australia*, 116–122.

Alonso, E., Vale, C., Vieytes, M. R., Laferla, F. M., Giménez-Llort, L., & Botana, L. M. (2011). 13-Desmethyl spirolide-C is neuroprotective and reduces intracellular Aβ and hyperphosphorylated tau in vitro. *Neurochemistry International, 59*(8), 1056–1065. https://doi.org/10.1016/j.neuint.2011.08.013

Alvarez, C., Soto, C., Cabezas, S., Alvarado-Mesén, J., Laborde, R., Pazos, F., Ros, U., Hernández, A. M., & Lanio, M. E. (2021). Panorama of the intracellular molecular concert orchestrated by actinoporins, pore-forming toxins from sea anemones. *Toxins, 13*(8), 567.

Anderson, D. M., Glibert, P. M., & Burkholder, J. M. (2002). Harmful algal blooms and eutrophication: Nutrient sources, composition, and consequences. *Estuaries, 25*(4), 704–726.

Aransiola, S. A., Oyewole, O. A., Maddela, N. R., Ijah, U. J. J., & Manjunatha, B. (Eds.). (2024). *Marine Greens: Environmental, Agricultural, Industrial and Biomedical Applications* (1st ed.). Boca Raton, FL: CRC Press, Taylor and Francis Group. https://doi.org/10.1201/9781003369738

Aransiola, S. A., Victor-Ekwebelem, M. O., Ikhumetse, A. A., & Abioye, O. P. (2021). Challenges and future prospects of biotechnology. In N. R. Maddela & L. C. García (Eds.), *Innovations in Biotechnology for a Sustainable Future*. Springer Nature, Switzerland AG. https://doi.org/10.1007/978-3-030-80108-3_20

Assunção, J., Guedes, A. C., & Malcata, F. X. (2017). Biotechnological and pharmacological applications of biotoxins and other bioactive molecules from dinoflagellates. *Marine Drugs, 15*(12), 393. https://doi.org/10.3390/md15120393

Baden, D. G., Abraham, W. M., & Bourdelais, A. J. (2008). Polyether brevetoxin derivatives as a treatment for cystic fibrosis, mucociliary dysfunction, and pulmonary diseases. U.S. Patent No. US7399782B2. U.S. Patent and Trademark Office.

Bala, S., Garg, D., Thirumalesh, B. V., Sharma, M., Sridhar, K., Inbaraj, B. S., & Tripathi, M. (2022). Recent strategies for bioremediation of emerging pollutants: A review for a green and sustainable environment. *Toxics, 10*(8), 484. https://doi.org/10.3390/toxics10080484

Brazzelli, M., Cruickshank, M., Tassie, E., et al. (2015). Collagenase clostridium histolyticum for the treatment of Dupuytren's contracture: Systematic review and economic evaluation. *Southampton (UK): NIHR Journals Library,* October (Health Technology Assessment, No. 19.90.). Chapter 1, Background. Available from: https://www.ncbi.nlm.nih.gov/books/NBK326592/

Carmichael, W. W. (1992). Cyanobacteria secondary metabolites—The cyanotoxins. *Journal of Applied Bacteriology, 72*(6), 445–459.

Chandra Sekhar, J., Sandhya, S., Vinod, K. R., Banji, D., Sudhakar, K., & Chaitanya, R. S. N. A. K. K. (2012). Plant toxins-useful and harmful effects. *HYGEIA - Journal for Drugs and Medicines, 4*(1), 79–90.

Chen, S., Wang, X., Yang, H., & Zhao, Q. (2017). Nanomaterial-based biosensors for detection of biotoxins. *Journal of Nanomaterials, 2017*(1), 1–11.

Cho, K., Heo, J., Han, J., Hong, H. D., Jeon, H., Hwang, H., Hong, C., Kim, D., Han, J. W., & Baek, K. (2020). Industrial applications of dinoflagellate phycotoxins based on their modes of action: A review. *Toxins, 12*(12), 805. https://doi.org/10.3390/toxins12120805

Flieger, M., Wurst, M., & Shelby, R. (2019). Ergot alkaloids—Sources, structures and biological effects. *Toxins, 1*(2), 95–142. https://doi.org/10.3390/toxins1020095

Fu, H., & Yang, S. T. (2022). Editorial: Development and application of clostridia as microbial cell-factories for biofuels and biochemicals production. *Frontiers in Bioengineering and Biotechnology, 9,* 831135. https://doi.org/10.3389/fbioe.2021.831135

Hallegraeff, G. M. (1993). A review of harmful algal blooms and their apparent global increase. *Phycologia, 32,* 79–99. https://doi.org/10.2216/i0031-8884-32-2-79.1

Hamad, G., Hafez, E. E., Sobhy, S. E., Mehany, T., Elfayoumy, R. A., Elghazaly, E. M., Eskander, M., Tawfik, R. G., Hussein, S. M., & Pereira, L. (2023). Detection of Clostridium botulinum in some Egyptian fish products, its control in vitro using Citrus leaves extracts, and applicability of Citrus limon leaf extract in tuna. *Foods, 12*(14), 1466. https://doi.org/10.3390/foods12071466

Harris, J. B. (2018). Cholera: Immunity and prospects in vaccine development. *The Journal of Infectious Diseases, 218*(Suppl_3), S141–S146. https://doi.org/10.1093/infdis/jiy414

Hölker, U., Höfer, M., & Lenz, J. (2004). Biotechnological advantages of laboratory-scale solid-state fermentation with fungi. *Applied Microbiology and Biotechnology, 64*(2), 175–186. https://doi.org/10.1007/s00253-003-1503-3

Huan, Y., Kong, Q., Mou, H., & Yi, H. (2020). Antimicrobial peptides: Classification, design, application, and research progress in multiple fields. *Frontiers in Microbiology, 11,* 582779. https://doi.org/10.3389/fmicb.2020.582779

Hudnell, H. K. (Ed.). (2008). *Cyanobacterial Harmful Algal Blooms: State of the Science and Research Needs*. Springer.

Ibrahim, M. A., Griko, N., Junker, M., & Bulla, L. A. (2010). Bacillus thuringiensis: A genomics and proteomics perspective. *Bioengineered Bugs, 1*(1), 31–50. https://doi.org/10.4161/bbug.1.1.10519

Ilgaz Aydinlar, E., Yalinay Dikmen, P., & Sağduyu Kocaman, A. (2013). Botulinum toxin in migraine treatment. *Noro Psikiyatri Arsivi, 50*(Suppl 1), S36–S40. https://doi.org/10.4274/npa.y7198

Jiang, L., Wang, W., Yang, S., & Yu, H. (2018). Genomic insights into the production of biotoxins by harmful algal blooms. *Marine Genomics, 40*, 1–12.

Kang, T. S., Georgieva, D., Genov, N., Murakami, M. T., Sinha, M., Kumar, R. P.,. . . Kini, R. M. (2011). Enzymatic toxins from snake venom: Structural characterization and mechanism of catalysis. *Toxicon, 58*(2), 120–131.

Kattimani, V., Tiwari, R. V. C., Gufran, K., Wasan, B., Shilpa, P. H., & Khader, A. A. (2019). Botulinum toxin application in facial esthetics and recent treatment indications (2013–2018). *Journal of International Society of Preventive & Community Dentistry, 9*(2), 99–105. https://doi.org/10.4103/jispcd.JISPCD_430_18

Kenworthy, A. K., Schmieder, S. S., Raghunathan, K., Tiwari, A., Wang, T., Kelly, C. V., & Lencer, W. I. (2021). Cholera toxin as a probe for membrane biology. *Toxins, 13*, 543. https://doi.org/10.3390/toxins13080543

Kimple, M. E., Brill, A. L., & Pasker, R. L. (2013). Overview of affinity tags for protein purification. *Current Protocols in Protein Science, 73*, 9.9.1–9.9.23. https://doi.org/10.1002/0471140864.ps0909s73

Kocyigit, E., Kocaadam-Bozkurt, B., Bozkurt, O., Ağagündüz, D., & Capasso, R. (2023). Plant toxic proteins: Their biological activities, mechanism of action, and removal strategies. *Toxins, 15*(6), 356. https://doi.org/10.3390/toxins15060356

Kovacs, J. A., Hiemenz, J. W., & Ebb, G. (2021). Immunosuppressive effects of cyclosporine and tacrolimus. *Clinical Microbiology Reviews, 15*(1), 134–148. https://doi.org/10.1128/CMR.15.1.134-148.2002

Liu, C.-C., Yang, H., Zhang, L.-L., Zhang, Q., Chen, B., & Wang, Y. (2014). Biotoxins for cancer therapy. *Asian Pacific Journal of Cancer Prevention, 15*(12), 4753–4758.

Llewellyn, L. E. (2006). Saxitoxin, a toxic marine natural product that targets a multitude of receptors. *Natural Product Reports, 23*(2), 200–222.

McGeachan, R. I., Schwarz, T., Gunn-Moore, D. A., & Marioni-Henry, K. (2020). Botulinum toxin type A for the treatment of muscle contractures secondary to acute spinal cord injury in a young cat. *JFMS Open Reports, 6*(1), 2055116920922648. https://doi.org/10.1177/2055116920922648

Meriluoto, J., & Spoof, L. (2008). Cyanotoxins: Sampling, sample processing and toxin uptake. In H. K. Hudnell (Ed.), *Cyanobacterial Harmful Algal Blooms: State of the Science and Research Needs* (pp. 483–499). Springer.

Moss, M. O. (2018). Fungi, quality assurance and safety of foods. *Food Science and Technology International, 13*(2), 153–157. https://doi.org/10.1177/1082013206070566

Nielsen, A. A., Der, B. S., Shin, J., Vaidyanathan, P., Paralanov, V., Strychalski, E. A.,. . . Voigt, C. A. (2016). Genetic circuit design automation. *Science, 352*(6281), aac7341.

Ochieng, P. E., Kemboi, D. C., Scippo, M. L., Gathumbi, J. K., Kangethe, E., Doupovec, B.,. . . Okoth, S. (2022). Maximizing laboratory production of aflatoxins and fumonisins for use in experimental animal feeds. *Microorganisms, 10*(12), 2385. https://doi.org/10.3390/microorganisms10122385

Pandey, M., Choudhury, H., Vijayagomaran, P. A., Lian, P. N. P., Ning, T. J., Wai, N. Z.,. . . Amin, M. C. I. M. (2022). Recent update on bacteria as a delivery carrier in cancer therapy: From evil to allies. *Pharmaceutical Research, 39*(6), 1115–1134. https://doi.org/10.1007/s11095-022-03240-y

Patocka, J., Gupta, R. C., Wu, Q.-h., & Kuca, K. (2015). Toxic potential of palytoxin. *Journal of Huazhong University of Science and Technology [Medical Sciences], 35*, 773–780. https://doi.org/10.1007/s11596-015-1506-3

Paton, J. C., & Paton, A. W. (1998). Pathogenesis and diagnosis of Shiga toxin-producing Escherichia coli infections. *Clinical Microbiology Reviews, 11*(3), 450–479. https://doi.org/10.1128/CMR.11.3.450

Pradhan, B., & Ki, J.-S. (2022). Phytoplankton toxins and their potential therapeutic applications: A journey toward the quest for potent pharmaceuticals. *Marine Drugs, 20*(4), 271. https://doi.org/10.3390/md20040271

Pradhan, B., Kim, H., Abassi, S., & Ki, J. S. (2022). Toxic effects and tumor promotion activity of marine phytoplankton toxins: A review. *Toxins, 14*(6), 397. https://doi.org/10.3390/toxins14060397

Rubiolo, J., López-Alonso, H., Martínez, P., Millán, A., Cagide, E., Vieytes, M., Vega, F., & Botana, L. (2014). Yessotoxin induces ER-stress followed by autophagic cell death in glioma cells mediated by mTOR and BNIP3. *Cellular Signalling, 26*(2), 419–432. https://doi.org/10.1016/j.cellsig.2013.10.004

Sellner, K. G., Doucette, G. J., & Kirkpatrick, G. J. (2003). Harmful algal blooms: Causes, impacts and detection. *Journal of Industrial Microbiology and Biotechnology, 30*(7), 383–406.

Shafiee, F., Aucoin, M. G., & Jahanian-Najafabadi, A. (2019). Targeted diphtheria toxin-based therapy: A review article. *Frontiers in Microbiology, 10*, 2340. https://doi.org/10.3389/fmicb.2019.02340

Singh, B., Sharma, R., Kanwar, S. S., & Chauhan, A. (2018). Applications of microbial enzymes in the food industry. *Enzyme Research, 2018*. https://doi.org/10.1155/2018/1875137

Tyagi, N., Tyagi, M., Pachauri, M., & Ghosh, P. C. (2015). Potential therapeutic applications of plant toxin-ricin in cancer: Challenges and advances. *Tumour Biology, 36*(11), 8239–8246. https://doi.org/10.1007/s13277-015-4028-4

Vinale, F., Sivasithamparam, K., Ghisalberti, E. L., Marra, R., Ritieni, A., & Woo, S. L. (2017). Trichoderma-plant-pathogen interactions. *Soil Biology & Biochemistry, 40*(1), 1–10. https://doi.org/10.1016/j.soilbio.2007.07.002

Wang, D. (2008). Neurotoxins from marine dinoflagellates: A brief review. *Marine Drugs, 6*, 349–371. https://doi.org/10.3390/md20080016

Wolosker, N. J. R., Milanez de Campos, J. R., & Fukuda, J. M. (2016). Management of compensatory sweating after sympathetic surgery. *Thoracic Surgery Clinics, 26*(4), 445–451.

Wu, S., Wang, Y., Zhang, M., & Liu, J. (2019). Regulatory considerations and safety assessment of biotoxins in food. *Food Control, 96*, 59–68.

Zhou, Y., Li, H., Wang, Z., & Liu, Y. (2017). Interdisciplinary approaches in biotoxin research: Perspectives and challenges. *Toxicon, 142*, 20–27.

Zhu, X., Zhao, Y., Wu, L., Gao, X., Huang, H., Han, Y., & Zhu, T. (2024). Advances in biosensors for the rapid detection of marine biotoxins: Current status and future perspectives. *Biosensors, 14*(4), 203. https://doi.org/10.3390/bios14040203

9

Applications of Animal Toxins: Traditional and Modern Techniques

Peace Abiodun Olajide, Babatunde Oluwafemi Adetuyi, Victoria Olufunmi Adeyemo-Eleyode, Charles Chinazaekpele Chidume, Oluwatosin Adefunke Adetuyi, and Ayobami Ifeoluwa Awe

9.1 Introduction

Natural selection poses a threat to all species; thus living things must adapt to their changing surroundings and compete with other living things (Darwin, 1859). Over the course of evolution, certain features conferring benefits related to basic necessities have given some species an advantage over others. Thus, poisons and venoms are the result of natural selection. As a result, poisons and venoms have developed separately over time and are present in a wide range of taxa, such as microorganisms, plants, mollusks, arthropods, and reptiles. These poisons can have a variety of negative effects, including hemorrhage, necrosis, and neurological toxicity. They are made up of several different substances, such as protein molecules, fragments of DNA, enzymatic components, and inorganic particles (Fry et al., 2009). In the majority of cases, venoms have developed through ongoing, long-term coevolution as defensive and predatory tactics in organisms. For example, over evolution, some snake prey or predators have developed resistance to snake venom multiple times (Biardi & Coss, 2011; Jansa & Voss, 2011). Given the high molecular diversity found in the targets of toxins, such as routes of transmission, enzymatic agents, receptors, and other physiological components, it is easy to understand how evolution can be responsible for the various chemical makeup of venomous substances that target these elements. These venoms contain highly concentrated and powerful toxins (Zhang, 2015). Furthermore, given the high metabolic cost of venom synthesis, their component effects are frequently synergistic, which is a crucial adaptation to limit the amount of venom discharged (Nisani et al., 2007, 2012).

Many animal toxins have coevolved with humans since we have evolved alongside venomous animals. Furthermore, animal envenomation is a major

DOI: 10.1201/9781003500605-11

source of mortality and morbidity and has historically affected the entire world (Kasturiratne et al., 2008; Balhara & Stolbach, 2014). Thus, the original goals of the study of animal venoms and toxins were to counteract the effects of venom and treat animal envenomation. Nonetheless, Felice Fontana, an Italian naturalist, began studying how snake venom affects blood coagulation in 1781. Eventually, by the 1890s, scientists Albert Calmette, Césaire Auguste Phisalix, and Gabriel Bertrand had created the first antivenom therapy (Calmette, 1894; Phisalix & Bertrand, 1894). But as our understanding of the physiology of poisons and venoms grew, these compounds turned from enemy to ally and became invaluable research tools. Natural poisons have been employed as research tools for a long time. Through tests using a pufferfish toxin, the significance of Na+ and K+ channels to the action potential was identified (Narahashi et al., 1969). Nicotinic receptors were successfully purified and cloned thanks to the extraction of toxins from snake venom, such as α-bungarotoxin and cobratoxin (Changeux et al., 1970). Subgroups of various toxins created by biotechnological engineering allowed studies of multiple subtypes of voltage-dependent Ca^{2+} channels (VDCCs), and the ω-conotoxin obtained from fish-eating marine snails, Conus snails, was also essential for N-type Ca^{2+} channel study (Olivera et al., 1987; McEnery et al., 1991).

Notably, a number of species' venoms are being studied for their potential to treat a wide range of pathologies, such as cancer, autoimmune diseases, cardiovascular disorders, and pain (Brunner et al., 1980; Ye et al., 2016). Because of the great diversity of compounds present in the venom of various kinds of animals and their exceptional sensitivity to cell targets, the pharmacological study of toxins is an exciting field. As a result, when our knowledge of neurological ailments advances and new therapeutic targets are identified, the likelihood of employing animal poisons as the main prospects for drug development increases.

9.1.1 Animal Toxins' Therapeutic Uses in Diseases

Animal venoms are complex mixtures. Ingredients in mixtures have the ability to pharmacologically affect pertinent human medical conditions in addition to acting efficiently and selectively on target proteins. In numerous studies, the components of venoms from different species have been examined. Numerous species' poisons frequently differ structurally and have minimal sequence homology. It is important to remember that different proteins or toxin peptides from various organisms can act on the same target; yet, depending on their unique properties and inhibitory effects on the target proteins, the effects of those toxins may vary. The foundation of drug design is composed of toxins possessing appropriate inhibitory activity, high potency, and high specificity. The following sections highlight toxins that have been linked to specific diseases or activities.

9.2 Anticancer Activity

Cancer is a disease that can arise from a variety of factors, such as genetic or environmental mutations, infections with pathogens, unhealthy lifestyle choices, or drug misuse. These factors can cause aberrant cells to divide uncontrollably in a particular portion of the body, which can have a direct impact on a person's quality of life or even cause death. Many treatments have been tried to inhibit the growth of cancerous cells or to eradicate tissue that has the potential to become cancerous. Radiation therapy and/or chemotherapy are frequently utilized in conjunction with surgical operations. Small molecular weight chemicals, which frequently lack target specificity and carry a higher risk of undesirable side effects like bone marrow toxicity, cardiotoxicity, and immunosuppression that increases the risk of infection, are the basis of chemotherapy. The development of antitumor drugs derived from natural animal venoms has emerged as a novel approach to address these issues. Toxins derived from natural resources generally show strong lethal effects on malignant cells through changes to the cell cycle, suppression of enzyme activity, impairment of cancer proliferation, and modulation of the apoptosis response pathway. Among these, snake venom is a plentiful supply of cytotoxins for research on cancer. A variety of snake venom components have been identified, including lectins, metalloproteinases, aggretin, disintegrins, rhodostomin, and cytotoxins (CT1, CT2, and CT3). Some of these components have been shown to be effective in treating different types of human cancers (Macedo et al., 2015; Calderon et al., 2014; Alabi et al., 2023).

It has been found that ion channel expression on the cell surface is changed or abnormal in illness and cancer processes. As a result, ion channels including Na^+, K^+, Ca^{2+}, and Cl^- that are targeted by animal venoms may have specific effects on cancer cells. Animal venoms, such as those from bees, scorpions, spiders, and other species, have been researched for their anticancer properties. They concentrate on ion channels in different kinds of cancer. Examples of mechanisms by which the anticancer effect of AGAP peptide from BmK scorpion venom is confirmed include alteration of the cell cycle and interaction with elements necessary for modifying signaling pathways related to cell viability and development, cell death, cell proliferation, and so forth. Voltage-gated sodium channels are selectively inhibited by AGAP peptide (Zhao et al., 2011). Other ion channel-related scorpion toxins, such as chlorotoxin, may also have anticancer effects (Ding et al., 2014). Additionally, anticancer actions have been reported for venom components from various animal taxa, such as the family Bufonidae, bees, and spiders (Mahadevappa et al., 2017; Oršolić, 2012).

9.3 Using Animal Venom to Treat Neurological Conditions

The degenerative illness known as neurodegeneration is what eventually leads to neurons' death, causing them to lose their structures or functions. Millions of people worldwide are impacted by neurodegenerative disorders, which include multiple sclerosis, amyotrophic lateral sclerosis, Parkinson's disease (PD), Alzheimer's disease (AD), Huntington's disease, epilepsy, and others. There is an urgent need to investigate effective medications because many diseases are now incurable and lack a particularly effective therapy for treatment. Neurodegeneration can result from a variety of mechanisms, including aging, aggregation formation, cellular death, mutations in genes, protein misfolding, and stress. Given the lengthy evolutionary history of humans and prey and predator animals, a number of animal venom components exhibit exceptional selectivity and affinity for various targets located in human central nervous systems. According to a recent study, there is a wealth of neuroactive chemicals found in animal venoms. These compounds are good prospects for the development of new medications and can be utilized as pharmacological therapy tools to study the pathological evolution of neurodegenerative disorders. For instance, a great deal of study has been conducted on the potential therapeutic applications of neuroactively rich snake venoms for neurodegenerative illnesses. Dendrotoxins are beneficial in treating AD caused by acetylcholine shortages because they have the ability to block the K+ channel and increase acetylcholine synthesis. These dendrotoxins are obtained from the venom of African mambas, namely from the *Dendroaspis* genus. In an animal model of AD, the amyloid b-protein (Ab), one of the constituents of amyloid plaques, can be broken down by metalloproteases derived from snake venom (Nalivaeva et al., 2012). Bee venom (*Apis mellifera*) has been shown to have an anti-inflammatory impact in a number of animal models of Parkinson's disease. It can also reduce oxidative stress, CD^{4+} T cell infiltration, and microglial activation while improving motor coordination and balance (Awad et al., 2017; de Souza et al., 2018).

9.4 Analgesic Action

Neuropathic discomfort is defined as a chronic pain syndrome resulting from injured or improperly functioning neurons (Hamad et al., 2018). In the course of pain signals traveling through neurons, presynaptic neurons produce excitatory or inhibitory neurotransmitters that either activate or inhibit neurons that are postsynaptic (Figure 9.1).

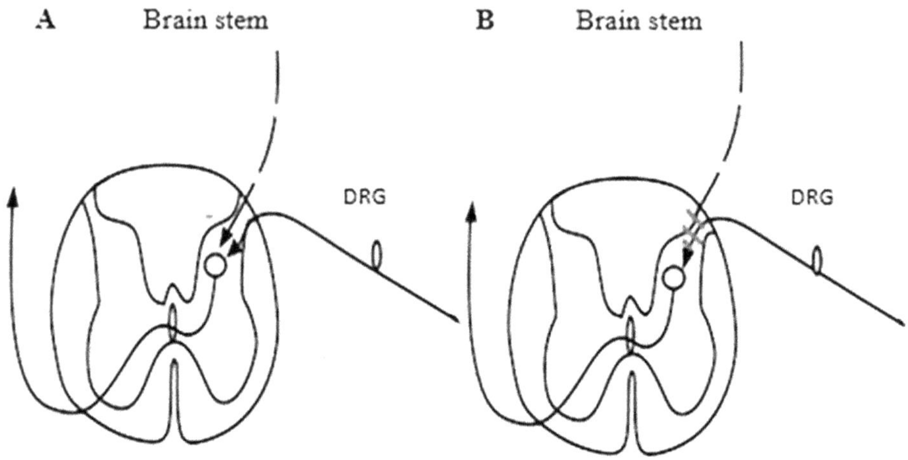

FIGURE 9.1
Neural mechanisms in the spinal cord that inhibit pain. The two methods whereby nociceptive primary afferent nerve fibers in the spinal cord can be inhibited from transmitting pain signals are shown in diagrams A and B. (A) The suppression of pain signaling at the postsynaptic level. (B) Indirect presynaptic suppression of pain signals through voluminously sent inhibitory neurotransmitter emanating from descending inhibitory axon in the brain stem.

Toxins that are permitted to alter the transmission of neuronal signals can target several channels and transporters that are involved in the release of neurotransmitters or Ca^{2+} fluxes. Promising treatment possibilities may include toxins with high selectivity and specificity towards their targets. One such is the 25 amino acid x-conotoxin MVII A found in cone snails, which blocks the N-type CaV2.2 voltage-gated calcium channel (VGCC) on the central synapses of the spinal cord's primary sensory dorsal root ganglion (DRG) neurons, or nociceptors (Adams & Berecki, 2013). The secondary pain sensory neuron's action potential generation is inhibited and the transmission of pain signals is stopped when the CaV2.2 channel in presynaptic neurons is blocked. Ziconotide, a synthetic form of x conotoxin MVII A, has been used as Prialt, a medication for treating neuropathic pain, due to its great potency. Moreover, the *Conus marmoreus*–isolated Chi-conotoxin MrIA noncompetitively inhibits the norepinephrine transporter (NET) on a terminal of descending axons in the brain stem. The neurotransmitter noradrenaline's reuptake is inhibited when Chi-conotoxin MrIA blocks NET in the presynaptic membrane; it raises the synaptic cleft's noradrenaline levels. Two methods are available for preventing the spread of pain impulses when descending axon terminals release the pain transmitter noradrenaline: the first is through postsynaptic inhibition, which involves hyperpolarizing cell membrane potentials and inhibiting spinal relay neurons' activity; the second is known as presynaptic inhibition, and it includes using noradrenaline volume transmission to block the nociceptive primary afferent fibers' ability to function end to end, delaying the generation of action potentials and preventing the upward propagation of signals that cause pain (Pertovaara & Almeida, 2006). Toxin-derived drugs are frequently evaluated using behavioral tests for the in vivo treatment of neuropathic pain, including the mouse allodynia model (Nielsen et al., 2005) and hypersensitivity (Gbata et al., 2005). According to Sharpe et al. (2003), clinical phase II trials have been conducted using Xen2174 (13 amino acids), the synthetic form of Chi-conotoxin MrIA, to treat neuropathic pain.

9.5 Cardiovascular Diseases

A group of illnesses known as cardiovascular disease includes thromboembolic disease, heart failure, hypertensive heart disease, stroke, and other conditions affecting the heart and blood arteries. Venom-based medications are used to successfully treat a number of cardiovascular conditions. Drawn from the venom of the cantil snake, the well-known toxin bradykinin-potentiating peptide b (BPPb) lowers blood pressure by preferentially attaching to an enzyme on tissue surfaces and blocking the human angiotensin-converting enzyme (ACE). Renin-angiotensin systems state that the enzyme ACE, which is found on the outside of kidney and lung endothelial cells, is necessary to produce angiotensin II (AngII), which raises blood pressure (Masuyer et al., 2012). The cleavage of bradykinin, a vasodilator that lowers blood pressure, is likewise accomplished by the enzyme ACE. As a result, blood pressure eventually drops because the suppressed ACE is unable to cleave bradykinin and create AngII, a vasoconstrictor. The small molecule medication Capoten (captopril), which was created based on structure-activity investigations of BPPs, has been used extensively to treat hypertension. However, because of the free thiol group in the captopril molecule, this medication may have a number of negative consequences. Therefore, peptide BPPs with optimal structural forms would be better for treating hypertension with fewer adverse effects.

Antithrombotics are also discovered to be beneficial from venoms. When a blood clot forms inside the blood vessels, thrombosis occurs, obstructing the blood vessels that supply the cardiovascular system. Platelet aggregation is a crucial step in the production of thrombus (Scarborough et al., 1991). Platelets bind to the sub-endothelial layer of collagen in blood vessels via binding with sticky proteins (fibrinogen and von Willebrand factor) and receptors (integrins). Collagen binding then causes platelets to become activated, which in turn causes intra-platelet signaling and downstream kinase cascades. In the meantime, the integrin superfamily member platelet receptor glycoprotein (GP)IIb-IIIa is transformed into its active state to initiate platelet aggregation (Scarborough et al., 1991). Tergeminin, echistatin, and eristicophin are among the other venom peptides that function as "disintegrins," preventing sticky proteins from attaching to integrins (Scarborough et al., 1991). According to Lewis and Garcia (2003), researchers are certain that disintegrins' ability to prevent platelet aggregation is what gives them their anti-thrombotic properties.

9.6 Autoimmune Diseases

An aberrant immune reaction to a healthy body part can result in an autoimmune illness. There is a need for medications that work on the target with reduced adverse effects and with selectivity and specificity. Previous studies have shown that during the T lymphocyte immune response, the voltage-gated potassium channel KV1.3 and the calcium-activated K+ channel (KCa) affect the membrane potential and calcium signaling in T cells (Shen et al., 2017). Autoimmune disorders are characterized by the up-regulated expression of KV1.3 in T and B cells (Wang et al., 2016). Certain poisons found in the venoms of sea anemones and scorpions have been shown to suppress the KV1.3 channel. This decreases the activation of effector memory T (TEM) and the release of associated cytokines, which in turn lessens the symptoms of autoimmune disorders. A small number of toxins, based on their potencies, specificities, and inhibitory activities (Kd and IC50, EC50) to this channel, can be used as treatments for autoimmune illnesses, despite the fact that several toxins, including ShK, BmKTX, OSK1, HsTX1, and others, can block the KV1.3 channel [39]. The chemically produced version of the toxin ShK (ShK-186) (Wang et al., 2016), which is produced using an artificial amino acid, is currently employed in phase II clinical studies and exhibits improved selectivity to the KV1.3 channel (Shen et al., 2017). In addition to the improvement of poisons through synthetic versions, a great deal of research focuses on toxin-antibody fusion proteins as therapeutics. Previous work reported good potency, specificity, and inhibitory action of toxin Vm24 fused in the CDR loop of an antibody (Wang et al., 2016). All things considered, the development of therapeutics for a range of illnesses could greatly benefit from research on animal poisons.

9.7 Conclusion

The wide range of animal toxins remains fascinating to practitioners and academics alike, providing a wealth of ideas for both conventional and cutting-edge methods. The wide range of uses for these toxins highlights their enormous potential, from traditional medicine-based cures to cutting-edge developments in biotechnology and medication research. Uncovering the mysteries hidden in animal venoms and poisons could help us solve a wide range of problems in agriculture, medicine, and other fields as we work to close the gap between tradition and innovation. Accepting the complementary nature of modern science and conventional wisdom creates new opportunities for using animal toxins for human benefit.

References

Adams DJ, Berecki G (2013). Mechanisms of conotoxin inhibition of N-type (Ca(v)2.2) calcium channels. *Biochim Biophys Acta* 1828:1619–1628.

Alabi MA, Arowolo MA, Na'Allah A, Prabhkar PK, Linus EG, Aransiola SA, et al. (2023). Phytochemicals and anticancer activity of methanol extract of *Trigonella foenum-greacum* seed on breast cancer cell lines. *S Afr J Bot* 160:273–281. https://doi.org/10.1016/j.sajb.2023.07.021

Awad K, Abushouk AI, AbdelKarim AH, Mohammed M, Negida A, Shalash AS (2017). Bee venom for the treatment of Parkinson's disease: How far is it possible? *Biomed Pharmacother* 91:295–302.

Balhara KS, Stolbach A. (2014). Marine envenomations. *Emerg Med Clin North Am* 32:223–243. doi: 10.1016/j.emc.2013.09.009

Biardi JE, Coss RG (2011). Rock squirrel (Spermophilus variegatus) blood sera affects the proteolytic and hemolytic activities of rattlesnake venoms. *Toxicon* 57: 323–331. doi: 10.1016/j.toxicon.2010.12.011

Brunner HR, Gavras H, Waeber B, Textor SC, Turini GA, Wauters JP (1980). Clinical use of an orally acting converting enzyme inhibitor: Captopril. *Hypertension* 2:558–566. doi: 10.1161/01.HYP.2.4.558

Calderon LA, Sobrinho JC, Zaqueo KD, de Moura AA, Grabner AN, Mazzi MV, et al. (2014). Antitumoral activity of snake venom proteins: New trends in cancer therapy. *Biomed Res Int* 2014:203639.

Calmette A (1894). L'immunisation artificielle des animaux contre le venin des serpents, et la thérapeutique expérimentale des morsures venimeuses. *C R Soc Biol* 46:120–124.

Changeux JP, Kasai M, Lee CY (1970). Use of a snake venom toxin to characterize the cholinergic receptor protein. *Proc Natl Acad Sci USA* 67:1241–1247. doi: 10.1073/pnas.67.3.1241

Darwin CR (1859). *On the origin of species*. John Murray, London.

de Souza JM, Goncalves BDC, Gomez MV, Vieira LB, Ribeiro FM (2018). Animal toxins as therapeutic tools to treat neurodegenerative diseases. *Front Pharmacol* 9:145.

Ding J, Chua PJ, Bay BH, Gopalakrishnakone P (2014). Scorpion venoms as a potential source of novel cancer therapeutic compounds. *Exp Biol Med (Maywood)* 239:387–393.

Fry BG, Roelants K, Champagne DE, Scheib H, Tyndall JD, King GF, et al. (2009). The toxicogenomic multiverse: Convergent recruitment of proteins into animal venoms. *Annu Rev Genomics Hum Genet* 10:483–511. doi: 10.1146/annurev.genom.9.081307.164356

Hamad MK, He K, Abdulrazeq HF, Mustafa AM, Luceri R, Kamal N, et al. (2018). Potential uses of isolated toxin peptides in neuropathic pain relief: A literature review. *World Neurosurg* 113(333–347):e335.

Jansa SA, Voss RS (2011). Adaptive evolution of the venom-targeted vWF protein in opossums that eat pitvipers. *PLoS One* 6:e20997. doi: 10.1371/journal.pone.0020997

Kasturiratne A, Wickremasinghe AR, de Silva N, Gunawardena NK, Pathmeswaran A, Premaratna R, et al. (2008). The global burden of snakebite: A literature analysis and modeling based on regional estimates of envenoming and deaths. *PLoS Med* 5:e218. doi: 10.1371/journal.pmed.0050218

Lewis RJ, Garcia ML (2003). Therapeutic potential of venom peptides. *Nat Rev Drug Discov* 2:790–802.

Macedo JKA, Fox JW, de Souza Castro M (2015). Disintegrins from snake venoms and their applications in cancer research and therapy. *Curr Protein Pept Sci* 16:532–548.

Mahadevappa R, Ma R, Kwok HF (2017). Venom peptides: Improving specificity in cancer therapy. *Trends Cancer* 3:611–614.

Masuyer G, Schwager SL, Sturrock ED, Isaac RE, Acharya KR (2012). Molecular recognition and regulation of human angiotensin-I converting enzyme (ACE) activity by natural inhibitory peptides. *Sci Rep* 2:717.

McEnery MW, Snowman AM, Snyder SH (1991). Evidence for subtypes of the omega-conotoxin GVIA receptor. Identification of the properties intrinsic to the high-affinity receptor. *Ann N Y Acad Sci* 635:435–437. doi: 10.1111/j.1749-6632.1991.tb36519.x

Nalivaeva NN, Beckett C, Belyaev ND, Turner AJ (2012). Are amyloid-degrading enzymes viable therapeutic targets in Alzheimer's disease? *J Neurochem* 120(Suppl 1):167–185.

Narahashi T, Moore JW, Frazier DT (1969). Dependence of tetrodotoxin blockage of nerve membrane conductance on external pH. *J Pharmacol Exp Ther* 169:224–228.

Nielsen CK, Lewis RJ, Alewood D, Drinkwater R, Palant E, Patterson M, et al. (2005). Anti-allodynic efficacy of the chi-conopeptide, Xen2174, in rats with neuropathic pain. *Pain* 118:112–124.

Nisani Z, Boskovic DS, Dunbar SG, Kelln W, Hayes WK (2012). Investigating the chemical profile of regenerated scorpion (Parabuthus transvaalicus) venom in relation to metabolic cost and toxicity. *Toxicon* 60:315–323. doi: 10.1016/j.toxicon.2012.04.343

Nisani Z, Dunbar SG, Hayes WK (2007). Cost of venom regeneration in Parabuthus transvaalicus (Arachnida: Buthidae). *Comp Biochem Physiol A Mol Integr Physiol* 147:509–513. doi: 10.1016/j.cbpa.2007.01.027

Olivera BM, Cruz LJ, de Santos V, LeCheminant GW, Griffin D, Zeikus R, et al. (1987). Neuronal calcium channel antagonists. Discrimination between calcium channel subtypes using omega-conotoxin from Conus magus venom. *Biochemistry* 26:2086–2090. doi: 10.1021/bi00382a004

Oršolić N (2012). Bee venom in cancer therapy. *Cancer Metastasis Rev* 31:173–194.

Ouyang C, Teng C-M, Huang T-F (1990). Characterization of snake venom principles affecting blood coagulation and platelet aggregation. In: Liu CY, Chien S (eds) *Fibrinogen, thrombosis, coagulation, and fibrinolysis*. Springer, Boston, pp. 151–163.

Pertovaara A, Almeida A (2006). Chapter 13 Descending inhibitory systems. In: Cervero F, Jensen TS (eds) *Handbook of clinical neurology*. Elsevier, New York, pp. 179–192.

Phisalix C, Bertrand G. (1894). Sur la propriété antitoxique du sang des animaux vaccinés contre le venin de vipère. *C R Acad Sci* 46:111–113.

Scarborough RM, Rose JW, Hsu MA, Phillips DR, Fried VA, Campbell AM, et al. (1991). Barbourin. A GPIIb-IIIa-specific integrin antagonist from the venom of Sistrurus m. barbouri. *J Biol Chem* 266:9359–9362.

Sharpe IA, Palant E, Schroeder CI, Kaye DM, Adams DJ, Alewood PF, Lewis RJ (2003). Inhibition of the norepinephrine transporter by the venom peptide chi-MrIA. Site of action, Na+ dependence, and structure-activity relationship. *J Biol Chem* 278:40317–40323

Shen B, Cao Z, Li W, Sabatier JM, Wu Y (2017). Treating autoimmune disorders with venom-derived peptides. *Expert Opin Biol Ther* 17:1065–1075

Wang RE, Wang Y, Zhang Y, Gabrelow C, Zhang Y, Chi V, et al. (2016). Rational design of a KV1.3 channel-blocking antibody as a selective immunosuppressant. *Proc Natl Acad Sci USA* 113:11501–11506.

Ye M, Chung HS, Lee C, Yoon MS, Yu AR, Kim JS, et al. (2016). Neuroprotective effects of bee venom phospholipase A2 in the 3xTg AD mouse model of Alzheimer's disease. *J Neuroinflammation* 13:10. doi: 10.1186/s12974-016-0476-z

Zhang Y. (2015). Why do we study animal toxins? *Dongwuxue Yanjiu* 36:183–222.

Zhao Y, Cai X, Ye T, Huo J, Liu C, Zhang S, Cao P (2011). Analgesicantitumor peptide inhibits proliferation and migration of SHG-44 human malignant glioma cells. *J Cell Biochem* 112:2424–2434.

10

The Potential of Biotoxins for Drug Discovery and Development

Adekunle Rowaiye, Lorretha Emenyeonu, Ezinne Janefrances Nwonu, Grace Onyukwo Abakpa, Doofan Bur, and Gordon Ibeanu

10.1 Introduction

Biotoxins are toxic substances produced by living organisms, including plants, animals, fungi, bacteria, aquatic species, insects, reptiles, and amphibians (El-Masry et al. 2015). These naturally occurring toxins can be harmful or lethal to other organisms, including humans, and often serve as a defense mechanism for the producing organism (Janik et al. 2019).

Biotoxins can affect biological systems in various ways, depending on their structure and the target organism. Some common mechanisms of action of biotoxins include enzymatic activity in which they disrupt cellular processes (Janik et al. 2019); membrane disruption, causing cell lysis and death (Sitprija and Sitprija 2019); binding to specific receptors on cells; and blocking normal cellular communication (Clark et al. 2019). Biotoxins also modulate signaling pathways by binding to receptors and altering downstream effects (Zhou et al. 2022).

Biotoxins, often associated with toxicity and harm, have garnered significant attention in recent years due to their potential medicinal properties. While traditionally viewed as harmful substances produced by living organisms, emerging research has unveiled a new perspective on biotoxins as therapeutic agents (Tariq et al. 2021). This paradigm shift has sparked exploration into harnessing the medicinal potential of biotoxins for various applications in healthcare and biotechnology (Wei and Zhang 2022).

The medicinal effect of biotoxins encompasses a wide range of bioactive compounds that exhibit diverse biological activities, including antimicrobial, anticancer, analgesic, anti-inflammatory, and immunomodulatory properties. Understanding and harnessing these properties have opened avenues for developing novel drugs, biologics, and therapeutic interventions with enhanced efficacy and reduced side effects compared to conventional treatments (Bordon et al. 2020).

DOI: 10.1201/9781003500605-12

This chapter explores the medicinal effect of biotoxins, delving into their mechanisms of action, pharmacological properties, and potential applications in disease management and biomedical research. By elucidating the therapeutic potential of biotoxins, this study aims to contribute to the growing body of knowledge in pharmacology and drug discovery, paving the way for innovative and sustainable healthcare solutions.

10.2 Materials and Methods

A search for relevant original research and review publications on the therapeutic effects of biotoxins, primarily published between 2018 and 2024, was conducted using the PubMed database and Google Scholar search engine. The search utilized keyword combinations such as "biotoxin AND anti-inflammatory," "biotoxin AND antimicrobial," "biotoxin AND anticoagulative," "biotoxin AND neuroregenerative," "biotoxin AND anti-diabetic," "biotoxin AND antihypertensive," and "biotoxin AND anticancer." All related articles were selected and reviewed, resulting in a total of 145 English-language articles.

10.3 Medicinal Effect of Biotoxins

The medicinal impact of biotoxins includes a variety of bioactive compounds that display a wide array of bioactivities (Figure 10.1 and Table 10.1).

10.4 Analgesic, Anti-Inflammatory, and Immunomodulatory Properties

Some biotoxins have been found to possess promising therapeutic properties, including analgesia, anti-inflammation, and immunomodulation (Upadhyay 2018). These natural compounds obtained from a broad spectrum of species are of significant interest to researchers because of their varying therapeutic prospects and distinctive modes of action in different models of pain (Zhou et al. 2022).

Analgesics, also known as painkillers or antinociceptives, are drugs used in the treatment and management of pain, and most analgesic agents currently in use centrally modulate the processing and transmission of pain

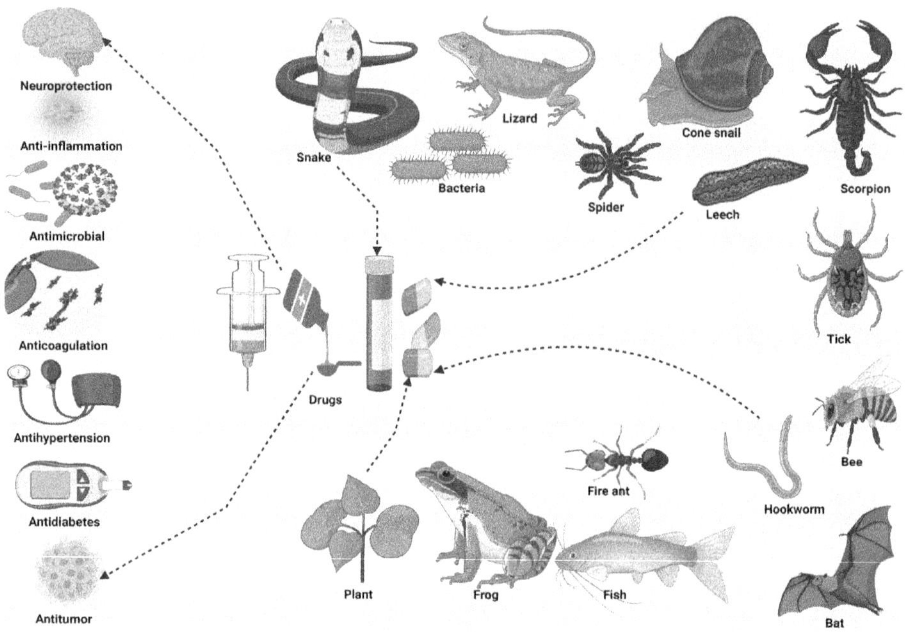

FIGURE 10.1
The medicinal effect of biotoxins. Created with Biorender.com.

TABLE 10.1
Biotoxins and Their Medicinal Effects

Organism	Scientific Name	Biotoxin	Medicinal Effect
Freshwater catfish	*Mystus gulio*	Spine sheath venom	Analgesic (Baskaradoss and Kumar 2018)
Spider (African rear-horned baboon tarantula)	*Ceratogyrus darlingi*	Biopeptide Cd1a	Analgesic (Sousa et al. 2017).
Spider	*Phoneutria nigriventer*	Venom	Analgesic (Pereira et al. 2023).
Bacteria	*Mycobacterium ulcerans*	Mycolactone	Analgesic (Guenin-macé et al. 2019).
Cone snails	*Conus virgo*	Crude venom	Anti-inflammatory (Mohamed et al. 2022)
Bee	*Apis mellifera*	Bee venom and apamin	Anti-inflammatory (Lee et al. 2020)
Egyptian scorpion	*Androctonus amoreuxi*	Crude venom	Anti-inflammatory (Hassan et al. 2019).

TABLE 10.1 ***(Continued)***

Biotoxins and Their Medicinal Effects

Organism	Scientific Name	Biotoxin	Medicinal Effect
Marine tunicate	*Phallusia nigra*	Tunic	Anti-inflammatory (Syed et al. 2021)
Zygophyllum-leaved heliotrope	*Heliotropium digynum*	pyrrolizidine alkaloid	Anti-inflammatory (Aboelmagd et al. 2018).
South American rattlesnake	*Crotalus durissus terrificus*	Crotoxin	Immunomodulation (Minutti-Zanella et al. 2021).
Sea anemone	*Stichodactyla helianthus*	Dalazatide	Immunomodulatory (Tarcha et al. 2017)
Hookworm	*Ancylostoma caninum*	Acan1	Immunomodulatory (Smallwood et al. 2021).
Hookworm	*Necator americanus*	Nak1	Immunomodulatory (Smallwood et al. 2021).
Marajó lancehead snake	*Bothrops marajoensis*	L-AAO	Antibacterial (Yacoub et al. 2020).
South American rattlesnake	*Crotalus durissus*	Crotamine	Antibacterial (Silva et al. 2015).
Bee	*Apis mellifera*	Propolis extracts	Antiviral (Ripari et al. 2021)
Black desert cobra	*Walterinnesia aegyptia*	PLA2	Antimicrobial (Bacha et al. 2018)
Large clawed scorpion	*Scorpio maurus palmatus*	Smp76	Antiviral (El-Bitar et al. 2019).
Spider	*Pardosa berivivulva*	Silk	Antimicrobial (Phartale et al. 2019)
Red-eyed tree frog	*Agalychnis callidryas*	Dermaseptin-AC	Antibacterial (Chen et al. 2021).
Vampire bat	*Desmodus rotundus*	Desmoteplase	Anticoagulative (Piechowski-Jozwiak et al. 2022).
Mexican leech	*Haementeria officinalis*	Antistasin	Anticoagulative (Theunis-sen et al. 1994)
Leech	*Poecilobdella manillensis*	Poecistasin	Anticoagulative (Tang et al. 2018).
Tropical bont tick	*Amblyomma variegatum*	Variegin	Anticoagulative (Koh et al. 2019).
Saw-scaled viper	*Echis carinatus*	Tirofiban	Anticoagulative (Yang et al. 2019).
Leech	*Hirudo medicinalis*	Hirudin	Anticoagulative (Junren et al. 2021).
Chinese moccasin snake	*Deinagkistrodon acutus*	Hemocoagulase agkistrodon	Anticoagulative (Li et al. 2018b)
Chinese moccasin snake	*Deinagkistrodon acutus*	Defibrase	Anticoagulative (Oliveira et al. 2022)
Brazilian pit viper	*Bothrops jararaca*	Botrocetin	Anticoagulative (Thomazini et al. 2021).

(*Continued*)

TABLE 10.1 ***(Continued)***
Biotoxins and Their Medicinal Effects

Organism	Scientific Name	Biotoxin	Medicinal Effect
Saw-scaled viper	*Echis carinatus*	Echistatin	Anticoagulative (Gan et al. 1988)
Malayan pit viper	*Calloselasma rhodostoma*	Ancrod	Anticoagulative (Moore et al. 1994)
Habu snake	*Trimeresurus flavoviridis*	IX/X-bp	Anticoagulative (Sekiya et al. 1993).
Brazilian pit viper	*Bothrops jararaca*	Captopril	Antihypertensive (Choi et al. 2019)
Brazilian pit viper	*Bothrops jararaca*	Bradykinin potentiating peptides	Antihypertensive (Lameu et al. 2013).
Mamba snake	Genus *Dendroaspis*	Dendrotoxin	Antihypertensive (AlShammari et al. 2024)
Cone snails	Genus *Conus*	Conotoxin	Antihypertensive (Mir et al. 2016).
Cobra	Genus *Naja*	Cardiotoxin	Antihypertensive (Averin and Utkin 2021).
Snakes	*Serpentes*	Snake venom metalloproteinases	Antihypertensive (Olaoba et al. 2020).
Texas coral snake	*Micrurus tener tener*	Wasabi receptor toxin	Antihypertensive (Robinson et al. 2022)
Gila monster lizard	*Heloderma suspectum*	Exendin-4	Antidiabetic (Coulter-Parkhill et al. 2021)
Bee	*Apis mellifera*	Melittin	Antidiabetic (Hossen et al. 2017)
Bacteria	*Clostridium botulinum*	BTX-A	Antidiabetic (Lakhan et al. 2015).
Bee	*Apis mellifera*	Melittin	Anticancer (Tariq et al. 2021).
Bacteria	*Klebsiella pneumoniae*	Microcin E492	Anticancer (Varas et al. 2020)
Bacteria	*Enterococcus faecium*	Enterocin-B	Anticancer (Ankaiah et al. 2018)
Bacteria	*Pseudomonas aeruginosa*	Exotoxin A	Anticancer (Khoshnood et al. 2022).
Bacteria	*Corynebacterium diphtheriae*	CRM197	Anticancer (Márquez-López and Fararragha 2023).
Bacteria	*Vibrio cholerae*	CtxA and CtxB	Anticancer (Márquez-López and Fararragha 2023).
Bacteria	*Clostridium perfrigens*	Pore-forming enterotoxin	Anticancer (Khoshnood et al. 2022)

TABLE 10.1 ***(Continued)***

Biotoxins and Their Medicinal Effects

Organism	Scientific Name	Biotoxin	Medicinal Effect
Bacteria	*Pseudomonas aeruginosa*	azurin	Anticancer (Ashu et al. 2019)
Bacteria	*Chromobacterium violaceum*	Romidepsin	Anticancer (Ashu et al. 2019)
Bacteria	*Bacillus subtilis*	Epsilon-poly-L-lysin	Anticancer (Ashu et al. 2019)
Fire ant	*Solenopsis invicta*	Solenopsis A	Anticancer (Noble et al. 2020)
Cecropia moth	*Hylaphora cecropha*	Cecropin A	Anticancer (Ziaja et al. 2020)
Chinese wolf spider	*Lycosia singoriensis*	Lycosin-1	Anticancer (Noble et al. 2020)
Chinese bird spider	*Haplopelma hainanum*	Venom	Anticancer (Lian et al. 2018)
Central Asian spider	*Lachesana tarabaevi*	Latarcin 2a	Anticancer (Wu et al. 2019).
Honduran curlyhair tarantula	*Brachypelma albopilosum*	Brachyin	Anticancer (Guo et al. 2024)
South American tarantula	*Psalmopoeus cambridgei*	Psalmotoxin	Anticancer (Wu et al. 2019)
Spider	*Macrothele raveni*	Venom	Anticancer (Noble et al. 2020)
Scorpion	*Androctonus australis*	Venom	Anticancer (Nafie et al. 2020)
Scorpion	*Leiurus quinquestriatus*	Chlorotoxin	Anticancer (Noble et al. 2020)
Snake	*Ophiophagus hannah*	Venom	Anticancer (Kerkkamp et al. 2018).
Snake	*Naja naja oxiana*	Crude venom	Anticancer (Offor and Piater 2023)
Snake	*Naja atra*	Cardiotoxin-3	Anticancer (Moga et al. 2018).
Snake	*Bathrops leucurus*	Leucurogin	Anticancer (Li et al. 2018b)
Snake	*Naja nigricollis*	Nigexine	Anticancer (Offor and Piater 2023)
Bacteria	*Clostridium botulinum*	Botulinum neurotoxin	Anticancer (Rosales et al. 2018).
Bacteria	*Clostridium tetani*	Tetanus neurotoxin	Anticancer (Xu and Ling 2020).

signals by targeting ion channels and receptors located in the brain and spinal cord. Analgesics include classes of medications such as opioids, acetaminophen, antiepileptics, and non-steroidal anti-inflammatory drugs (NSAIDs), amongst others (Maatuf et al. 2019; Milani and Davis 2023). Although various classes of analgesic drugs have been in use, they pose significant side effects to some body organs such as the kidney and liver and thus intensify the need for developing less toxic and more effective ones (Abbas et al. 2020).

Baskaradoss and Kumar (2018) investigated the analgesic activity of crude petroleum ether extracts of the spine sheath and epidermal mucus of freshwater catfish, *Mystus gulio*. When injected intraperitoneally in albino mice, the analgesic activity of the spine sheath venom showed moderate toxicity compared to paracetamol, primarily affecting the cardiovascular system and peripheral neuromuscular transmission.

The analgesic potential of the biopeptide Cd1a was explored by Sousa et al. (2017). From their report, Cd1a, a venom isolated from the spider *Ceratogyrus darlingi* (African rear-horned baboon tarantula), demonstrated analgesic characteristics by reversing spontaneous pain induced in mice when injected with OD1, a scorpion toxin. The analgesic activity of Cd1a (400 pmol) was observed to be dose dependent and had no off-target effects. Studies on some other spider species such as *Phoneutria nigriventer* with promising analgesic activities have been highlighted in a recent review on animal venoms (Pereira et al. 2023).

The polyketide toxin, mycolactone, is produced by *Mycobacterium ulcerans* and is widely known to be the causative agent of the Buruli ulcer, which is characterized by an infectious, ulcerative, and painless skin lesion (Guenin-macé et al. 2019). Furthermore, mycolactone has been suggested to possess analgesic properties. In vitro, mycolactone was observed to target angiotensin II (AT_2) type 2 receptors, which led to potassium-dependent hyperpolarization, thereby inducing analgesia in dorsal root ganglion neurons obtained from adult male mice (Song et al. 2017). In another investigation, Babonneau et al. (2019) revealed that mycolactone levels in mouse tissue decreased rapidly and induced hypoesthesia in very small amounts.

Some models of pain are accompanied by inflammation, which has been described as the body's defense mechanism against injury, pathogenic infection, and metabolic stress and is characterized by redness, swelling, warmth, and loss of function (Antonelli and Kushner 2017). Although there are several commercially available anti-inflammatory drugs, certain biotoxins have demonstrated the potential to be used as anti-inflammatory agents. Conotoxins are a complex mixture of toxins produced by cone snails (genus *Conus*), which are targeted at the cellular receptors of their predators and prey and are used to immobilize them (Jin et al. 2019).

The crude venom obtained from *Conus virgo* has been reported by Mohamed et al. (2022) to exhibit anti-inflammatory potential in addition to analgesia and antipyresis in carrageenan-induced paw edema in male albino mice at a dose of 9.1 mg/kg. However, the anti-inflammatory effect was observed to be lower than the control group treated with ketoprofen at 0.5 mg/kg after

3 hours post-treatment. In addition, a significant reduction in abdominal writhing of the mice (injected peritoneally with acetic acid) was indicative of the analgesic potential of the conotoxins. These findings corroborate the results of previous studies, which also suggest that venom from cone snails possesses the potential to be used as both an anti-inflammatory and analgesic agent (Shwtar et al. 2017).

Bee venom and apamin (a component of bee venom) have both been shown to possess the ability to ameliorate monosodium urate crystal-induced inflammation in gouty arthritis in male mice. The investigations of Lee et al. (2020) revealed a significant decrease in paw edema at 1 mg/kg each of bee venom and apamin, as well as a reduction in the production of the proinflammatory cytokines TNF-α, IL-1β, and IL6.

The study by Hassan et al. (2019) indicates that crude venom extracted from the Egyptian scorpion *Androctonus amoreuxi* exhibits both analgesic and anti-inflammatory properties in the context of rheumatoid arthritis. Rheumatoid arthritis was induced in the hind paws of adult male albino rats using 0.1 ml of complete Freund's adjuvant. Subsequently, doses of 0.24 and 0.48 mg/kg of the crude scorpion venom were administered, resulting in pain relief, reduced paw edema, and increased mobility in the rats.

In the inquiry by Syed et al. (2021), male Wister albino mice with carrageenan-induced edema in their paws (500 µg/paw) were injected peritoneally with crude methanol, acetone, and acetonitrile extracts (tunic) of the solitary marine tunicate *Phallusia nigra* and their fractions at 50 mg/kg. Results from the tail-flick test indicated analgesic activity, which peaked after 60 minutes and declined gradually after 120 minutes. Furthermore, these extracts decreased the paw edema in a manner dependent on time and comparable to indomethacin at 10 mg/kg, which suggests the potential to be used as an anti-inflammatory agent.

Alkaloids form another group of interesting biotoxins and are toxic amines that are naturally produced by plants as a means of defense against herbivores. The pyrrolizidine alkaloid, 7-angelyolsincamidine N-oxide, isolated from the Zygophyllum-leaved heliotrope *Heliotropium digynum* (Forssk.) C. Chr., has demonstrated the ability to exert an anti-inflammatory effect on lipopolysaccharide-induced macrophage RAW 264.7 cells derived from mice by suppressing the production of nitric oxide (Aboelmagd et al. 2018).

Several biotoxins such as venoms and their derivatives, including venom-derived synthetic peptides, have been implicated in immunomodulation (Minutti-Zanella et al. 2021). Crotoxin (CTX), the primary neurotoxin derived from *Crotalus durissus terrificus* (South American rattlesnake), has been suggested to have the potential to exert anti-inflammatory and analgesic as well as immunomodulatory effects. In their study, Sant'Anna et al. (2019) demonstrated that conjugating crotoxin with nanostructured mesoporous silica (SBA-15) to reduce toxicity resulted in a prolonged antinociceptive effect in neuropathic pain induced by partial sciatic nerve ligation (PSNL) compared to crotoxin alone. In addition, the production of the spinal cytokine IL-6 was reduced, while that of IL-10 was upregulated.

Tarcha et al. (2017) assessed the safety and efficacy of dalazatide in adult patients with mild-to-moderate plaque psoriasis. Dalazatide is a 37-amino acid synthetic peptide that specifically inhibits the voltage-gated Kv1.3 potassium channel, a derivative of ShK, initially found in the venom of the sea anemone *Stichodactyla helianthus*. The function and expression of Kv1.3 channels are crucial for chronically activated memory T cells, which play a significant role in autoimmune diseases such as psoriasis. The study found that dalazatide treatment lowered plasma levels of various inflammation markers (IL-1 receptor antagonist, IL-8, IL-17A, IL-18, and soluble TNF-a receptor 2) and decreased the expression of T cell activation markers on peripheral blood memory T cells. The findings suggest that dalazatide is generally well tolerated and can improve psoriatic skin lesions by modulating T cell activation and reducing inflammation.

Acan1 and Nak1 are small molecular weight peptides synthetically derived from the excretory secretion of the hookworms *Ancylostoma caninum* and *Necator americanus*, respectively. These peptides have been shown to suppress cytokine production and T-cell proliferation. Specifically, they demonstrated immunomodulatory potential by inhibiting the proliferation of human CD^{4+} T cells in vitro and exhibited anti-colitic activity in in vivo experiments using mice with colitis induced by 2,4,6-trinitrobenzene sulphonic acid (TNBS) (Smallwood et al. 2021).

Avalo et al. (2022) have summarized the effects of venom from various animal species on the human immune system. These venoms impact different cells, cellular structures, and tissues, including the skin, nervous, hematological, digestive, excretory, and immune systems, as well as the heart. Components of the innate immune system, such as phagocytes, mast cells, complements, cytokines, inflammasomes, and transcription factors, can be either stimulated or suppressed by these venoms. Similarly, the adaptive immune system can also be modulated.

Many plants are known to naturally defend themselves against herbivores by producing cyanogenic glycosides. In addition to being implicated in cancer therapy, amygdalin, which is a cyanogenic glycoside, has been suggested to have other medicinal properties, including analgesia, anti-inflammation, and immunomodulation (Soto-Blanco 2022). Intraperitoneal administration of amygdalin inhibited the expression of the pro-inflammatory cytokines IL-6, TNF-α, and IL-1β in acetaminophen-induced liver injury in mice and reduced liver necrosis (Zhang et al. 2022). Furthermore, the results of previous research indicated the ability of amygdaline to impede NF-κB and NLRP3 signaling pathways and hinder the production of TNF-α, IL-1β, and IL-6 in the bronchoalveolar lavage fluid in mice with lipopolysaccharide-induced acute lung injury (Zhang et al. 2017).

The potential of biotoxins to induce analgesia, anti-inflammatory, and immunomodulatory effects presents exciting prospects for the development of novel therapeutics with enhanced safety and efficacy profiles.

10.5 Antimicrobial Properties

Microbial infections pose a significant threat to public health, resulting in substantial morbidity and mortality globally, which is exacerbated by the growing issue of antimicrobial resistance (Rincón-Cortés et al. 2022). The rise of antimicrobial resistance has become a major public health concern, causing at least 70,000 deaths annually and projected to increase to 10 million deaths per year by 2050 (Chen et al. 2021; Yacoub et al. 2020). This critical situation necessitates the development of novel, natural agents with diverse mechanisms of action that are less toxic and more effective against microbial infections (Yacoub et al. 2020).

Nature offers a wide range of antimicrobial compounds that could replace conventional over-the-counter antimicrobials. Antimicrobial peptides (AMPs) have been shown to be a promising alternative and demonstrated effectiveness against various microorganisms, including bacteria, fungi, viruses, and parasites (Parente et al. 2018). These short peptides, composed of fewer than 100 amino acids, can adopt different structures and charge properties and serve as a natural defense mechanism in various organisms (Dan et al. 2020).

AMPs exhibit bactericidal activity by interacting with and permeating microbial membranes, inhibiting intracellular targets, inhibiting microbial metabolic processes, and modulating the immune response through toll-like receptor activation, ultimately stimulating the innate immune system (Zhang and Yang 2022; Mwangi et al. 2019). Animal venom, containing a variety of biological components and AMPs, is utilized for predation and defense, including protection against pathogens (Diaz-Gomez et al. 2024).

Studies reveal that AMPs have several advantages, such as a potent bactericidal effect, low potential to induce antimicrobial resistance, absence of residue formation in biological fluids, anti-biofilm effects, and synergistic activity when combined with bactericidal antimicrobials (Li et al. 2022). AMPs are considered potential drugs against drug-resistant organisms, as they are mainly broad spectrum and are unlikely to cause resistance (Chen et al. 2021). However, because these AMPs are isolated in small quantities, chemical synthesis is essential. This process enhances the potency, selectivity, and stability of AMPs, making it crucial in combating antimicrobial resistance and advancing drug development (Boto et al. 2018).

Animal venom-derived peptides, as part of AMPs, have emerged as promising alternatives to combat antimicrobial-resistant infections (Lima and Lima 2023). These peptides have garnered significant attention for their potential to be developed into synthetic peptides or analogs as new antimicrobial agents. Animal venoms and secretions have long been recognized as rich sources of bioactive molecules, exhibiting various biological effects, including antimicrobial activities, and are being explored for developing new drugs (Park et al. 2018). Also, venom from plants and algae extracts has been extensively investigated for its antimicrobial properties, which are used for self-defense or prey immobilization (Yacoub et al. 2020).

10.5.1 Antimicrobial Agents from Snakes

Reported as the animal with the most complex venoms, snakes have been one of the most studied, especially those belonging to the family *Viperidae, Crotalidae*, and *Elapidae*. Snake venom has also been reported to contain mostly enzymes and non-enzymatic proteins and peptides, which, despite its toxic nature, could have other desirable pharmacological effects (Munawar et al. 2018).

Snake venom is a complex mixture of various protein-based components, categorized into four groups. The first group consists of three-finger toxins (3FTx), phospholipases A2 (PLA2), snake venom metalloproteases (SVMP), and snake venom serine proteases (SVSP). The second group includes smaller amounts of proteins like Kunitz peptides (KUN), cysteine-rich secretory proteins (CRiSP), and others. The third group comprises less common proteins, such as venom nerve growth factor (VNGF) and vascular endothelial growth factor (VEGF). The fourth group contains rare proteins, including cobra venom factors (CVF) and galactose-binding proteins (Bocian and Hus 2020).

Research has identified that snake venom's bactericidal properties are primarily attributed to PLA2, L-amino acid oxidase (LAAO), and enzyme fragments, as well as fragments of three-finger toxins (Bocian and Hus 2020). Specifically, L-AAO from *Bothrops marajoensis* venom has been shown to inhibit the growth of various microorganisms, including *Pseudomonas aeruginosa, Candida albicans,* and *Staphylococcus aureus,* as well as the parasitic growth of *Leishmania chagasi* and *Leishmania amazonensis* (Yacoub et al. 2020). Notably some snake venom produces AMPs like human defensins and cathelicidins. For instance, *Crotalus durissus* venom contains crotamine, a small basic myotoxin that targets bacteria through membrane permeabilization (Silva et al. 2015). Similarly, another study by Bacha et al. (2018) reported that PLA2 from *Walterinnesia aegyptia* venom showed antimicrobial properties against various human pathogenic strains, highlighting the potential of venom-derived compounds as antimicrobial agents.

10.5.2 Antimicrobial Agents from Insects

Wasps and bees, both flying insects belonging to the order Hymenoptera and suborder Apocrita, share a close relationship (Yacoub et al. 2020). Their venom is a complex mixture of proteins, enzymes, peptides, and smaller molecules. Additionally, bees (*Apis mellifera*) collect a resinous substance called propolis, which possesses various biological properties with potential as a safe therapeutic option (Cruz et al. 2020; Norma et al. 2023),

According to Norma et al. (2023), in vitro studies revealed that propolis extracts from Mexico and Brazil, as well as their phenolic compounds (quercetin, caffeic acid, and rutin), exhibited antiviral effects against HCoV-229E infection in human lung cells (MRC-5). The study demonstrated the antiviral activity of propolis extracts and their potential for developing natural therapeutic formulations against other coronavirus strains.

Consisting of mixtures of peptides, enzymes, mucoproteins, free amino acids, amines, nucleotides, lipids, heterocyclic components, inorganic salts, and other unknown substances, scorpion venoms have also been reported to have antimicrobial peptides (Yacoub et al. 2020). AMPs from scorpion venoms are cationic, amphipathic, and alpha-helical peptides with significant activity against bacteria and fungi by causing membrane lysis. Smp76 is a peptide purified from the venom of *Scorpio maurus palmatus* that has demonstrated activity against Hepatitis C virus (HCV), dengue virus (DENV), and viruses belonging to the *Flaviviridae* family (El-Bitar et al. 2019).

Spiders are known to produce silk that is known for its strength and toughness and thus has been an interesting material for scientists. In fact, many studies have shown that spider webs significantly exhibit antimicrobial activities (Yacoub et al. 2020). Phartale et al. (2019) demonstrated that *Pardosa berivivulva* silk has useful bactericidal and fungicidal properties. In another study, various full and partial sequences of transcriptome data from the spider *Pardosa astrigera* were tested against *Bacillus subtilis, Escherichia coli, Pseudomonas aeruginosa, Staphylococcus aureus,* and *Staphylococcus epidermidis*. The sequences showed strong antimicrobial activity against all five bacterial strains, demonstrating high potency and cytocompatibility (Lee et al. 2022).

10.5.3 Antimicrobial Agents from Frogs

After several studies, the amphiphilic α-helical cationic AMPs found in many frog species have been reported to have withstood the test of antimicrobial resistance during long-term evolution (Varga et al. 2018). AMPs of the dermaseptin family have shown effectiveness against bacteria, parasites, fungi, protozoa, viruses, and several human cancer cells *in vitro,* as well as demonstrating immune-modulatory effects (Bartels et al. 2019). Dermaseptin-AC, a new antimicrobial peptide, was discovered from the skin secretion of the red-eyed tree frog *Agalychnis callidryas* with effective broad-spectrum antibacterial activity and inhibited the formation of methicillin-resistant *Staphylococcus aureus* (MRSA) biofilm, showing appropriate selectivity to microorganisms and cancer cells *in vitro*. Furthermore, in in vivo studies Dermaseptin-AC demonstrated a similar efficacy to that of vancomycin in immunosuppressed mice with MRSA pneumonia (Chen et al. 2021).

10.6 Anticoagulative Properties

Several biotoxins possess anticoagulative properties, which means they can inhibit blood clotting and could be potential sources of drugs. Blood coagulation involves the activation of either the intrinsic or extrinsic pathway, which results in the formation of factor Xa, culminating in the activation of thrombin. Thrombin then catalyzes the conversion of fibrinogen to fibrin, the final step in blood clot formation. Additionally, thrombin plays a crucial role in altering platelet morphology, releasing ADP, and producing thromboxane A2 (TXA2) and chemokines, all of which promote thrombus formation (Zhang et al. 2021).

Desmoteplase: Desmoteplase (DSPA), a fibrinolytic enzyme from the saliva of vampire bat *Desmodus rotundus,* activates plasminogen to plasmin to degrade fibrin clots. Intravenously administered DSPA is safe and well tolerated, with plasma fibrinolytic activity correlating with blood concentration. It has shown promising results in myocardial infarction and pulmonary embolism compared to alteplase. DSPA is theoretically superior due to its high fibrin specificity, no beta-amyloid activation, and lack of neurotoxicity and has improved outcomes in patients with significant stenosis or occlusion of proximal precerebral vessels. Its inclusion in ischemic stroke treatment could extend the intervention time window, benefiting patients outside the 4.5-hour thrombolysis window, including those with wake-up strokes or strokes of unknown onset (Piechowski-Jozwiak et al. 2022).

In an in vivo study using rabbit eyes, DSPA was compared to tissue plasminogen activator (t-PA) for its intraocular fibrinolytic effect and short-term toxicity. Topical DSPA showed no significant differences compared to the vehicle-treated group. Intracameral t-PA demonstrated higher fibrinolytic efficacy than DSPA at early time points, but by 24 hours post-application, there was no significant difference between the two. Animals treated with t-PA had significantly more side effects than those treated with DSPA, which exhibited no-to-mild side effects after both topical and intracameral treatments. DSPA appears to be a promising drug with fewer side effects and similar fibrinolytic efficacy to t-PA 24 hours after intracameral application in rabbit eyes at the tested concentration, and increasing the intracameral DSPA doses might improve its efficacy (Voelter et al. 2019).

Antistasin: Antistasin belongs to a novel family of serine protease inhibitors; is derived from the salivary gland of the Mexican leech (*Haementeria officinalis*); and is a potent inhibitor of blood coagulation factor Xa, a crucial enzyme in the coagulation cascade. By inhibiting factor Xa, Antistasin prevents the conversion of prothrombin to thrombin, thereby inhibiting clot formation (Theunissen et al. 1994).

Similarly, a new antistasin-type inhibitor from the leech *Poecilobdella manillensis,* named poecistasin, has been identified. Poecistasin is a 48-amino-acid protein with a single domain. Poecistasin inhibited factor XIIa(from the intrinsic pathway), kallikrein, trypsin, and elastase but had no inhibitory effect on factor Xa and thrombin. Poecistasin demonstrated anticoagulant activities by prolonging activated partial thromboplastin time and inhibiting FeCl3-induced carotid artery thrombus formation, suggesting its significant role in aiding *Poecilobdella manillensis* to feed on blood by inhibiting coagulation. Additionally, poecistasin alleviated symptoms of ischemic stroke in a transient middle cerebral artery occlusion mouse model. These findings indicate that poecistasin plays a vital role in blood-feeding and may be a promising candidate for developing clinical anti-thrombosis and anti-ischemic stroke therapies (Tang et al. 2018).

Variegin: Variegin is obtained from the saliva of tropical bont tick (*Amblyomma variegatum*). Variegin is a unique direct thrombin inhibitor (DTI) preventing the formation of fibrin clots. Variegin is a potent inhibitor of thrombin, targeting its active site and exosite-1 with a remarkable inhibitory constant of 0.3 nM, making it nine times more effective than bivalirudin. It exhibits exceptional selectivity for thrombin over other blood coagulation serine proteases, with a plasma half-life of 50 minutes, contrasting with bivalirudin's 25 minutes and heparin's longer duration. In preclinical models of percutaneous coronary intervention (PCI) with aspirin and ticagrelor, a low dose of variegin demonstrated superior antithrombotic effects and significantly lower bleeding risk compared to heparin or bivalirudin (Koh et al. 2019).

Tirofiban: Derived from the venom of the saw-scaled viper *Echis carinatus*, tirofiban is a non-peptide selective glycoprotein (GP) IIb/IIIa receptor inhibitor that reversibly inhibits fibrinogen-dependent platelet aggregation and subsequent thrombus formation, which are key factors in the major atherosclerotic complications of ischemic stroke. Its adjunctive use has been extensively evaluated in progressive stroke, combined intravenous thrombolysis (IVT), and endovascular treatment (EVT) through both preclinical and clinical studies. Tirofiban's ability to specifically inhibit ongoing platelet aggregation and thrombus formation, rather than absolute thrombolysis, suggests that this widely used GP IIb/IIIa inhibitor, with high affinity and a short plasma/biologic half-life, holds significant potential for acute ischemic stroke treatment (Yang et al. 2019).

Hirudin: Hirudin is an acidic polypeptide secreted by the salivary glands of the medicinal leeches *Hirudo medicinalis*. It is the most potent natural specific inhibitor of thrombin. By binding thrombin, hirudin prevents the conversion of fibrinogen to fibrin, effectively inhibiting clot formation (Junren et al. 2021). In elderly patients with unilateral intertrochanteric fractures undergoing proximal femoral nail antirotation (PFNA) and anticoagulant therapy, the combination of natural hirudin and low molecular weight heparin (LMWH) proved to be more effective in preventing perioperative deep venous thrombosis (DVT) than LMWH-calcium alone, with no significant difference in safety (Zhang et al. 2018).

Hemocoagulase Agkistrodon and Defibrase: Hemocoagulase agkistrodon (HCA), a thrombin-like enzyme (TLE) derived from the venom of the Chinese moccasin snake (*Deinagkistrodon acutus*), has been utilized in clinical practice as a hemostatic agent. HCA, as a distinctive and novel member of the TLE family, has potential as a clinical drug for the prevention and treatment of hemorrhage due to its complex and unique interactions with the blood system (Li et al. 2018a). Similarly, defibrase, also found in *Deinagkistrodon acutus*, breaks down fibrinogen, reducing the ability of blood to clot (Oliveira et al. 2022). The combination of naoxintong capsules and defibrase injection is clinically effective in treating acute cerebral thrombosis, as it reduces hemorheological indexes, improves coagulation function, and enhances neurological function, demonstrating considerable clinical application value (Jia et al. 2019).

Botrocetin: Botrocetin from venom of the snake *Bothrops jararaca* enhances the interaction between von Willebrand factor (vWF) and platelets, which can lead to platelet aggregation (Thomazini et al. 2021). Patients bitten by snakes frequently exhibit a bleeding tendency, characterized by thrombocytopenia, consumption coagulopathy, mucous bleeding, and occasionally thrombotic microangiopathy. The von Willebrand factor (VWF) is essential for primary hemostasis, and certain venom proteins, like botrocetin (a C-type lectin-like protein) and snake venom metalloproteinases (SVMP), can disrupt the normal interaction between platelets and VWF, potentially contributing to snakebite-induced bleeding. A study investigated the relationship between plasma VWF, platelets, botrocetin, and SVMP from *Bothrops jararaca* snake venom (BjV) in the development of thrombocytopenia. The results revealed that BjV induced rapid and severe thrombocytopenia. The findings indicated that while botrocetin in BjV did not significantly influence the extent or duration of thrombocytopenia caused by envenomation, it did contribute to reduced levels and functionality of plasma VWF. Therefore, VWF alterations during *B. jararaca* envenomation are a secondary event and not the primary mechanism for decreased platelet counts (Thomazini et al. 2021).

Echistatin: Echistatin, a 49-residue protein that inhibits platelet aggregation, was purified from the venom of the saw-scaled viper (*Echis carinatus*). A 10-residue segment of echistatin shares 90% identity with a sequence in trigramin, another platelet aggregation inhibitor from the green tree viper (*Trimeresurus gramineus*). Echistatin effectively inhibits fibrinogen-dependent platelet aggregation initiated by adenosine diphosphate, with an IC50 of 3×10^{-8} M, and prevents platelet aggregation triggered by thrombin, epinephrine, collagen, or platelet-activating factor. As a disintegrin, echistatin achieves this by blocking the glycoprotein IIb/IIIa receptor on platelets, which is crucial for platelet cross-linking and clot formation (Gan et al. 1988).

Others: Ancrod, a rapid-acting defibrinogenating agent sourced from the venom of the Malayan pit viper (*Calloselasma rhodostoma*), has been effectively used as an alternative to heparin sulfate for anticoagulation in peripheral vascular procedures and coronary artery bypass surgery. As an enzyme, ancrod breaks down fibrinogen, thereby reducing its availability for clot formation. This degradation results in lower blood viscosity and prevents the formation of clots (Moore et al. 1994).

Another anticoagulant protein, named IX/X-bp (factor IX/factor X-binding protein), was isolated from the venom of the habu snake (*Trimeresurus flavoviridis*) and found to be homologous to botrocetin from the venom of *Bothrops jararaca*. This protein has a structure similar to the carbohydrate-recognition domains of C-type lectins (Sekiya et al. 1993).

These biotoxins have significant potential for therapeutic use in preventing and treating thrombotic disorders.

10.7 Antihypertensive Properties

Several biotoxins exhibit anti-hypertensive properties, often through mechanisms such as inhibiting enzymes involved in blood pressure regulation or interacting with receptors that control vascular tone.

Captopril: Derived from the venom of the Brazilian pit viper (*Bothrops jararaca*), captopril was the first ACE inhibitor developed. Captopril is an angiotensin-converting enzyme (ACE) inhibitor primarily used in the treatment of hypertension and certain types of congestive heart failure. It works by blocking the conversion of angiotensin I to angiotensin II, a potent vasoconstrictor, thereby lowering blood pressure and reducing strain on the heart. Pharmacodynamically, captopril's inhibition of ACE also reduces the degradation of bradykinin, contributing to vasodilation (Choi et al. 2019).

A study by Mayasari (2020) was conducted at a puskesmas (community health center) in the Banyuwangi district to analyze the impact of captopril on blood pressure in hypertension patients. The results indicated that captopril significantly reduced blood pressure in hypertension patients. Endogenous kinins and other substances inhibited by aprotinin contribute to captopril's antihypertensive effect in patients with angiotensin-dependent hypertension (Mimran et al. 1980).

Several other studies highlight captopril's significance in managing cardiovascular diseases, demonstrating its wide range of therapeutic uses. Long-term follow-up research has also assessed captopril's effectiveness in treating heart failure and post-myocardial infarction, affirming its advantages in enhancing cardiac function and increasing survival rates (Andrès et al. 2019).

Bradykinin Potentiating Peptides: Bradykinin potentiating peptides (BPPs) from the venom of the Brazilian pit viper *Bothrops jararaca* enhance the effects of bradykinin, a peptide that causes blood vessels to dilate, thereby reducing blood pressure (Lameu et al. 2013).

BPPs function by inhibiting the angiotensin-converting enzyme, which prevents the breakdown of bradykinin and extends its vasodilatory effects. Initially identified in the venom of Bothrops jararaca, BPPs are proline-rich oligopeptides consisting of 5–13 amino acid residues. Structurally, many of these peptides feature a pyroglutamic acid at the N-terminal and a distinctive C-terminal sequence ending in IPP, which is crucial for binding to the ACE catalytic site (Pinheiro-Júnior et al. 2018).

BPP has a similar mechanism of action as the hypotensive drug captopril, which is widely used in the treatment of hypertension (Sciani and Pimenta, 2017). They target the renin-angiotensin-aldosterone system by inhibiting ACE, potentially contributing to the hypotensive shock seen during envenomation by this species. The LmrBPP9 peptide was synthesized with an automated solid-phase peptide synthesizer and purified using reversed-phase fast protein liquid chromatography (FPLC). The synthetic peptide demonstrated a strong ACE inhibition with an in vitro IC50 of 4.25 ± 0.10 μM. In vivo studies indicated that LmrBPP9 effectively reduced blood pressure in both normotensive and hypertensive rats, with a more pronounced effect in the hypertensive group. These findings support the in vitro results, suggesting that the synthetic peptide LmrBPP9 has potential as a new antihypertensive drug (Pinheiro-Júnior et al. 2018).

Dendrotoxin: Dendrotoxin is a potent neurotoxin found in the venom of mamba snakes (genus *Dendroaspis*). These toxins are known for their ability to bind and block voltage-gated potassium (Kv) channels, which play a critical role in regulating neuronal excitability and neurotransmitter release. This blockade results in prolonged depolarization of the neuronal membrane, leading to an increase in neurotransmitter release. The enhanced release of neurotransmitters can cause various neurological effects, including convulsions and paralysis, which are characteristic of dendrotoxin poisoning (AlShammari et al. 2024).

Though primarily neurotoxic, dendrotoxin can affect blood pressure regulation by blocking potassium channels particularly Kv1 family channels, in vascular smooth muscle cells (VSMCs). (Jackson 2018; Daghbouche-Rubio et al. 2022). Kv channels play an important role in regulating VSMC membrane potential and vascular tone. They contribute to the negative feedback regulation of VSMC membrane potential and myogenic tone (Jackson 2018). By blocking Kv channels, dendrotoxin can cause depolarization of VSMCs. This leads to activation of voltage-dependent calcium channels, increasing intracellular calcium and promoting vasoconstriction (Daghbouche-Rubio et al. 2022; Austin and Wray 2000).

The vasoconstriction induced by dendrotoxin can increase vascular resistance and potentially raise blood pressure (Daghbouche-Rubio et al. 2022). Kv channels are involved in the vasodilatory effects of some compounds like cAMP-related vasodilators, hydrogen sulfide, and hydrogen peroxide. Blocking these channels with dendrotoxin could impair these vasodilatory mechanisms (Jackson 2018). However, the exact contribution of Kv channels blocked by dendrotoxin to blood pressure control may vary depending on the specific vascular bed and physiological conditions (Jackson 2018; Tykocki et al. 2017).

Conotoxins: Conotoxins are small peptides derived from the venom of cone snails (genus *Conus*). These peptides are highly potent and selective inhibitors or modulators of various ion channels, receptors, and transporters, making them valuable tools in neuropharmacology and potential therapeutic agents for several medical conditions (Mir et al. 2016).

Each type of conotoxin has a unique target, and they are classified based on their molecular targets and mechanisms of action. α-conotoxins target nicotinic acetylcholine receptors (nAChRs), which are involved in neuromuscular transmission and modulation of neurotransmitter release (Tae and Adams 2023); ω-conotoxins inhibit voltage-gated calcium channels (VGCCs), affecting neurotransmitter release and synaptic plasticity (Trevisan and Oliveira 2022); δ-conotoxins block voltage-gated sodium channels (VGSCs), altering neuronal excitability (Mackieh et al. 2021); μ-conotoxins also target VGSCs, but with different specificity compared to δ-conotoxins excitability (Mackieh et al. 2021); and κ-conotoxins target potassium channels, influencing action potential duration and neuronal excitability (Groome 2023).

Voltage-gated channels are important targets for antihypertensive drugs. Calcium channel blockers are widely used to treat hypertension by inhibiting L-type Ca^{2+} channels. Kv channels are being explored as potential therapeutic targets for hypertension. In summary, voltage-gated channels, particularly Ca^{2+} and K^{+} channels, play a critical role in regulating vascular tone and blood pressure. Their altered function or expression can contribute to hypertension, making them important targets for both understanding the pathophysiology of hypertension and developing therapeutic interventions (Nieves-Cintrón et al. 2018; Daghbouche-Rubio et al. 2022; Baker 2000).

Cardiotoxins: Cardiotoxins (CTs) are a group of toxic proteins found in snake venoms, particularly those of cobras (*Naja* species). They are three-finger toxins that consist of about 60 amino acid residues and contain four disulfide bonds. CTs reduce blood pressure primarily through their interaction with cell membranes to form ionic pores, leading to cell depolarization and death (Averin and Utkin 2021).

CTs interact directly with cell membranes, forming ionic pores that cause cell depolarization. The initial depolarization caused by CTs results in an increase in intracellular calcium concentration. This calcium influx comes from both intra- and extracellular sources and can vary depending on the type of myocardial tissue. The increased intracellular calcium concentration activates peptidases and leads to the disintegration of cardiomyocyte structures, ultimately resulting in cell death through a necrotic mechanism (Averin and Utkin 2021).

In muscle tissues, including blood vessels, CTs cause contracture. This contractile response involves the influx of extracellular calcium and its release from intracellular stores. In phenylephrine-precontracted aortic rings, a transient relaxation effect is observed, likely due to the activation of endothelial cells. The interaction of CTs with smooth muscle and endothelial cells in blood vessels leads to contracture and subsequent cell death, which can affect vascular tone and blood pressure regulation. The depolarization and subsequent cell death caused by CTs can lead to a reduction in vascular resistance. This reduction in resistance can lower blood pressure. Additionally, the transient relaxation effect observed in blood vessels could also contribute to a temporary decrease in blood pressure (Averin and Utkin 2021).

Snake venom metalloproteinases: Snake venom metalloproteinases (SVMPs) are a class of zinc-dependent enzymes found in the venom of many snake species, particularly vipers. These enzymes can degrade extracellular matrix components and affect blood vessel stability and function (Olaoba et al. 2020).

Some SVMPs have been found to influence blood pressure regulation indirectly. BmooMPα-I, a metalloproteinase isolated from *Bothrops moojeni* venom, has been shown to lower blood pressure, reverse left ventricular remodeling, and enhance cardiac electrical conduction in rats with renovascular hypertension. This enzyme exhibits kininogenase activity, cleaving kininogen to release bradykinin and hydrolyzing angiotensin I at post-proline and aspartic acid positions to produce an inactive peptide. A study evaluating the antihypertensive effects of BmooMPα-I in a two-kidney, one-clip (2K1C) model concluded that BmooMPα-I effectively improved blood pressure levels and cardiac remodeling, demonstrating a cardioprotective effect (Estrada et al. 2022).

Wasabi Receptor Toxin: Wasabi receptor toxin (WaTx) is a toxin from the venom of the Texas coral snake (*Micrurus tener tener*) that targets the TRPA1 receptor (wasabi receptor), involved in pain and inflammation pathways. Modulation of TRPA1 has been linked to cardiovascular effects, including blood pressure regulation (Robinson et al. 2022).

The TRPA1 channel is a calcium-permeable, nonselective cation channel in the plasma membrane, part of the transient receptor potential (TRP) channel superfamily. Activation of the TRPA1 channel triggers peripheral vasodilation and causes a biphasic blood pressure response. Conversely, the absence of channel expression or inhibition of its activation has been shown to mitigate heart failure, myocardial ischemia–reperfusion injury, myocardial fibrosis, and arrhythmia. Due to its association with various cardiovascular diseases, the TRPA1 channel presents an attractive target for therapeutic interventions (Wang et al. 2019)

10.8 Antidiabetic Properties

Since diabetes mellitus (DM) is one of the most common and serious endocrine metabolic disorders, it is important to elucidate novel antidiabetic therapeutic agents from various sources, including natural products.

Exendin-4, originating from the saliva of the Gila monster lizard *Heloderma suspectum*, stands as a pioneering example in diabetes drug discovery, providing insights into cell signaling pathways related to insulin release and metabolism (Coulter-Parkhill et al. 2021). Research by Hadjiyanni et al. (2008) demonstrated that exendin-4 modifies the onset of diabetes in nonobese diabetic mice. As a glucagon-like peptide-1 (GLP-1) mimic that is resistant to dipeptidyl peptidase IV (DPP-IV), its synthetic version, exenatide, is utilized in the treatment of type 2 diabetes (T2DM). A study conducted by Lupi et al. (2008) involved treating pancreatic islets from both non-diabetic and T2DM subjects with exendin-4 for 48 hours, revealing several direct beneficial effects on insulin secretion and the expression of genes essential for beta-cell function and differentiation.

Bee venom (BV) is a complex blend of proteins, peptides, and low molecular weight components, with melittin being its primary component. Melittin is a peptide made up of 26 amino acids, specifically with the sequence GIGAVLKVLTTGLPALISWIKRKRQQ. It possesses several significant biological effects and has relatively low toxicity. Recent animal studies have demonstrated that melittin has notable glucose and lipid-lowering activities through various mechanistic pathways. The primary antidiabetic effect of melittin is the enhancement of insulin secretion via depolarization of pancreatic β-cells. Additional mechanisms may include stimulation of phospholipase A2, increased glucose uptake, improved lipid profiles, and reduced inflammation (Hossen et al. 2017).

T2DM is plagued by numerous complications, including painful diabetic neuropathy (PDN), which significantly impacts the quality of life of affected individuals. Numerous treatments exist for neuropathic pain, and recent studies have highlighted the potential analgesic benefits of botulinum toxin-A (BTX-A) for such pain. A meta-analysis of two studies on PDN revealed an improvement of 1.96 Visual Analog Scale (VAS) points following BTX-A treatment, indicating a clinically meaningful reduction in pain (Lakhan et al. 2015). The efficacy and safety of intramuscular BTX-A injections for treating cramps in PDN was also evaluated in a single-center, double-blind, placebo-controlled study of diabetic patients. All outcome measures showed significant improvement with BTX-A compared to placebo, with significant changes from baseline observed after just 1 week and lasting up to 14 weeks (Restivo et al. 2018).

In another study involving 42 diabetic patients, the therapeutic potential of BTX-A to manage PDN was investigated. The results revealed a significant reduction in VAS scores at 1, 4, and 12 weeks after Botox injections compared to the placebo group. However, there was no notable improvement in Pittsburgh Sleep Quality Index (PSQI) scores among patients who received Botox compared to those who received the placebo. These findings indicate that BTX-A shows efficacy in severe diabetic neuropathy and may present an alternative approach in managing this condition (Hossam Egila et al. 2020).

10.9 Anticancer/Antitumor Properties

Several studies have reported some of the biotoxin receptors to be overexpressed in the endothelial cells found in the neovasculature of both solid tumors and malignant cells. This ability to recognize and bind to their targets specifically implies that biotoxins can be beneficial sources of ligands for use in developing molecular-based therapeutic interventions (Márquez-López and Fararragha. 2023).

Cancer is a debilitating disease that occurs worldwide with various complications and high mortality rates. Conventional cancer therapies involve the use of chemotherapy, radiotherapy, surgery, or a combination of any of these therapies to target and destroy tumor cells and improve patient outcomes (Răileanu and Bacalum 2023). However, there are several adverse effects of these conventional therapies that limit their efficacy at curbing tumor growth. They include drug resistance, poor targeting, and toxicity to normal cells due to inability to distinguish between normal and tumor cells (Márquez-López and Fararragha 2023; Răileanu and Bacalum 2023). This implies that there is a need for more novel drugs and therapeutic interventions that can provide solutions to these limitations (Răileanu and Bacalum 2023).

Numerous studies in recent times have shown that a variety of toxins such as scorpion venom, bee venom, sea anemone venom, and snake venom exhibit extraordinary anticancer activity (Tariq et al. 2021).

10.9.1 Antitumor Activity of Bee Venom

Bee venom produced by honeybees has demonstrated great potential in the treatment of various types of cancers (Tariq et al. 2021). Eighteen bioactive compounds consisting of peptides, enzymes, and other amines and non-peptide components are found in bee venom (Ullah et al. 2023; Tariq et al. 2021). The most essential active constituent is melittin, which makes up 40–60% of dried bee venom. Several studies have reported its antitumor activity in non-small cell lung cancer, pancreatic cancer, glioblastoma, lung cancer, cervical cancer, and leukemia. Melittin prevented invasion and spread of liver cancer cells by inhibiting the Rac1-dependent pathway (Badawi 2021). Also, melittin was able to target triple negative breast cancer and HER-2 enriched tumors, which are the most aggressive and treatment-resistant types of breast cancer. The cytotoxic effect of melittin was greater in tumor cells compared to normal cells (Tariq et al. 2021). Nonetheless, it exhibits non-specific cytotoxic effects which can be detrimental to normal cells. This means that an appropriate delivery vehicle in addition to a controlled dosage is essential to achieving the desired therapeutic results with melittin therapy (Kwon et al. 2022).

Bee venom and melittin inhibited proliferation of prostate cancer cell (LNCap, PC-s, and DU145) lines. Previous in vivo studies revealed that tumor growth diminished gradually in a time-dependent manner in PC-3 prostate cancer cells after administering subcutaneous injections of the venoms to male xenograft nude mice (Badawi 2021). Melittin induced apoptotic effects in leukemia (U937) cells by inhibiting protein kinase B signaling (Ullah et al. 2023).

Melittin may therefore be a great alternative for cancer therapy due to its observed ability to significantly inhibit tumor cell growth and clonogenicity, induce apoptosis, and inhibit tumor metastasis (Tariq et al. 2021).

10.9.2 Antitumor Activity of Bacterial Peptides

Peptides such as bacteriocins produced by bacteria are one of the promising biotoxins for cancer treatment. One such bacteriocin is Microcin E492 produced by *Klebsiella pneumoniae,* which has been found to be toxic to various cancer lines, including HeLa, Jurkat, and RJ2.25 (Varas et al. 2020). Its anticancer property was evaluated in a recent study using the HT29 human colorectal cancer cell line and an animal model of zebrafish larvae bearing xenografts of human cancer cells. In vitro experiments revealed that the peptide was significantly cytotoxic against HT29 colorectal cancer cells in vitro. Similarly, in vivo tests involving intratumor injection of microcin E492 into the zebrafish xenograft model bearing same colorectal cancer cells resulted in significant reduction of the tumor cell mass (Varas et al. 2020).

Enterococcus faecium por1 produces a bacteriocin known as enterocin-B, which has also been demonstrated to induce cytotoxicity in HeLa, HT29, and AGS human cancer cell lines. This bacteria species also produces enterocin-A, which, when combined with enterocin-B to treat these cancer cell lines, significantly increased the anti-proliferative activity of the bacteriocins (Ankaiah et al. 2018).

A class of bacterial toxins known as AB toxins have also demonstrated anticancer potential. The toxins are composed of two distinct parts—the active catalytic domain (A) and the receptor binding domain (B). The less toxic B subunit is preferred for use in cancer therapies over the toxic A subunit, which has negative consequences. Examples of AB toxins include botulinum neurotoxin, tetanus neurotoxins, diphtheria toxin, ricin toxin, and exotoxin A (Márquez-López and Fararragha 2023).

Exotoxin A secreted by *Pseudomonas aeruginosa* induces cytotoxicity in cancer cells by altering mRNA translation. Other anti-cancer mechanisms of the toxins observed in melanoma cells include inactivation of poly ADP-ribose polymerase (PARP), stimulating caspase 3-dependent apoptosis and DNA fragmentation, impaired endoplasmic reticulum function, and increased intracellular calcium levels (Khoshnood et al. 2022).

In a mouse model of ovarian cancer, it was observed that a mutant form of diphtheria toxin, CRM197, strongly inhibited tumorigenesis when injected intraperitoneally and when given alongside the chemotherapy drug Paclitaxel. CRM197 also produced similar effects in mouse models of adrenocortical carcinoma and pancreatic cancer. Subcutaneous injections of CRM197 administered to cancer patients also resulted in some level of antitumor activity (Márquez-López and Fararragha 2023).

Cholera toxin is used for immunotherapy used of cancers with mucus membrane origin such as pancreatic and colon cancer. An in vitro study performed with human small-cell lung carcinoma cell lines showed that cholera toxin can inhibit tumor growth. CtxA and CtxB fusion protein was also found to retard prostate tumor growth, stimulate dendritic cell maturation, and enhance cytotoxic T cell response (Márquez-López and Fararragha 2023).

The pore-forming enterotoxin produced by *Clostridium perfrigens* has been observed in previous studies to induce necrosis of cancer cells, inhibit tumor growth, and prevent tumorigenesis (Khoshnood et al. 2022).

Ashu et al. (2019) described several other bacterial peptides with anticancer properties. An example is azurin from *Pseudomonas aeruginosa*, which is effective against various breast cancer cell lines such as MCF-7, MDA-MB-157, T47D, and ZR-75–1; colon cancer HCT-116; and melanoma Mel-2. Romidepsin from *Chromobacterium violaceum* exhibits anticancer activity in over 20 cell lines such as neuroblastoma, T-cell lymphoma, lung, and mammary and colon adenocarcinomas. Also, epsilon-poly-L-lysin secreted by *Bacillus subtilis* and *Streptomyces albulus* exerts its anticancer properties on the HeLa cervical cancer cell line and HepG2 hepatocellular carcinoma (Ashu et al. 2019).

10.9.3 Antitumor Activity of Insect Venoms

Insects secrete a variety of toxic bioactive compounds for protection against harmful predators, but some of these compounds have been exploited for medicinal purposes. The fire ants *Solenopsis invicta* and *Solenopsis germinate* produce an active alkaloid known as solenopsis A which is a potential anticancer agent that inhibits angiogenesis (Noble et al. 2020) by delaying formation of angiogenesis precursor in vivo (Mo et al. 2023).

Cecropins isolated from *Hylaphora cecropha* pupae possess some selective antitumor activity, as demonstrated in in vitro studies using various cancer cell lines. Cecropin A inhibited tumor growth in leukaemia cell lines K562, U937, THP1, and HL-60 without inducing any cytotoxicity in human embryonic kidney 293 and peripheral blood mononuclear cells used as non-cancer control cell lines. However, the mechanism of action behind this selectivity property is yet to be deciphered (Ziaja et al. 2020). A synthetic peptide combining cecropin A and melittin showed anticancer activity against murine melanoma cells through mechanisms such as inhibition of ATP synthesis, altered mitochondrial activity, and cell lysis (Răileanu and Bacalum 2023).

Cecropin B is considered a promising cancer treatment due to its unique ability to selectively destroy cancer cells without causing any damage to normal cells such as erythrocytes, lymphocytes, or fibroblasts (Ziaja et al. 2020). In vivo studies using mammalian models showed that cecropin B and a synthetic analog known as *B. mori Cec XJ* increased the survival rate of mice with malignant ascites, suggesting that these peptides have anticancer potential (Brady et al. 2019).

Venoms produced by various species of spiders are promising candidates for cancer therapy. The spider *Lycosia singoriensis* produces a peptide known as lycosin-1 which caused more than 90% cell death in six human cancer cell lines treated with 40 μM of the venom. In contrast, the same concentration of the venom induced only about 25% death in healthy liver cells, mouse skin epidermal cells, and erythrocytes, indicating that it is mostly cancer specific (Noble et al. 2020).

In studies by Lian et al. (2018), the venom secreted by *Haplopelma hainanum* significantly suppressed cell growth and induced apoptosis via the mitochondrial-dependent pathway in human hepatocellular carcinoma cell line HepG2. Latarcin 2a obtained from the Central Asian spider *Lachesana tarabaevi* demonstrated cytotoxic effects on human erythroleukemia (K562) cells in vitro. Its mechanism of action on K562 cells included disruption of cell membrane integrity by forming membrane blebs and pores, inactivation of mitochondrial function, cell swelling, and finally cell death (Wu et al. 2019). A neutrotoxin, brachyin, which is a component of the venom of *Brachypelma albopilosum*, strongly inhibited cell growth in C8166, Molt-4, A549, BIU-87, T24, and Calu-6 cancer cell lines, with IC_{50} values between 1.5 and 24 μg/mL (Guo et al. 2024).

Psalmotoxin isolated from the South American tarantula spider species *Psalmopoeus cambridgei* significantly inhibited basally active cation currents in malignant astroglioma cells and freshly resected glioblastoma multiforme without any damage to normal human astrocytes. Patients suffering from glioblastoma multiforme have a poor prognosis. Therefore, these results offer hope for effective treatment of glioma because they are very invasive, and ion transport plays a critical role in the growth and metastasis of glioma cells (Wu et al. 2019).

Macrothele raveni spider venom stimulated apoptotic and necrotic effects in a human cervical cancer cell line (HeLa) in a time and dose-dependent manner. *M. raveni* venom also had anticancer effects on human breast carcinoma (MCF-7) cells. The mechanism of action in MCF-7 involved inhibition of DNA synthesis, reduced cell viability, and inducing apoptosis and cell necrosis (Wu et al. 2019; Noble et al. 2020).

The scorpion species *Androctonus crassicauda, Androctonus bicolor, Leiurus quinquestriatus, Odontobuthus doriae,* and *Rhopalurus junceus* produce venoms that have been studied and observed to decrease cell proliferation in human brain, breast, lungs, larynx, colorectal, and cervix carcinoma cell lines. A reduced proliferative effect occurred as result of the venom's ability to upregulate expression of apoptotic gene *bax* and *bax/bcl* (anti-apoptotic gene) ratio; decrease expression of the *bcl* gene; increase activities of caspase enzymes 3, 8, and 9; and stimulate expression of Fas-L (Mikaelian et al. 2020).

Nafie et al. (2020) investigated and validated the antitumor potential of venom from the scorpion species *Androctonus australis*. This venom exhibited selective antitumor activity in a MCF-7 breast carcinoma cell line in vitro with an IC_{50} value of 19.71 μg/mL. This may be attributed to the anti-proliferative, anti-metastatic, and anti-apoptotic property of scorpion venoms both in vitro and in vivo (Nafie et al. 2020).

Chlorotoxin is a neurotoxic peptide isolated from the venom of the *Leiurus quinquestriatus* scorpion with anticancer properties. It has the extraordinary ability to bind to cancer cells without damaging normal cells. This may be due to the overexpression of its targets, mainly certain ion channels and membrane proteins in cancer cells. In a previous study, chlorotoxin was able to target melanoma, glioma, neuroblastoma, small-cell lung cancer, and medulloblastoma cell lines. Its remarkable ability to bind glioma cells without accumulating in normal brain cells makes it a promising delivery vehicle for chemotherapeutic drugs, cancer imaging, and treatment of glioma (Noble et al. 2020).

10.9.4 Antitumor Activity of Snake Venoms

Crude extracts of snake venom are a source of various components with promising anticancer potential (Offor and Piater 2023). These components include phospholipase A_2, metalloproteases, L-amino acid oxidases, and disintegrins (Li et al. 2018b). Whole snake venom produced by *Ophiophagus hannah* and *Echis carinatus* exerted strong anticancer effects on pancreatic tumor cells in vitro. On the other hand, in vivo tests showed that *O. hannah* venom very significantly inhibited angiogenesis (Kerkkamp et al. 2018).

Crude venom extracted from *Naja naja oxiana* had apoptotic effects on human breast cancer (MCF-7), human hepatocellular carcinoma (HepG2), and human prostate carcinoma (DU145) cell lines, with IC_{50} values of 26.59, 28.85, and 21.17 μg/ml, respectively, compared to a normal dog kidney cell line (MDCK), which had an IC_{50} of 47.1 μg/ml (Offor and Piater 2023). Also, cardiotoxin-3 (CTX-3) isolated from the venom of *Naja atra* induced apoptosis in breast carcinoma MDA-MB-231 and MCF-7 cell lines. In breast cancer cells, CTX-3 reduced the expression of matrix metalloproteinase MMP-9 by inhibiting PI3K/Akt signaling pathways and p38 MAPK and NF-κB activity, resulting in the prevention of metastasis (Moga et al. 2018).

Leucurogin, a disintegrin derived from the *Bathrops leucurus* snake, exhibited significant antitumor effects against Ehrlich tumors in a mice xenograft model following the administration of 10 μg/day. Another study on the sponge implant mouse model confirmed the ability of leucurogin to inhibit angiogenesis in a tumor (Li et al. 2018a).

Nigexine, a phospholipase A_2 from the venom of *Naja nigricollis*, was observed to reduce cell viability and inhibit proliferation of epithelial FL cells, C-133 T neuroblastoma cells, and promyelocytic leukaemia HL 60 cells (Offor and Piater 2023).

10.10 Neuroprotective Activity

Researchers have been enthralled by the interesting but complex relationship between poisons and the neurological system, which reveals both their harmful and unexpectedly healing potential (Pirazzini et al. 2022; Sharma and Singh 2019). The effects of botulinum and tetanus toxins on neuronal function are particularly notable among the wide range of toxins. Though historically known for their paralyzing effects, new findings have shown their complex roles in neurodegeneration and neuroprotection, opening exciting new treatment options (Pellett and Tepp 2019).

Botulinum neurotoxin (BoNT) is a biotoxin produced by the bacterium *Clostridium botulinum*. This toxin has revolutionized medical practice with its remarkable efficacy in treating neuromuscular disorders (Rosales et al. 2018). Its mechanism of action involves cleaving to soluble n-ethylmaleimide-sensitive factor attachment receptor (SNARE) proteins, and inhibiting neurotransmitter release underlies its potent muscle-relaxing effects. Despite its well-established neuromuscular blockade, emerging evidence reveals unexpected neuroprotective properties (Pirazzini et al. 2022; Zhou and Dong 2019).

Studies have also shown the potential of BoNT in mitigating neurodegenerative processes. It exerts neuroprotective effects in conditions like Alzheimer's and Parkinson's diseases by the modulation of neurotransmitter release especially acetylcholine (Zhou and Dong 2019; Rosales et al. 2018). Experimental models and studies have revealed the potential of administering BoNT, and they include reduction of oxidative stress, promotion of neural survival, and attenuation of neuroinflammation, thus offering promising avenues for new therapeutic strategies (Dressler 2012; Pirazzini et al. 2017).

Postherpetic neuralgia, posttraumatic neuralgia, and severe diabetic neuropathy are the three main prevalent types of neuropathic pain for which studies on BoNT/A1 are promising and show efficacy or potential benefit (Betancor et al. 2021). This type of human pain is caused by injury to or malfunctions in the peripheral or central nerve systems, and it is not unusual for them not to respond to analgesic drugs (Ri et al. 2021; Dressler 2012). According to a systematic assessment of the therapeutic value of subcutaneous or intradermal injection of BoNT/A1 for the treatment of trigeminal neuralgia, this treatment should be taken into consideration as a surgical alternative (Morra et al. 2016). In a recent trial, repeated intra/subcutaneous injections of BoNT/A1 (up to six times) for 2 years were used to treat severe post-herpetic neuralgia; the injections significantly reduced pain and had no negative side effects. According to Ri et al. (2021), adjunctive local BoNT/A1 injection appears to be a secure and successful treatment for the long-term control of chronic neuropathic pain. A systematic review and meta-analysis of randomized controlled trials by Datta Gupta et al. (2022) provided more proof that BoNT-A1 is safe, long-lasting, and effective in treating neuropathic pain; it also showed no significant adverse effects.

The role of BoNT also transcends targeting traditional neurodegenerative disorders, as revealed from research. It combats conditions like migraine headaches and improves neuropathic pain and psychiatric conditions like anxiety and depression (Pirazzini et al. 2022; Zhou and Dong 2019). These diverse applications of BoNT emphasize its complex and versatile interactions with the nervous system, necessitating further research into the neuroprotective mechanisms and clinical implications (Pirazzini et al. 2017).

Another intriguing key player in the neurotoxin realm is the tetanus neurotoxin (TeNT). This is a biotoxin produced by the bacterium *Clostridium tetani* and is the causal agent of the often-fatal disease known as tetanus, which causes severe muscle spasms and respiratory failure (Xu and Ling 2020). The toxicity of TeNT is influenced by the presence of an L chain with metalloprotease activity (Schiavo et al. 2000), but only a 50 kDa non-toxic carboxy-terminal fragment called TTC is needed for TeNT to be targeted to neuronal synapses. Studies have revealed that TTC is sufficient for neuron internalization and binding, retrograde transport, and trans-synaptic transport (Betancor et al. 2021; Herreros et al. 2000).

Consequently, TTC has been used to target therapeutic molecules to the central nervous system (Toivonen et al. 2010). By attaching these molecules to TTC, various molecules, including insulin-like growth factor 1 (IGF-1), glial-derived neurotrophic factor (GDNF), and brain-derived neurotrophic factor (BDNF), have been successfully transported into neurons (Ciriza et al. 2008; Betancor et al. 2021).

Additionally, further research has also shown that TTC possesses neurotrophic qualities besides being a carrier. By attaching to Trk receptors and initiating Trk-dependent signaling, which triggers the activation of neuronal survival pathways and the prevention of apoptosis, TTC imitates the activity of endogenous neurotrophic ligands (Toivonen et al. 2010). Although the precise method by which TTC activates Trk receptors is unknown, investigations conducted in vitro and in vivo have shown that TTC binding to these receptors activates neuroprotective pathways (Betancor et al. 2021). In mouse models of spinal muscular atrophy (SMA), TTC alone delays the onset of symptoms and functional deficits, reducing motoneuron death and extending the lifespan of the mice. In mouse models of amyotrophic lateral sclerosis (ALS), it also modifies autophagy markers and lowers apoptosis (Olivan et al. 2016).

TTC has been dubbed a neuroprotective molecule because it binds to Trk receptors and triggers Trk-dependent signaling, which in turn stimulates neuronal survival pathways and prevents apoptosis (Sharma and Singh 2019). This has been shown in earlier *in vivo* investigations to improve mouse lifespan, suppress apoptosis, and control autophagy in murine models of neurodegenerative illnesses such SMA and ALS (Betancor et al. 2021).

Interestingly, while tetanus toxin's primary action induces neurotoxicity, researchers are exploring its therapeutic potential in targeted neuronal modulation (Sharma and Singh 2019). Engineered derivatives of tetanus toxin, such as TeNT-Hc fragment, have shown promise in selectively targeting and modulating specific neuronal populations (Xu and Ling 2020). This selective manipulation opens doors to innovative therapeutic strategies, including targeted drug delivery, neuronal tracing, and potentially neuroprotection in conditions characterized by aberrant neuronal activity (Rossetto and Montecucco 2019).

The complex relationship of these neurotoxins with the central nervous system reveals their neuroprotective potential. While being associated with paralytic effects, these toxins offer interesting insights into neurobiological and therapeutic interventions. A deeper dive into the realm of toxin-mediated neuroprotection will bring about a better understanding of how to harness the capabilities of these toxins in protecting and preserving neural health and function.

10.11 Future Perspectives and Conclusion

Further investigation into the mechanisms of action and remedial applications of these natural alternatives is crucial to unlock their full potential in addressing various health conditions and improving clinical outcomes. The medicinal use of biotoxins is a rapidly evolving field with promising implications for future therapeutics. Continued research into the molecular mechanisms of biotoxins can uncover new pathways and targets for drug development, potentially leading to innovative treatments for a wide range of diseases. The specificity and potency of biotoxins make them attractive candidates for addressing conditions that are currently difficult to treat with conventional pharmaceuticals.

Advancements in biotechnology and molecular engineering are expected to enhance the ability to harness and modify biotoxins, increasing their safety and efficacy. The development of recombinant technologies and synthetic analogs will likely facilitate the production of biotoxin-based drugs, making them more accessible and cost effective. Furthermore, personalized medicine approaches could optimize the therapeutic application of biotoxins, tailoring treatments to individual genetic profiles and disease states.

Interdisciplinary collaborations among biologists, chemists, pharmacologists, and clinicians will be crucial in driving forward the clinical translation of biotoxins. Additionally, regulatory frameworks will need to adapt to ensure the safe and ethical development of biotoxin-based therapies.

With sustained investment in research and development, biotoxins hold the potential to revolutionize the treatment landscape for numerous medical conditions.

Biotoxins, derived from a diverse array of organisms, offer unique therapeutic properties that have been exploited in traditional medicine for centuries and are now being rigorously studied in modern biomedical research. Their ability to target specific biological pathways with high precision makes them valuable tools in the development of new drugs. From managing chronic pain and neurodegenerative diseases to combating cancer and infections, biotoxins have shown significant medicinal potential. This chapter has highlighted various biotoxins and their mechanisms of action, showcasing their broad applicability in treating different ailments. Despite their potent biological activities, the therapeutic use of biotoxins must carefully balance efficacy with safety, necessitating thorough preclinical and clinical evaluations.

In summary, the medicinal effects of biotoxins represent a frontier in pharmaceutical sciences, offering promising avenues for future drug discovery and development. As our understanding of these complex molecules grows, so will our ability to harness their power for the benefit of human health. The integration of biotoxins into mainstream medicine could mark a significant advancement in our approach to treating a myriad of health conditions, ultimately improving patient outcomes and quality of life.

References

Abbas, R. N., Jouda, J., Alshammary, A. G., & Jumaa, M. S. (2020). Toxicity of liver and kidney induced by different concentrations of tramadol in young and adult mice. *Annals of Tropicals Medicine Health*, 23, 128–133.

Aboelmagd, M., Elokely, K., Zaki, M. A., Said, A., Haggag, E. G., & Ross, S. A. (2018). Anti-inflammatory of pyrrolizidine alkaloids from *Heliotropium digynum*. *Medicinal Chemistry Research*, 27, 1066–1073.

AlShammari, A. K., Abd El-Aziz, T. M., & Al-Sabi, A. (2024). Snake venom: A promising source of neurotoxins targeting voltage-gated potassium channels. *Toxins*, 16, 12.

Andrès, E., Lorenzo Villalba, N., Zulfiqar, A. A., Serraj, K., Mourot-Cottet, R., & Gottenberg, J. E. (2019). State of art of idiosyncratic drug-induced neutropenia or agranulocytosis, with a focus on biotherapies. *Journal of Clinical Medicine*, 8(9), 1351.

Ankaiah, D., Palanichamy, E., Antonyraj, C. B., Ayyanna, R., Perumal, V., Ahamed, S. I. B., & Arul, V. (2018). Cloning, overexpression, purification of bacteriocin enterocin-B and structural analysis, interaction determination of enterocin-A, B against pathogenic bacteria and human cancer cells. *International Journal of Biological Macromolecules*, 116, 502–512.

Antonelli, M., & Kushner, I. (2017). It's time to redefine inflammation. *FASEB Journal: Official Publication of the Federation of American Societies for Experimental Biology*, 31(5), 1787–1791.

Ashu, E. E., Xu, J., & Yuan, Z. C. (2019). Bacteria in cancer therapeutics: A framework for effective therapeutic bacterial screening and identification. *Journal of Cancer*, 10(8), 1781–1793.

Austin, C., & Wray, S. (2000). Interactions between Ca2+ and H+ and functional consequences in vascular smooth muscle. *Circulation Research*, 86(3), 355–363.

Avalo, Z., Barrera, M. C., Agudelo-Delgado, M., Tobón, G. J., & Cañas, C. A. (2022). Biological effects of animal venoms on the human immune system. *Toxins*, 14(5), 344.

Averin, A. S., & Utkin, Y. N. (2021). Cardiovascular effects of snake toxins: Cardiotoxicity and cardioprotection. *Acta Naturae*, 13(3), 4.

Babonneau, J., Bréard, D., Reynaert, M.-L., Marion, E., Guilet, D., Saint André, J.-P., Croué, A., Brodin, P., Richomme, P., & Marsollier, L. (2019). Mycolactone as analgesic: Subcutaneous bioavailability parameters. *Frontiers in Pharmacology*, 10, 378.

Bacha, B., Alonazi, A., Elshikh, M. A., & Karray, A. (2018). A novel bactericidal homodimeric PLA2 group-I from Walterinnesia aegyptia venom. *International Journal of Biological Macromolecules*, 117, 1140–1146.

Badawi, J. K. (2021). Bee venom components as therapeutic tools against prostate cancer. *Toxins*, 13, 337.

Baker, E. H. (2000). Ion channels and the control of blood pressure. *British Journal of Clinical Pharmacology*, 49(3), 185–198.

Bartels, E. J. H., Dekker, D., & Amiche, M. (2019). Dermaseptins, multifunctional antimicrobial peptides: A review of their pharmacology, effectivity, mechanism of action, and possible future directions. *Frontiers in Pharmacology*, 10, 1421. https://doi.org/10.3389/fphar.2019.01421.

Baskaradoss, K., & Kumar, P. (2018). Observation of acanthotoxicity effect of freshwater catfish Mystus gulio from spine and mucus extract. *International Journal of Fisheries and Aquatic Studies*, 6(3), 31–37.

Betancor, M., Moreno-Martínez, L., López-Pérez, Ó. et al. (2021). Therapeutic assay with the non-toxic C-terminal fragment of tetanus toxin (TTC) in transgenic murine models of prion disease. *Molecular Neurobiology*, 58, 5312–5326.

Bocian, A., & Hus, K. K. (2020). Antibacterial properties of snake venom components. *Chemical Papers*, 74, 407–419. https://doi.org/10.1007/s11696-019-00939-y.

Bordon, K. D. C. F., Cologna, C. T., Fornari-Baldo, E. C., et al. (2020). From animal poisons and venoms to medicines: Achievements, challenges and perspectives in drug discovery. *Frontiers in Pharmacology*, 11, 1132.

Boto, A., Pérez de la Lastra, J. M., & González, C. C. (2018). The road from host-defense peptides to a new generation of antimicrobial drugs. *Molecules*, 23(2), 311.

Brady, D., Grapputo, A., Romoli, O., & Sandrelli, F. (2019). Insect cecropins, antimicrobial peptides with potential therapeutic applications. *International Journal of Molecular Sciences*, 20(23), 5862.

Chen, J., Hao, D., Mei, K., et al. (2021). In vitro and in vivo studies on the antibacterial activity and safety of a new antimicrobial peptide dermaseptin-AC. *Microbiology Spectrum*, 9(3), e01318–21.

Choi, S., Han, S., Jeon, S., & Yim, D. S. (2019). Quantitative prediction of human pharmacokinetics and pharmacodynamics of CKD519, a potent inhibitor of cholesteryl ester transfer protein (CETP). *Pharmaceutics*, 11(7), 336.

Ciriza, J., García-Ojeda, M., Martín-Burriel, I., et al. (2008). Antiapoptotic activity maintenance of brain derived neurotrophic factor and the C fragment of the tetanus toxin genetic fusion protein. *Open Life Science*, 3.

Clark, G. C., Casewell, N. R., Elliott, C. T., Harvey, A. L., Jamieson, A. G., Strong, P. N., & Turner, A. D. (2019). Friends or foes? Emerging impacts of biological toxins. *Trends in Biochemical Sciences*, 44(4), 365–379.

Coulter-Parkhill, A., McClean, S., Gault, V. A., & Irwin, N. (2021). Therapeutic potential of peptides derived from animal venoms: Current views and emerging drugs for diabetes. *Clinical Medicine Insights: Endocrinology and Diabetes*, 14, 11795514211006071.

Cruz, J. N., da Silva, A. G., da Costa, W. A., et al. (2020). Volatile compounds, chemical composition and biological activities of Apis mellifera bee propolis. In *Essential Oils-Bioactive Compounds, New Perspectives and Applications*. IntechOpen.

Daghbouche-Rubio, N., López-López, J. R., Pérez-García, M. T., & Cidad, P. (2022). Vascular smooth muscle ion channels in essential hypertension. *Frontiers in Physiology*, 13, 1016175.

Dan, X., & Wuyuan, L. (2020). Defensins: A double-edged sword in host immunity. *Frontiers in Immunology*, 11, 764.

Datta Gupta, A., Edwards, S., Smith, J., et al. (2022). Systematic review and meta-analysis of efficacy of botulinum toxin A for neuropathic pain. *Toxins (basel)*, 14, 36.

Diaz-Gomez, J. L., Martin-Estal, I., Rivera-Aboytes, E., Gaxiola-Muniz, R. A., Puente-Garza, C. A., Garcia-Lara, S., & Castorena-Torres, F. (2024). Biomedical applications of synthetic peptides derived from venom of animal origin: A systematic review. *Biomedicine & Pharmacotherapy*, 170, 116015.

Dressler, D. (2012). Clinical applications of botulinum toxin. *Current Opinion in Microbiology*, 15(3), 325–336.

El-Bitar, A. M. H., Sarhan, M., Abdel-Rahman, M. A., et al. (2019). Smp76, a scorpine-like peptide isolated from the venom of the scorpion scorpio maurus palmatus, with a potent antiviral activity against hepatitis C virus and dengue virus. *International Journal of Peptide Research and Therapeutics*, 26, 811–821.

El-Masry, E. M., & Abou-Donia, M. B. (2015). Naturally occurring toxins. *Mammalian Toxicology*, 605–640.

Estrada, J. E. C., Rodrigues, K. E., Maciel, A., et al. (2022). BmooMPα-I, a metalloproteinase isolated from bothrops moojeni venom, reduces blood pressure, reverses left ventricular remodeling and improves cardiac electrical conduction in rats with renovascular hypertension. *Toxins*, 14(11), 766.

Gan, Z. R., Gould, R. J., Jacobs, J. W., Friedman, P. A., & Polokoff, M. (1988). Echistatin. A potent platelet aggregation inhibitor from the venom of the viper, Echis carinatus. *Journal of Biological Chemistry*, 263(36), 19827–19832.

Groome, J. R. (2023). Historical perspective of the characterization of conotoxins targeting voltage-gated sodium channels. *Marine Drugs*, 21(4), 209.

Guenin-macé, L., Ruf, M.-T., Pluschke, G., & Demangel, C. (2019). Mycolactone: More than just a cytotoxin. *Buruli Ulcer: Mycobacterium Ulcerans Disease*, 117–134.

Guo, R., Guo, G., Wang, A., Xu, G., Lai, R., & Jin, H. (2024). Spider-venom peptides: Structure, bioactivity, strategy, and research applications. *Molecules*, 29(1), 35.

Hadjiyanni, I., Baggio, L. L., Poussier, P., & Drucker, D. J. (2008). Exendin-4 modulates diabetes onset in nonobese diabetic mice. *Endocrinology*, 149(3), 1338–1349.

Hassan, A. K., Elfeky, E. M., Abbas, O. A., & Hefny, M. A. (2019). Potential Anti-Inflammatory Effects of the Egyptian scorpion (Androctonus amoreuxi) venom in rheumatoid rat model. *Egyptian Academic Journal of Biological Sciences. C, Physiology and Molecular Biology*, 11(2), 85–102.

Herreros, J., Lalli, G., & Schiavo, G. (2000). C-terminal half of tetanus toxin fragment C is sufficient for neuronal binding and interaction with a putative protein receptor. *Biochemical Journal*, 347(1), 199–204.
Hossam Egila, H. E., Gomaa, M., Abdel-naby, A., & Shehab El-din, M. (2020). Botulinum toxin type A in severe diabetic neuropathy. *Benha Medical Journal*, 37(3), 723–730.
Hossen, M. S., Gan, S. H., & Khalil, M. I. (2017). Melittin, a potential natural toxin of crude bee venom: Probable future arsenal in the treatment of diabetes mellitus. *Journal of Chemistry*, 2017(1), 4035626.
Jackson, W. F. (2018). KV channels and the regulation of vascular smooth muscle tone. *Microcirculation (New York, N.Y.: 1994)*, 25(1), 10.1111/micc.12421.
Janik, E., Ceremuga, M., Saluk-Bijak, J., & Bijak, M. (2019). Biological toxins as the potential tools for bioterrorism. *International Journal of Molecular Sciences*, 20(5), 1181.
Jia Min, J. M., Liu HuiChun, L. H., & Wang CongPing, W. C. (2019). Clinical study on Naoxintong Capsules combined with defibrase in treatment of acute cerebral thrombosis. *Drugs and Clinic*, 34(9), 2686–2689.
Jin, A. H., Muttenthaler, M., Dutertre, S., et al. (2019). Conotoxins: Chemistry and biology. *Chemical Reviews*, 119(21), 11510–11549.
Junren, C., Xiaofang, X., Huiqiong, Z., et al. (2021). Pharmacological activities and mechanisms of hirudin and its derivatives-a review. *Frontiers in Pharmacology*, 12, 660757.
Kerkkamp, H., Bagowski, C., Kool, J., van Soolingen, B., Vonk, F. J., & Vlecken, D. (2018). Whole snake venoms: Cytotoxic, anti-metastatic and antiangiogenic properties. *Toxicon: Official Journal of the International Society on Toxinology*, 150, 39–49.
Khoshnood, S., Fathizadeh, H., Neamati, F., Negahdari, B., Baindara, P., Abdullah, M. A., & Haddadi, M. H. (2022). Bacteria-derived chimeric toxins as potential anticancer agents. *Frontiers in Oncology*, 12, 953678.
Koh, C. Y., Shih, N., Leong, E. J. E., Amran, F. S., Li, A. W. L., Kini, R. M., & Chan, M. Y. Y. (2019). 2348 Novel direct thrombin inhibitor achieves superior antithrombotic effect with lower bleeding risk than heparin or bivalirudin. *European Heart Journal*, 40(Supplement_1), ehz748–0135.
Kwon, N.-Y., Sung, S.-H., Sung, H.-K., & Park, J.-K. (2022). Anticancer activity of bee venom components against breast cancer. *Toxins*, 14, 460.
Lakhan, S. E., Velasco, D. N., & Tepper, D. (2015). Botulinum toxin-A for painful diabetic neuropathy: A meta-analysis. *Pain Medicine*, 16(9), 1773–1780.
Lameu, C., Neiva, M., & Hayashi, M. (2013). Venom Bradykinin-related peptides (BRPs) and its multiple biological roles. *An Integrated View of the Molecular Recognition and Toxinology—From Analytical Procedures to Biomedical Applications*, 119–151.
Lee, B., Shin, M. K., Yoo, J. S., Jang, W., & Sung, J-S. (2022). Identifying novel antimicrobial peptides from venom gland of spider Pardosa astrigera by deep multi-task learning. *Frontiers in Microbiology*, 13, 971503.
Lee, Y. M., Cho, S.-N., Son, E., Song, C.-H., & Kim, D.-S. (2020). Apamin from bee venom suppresses inflammation in a murine model of gouty arthritis. *Journal of Ethnopharmacology*, 257, 112860.
Li, H., Huang, Y., Wu, X., et al. (2018a). Effects of hemocoagulase agkistrodon on the coagulation factors and its procoagulant activities. *Drug Design, Development and Therapy*, 12, 1385–1398.
Li, L., Huang, J., & Lin, Y. (2018b). Snake venoms in cancer therapy: Past, present and future. *Toxins*, 10(9), 346.

Li, X., Zuo, S., Wang, B., Zhang, K., & Wang, Y. (2022). Antimicrobial mechanisms and clinical application prospects of antimicrobial peptides. *Molecules*, 27, 2675.

Lian, W., Lian, H., Li, Q., Hu, A., & Liu, S. (2018). The venom of spider Haplopelma hainanum suppresses proliferation and induces apoptosis in hepatic cancer cells by caspase activation in vitro. *Journal of Ethnopharmacology*, 225, 169–177.

Lima, W. G., & Lima, M. E. (2023). Therapeutic prospection of animal venoms-derived antimicrobial peptides against infections by multidrug-resistant Acinetobacter baumannii: A systematic review of pre-clinical studies. *Toxins*, 15, 268.

Lupi, R., Mancarella, R., Del Guerra, S., et al. (2008). Effects of exendin-4 on islets from type 2 diabetes patients. *Diabetes, Obesity and Metabolism*, 10(6), 515–519.

Maatuf, Y., Geron, M., & Priel, A. (2019). The role of toxins in the pursuit for novel analgesics. *Toxins*, 11(2), 131.

Mackieh, R., Abou-Nader, R., Wehbe, R., Mattei, C., Legros, C., Fajloun, Z., & Sabatier, J. M. (2021). Voltage-gated sodium channels: A prominent target of marine toxins. *Marine Drugs*, 19(10), 562.

Márquez-López, A., & Fanarraga, M. L. (2023). AB toxins as high-affinity ligands for cell targeting in cancer therapy. *International Journal of Molecular Sciences*, 24, 11227.

Mayasari, S. (2020). Analysis of the used of captopril drug with blood pressure of hypertension patients. *Jurnal Kesehatan Dr. Soebandi*, 8(2), 123–127.

Mikaelian, A. G., Traboulay, E., Zhang, X. M., Yeritsyan, E., Pedersen, P. L., Ko, Y. H., & Matalka, K. Z. (2020). Pleiotropic anticancer properties of scorpion venom peptides: *Rhopalurus princeps* venom as an anticancer agent. *Drug Design, Development and Therapy*, 14, 881–893.

Milani, D. A. Q., & Davis, D. D. (2023). Pain management medications. In *StatPearls [Internet]*. StatPearls Publishing.

Mimran, A. L. B. E. R. T., Targhetta, R., & Laroche, B. E. R. N. A. D. E. T. T. E. (1980). The antihypertensive effect of captopril. Evidence for an influence of kinins. *Hypertension*, 2(6), 732–737.

Minutti-Zanella, C., Gil-Leyva, E. J., & Vergara, I. (2021). Immunomodulatory properties of molecules from animal venoms. *Toxicon*, 191, 54–68.

Mir, R., Karim, S., Amjad Kamal, M., M Wilson, C., & Mirza, Z. (2016). Conotoxins: Structure, therapeutic potential and pharmacological applications. *Current Pharmaceutical Design*, 22(5), 582–589.

Mo, Y., Shi, Q., Qi, G., & Chen, K. (2023). Potential anti-tumor effects of Solenopsis invicta venom. *Frontiers in Immunology*, 14, 1200659.

Moga, M. A., Dimienescu, O. G., Arvătescu, C. A., Ifteni, P., & Pleş, L. (2018). Anticancer activity of toxins from bee and snake venom—an overview on ovarian cancer. *Molecules*, 23(3), 692.

Mohamed, A. A., Nabil, Z. I., & El-Naggar, M. S. (2022). Prospecting for candidate molecules from Conus virgo toxins to develop new biopharmaceuticals. *The Journal of Venomous Animals and Toxins Including Tropical Diseases*, 28, e20220028.

Moore, J. A., Burket, M. W., Puri, S., Temesy-Armos, P., Lachant, N., & Skeel, R. (1994). Ancrod infusion for anticoagulation during and after PTCA in a patient with heparin-induced thrombocytopenia. *Catheterization and Cardiovascular Diagnosis*, 32(3), 286–287.

Morra, M. E., Elgebaly, A., Elmaraezy, A., et al. (2016). Therapeutic efficacy and safety of Botulinum Toxin A Therapy in Trigeminal Neuralgia: A systematic review and meta-analysis of randomized controlled trials. *Journal of Headache Pain*, 1, 63.

Munawar, A., Ali, S. A., Akrem, A., & Betzel, C. (2018). Snake venom peptides: Tools of biodiscovery. *Toxins*, 10, 474.

Mwangi, J., Hao, X., Lai, R., & Zhang, Z. Y. (2019). Antimicrobial peptides: New hope in the war against multidrug resistance. *Zoological Research*, 40, 488–505.
Nafie, M. S., Abdel Daim, M. M., Ali, I. A. I., et al. (2020). Antitumor efficacy of the Egyptian Scorpion Venom *Androctonus Australis:* In vitro and in vivo study. *JoBAZ*, 81, 8.
Nieves-Cintrón, M., Syed, A. U., Nystoriak, M. A., & Navedo, M. F. (2018). Regulation of voltage-gated potassium channels in vascular smooth muscle during hypertension and metabolic disorders. *Microcirculation (New York, N.Y.: 1994)*, 25(1), 10.1111/micc.12423.
Noble, K., Rohaj, A., Abegglen, L. M., & Schiffman, J. D. (2020). Cancer therapeutics inspired by defense mechanisms in the animal kingdom. *Evolutionary Applications*, 13, 1681–1700.
Norma, P. S., Juan, C. G., Ikner, L. A., & Gerba, C. P. (2023). In vitro antiviral effect of Mexican and Brazilian propolis and phenolic compounds against human coronavirus 229E. *International Journal of Environmental Health Research*, 33(12), 1591–1603.
Offor, B. C., & Piater, L. A. (2023). Snake venom toxins: Potential anticancer therapeutics. *Journal of Applied Toxicology: JAT*, 10.1002/jat.4544. Advance online publication.
Olaoba, O. T., Dos Santos, P. K., Selistre-de-Araujo, H. S., & de Souza, D. H. F. (2020). Snake venom metalloproteinases (SVMPs): A structure-function update. *Toxicon: X*, 7, 100052.
Olivan, S., Calvo, A. C., Rando, A., et al. (2016). Neuroprotective effect of non-viral gene therapy treatment based on tetanus toxin c-fragment in a severe mouse model of spinal muscular atrophy. *Frontiers in Molecular Neuroscience*, 9.
Oliveira, A. L., Viegas, M. F., da Silva, S. L., Soares, A. M., Ramos, M. J., & Fernandes, P. A. (2022). The chemistry of snake venom and its medicinal potential. *Nature Reviews Chemistry*, 6(7), 451–469.
Parente, A., Daniele-Silva, A., Furtado, A. A., et al. (2018). Analogs of the scorpion venom peptide stigmurin: Structural assessment, toxicity, and increased antimicrobial activity. *Toxins*, 10, 161.
Park, J., Kwon, O., An, H.-J., & Park, K. K. (2018). Antifungal effects of bee venom components on Trichophyton rubrum: A novel approach of bee venom study for possible emerging antifungal agent. *Annals of Dermatology*, 30, 202–210.
Pellett, S., & Tepp, W. H. (2019). Toxins as tools in the study of synaptic function. *Toxins*, 11(11), 673.
Pereira, A., Cavalcante, J., Angstmam, D., Almeida, C., Soares, G., Pucca, M., & Ferreira Junior, R. (2023). Unveiling the pain relief potential: Harnessing analgesic peptides from animal venoms. *Pharmaceutics*, 15, 2766.
Phartale, N. N., Kadam, T. A., Bhosale, H. J., Karale, M. A., & Gyananath, G. (2019). Exploring the antimicrobial potential of Pardosa brevivulva silk. *The Journal of Basic and Applied Zoology*, 80, 31.
Piechowski-Jozwiak, B., Abidi, E., El Nekidy, W. S., & Bogousslavsky, J. (2022). Clinical pharmacokinetics and pharmacodynamics of desmoteplase. *European Journal of Drug Metabolism and Pharmacokinetics*, 47(2), 165–176.
Pinheiro-Júnior, E. L., Boldrini-França, J., de Campos Araújo, L. M. P., Santos-Filho, N. A., Bendhack, L. M., Cilli, E. M., & Arantes, E. C. (2018). LmrBPP9: A synthetic bradykinin-potentiating peptide from Lachesis muta rhombeata venom that inhibits the angiotensin-converting enzyme activity in vitro and reduces the blood pressure of hypertensive rats. *Peptides*, 102, 1–7.
Pirazzini, M., Montecucco, C., & Rossetto, O. (2022). Toxicology and pharmacology of botulinum and tetanus neurotoxins: An update. *Archives of Toxicology*, 96, 1521–1539.

Pirazzini, M., Rossetto, O., Eleopra, R., & Montecucco, C. (2017). Botulinum neurotoxins: Biology, pharmacology, and toxicology. *Pharmacological Reviews*, 69, 200–235.
Răileanu, M., & Bacalum, M. (2023). Cancer wars: Revenge of the AMPs (Antimicrobial Peptides), a new strategy against colorectal cancer. *Toxins*, 15, 459.
Restivo, D. A., Casabona, A., Frittitta, L., Belfiore, A., Le Moli, R., Gullo, D., & Vigneri, R. (2018). Efficacy of botulinum toxin A for treating cramps in diabetic neuropathy. *Annals of Neurology*, 84(5), 674–682.
Ri, S., Kivi, A., & Wissel, J. (2021). The safety and effect of local botulinum toxin A injections for long-term management of chronic pain in post-herpetic neuralgia: Literature review and cases report treated with incobotulinumtoxin A. *Journal of Personalized Medicine*, 11, 758.
Rincón-Cortés, C. A., Bayona-Rojas, M. A., Reyes-Montaño, E. A., & Vega-Castro, N. A. (2022). Antimicrobial activity developed by scorpion venoms and its peptide component. *Toxins*, 14, 740.
Ripari, N., Sartori, A. A., da Silva Honorio, M., Conte, F. L., Tasca, K. I., Santiago, K. B., & Sforcin, J. M. (2021). Propolis antiviral and immunomodulatory activity: A review and perspectives for COVID-19 treatment. *Journal of Pharmacy and Pharmacology*, 73(3), 281–299.
Robinson, S. D., Deuis, J. R., Klasfauseweh, T., Schendel, V., & Vetter, I. (2022). Venom-derived pain-causing toxins: Insights into sensory neuron function and pain mechanisms. *Pain*, 163(S1), S46–S56.
Rosales, R. L., Bigalke, H., Dressler, D., & Botulinum Neurotoxin for Head and Neck Disorders Consensus Statement Collaboration Group. (2018). Expert consensus recommendations for the use of botulinum toxin type A in the management of cervical dystonia. *Expert Review of Neurotherapeutics*, 18(6), 513–525.
Rossetto, O., & Montecucco, C. (2019). Tables of toxicity of botulinum and tetanus neurotoxins. *Toxins*, 11(12), 686.
Sant'Anna, M. B., Lopes, F. S. R., Kimura, L. F., Giardini, A. C., Sant'Anna, O. A., & Picolo, G. (2019). Crotoxin conjugated to SBA-15 nanostructured mesoporous silica induces long-last analgesic effect in the neuropathic pain model in mice. *Toxins*, 11(12), 679.
Schiavo, G., Matteoli, M., & Montecucco, C. (2000). Neurotoxins affecting neuroexocytosis. *Physiological Reviews*, 80, 717–766.
Sciani, J. M., & Pimenta, D. C. (2017). The modular nature of bradykinin-potentiating peptides isolated from snake venoms. *Journal of Venomous Animals and Toxins Including Tropical Diseases*, 23, 45.
Sekiya, F., Atoda, H., & Morita, T. (1993). Isolation and characterization of an anticoagulant protein (homologous to botrocetin from the venom of Bothrops jararaca. *Biochemistry*, 32(27), 6892–6897.
Sharma, S., & Singh, B. R. (2019). Tetanus toxin: Toxicokinetics, pathophysiology, and management strategies. *Journal of Pharmacy & Bioallied Sciences*, 11(4), 275.
Shwtar, N. S., Nabil, Z. I., Abdel-Daim, M. M., & El-Naggar, M. S. (2017). Analgesic, antipyretic, and anti-inflammatory activities of Conus vexillum venom. *Egyptian Academic Journal of Biological Sciences, C Physiology & Molecular Biology*, 9(1).
Silva, O. N., Fensterseifer, I. C., Rodrigues, E. A., et al. (2015). Clavanin A improves outcome of complications from different bacterial infections. *Antimicrobial Agents and Chemotherapy*, 59, 1620–1626.
Sitprija, V., & Sitprija, S. (2019). Marine toxins and nephrotoxicity: Mechanism of injury. *Toxicon*, 161, 44–49.

Smallwood, T. B., Navarro, S., Cristofori-Armstrong, B., Watkins, T. S., Tungatt, K., Ryan, R. Y., Haigh, O. L., Lutzky, V. P., Mulvenna, J. P., & Rosengren, K. J. (2021). Synthetic hookworm-derived peptides are potent modulators of primary human immune cell function that protect against experimental colitis in vivo. *Journal of Biological Chemistry*, 297(1), 100834.

Song, O.-R., Kim, H.-B., Jouny, S., et al. (2017). A bacterial toxin with analgesic properties: Hyperpolarization of DRG neurons by mycolactone. *Toxins*, 9(7), 227.

Soto-Blanco, B. (2022). Herbal glycosides in healthcare. In *Herbal Biomolecules in Healthcare Applications* (pp. 239–282). Elsevier.

Sousa, S., Wingerd, J., Brust, A., Bladen, C., Ragnarsson, L., & Herzig, V. (2017). Discovery and mode of action of a novel analgesic β-toxin from the African spider Ceratogyrus darlingi. *PLoS ONE*, 12(9), e0182848.

Syed, M. H., Gnanakkan, A., & Pitchiah, S. (2021). Exploration of acute toxicity, analgesic, anti-inflammatory, and anti-pyretic activities of the black tunicate, Phallusia nigra (Savigny, 1816) using mice model. *Environmental Science and Pollution Research*, 28, 5809–5821.

Tae, H. S., & Adams, D. J. (2023). Nicotinic acetylcholine receptor subtype expression, function, and pharmacology: Therapeutic potential of α-conotoxins. *Pharmacological Research*, 191, 106747.

Tang, X., Chen, M., Duan, Z., Mwangi, J., Li, P., & Lai, R. (2018). Isolation and characterization of poecistasin, an anti-thrombotic antistasin-type serine protease inhibitor from leech Poecilobdella manillensis. *Toxins*, 10(11), 429.

Tarcha, E. J., Olsen, C. M., Probst, P., Peckham, D., Muñoz-Elías, E. J., Kruger, J. G., & Iadonato, S. P. (2017). Safety and pharmacodynamics of dalazatide, a Kv1. 3 channel inhibitor, in the treatment of plaque psoriasis: A randomized phase 1b trial. *PLoS ONE*, 12(7), e0180762.

Tariq, R., Liaqat, A., & Khalid, U. A. (2021). An insight into the role of bee venom and melittin against tumor cells: A review of breast cancer therapy. *Archives of Breast Cancer*, 8(4), 267–276.

Theunissen, H. J., Dijkema, R., Swinkels, J. C., de Poorter, T. L., Vink, P. M., & Dinther, T. G. (1994). Mutational analysis of antistasin, an inhibitor of blood coagulation factor Xa derived from the Mexican leech Haementeria officinalis. *Thrombosis Research*, 75(1), 41–50.

Thomazini, C. M., Sachetto, A. T. A., de Albuquerque, C. Z., et al. (2021). Involvement of von Willebrand factor and botrocetin in the thrombocytopenia induced by Bothrops jararaca snake venom. *PLoS Neglected Tropical Diseases*, 15(9), e0009715.

Toivonen, J. M., Olivan, S., & Osta, R. (2010). Tetanus toxin C-fragment: The courier and the cure? *Toxins (Basel)*, 2, 2622–2644.

Trevisan, G., & Oliveira, S. M. (2022). Animal venom peptides cause antinociceptive effects by voltage-gated calcium channels activity blockage. *Current Neuropharmacology*, 20(8), 1579.

Tykocki, N. R., Boerman, E. M., & Jackson, W. F. (2017). Smooth muscle ion channels and regulation of vascular tone in resistance arteries and arterioles. *Comprehensive Physiology*, 7(2), 485–581.

Ullah, A., Aldakheel, F. M., Anjum, S. I., Raza, G., Khan, S. A., & Tlak Gajger, I. (2023). Pharmacological properties and therapeutic potential of honey bee venom. *Saudi Pharmaceutical Journal: SPJ: The Official Publication of the Saudi Pharmaceutical Society*, 31(1), 96–109.

Upadhyay, R. K. (2018). Animal venom derived toxins are novel analgesics for treatment of arthritis. *Journal of Molecular Sciences*, 2(1), 6.

Varas, M. A., Muñoz-Montecinos, C., Kallens, V., Simon, V., Allende, M. L., Marcoleta, A. E., & Lagos, R. (2020). Exploiting zebrafish xenografts for testing the in vivo antitumorigenic activity of microcin E492 against human colorectal cancer cells. *Frontiers in Microbiology*, 11, 405.
Varga, J. F. A., Bui-Marinos, M. P., & Katzenback, B. A. (2018). Frog skin innate immune defences: Sensing and surviving pathogens. *Frontiers in Immunology*, 9, 3128.
Voelter, K., Tappeiner, C., Klein, K., Borel, N., Bruetsch, D., Laguna Sanz, F., & Pot, S. A. (2019). Fibrinolytic capacity of desmoteplase compared to tissue plasminogen activator in rabbit eyes. *Journal of Ocular Pharmacology and Therapeutics*, 35(1), 66–75.
Wang, Z., Ye, D., Ye, J., et al. (2019). The TRPA1 channel in the cardiovascular system: Promising features and challenges. *Frontiers in Pharmacology*, 10, 1253.
Wei, D., & Zhang, X. (2022). Biosynthesis, bioactivity, biotoxicity and applications of antimicrobial peptides for human health. *Biosafety and Health*, 4(02), 118–134.
Wu, T., Wang, M., Wu, W., Luo, Q., Jiang, L., Tao, H., & Deng, M. (2019). Spider venom peptides as potential drug candidates due to their anticancer and antinociceptive activities. *The Journal of Venomous Animals and Toxins Including Tropical Diseases*, 25, e146318.
Xu, H., & Ling, Q. (2020). Advances in the research of tetanus toxin and its derivative fragments in the treatment of neurological diseases. *Chinese Journal of Pharmacology and Toxicology*, 34(2), 157–163.
Yacoub, T., Rima, M., Karam, M., Sabatier, J., & Failoun, Z. (2020). Antimicrobials from venomous animals: An overview. *Molecules*, 25(10), 2402.
Yang, M., Huo, X., Miao, Z., & Wang, Y. (2019). Platelet glycoprotein IIb/IIIa receptor inhibitor tirofiban in acute ischemic stroke. *Drugs*, 79(5), 515–529.
Zhang, A., Pan, W., Lv, J., & Wu, H. (2017). Protective effect of amygdalin on LPS-induced acute lung injury by inhibiting NF-κB and NLRP3 signaling pathways. *Inflammation*, 40, 745–751.
Zhang, C., Lin, J., Zhen, C., Wang, F., Sun, X., Kong, X., & Gao, Y. (2022). Amygdalin protects against acetaminophen-induced acute liver failure by reducing inflammatory response and inhibiting hepatocyte death. *Biochemical and Biophysical Research Communications*, 602, 105–112.
Zhang, C., & Yang, M. (2022). Antimicrobial peptides: From design to clinical application. *Antibiotics*, 11, 349.
Zhang, L., Li, Z., Ye, X., Chen, Z., & Chen, Z. S. (2021). Mechanisms of thrombosis and research progress on targeted antithrombotic drugs. *Drug Discovery Today*, 26(10), 2282–2302.
Zhang, Z., Li, Z., Li, J., & Liu, L. (2018). Effects of natural hirudin and low molecular weight heparin in preventing deep venous thrombosis in aged patients with intertrochanteric fracture. *Scientific Reports*, 8(1), 8847.
Zhou, H., & Dong, X. (2019). Botulinum neurotoxin serotype A and its potential relief in neurodegenerative diseases. *Current Pharmaceutical Design*, 25(31), 3324–3334.
Zhou, K., Luo, W., Liu, T., Ni, Y., & Qin, Z. (2022). Neurotoxins acting at synaptic sites: A brief review on mechanisms and clinical applications. *Toxins*, 15(1), 18.
Ziaja, M., Dziedzic, A., Szafraniec, K., & Piastowska-Ciesielska, A. (2020). Cecropins in cancer therapies-where we have been? *European Journal of Pharmacology*, 882, 173317.

11

Harmful Algal Blooms: Threat to Marine Life

Peace Abiodun Olajide, Babatunde Oluwafemi Adetuyi, Charles Chinazaekpele Chidume, Victoria Olufunmi Adeyemo-Eleyode, Peter Gbenga Oni, and Oluwatosin Adefunke Adetuyi

11.1 Introduction

Photosynthetic organisms, such as macrophytes, benthic and planktonic microalgae, and cyanobacteria, are what sustain aquatic ecosystems by fixing carbon, producing oxygen, and serving as the foundation of food webs. However, under some situations, the abundance of some taxa can increase to the point where it could be harmful to people as well as other living things. The phrase "harmful algal blooms" (HABs), which encompasses a range of species and consequences that are deemed undesirable by humans, is frequently used to describe these proliferations. All aquatic ecosystems, including freshwater, brackish, and marine ones (Aransiola et al., 2024), as well as all latitudes, are home to HABs. The benefits that aquatic ecosystems provide to human wellness and welfare—food supply, revenue generation, tourism, and recreation—are specifically threatened by lethal microalgal blooms in this work (Figure 11.1).

There are thousands of microalgal taxa known to exist; only about 300 of them are known to be harmful. More than 100 diverse species produce potent, long-lasting natural poisons that are hazardous or even lethal to humans and other animals, with no obvious physiological, evolutionary, or structural commonalities (Moestrup et al., 2009). Many human syndromes have been linked to the chemically varied substances produced by poisonous HAB species, and many of these compounds may also have negative effects on specific fish, seabirds, reptiles, and marine mammals.

Toxins can be inhaled by people through aerosolized toxins or toxic chemicals, skin contact with polluted water, or consumption of infected seafood items (fish or shellfish). HAB toxins are bio-concentrated in foodborne poisoning cases (Figure 11.2). They are often transferred up the food network to humans without harming the vector aquatic creature that first ingested

DOI: 10.1201/9781003500605-13

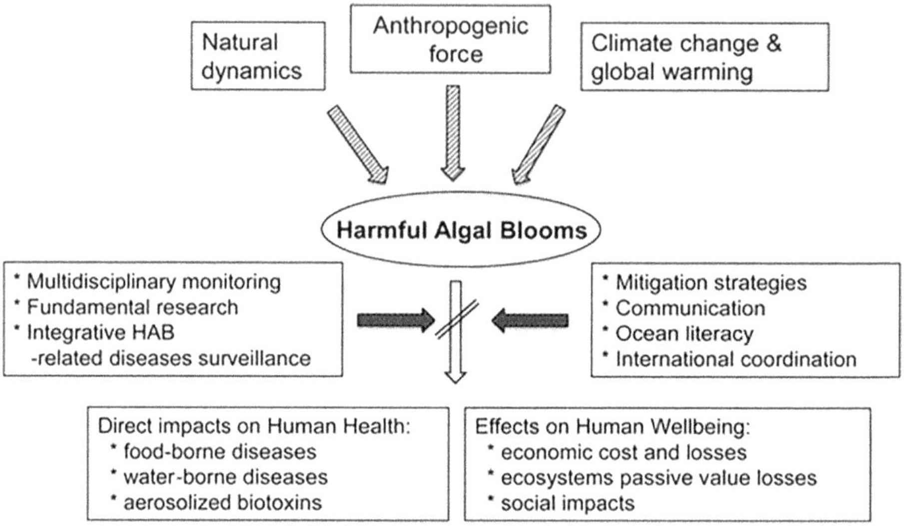

FIGURE 11.1
Conceptual connections between the primary factors that contribute to HAB incidence.

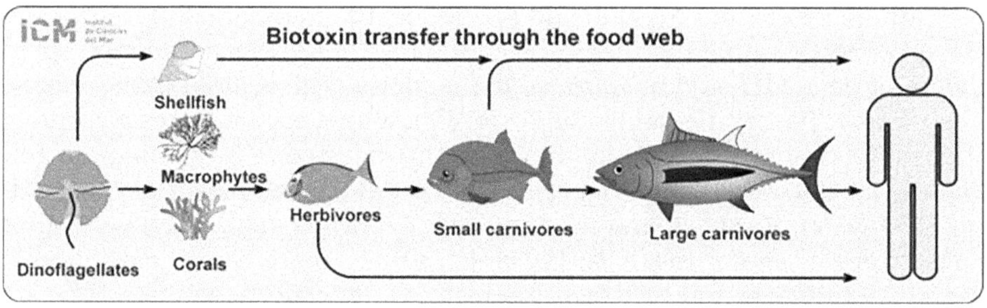

FIGURE 11.2
Humans are exposed to biotoxins via the marine food web.

the toxin. While modest abundances of extremely toxic microalgae can also cause seafood poisoning, high abundances of the HAB species that produce the toxin are typically associated with harmful effects. These hazardous epidemics have direct effects on human health; however, they also have unintended consequences in terms of costs and macroeconomic impact on other facets of the well-being of people. Specifically, HAB events may result in the closure of significant shellfisheries (Jin et al., 2008) and raise monitoring and management expenses (Hoagland et al., 2002).

The production of excess algal biomass is another dangerous consequence of various HAB taxa since it can have varying effects on ecosystems and individual organisms. Large blooms can lead to hypoxia and lower oxygen concentrations in marine waters when their accreted biomass is broken down by bacteria. This is particularly true in bottom waters that are isolated from surface waters by density gradients. Apart from the mortality of benthic animals due to oxygen depletion, some HABs can cause unpleasant surface scum and foul odors that deter visitors from visiting coastal leisure areas (Scatasta et al., 2003). Phytotoxins have the potential to induce chronic conditions and fatalities in untamed and domesticated fish (gill injury), birds (hypothermia), mammals of the sea, or particular invertebrates, in addition to generating financial losses in finfish farming and sightseeing. They can also cause losses in the non-market, "passive" values that people may have for exceptional ecosystems or protected species. These examples demonstrate how HABs may diminish the non-market, inadvertent benefits of aquatic environments and their services, limiting how aquatic environments may enhance human health and well-being (Hoagland & Scatasta, 2006).

Microalgae blooms, even those that are considered detrimental by humans, are a natural occurrence (Gowen et al., 2012), and many coastal human cultures have ingrained awareness of HAB episodes in their cultural history. In the past, this knowledge has assisted in reducing some of the negative consequences of HABs. Nonetheless, it may still be helpful to expand knowledge about public health hazards and methods that researchers and decision-makers can collaborate to solve to lessen the effects of HABs on human health and welfare. It is crucial to understand that while HABs are caused by intricate interactions between physical, chemical, and biological processes that operate in the marine environment at various spatiotemporal scales, prevention of their occurrence is not a practical option. The frequency of HABs in particular places may have been impacted by human changes to the marine environment during the past 50 years, particularly those that occur near the land-sea border. These alterations include the development of human-made beaches, modifications to the circulation of harbor water, and the dispersal of species through enriching nutrients and ship ballast waters (Davidson et al., 2014).

In addition to these stressors, climate change is already raising ocean temperatures in some regions, which may have an impact on the frequency of HABs (Gowen et al., 2012). More specifically, there may be fluctuations in the magnitude, intensity, and spatial spread of HABs, but considering the wide range of toxicological, physicochemical, biological, and ecological characteristics of HAB creatures, potential reactions are probably going to be very species specific. As a result, predicting such changes is still highly conjectural and needs a longer time series of ecological processes in addition to more specialized research (including modeling).

11.2 The Immediate Effects of HABS on Human Health

In maritime habitats, HABs can directly impact human health through foodborne illnesses linked to the eating of infected seafood (Figure 11.2), cutaneous contact with polluted water, and/or inhalation of airborne biotoxins. Apart from recognized health issues linked to microalgal toxins, there are also newly discovered phytotoxins and potential hazards of biotoxin contamination in desalinated drinking water. Toxic substances produced by marine microalgae will be referred to as "biotoxins," "phycotoxins," or "toxins" in the text that follows.

11.3 Foodborne Diseases: Overview

The most well-documented effect of HABs on humans is poisoning from consuming seafood contaminated with biotoxins (Figure 11.2). The poisoning process is caused by the bioconcentration of the biotoxins in filter-feeding fauna, primarily bivalve mollusks like *Mytilus* spp., which are ordinarily immune to these compounds. Additional vectors include fish (such as some planktivorous fish or members of the Tetraodontidae family), some crustaceans (such as crabs), some marine gastropods (such as whelks and moon snails), and echinoderms that absorb biotoxins through the food chain (Deeds et al., 2008). Long after the bloom in the saltwater has subsided, toxins deposited in fish tissues may persist. Furthermore, because these biotoxins lack a characteristic taste or odor, they cannot be identified except by using specialist laboratory testing. They are also not removed by boiling or processing seafood products (Zaias et al., 2010).

Although they can also have other effects on human health (e.g., okadaic acid altering phosphatase activity), the majority of algae toxins are principally neurotoxins (e.g., brevetoxins damaging the Na^{+} channels). Depending on the primary symptomatic mode, a variety of indications can be brought on by the various poisonous substances, which is why they have been linked to several clinically described syndromes: amnesic (ASP), azaspirazid (AZP), diarrheic (DSP), neurotoxic (NSP), and paralytic (PSP) shellfish poisonings, as well as ciguatera fish poisoning (CFP). According to Baden and Trainer (1993), among others, the disorders may manifest as symptoms from the neurological, digestive, respiratory, hepatic, dermatological, or cardiac systems. The effects can range from weeks to months (Friedman et al., 2008) and can be acute (Medcof, 1985). Many of the toxicological mechanisms behind the acute health impacts of HAB biotoxins remain poorly understood, despite a wealth of information regarding these effects. Furthermore, nothing is known about these biotoxins' long-term consequences, whether they result from acute exposure that causes permanent harm or from low-level exposure over an extended period.

At the moment, the only practical way to protect the general population from illnesses linked to food is to stop tainted shellfish from entering market sectors by continuously monitoring the species at fault and/or the level of biotoxin in seafood. In actuality, human exposure to biotoxins has been successfully reduced in many regions of the world by well-designed monitoring programs that concentrate on the toxic chemicals and causative organisms in commercial seafood connected to clinical syndromes. The Working Group on Harmful Algal Blooms Dynamics of the ICES (International Council for the Exploration of the Sea) UNESCO IOC compiles information regarding active HAB monitoring programs only at regional levels, such as for the North Atlantic. Monitoring, however, might be improved by supplementing it with other measures, including educating the public in non-commercial regions impacted by HABs (Reich et al., 2015) and raising awareness of the intricate mechanisms underlying detrimental events (Whyte et al., 2014).

Regrettably, dangerous blooms may happen in places where they haven't been seen before as a result of rising human impact on coastal marine ecosystems and global warming (Trainer et al., 2013). Furthermore, novel biotoxins are always being discovered. According to Turner et al. (2015), in these situations, identifying the causal organism and detecting toxins provide new difficulties for monitoring and management protocols. Notably, the most prevalent form of HAB-associated poisoning in tropical environments is ciguatera fish poisoning, for which there are no effective guidelines in place to safeguard human populations. According to Mattei et al. (2014), there is a risk of food poisoning in regions distant from the fishery due to the rise in international tourism and seafood trade.

11.4 Most Common Temperature-Related Biotoxin Syndromes

The most prevalent HABs in temperate latitudes of North America, South America, Asia, Europe, and South Africa result in shellfish poisonings.

Numerous species of Nitzschia and Pseudo-nitzschia produce the neurotoxin domoic acid. Consuming blue mussels from the island of Prince Edward, Canada, in 1987 caused a human epidemic of amnesic shellfish poisoning that left 107 people sick and 3 people dead (Bates et al., 1989). Since then, humans and other large vertebrates have been affected by a variety of shellfish toxicity episodes that are frequently caused by blooms of these pennate diatoms.

The small-plated dinoflagellate *Azadinium spinosum* produces a distinct class of polyether biotoxins known as azaspiracids (Tillmann et al., 2009). They were initially discovered in Irish mussels in 1995 (Satake et al., 1998). This biotoxin produces symptoms resembling those of DSP (Twiner et al., 2008), while in mouse experiments, slowly developing paralysis has also been reported. Nowadays, azaspiracids have been discovered in several more EU nations, with about 20 distinct AZA analogues being identified.

Diarrhetic shellfish poisoning (DSP) was first identified in association with *Dinophysis fortii* in Japan (Yasumoto et al., 1980) and *D. acuminata* in coastal waters of the Netherlands (Kat, 1983). In 1989, DSP-containing mussels were consumed, resulting in DSP poisoning (Boni et al., 1992). As a result of the production of okadaic acid or its derivative dinophysis toxins by ten species of the genus Dinophysis, two species of the genus Phalachroma (Reguera et al., 2012), and *Prorocentrum lima* (Koike et al., 1998), diarrheagenic shellfish poisoning is triggered. Severe (rapidly onset) but typically nonfatal digestive problems are caused by human DSP biotoxins binding to phosphatase receptors. In Europe, DSP outbreaks are frequent and impact shellfish consumers in ten or more nations. Occasionally, outbreaks have led to widespread illness and up to a 10-month closure of shellfish harvesting areas (Reguera et al., 2014).

The more recently identified yessotoxins and pectenotoxins are categorized in the DSP category for regulatory purposes. Some Dinophysis species produce pectenotoxins (Paz et al., 2004). In light of recent studies showing that oral administration of pectenotoxins and yessotoxins in mice had no harmful effects, experts have recently advocated for the deregulation of these chemicals (ICES, 2006).

A class of biotoxins known collectively as "brevetoxin" is responsible for neurotoxic shellfish poisoning (NSP). *Karenia brevis*, a naked dinoflagel, is the main producer of brevetoxins (Fleming et al., 2011). Interestingly, NSP has not been connected to any human deaths (Van Dolah, 2000). As early as 1648, toxic K. *brevis* red tides were observed in the Western Gulf of Mexico; reports of these events date back to the 1840s in Florida (Kirkpatrick et al., 2004).

Strong neurotoxins called saxitoxin and its derivatives are the cause of paralytic shellfish poisoning (PSP), which can result in facial numbness, headaches, nausea, and, in extreme situations, respiratory failure and even death. According to Ayres (1975), the earliest probable occurrences in the UK were in Leith in 1827 and Liverpool in 1888. The earliest known PSP epidemics were in 1901 and 1793, respectively, in Norway (Yndestad et al., 1985) and British Columbia (Gaines & Taylor, 1985). Events involving hazardous shellfish from the 1930s and 1940s were documented by Medcof (1985). PSP is mostly linked to blooms of the thecate (armored) dinoflagellate genus *Alexandrium* in Europe and North America, specifically *A. minutum* and *A. tamarense/funyense/catenella* group (Touzet et al., 2007). However, other species and strains of *Alexandrium* are not harmful.

11.5 Ciguatera Fish Poisoning

Ciguatera fish poisoning (CFP) is a common food poisoning that is connected to a natural, non-bacterial toxin and is found throughout the tropics, with a higher prevalence in susceptible island cultures. Several species of the benthic dinoflagellate genus *Gambierdiscus* (mostly G. *toxicus*) produce ciguatoxins or their precursors. The biotoxins are typically associated with fish, especially larger carnivorous species like barracuda (Heymann, 2004), though they have been detected in over 400 different fish species as well. A variety of acute neurological, gastrointestinal, and cardiac symptoms have been documented following the consumption of ciguatoxin-contaminated fish. Acute neurological symptoms can also linger for weeks or months in certain cases (Skinner et al., 2011). Acute ciguatera symptoms are made worse by repeated exposure to ciguatoxins (Pottier et al., 2001).

Regretfully, misdiagnosis and underreporting have left the true prevalence of the condition poorly recorded (Radke et al., 2015). Therefore, little is known about how it affects the health of ecosystems and human communities. According to data from the 17 PICTs' Health and Fisheries Authorities, the region's mean annual incidence rate from 1973 to 1983 was estimated by Skinner et al. (2011) to be 104 cases per 100,000 inhabitants. These estimations suggest that between 1998 and 2008, the South Pacific's documented CFP incidence should have grown by 60%, or up to 194 cases per 100,000 persons.

The incidence of CFP disease is highly variable, with certain locations experiencing particularly high rates. For example, between 2000 and 2008, there were as many as 497 cases per 10,000 people annually in French Polynesia (Chateau-Degat et al., 2009; Chinain et al., 2010). Similarly, between 1996 and 2006, there were as many as 440 cases per 10,000 people annually in the Caribbean (Tester et al., 2010). Data indicate that CFP constitutes an acute and chronic condition with significant public health significance at both local and global levels, despite uncertainty over the true frequency. Future anthropogenic pressures, such as rising coastal zone development; ocean warming (Villareal et al., 2007; Kibler et al., 2015); or natural disasters, such as hurricanes, may make the health issue worse. Coral reefs may be harmed by these stresses because they favor more resilient macroalgae that offer fresh surfaces for the development of the toxicogenic benthic dinoflagellates involved (Tester et al., 2010; Chateau-Degat et al., 2005).

It is difficult to address CFP as a health problem for the public by definition. For instance, local fishermen have traditionally used their traditional knowledge to "manage" the dangers associated with CFP. They may alert one another to places where fish that are known to be contaminated with ciguatoxin are found. Ciguatera generally goes undiagnosed or is only discovered after costly examination, so CFP cases could arise in non-tropical places due to increased trade and seaside tourism (Mattei et al., 2014; Epelboin et al., 2014). There is no biomarker to identify the sickness in humans, nor is there a dependable, economical way to identify the biotoxin.

11.6 Alternatives and Palytoxin-Related Poisoning

Ostreopsis has been linked to poisoning by consuming palytoxin (PLTX)-infected clupeid fish, crabs, or sea urchins (Deeds & Schwartz, 2010). Among the most potent marine-derived biotoxins are this chemical and its analogues (Ciminiello et al., 2015; Brissard et al., 2015). It is difficult to ascertain the actual threat of PLTX poisoning for individuals who eat seafood, despite the well-recorded but minuscule amount of acute PLTX-related incidents of poisoning in these tropical locales. This is because PLTX is often found in reef species that are not harvested for commercial purposes, it is distributed primarily in tropical regions of developing countries with minimal surveillance and reporting, and it co-occurs with other seafood biotoxins.

According to Rhodes (2011), Ostreopsis appears to be spreading to temperate latitudes, and during the past 20 years, there have been repeated blooms in the Mediterranean seas (Mangialajo et al., 2011; Illoul et al., 2012). Aerosol exposure at swimming beaches has been linked to Ostreopsis proliferation in this location (Brissard et al., 2014). The Panel on Contaminants in the Food Chain (CONTAM Panel) of the European Food Safety Authority (2009) assessed the health hazards to humans posed by PLTX-group biotoxins found in shellfish. The European policy to keep an eye on PLTX hasn't been formed yet, though.

Due to its ability to show both benthic and planktonic phases, Ostreopsis is easily dispersed, which increases the variety of seafood that may become infected and makes monitoring it more difficult (Bravo et al., 2012).

11.7 New Biotoxins Rising

11.7.1 Cyclic Imines

Numerous dinoflagellates have purportedly been claimed to create cyclic imines, such as spirolides, pinnatoxins, and gymnodimine. Due to the rapid death that takes place in the lipid-soluble biotoxin mice biological experiments, they are usually classified as fast-acting biotoxins (Molgo et al., 2014). Acute human food poisoning episodes had originally been linked to both gym nodimine and pinnatoxins (Seki et al., 1995; Uemura et al., 1995). Subsequent investigations revealed that the actual cause of the poisonings was not pinnatoxins but rather bacterial (Vibrio) contamination or other biotoxins. A Mediterranean lagoon in the south of France was discovered to have the highest levels of pinnatoxin-G, according to reports from all around the world (Hess et al., 2013). However, it should be noted that no incidents of food poisoning have been reported as of yet. Because of the biotoxin's strong affinity for the nicotinic acetylcholine (nACh) channel and its chemically inert nature against both acids and bases, there is a chance that prolonged exposure to even low concentrations of pinnatoxins may be harmful to people's health (Jackson et al., 2012).

11.8 BMAA

Recently, it has been confirmed that certain cyanobacteria that proliferate in freshwater habitats produce b-N-methylamino-L-alanine (BMAA), a non-protein amino acid. Seafood as well as marine diatoms have been shown to exhibit this (Jiang et al., 2014a; Brand et al., 2010; Reveillon et al., 2015). According to Bradley et al. (2013), there is a correlation between exposure to BMAA and a higher chance of developing neurodegenerative disorders like Parkinson's, Alzheimer's, and amyotrophic lateral sclerosis (ALS). Unknown acute food poisoning cases may be related to marine cyanotoxins in general (Golubic et al., 2010; Roue et al., 2014). Further investigation is required to validate these results as well as any potential epidemiological connections between BMAA and neurodegenerative illnesses.

11.9 Macro-Algae

There have been reports of macroalgal food poisoning from Asian nations where these items are customarily consumed. The polycavernosides present in *Gracilaria edulis* are particularly significant (Louzao et al., 2014). The metabolite domoic acid has been confirmed in *Chondria armata* after these macroalgae were grown in a lab (Daigo, 1959; Jiang et al., 2014b). Macroalgae contain domoic acid along with various glutamate receptor agonists, which may be important for studies on the effects of chronic exposure to subacute biotoxin doses.

11.10 Chronic and Subacute Exposure's Impact

The acute effects of marine biotoxins have long been recognized. As a result, international legislation (FAO, Codex alimentarius) has prioritized the avoidance of acute poisoning incidents (Lawrence et al., 2011). Few researchers have looked at long-term human exposure to sub-acute levels or the chronic impact of an acute exposure incident. Some studies have shown that minimal exposures to certain chemicals, including domoic acid, may have some negative effects on health when using in vivo models. Domoic acid exposure during pregnancy produced effects on the rat offspring (Levin et al., 2005). In this study, rats were exposed to domoic acid at a single low dose early in the period following delivery. The rats developed chronic hypo-activity, with the female progeny performing particularly badly in a labyrinth. According to Baron et al. (2011), rats exposed to modest doses of domoic acid developed locomotor abnormalities. Finally, gene alteration and impaired cellular mitochondrial function were also observed in zebrafish subjected to minimal exposure repeatedly over 36 weeks (Lefebve et al., 2012; Hiolski et al., 2014).

When small amounts of saxitoxins are repeatedly or chronically consumed through drinking water made from desalinated saltwater, sub-acute effects could also be an issue. Up until now, saxitoxins have only been restricted based on their acute effects; in Australia, Brazil, and New Zealand, drinking water is allowed to have up to 3 μg/L. However, recent research indicates that long-term use of saxitoxins may affect antioxidant defenses and cause oxidative stress in mammal livers and brains (Ramos et al., 2014; Silva et al., 2014). According to Molgo et al. (2014), cyclic imine biotoxins are capable of binding with receptors associated with Parkinson's and Alzheimer's disease, among other neurodegenerative diseases. Interestingly, studies using both in vitro and in-animal models showed certain benefits against Alzheimer's disease for gymnodimine and 13-desmethyl spirolide C. These substances ought to be investigated further to see whether they have any medicinal uses (Alonso et al., 2013).

11.11 Exposure to Mixtures Both in Combination and Separately

Patients may experience confusing diagnoses as a result of co-exposure to various agents. For instance, gastroenteritis (vomiting and diarrhea) induced by bacterial infection in shellfish may resemble the degree of disease brought on by okadaic acid. Because bacteria usually need to incubate in the patient for a while before producing their full effect, diseases from eating shellfish compromised with biotoxins typically appear a few hours after consumption, whereas bacterial pathogen-contaminated shellfish can take 12 to 24 hours to show symptoms.

Another poorly researched topic is exposure to mixtures of various biotoxin groups. Numerous studies have shown that biotoxins can co-occur in a single algal species or in shellfish that has been contaminated simultaneously by various algal species, so this is a severe issue (Reguera et al., 2014; Suikkanen et al., 2013). Specifically, there is the worry that certain substances—like yessotoxins, which frequently do not cause severe shellfish poisoning in people—possibly absorbed after other biotoxins—like azaspiracids and okadaic acid—damage the digestive system. Just a small number of researchers have looked into this possible risk because pure biotoxin supplies for the majority of HAB biotoxins are extremely scarce. When administered sub-acutely orally to mice, azaspiracids and yessotoxins did not show any potentiation (Aasen et al., 2011). Similarly, when ingested by mice at subacute dosages, even azaspiracids and okadaic acid—two biotoxins recognized for their capacity to injure the human digestive tract—did not produce synergistic effects (Aune et al., 2012). Yessotoxins and okadaic acid together did not produce any toxic effects in the oral mouse model (Sosa et al., 2013). Nevertheless, since the pH of the mouse and human digestive tracts differs greatly, more research (maybe with primates) could be required to rule out the possibility of synergistic harm. Last, a fly larval model demonstrated some domoic acid potentiation by the fungal metabolite peptaibols (Ruiz et al., 2010). These diverse results should be regarded as quite preliminary because they heavily depend on the biological model that was employed. We need longitudinal studies of people exposed to naturally occurring combinations of biotoxins over extended periods at individually modest amounts.

11.12 Waterborne Diseases

The primary threat to human and animal health in freshwater environments is cyanobacteria blooms, which are mostly caused by cyanotoxins such as microcystins contaminating drinking water supplies (Stewart et al., 2008). Health issues can also result from direct skin contact, aerosol exposure, or water ingestion during work or play in freshwater habitats where cyanobacteria blooms are present. On the other hand, while there is currently no published evidence to support the idea that ingesting seawater containing toxic marine microalgae poses a risk to human health, it is nevertheless a possibility.

The possibility of toxic HABs contaminating drinking water from desalination plants has lately come to light. Desalination is a fast-expanding global process that produces water for industrial and residential usage. More than 14,000 desalination facilities might be found in 150 countries in 2012 (Anderson & McCarthy, 2012). The West Asia Gulf region accounted for around half of this capacity, followed by North America (17%), Asia (without the Gulf) (10%), North Africa (8%), and Europe (7%). The installed capacity stood at 52.3 million m^3 per day in 2008. By 2015, the desalination process will have produced 94 million m^3 of freshwater per day globally, assuming an annual growth rate of 12%.

Chemical and physical characteristics indicate that reverse osmosis should be used in the desalination process to effectively remove them. Seubert et al.

(2012) supported this notion with a study that combined laboratory testing with a five-year observation of a Californian operating plant. Nevertheless, it has been noted that some taste and odor chemicals can penetrate preliminary processing and reverse osmosis barriers. One such compound is geosmin, which has a low molecular weight and is similar to the biotoxins previously addressed (Reiss et al., 2006). Furthermore, in membranes containing micro-fissures brought on the total removal of biotoxins is not guaranteed. High-biomass blooms can clog intake filters and result in excessive pressures (Richlen et al., 2010). However, there are just a few studies (Seubert et al., 2012) from plants operating during blooms of biotoxin-producing HAB species, and the data are still sparse (Laycock et al., 2012), based mostly on laboratory research (without the necessary up-scaling). Thus, more investigation is required to determine what happens to biotoxins throughout the desalination process. Biotoxins in drinking water from desalination facilities need to be monitored due to the possibility of long-term exposure.

11.13 HABS and Biotoxins in Aerosol Form

11.13.1 *Karenia brevis* and Brevetoxins

For more than 30 years, studies involving multiple institutions and disciplines have investigated how respiratory symptoms can be brought on by breathing in aerosols containing brevetoxins during high-biomass, toxic *Karenia brevis* blooms in the Gulf of Mexico and along Florida's coast (Fleming et al., 2011). Studies have shown that people with asthma (and perhaps other lung conditions) were more vulnerable to experiencing more severe and persistent symptoms (Bean et al., 2011). Respiratory disorders have been reported by beachgoers and full-time lifeguards (Backer et al., 2005). The health consequences of these effects have been modeled by more recent research (Hoagland et al., 2014).

To reduce the negative effects that *Karenia* blooms have on society and public health, the research's findings have been utilized to collaborate with relevant parties in the creation of local response management plans [93]. Decisions regarding one's health have also been influenced by information about their possibility.

11.14 Inflammatory Responses to *Ostreopsis*

Large-scale *Ostreopsis* spp. blooms have taken place in the Mediterranean during the last 20 years. During these blooms, beachgoers have gone for treatment in medical facilities and basic medical care clinics for upper respiratory illnesses (rhinorrhoea), fever, eye and nose irritation, and general malaise (Illoul et al., 2012). There's a chance that several Brazilian beaches are experiencing something similar (Proenca et al., 2010). Exposure to aerosols containing biotoxins or allergenic chemicals produced by fragments of Ostreopsis cells or associated microbiota may be the cause of the health impacts (Casabianca et al., 2013; Ciminiello et al., 2014). It has not been verified, however, it has been suggested that skin irritation results from direct skin contact with saltwater that has a high concentration of Ostreopsis cells. Currently, research is being conducted in both epidemiological and ecological domains to enhance comprehension of the dynamics of Ostreopsis blooms and potential connections to human health consequences (Vila et al., 2014; Berdalet et al., 2015).

11.15 Effects of HABS on Human Wellbeing

Along with the health hazards that come with being exposed to biotoxins, marine HABs can also have an impact on human health. They encompass the commercial and recreational uses of the coastal and marine areas by humans as well as the non-commercial, passive uses of the ocean. Furthermore, because of misunderstandings and insufficient communication of health hazards, marine HABs may cause complicated societal reactions in the impacted human communities.

11.16 Economic Effects of HABs Linked to Food Security and Seafood-Related Activities

Some HABs pose a threat to aquaculture food production, which has grown to be a significant source of nutrition for growing human populations, especially in coastal areas of emerging nations (related to declining wild fish stocks). Similar to farming, and occasionally in addition to it, aquaculture contributes to the support of numerous local and regional economies (FAO, 2006). The best methods for currently shielding people from HAB-related seafood poisoning associated with shellfish farming are to periodically close business-related and leisurely harvesting or growing areas and to check for the existence of HAB species or biotoxins (and wild harvest). Economic losses can arise from the collection and growth of shellfish as well as from the aquaculture of specific finfish when seafood products are contaminated. Ancillary businesses such as seafood processing, distribution, wholesaling, and retailing may also experience losses (Larkin & Adams, 2007; Morgan et al., 2010).

It is difficult to estimate the total economic expenses related to HAB occurrences. Geographical location, type of seafood, frequency, and severity of HAB-related incidents, length of fisheries closures, and healthcare expenses all significantly affect these expenditures. Hoagland et al. (2002), for instance, calculated the yearly economic effects of HABs in the USA from 1987 to 1992. The economic consequences were estimated to be worth US$50.0 million per year at the time; this amount has since been adjusted for inflation to US$100.0 million annually (Hoagland & Scatasta, 2006). It is noteworthy that the anticipated impacts vary significantly from one year to the next. This estimate was derived from a compilation of evaluations of the economic impacts in the areas of monitoring and management, commercial fisheries, public health, and recreation and tourism. Remarkably, the majority of the effects over that period—roughly 42% of the average nationwide effects—are related to public health.

There aren't many studies that address the precise economic impact of illnesses caused by HAB. According to UNEP Global Environmental Outlook estimates, the yearly global economic burden of algal biotoxins on individuals from seafood alone is US$4.0 billion (GESAMP, 2001). In contrast, the annual cost of infectious hepatitis caused by seafood eating was calculated to be US$7.2 billion. Depending on the severity of the occurrence, the annual direct medical care expenses for the respiratory and digestive disorders brought on by *K. brevis* blooms varied from US$0.1 to US$0.7 million (Hoagland et al., 2014). However, huge, long-lasting blooms, like the one that occurred in 2005–06, may result in illness expenses exceeding US$1.0 million annually. With a discount rate of 3% and the assumption that *K. brevis* blooms would continue to cause disease costs on average each year, future medical expenses would be marked up at a rate between US$2.0 and US$24.0 million.

Fleming et al. (2002) calculated that in traditionally non-endemic countries, such as Canada, the average medical expenditures of screening and therapy for ciguatera fish poisoning were about CA$2470 per case. In 1990, there were approximately 1000 cases annually associated with tourism and food importation. According to Pennotti et al. (2013), precise calculations of the human costs associated with these illnesses require sufficient knowledge of their incidence and prevalence as well as an awareness of the short- and long-term impacts on human health.

A review of the costs associated with monitoring and management—such as sampling programs or approaches to lessen the likelihood of HAB occurrences or their effects—has to be considered in any evaluation of the financial impacts of HABs (Hoagland et al., 2002). Strategies to lessen the effects of HABs could include, for example, restricting the closures of shellfish harvesting or changing the timing of harvesting shellfish or finfish, although these activities might also come with costs related to the marketability of the final product. Wessells et al. (1995) state that paralytic shellfish poisoning in blue mussels from the Canadian Maritimes caused illnesses and consequent harvest limits, which hurt the market for mussels from Maine. Following the market's demand for seafood declined upon discovering a HAB-induced fish death, Whitehead et al. (2003) found that mandatory seafood inspection systems were more effective in regaining customer confidence and driving demand than broad public assurances of seafood safety.

Despite causing short-term losses, experience indicates that closure tactics in areas that produce shellfish may be advantageous in the long run. For instance, there have been some advantages to using this strategy in the northern Japanese regions. Over 60% of Japan's scallop aquaculture is sourced from this region; annually, it produces approximately 500,000 tons, valued at approximately US$700.0 million. The 1980s saw the total shutdown of shellfish harvesting due to paralytic and diarrheal shellfish poisoning incidents, which had severe economic effects (Imai et al., 2014). Another illustration comes from Northwest Spain's Galician region. The Rías is an extremely productive ecosystem that produces between 0.2 and 0.3 million tons of mussels (*Mytilus edulis*) annually. As DSP biotoxin concentrations exceed EU regulatory thresholds, harvesting prohibitions can extend up to nine months (Blanco et al., 2013). With the greatest rate of diarrheic shellfish poisoning in the world, Europe is closely watching biotoxins to make sure that any restrictions on shellfish harvesting are only temporary.

The majority of HAB species that kill fishes release biotoxins that are cytotoxic, neurotoxic, or hemolytic. Large-scale fish kills, frequently at aquaculture locations, have been directly connected to certain HAB species. Fisheries linked to HABs were projected to have lost more than E800 million in European coastal waters in 2003 (Scatasta et al., 2003). Kim (2006) estimated that Japan suffers yearly losses from aquaculture attributable to HAB of more than US$1.0 billion. At the Workshop on Economic Impacts of Harmful Algal Blooms and Aquaculture hosted by PICES (North Pacific Science Organization), recent estimates were given (Trainer & Yoshida, 2014). The combined economic losses from the production of farmed fish and shellfish in Korea, Japan, and China between 2006 and 2012 were projected to be US$94.0 million. Numerous estimates of real economic losses should be considered overstated, as they fail to account for the saved expenditures related to not fishing. Remember that a large number of these estimations represent missed gross revenues (sales). In instances where commercial wild harvest fisheries are not well managed, leading to economic or biological overexploitation—a frequent occurrence—loss of net economic values, which indicate true declines in human welfare, are probably not going to account for a significant portion of reported lost sales.

The functioning of desalination plants may be particularly impacted by high biomass HABs, which would disrupt water production and cause large financial losses (Andderson & McCarthy, 2012; Richlen et al., 2010).

11.17 Social Impacts of the Health Risks Caused by Toxic HABs: The Case of Ciguatera Fish Poisoning

HABs may have detrimental social effects on human populations whose income is derived from shellfish and aquaculture operations. Reputational damage, decreased earnings, layoffs, and long-term changes in seafood eating patterns are a few examples of these consequences (Magnien, 2001). These additional human components have received relatively little research, and many of the social effects are still mostly speculative and unknown (Bauer et al., 2009).

Ciguatera fish poisoning has been associated with several unfavorable consequences, such as the disappearance of a traditional food source, loss of revenue in fishing industry operations, a drop in tourism, increased medical costs, and substantial control and surveillance costs (Epstein & Rapport, 1996). Research indicates that apprehension over CFP leads to a reduction in coral lagoon fishing (Dewailly et al., 2008), hence heightening dependence on pelagic fish or less nutritious imported canned fish or red meat. This new diet may contribute to the increasing weight gain pattern among those from the Pacific Islands, along with decreased levels of cardiovascular activity. Chronic diseases, such as diabetes, hypertension, and cardiovascular diseases, are also becoming more common in indigenous Pacific populations (Lewis & Ruff, 1993).

The financial status of tropical islands, especially those that mostly rely on the local reef fisheries for tourism, export commodities, and food, may suffer from outbreaks of ciguatera fish poisoning. The gradual decline of indigenous fishing abilities has been attributed to decreased fishing attempts caused by the endemic ciguatera, as younger generations give up on artisanal or commercial fishing. One such instance is Rarotonga, an island in the southern Cook Islands with the highest incidence of ciguatera toxicity worldwide (Rongo & van Woesik, 2012).

When discussing how HABs impact the general population, it is important to note that tropical waterways are not adequately maintained to prevent ciguatera fish poisoning. Because finfish in these areas may contain deposited ciguatoxin, fishermen may usually get to regions where CFP illnesses could spread widely. In light of this, scientists and managers might want to give priority to defining the scope of the CFP issue in tropical areas and creating solutions.

11.18 Present and Future Challenges, Strategies, and Opportunities

HABs are natural occurrences that most likely started thousands of years ago before history was written (Mudie et al., 2002). HABs are an international problem for humans, yet it is not practical to think that HABs might be avoided. However, during the past 40 years, advances in our knowledge of HAB dynamics have provided new perspectives for developing mitigation solutions. Effective approaches take into account both the current state of affairs and the likelihood that HAB will spread and become more common in the future due to climatic and other environmental changes. Across the globe, common tactics might be modified to address particular, regional issues. Notwithstanding certain drawbacks, recent technological developments and concerted global research initiatives should contribute to better management of the effects of HABs.

11.19 Enhancing Surveillance and Investigating Requirements to Anticipate and Identify HAB Occurrences

Fewer fatal human poisonings have occurred since HAB taxa and their toxins have been monitored in different parts of the world (Davidson & Bresnan, 2009). There are regional variations in how these monitoring operations are carried out since different entities have varying capacities for conducting local risk assessments. These initiatives have, for the most part, been successful in protecting public health; nevertheless, as environmental conditions—particularly those related to climate change—and human activities in coastal oceans evolve, further development will be required.

There are presently no efficient surveillance systems in developing nations, where they are usually at best rudimentary, despite the increasing shipment of marine-based goods to other countries (Reich et al., 2015). Established monitoring programs have constraints relating to technology, logistics, and cost even if they have been successful (DeGrasse & Martinez-Diaz, 2012; Hess, 2012; Suzuki & Watanabe, 2012).

The most popular method of monitoring dangerous algal species is light microscopy, although using it takes time and requires certain knowledge and experience. The creation of quantitative biomolecular instruments to aid in monitoring may enhance it. With so many different creatures to follow and no truly quantitative molecular technologies for determining their number, monitoring groups are now unable to replace optical microscopy as the primary tool. Sustaining and assisting microscopists in their detection and measurement of HAB species is necessary to achieve successful surveillance.

Although it is possible to identify hazardous microalgal species in coastal waters and use this information to predict the likelihood of biotoxins developing in, say, shellfish, there are still a lot of unknowns (Trainer & Suddleson, 2005). Among these is the fact that toxicity in shellfish is not always correlated with the presence of potentially hazardous organisms. For instance, it has been reported that simultaneously occurring, morphologically identical, poisonous, and non-toxic *Alexandrium tamarense* cells can be found in Scottish waters (Touzet et al., 2010). Furthermore, the benthic nature, fragility in preservation, or small size of recognized hazardous creatures can make them difficult to discover. For instance, the creator of azaspiracids, *Azadinium spinosum*, is barely 7 × 12 mm in size. The connection with the organism's produced biotoxin was established in 2007 (Tillmann et al., 2009), following the development of biomolecular methods for monitoring the organism in water (Kilcoyne et al., 2014) as well as guidelines for biotoxin analysis being separated (Kilcoyne et al., 2012). Toxicology itself is also not always adequately described. It is possible to connect toxicity to unknown or new species or vectors. For instance, in 2002, 21 persons developed neurological illnesses as a result of consuming pufferfish from Florida (Centers for Disease Control and Prevention (CDCP), 2002). At first, tetrodotoxin was thought to be the cause of the outbreak based on patient symptoms and reports of pufferfish intake. The existence of a Na^+ channel-blocking toxin in the unconsumed portions of fish was confirmed by a mouse bioassay. This toxin is tentatively identified as tetrodotoxin, which is typically associated with pufferfish. Tests using simple methods verified the unanticipated detection of saxitoxin in the fish samples, but not tetrodotoxin. Analysis of specimens of urine collected from the epidemic's recipients confirmed these findings. This was North America's first verified report of saxitoxin poisoning linked to pufferfish consumption (Landsberg et al., 2006).

Bioassays are widely utilized in the biotoxin investigation field providing a rapid way to find toxins in potentially contaminated seafood, setting off alarms, and halting the harvesting of contaminated shellfish. However, due to several ethical and technological concerns (Hess et al., 2006), bioassays have recently been replaced in several countries, especially in Europe (European Commission, 2011), by non-animal alternatives including cell tissue cultures (Van Dolah et al., 2012). Currently, research efforts are concentrated on developing multi-toxin techniques for identifying multiple types of chemicals in biosensor systems (Campbell et al., 2014).

Using resins to passively trap biotoxins, MacKenzie et al. (2004) developed a conceivably useful method for collecting samples. When the generating organisms, like *Azadinium* spp., are small or have a benthic lifestyle, like *Prorocentrum lima* and *Vulcanodinium rugosum*, it is challenging to monitor them. In these cases, this method has been successfully utilized to trace biotoxins (Fux et al., 2009; Zendong et al., 2014). However, the method has not been standardized, and further work will be required to make it suitable for hydrophilic biotoxins. Currently, it is difficult to automate or modify passive biotoxin capture for in situ detection. Moreover, to address the challenges posed by developing biotoxins, continuous improvement of its analytical techniques would be necessary (Turner et al., 2015).

Increased frequency sample collection might be beneficial in certain coastal environments; however, existing technologies have issues with representative sampling of in situ biotoxins and toxin-producing microalgae, which seldom happens more than once a week. It is necessary to develop and standardize sample methodologies when dealing with benthic hazardous species, such as *Gambierdiscus*, *Ostreopsis*, and *Prorocentrum lima* (Tester et al., 2014). There are currently insufficient automated, trustworthy, and reasonably priced techniques for identifying dangerous species or their biotoxins for regular in-situ monitoring. Although there have been some promising approaches lately established (Hess et al., 2012; ICES, 2015) for detecting species that produce biotoxins, these methods are still primarily considered research tools and are rarely used for elevated frequency in situ surveillance. The Environmental Sample Processor (ESP) and the Imaging Flow Cytobot (IFCB) (Olson & Sosik, 2007) are two examples of automated in situ monitoring platforms. The ESP gathers, treats, and transmits water samples in real time to the laboratory. It then uses precise and sensitive molecular assays to identify toxins and target HAB cells. All plankton cells (with sizes between 5 and 150 mm) can have their fluorescence properties and high-resolution photos are recorded at a high frequency of three samples per hour using the IFCB imaging flow cytometer. The data can also be sent in virtually real time to a laboratory (Campbell et al., 2013). However, they are currently quite expensive and cannot be used to monitor specific locations that produce shellfish. While they can't take the place of more established monitoring methods, attempts are currently being undertaken to make it easier for them to be used for this purpose. Thankfully, these complex systems are valuable resources for expanding our knowledge of the connections between HABs and ocean dynamics.

Economic expenses have a significant impact on the adoption of monitoring technology (Frolov et al., 2013). Certain techniques are rather basic and involve the microscopic examination of water samples to identify specific HAB species and the detection of biotoxins in shellfish tissues. Other programs include model-based bloom occurrence projections and in situ phytoplankton monitoring, such as those conducted in California Bay (Ryan et al., 2011) and the Gulf of Maine (McGillicuddy et al., 2005). Bernard et al. (2014) estimate that the annual expenses of monitoring might be as much as $1 billion, which would represent 10% of the total expenditures associated with HABs worldwide, which are expected to be $10 billion for freshwater and marine environments. Enhancing global collaboration for the collection, analysis, and dissemination of data from earth observations could potentially improve the effectiveness of a satellite-based monitoring system (Fritz et al., 2008).

Forecasts, warning signs, and finally hypotheses of HAB episodes can be provided by integrating monitoring with modeling, operational oceanography, and other resources (GEOHAB, 2011; Davidson, 2014). But to develop a predictive capability, one must know the ecophysiology of HAB species as well as the molecular and physical processes affecting bloom production.

One issue is that HAB species lack traits that set them apart from other phytoplankters in various situations, such as satellite remote sensing. The several processes (biological, ecological, physical, chemical, and climatic) that govern the dynamics of HAB and microalgae, in general, are not fully understood by us, which makes parameterizing them in numerical models quite challenging. The intricacy of biological relationships and the difficulties that come with building ecological models have hindered development thus far. HAB-OFS, the HAB operational prediction for Florida and Texas produced by NOAA (Stumpf et al., 2008), is one example. To forecast *K. brevis* blooms, HAB-OFS combines buoy data, public health reports, field observations, models, and satellite imagery. Washington's stakeholder communities have contributed to another NOAA attempt to forecast Pseudo-nitzschia (Brown et al., 2012). According to a linked physical/biological model (He et al., 2008), wind forcing and plume advection govern the movement of *Alexandrium fundyense* cells in the Gulf of Maine. The Monterey Bay and Chesapeake Bay Pseudo-nitzschia blooms have been effectively hindcast by statistically based models (Anderson et al., 2009; Lane et al., 2009). In summary, conceptual models have been useful in understanding the dynamics of blooms and developing preventive interventions. Examples of these include the *Phaeocystis* blooms in Vietnam (Hai et al., 2010) and the *Dinophysis acuminata* (Velo-Suarez et al., 2014) in the Rías of northwest Spain.

A deeper comprehension of HAB dynamics, enhanced monitoring programs, and the development of strategies to lessen the negative effects of HABs on human health and welfare could all result from ongoing basic research.

11.20 Public Outreach and Raising Awareness of Oceans and HABs in the Classroom

Humans have evolved coping mechanisms for dealing with various natural events, such as HABs, over time. Certain regions, including the Pacific Islands, have functionally accurate traditional knowledge concerning ciguatera, although lacking scientific evidence (Chinain et al., 2010).

In the Gulf of Mexico, close to Apalache Bay, the indigenous peoples could not tell the time by the phases of the moon and sun. Instead, they determined the seasons by fishkills (Ferrando, 1984), which may have been caused by *Karenia brevis* blooms during that period. This information was reported by Spanish explorer Alvar Nuñez Cabeza de Vaca, who lived from 1490 to 1558.

Red tides, also known as "purgas de mar," are a common occurrence for the people who live in the Galician Rías. They are thought to be similar to menstruation because they purify the local waters and typically occur in the fall. It was common knowledge that eating shellfish collected when the ocean was reddish-brown was dangerous. When developers began mass-cultivating mussels in the Galician Rías without knowledge of the blooms, the spread of deadly mussels increased. In the fall of 1976, there was one exceptionally severe instance (Estrada et al., 1984).

According to local folklore in northern Japan, eating shellfish during the early spring snowmelt flow into the sea is discouraged (Fukuyo et al., 2002). Similar myths are prevalent in the UK and the USA (O'Connor, 2008; Whyte, 2013) and proclaim that one should only eat shellfish during months that end with the letter "r," that is, avoid eating shellfish from May to August when HABs are most likely to happen (although food contamination by bacteria cannot be ruled out). Fukuyo et al. (2002) speculate that the reason for the emergence of this kind of folklore could be that the toxic contamination of shellfish has been a recurring event for a considerable amount of time, resulting in numerous tragedies for the local population. Self-regulating behavior to stay away from high-risk fish species and certain fishing spots was the outcome of community education.

There are a variety of reasons effective communication regarding HABs and their impacts can be difficult. This is partly because HAB occurrences are complex and hard to forecast, avoid, or regulate at the moment. The majority of medical and public health professionals lack an in-depth understanding of HABs and how they may affect people's health and well-being. But when many coastal populations are not properly informed about the public health concerns of HABs nowadays, a phenomenon called the "halo effect" can occur (Parsons et al., 2006). One common way that the halo effect manifests itself is as a reduction in consumption of all seafood, regardless of the actual risks posed by phycotoxins. Additional manifestations of the halo effect may have an impact on coastal tourism and commercial and recreational fishing practices. To better reach the diverse spectrum of end users and stakeholders, it would be beneficial to improve the scientific messaging on HABs.

Thankfully, there are currently instances of intriguing and maybe effective early warning systems and distribution connected to protecting human health from hazardous episodes caused by HAB. The United States National Oceanographic and Atmospheric Administration (NOAA), for instance, creates HAB Bulletins that forecast HABs for managers in the Great Lakes (for cyanobacteria), the Pacific Northwest (for toxic *Pseudo-nitzchia*), and the Gulf of Mexico (for *Karenia brevis*). Along with information from satellite imagery, oceanic modeling, and on-the-ground monitoring, the bulletins provide real-time updates from lifeguards and management. These resources were created with feedback and involvement from stakeholders, ensuring that the end products are truly helpful to and utilized by those (such as beach managers) who want current information.

11.21 Conclusion

Harmful algal blooms are becoming a more serious concern, which calls for quick response and preventative measures. Consuming contaminated seafood puts human populations at risk from the poisons released during these blooms, which also endanger the health of marine life. Comprehensive monitoring procedures and efficient management strategies are required since the incidence and severity of HABs are expected to rise in response to intensifying environmental changes and fertilizer runoff. Because unregulated hazardous algal blooms have consequences that go beyond immediate ecological impacts to include wider environmental and public health concerns, it is imperative to preserve the delicate balance of marine ecosystems. To lessen the negative effects of HABs and ensure the welfare of both human communities and marine species, sustainable practices must be combined with continuous study and close monitoring.

References

Aasen J.A.B., Espenes A., Miles C.O., Samdal I.A., Hess P. and Aune T. (2011) Combined oral toxicity of azaspiracid-1 and yessotoxin in female NMRI mice. *Toxicon* 57, 909–917.

Alonso E., Otero P., Vale C., Alfonso A., Antelo A., Giménez-Llort L., Chabaud L., Guillou C. and Botana L.M. (2013) Benefit of 13-desmethyl spirolide C treatment in triple transgenic mouse model of Alzheimer disease: ß-Amyloid and neuronal marker improvement. *Current Alzheimer Research* 10, 279–289.

Anderson C.R., Siegel D.A., Kudela R.M. and Brzezinski M.A. (2009) Empirical models of toxigenic pseudo-nitzschia blooms: Potential use as a remote detection tool in the Santa Barbara channel. *Harmful Algae* 8, 478–492.

Anderson D.M. and McCarthy S. (2012) *Red tides and harmful algal blooms: Impacts on desalination operations.* Muscat Oman: Middle East Desalination Research Center (Report).

Aransiola S.A., Oyewole O.A., Maddela N.R., Ijah U.J.J. and Manjunatha B. (Eds.). (2024). *Marine greens: Environmental, agricultural, industrial and biomedical applications.* (1st ed.). Boca Raton, FL: CRC Press, Taylor and Francis Group. https://doi.org/10.1201/9781003369738.

Aune A., Espenes A., Aasen J.A.B., Quilliam M.A., Hess P. and Larsen S. (2012) Study of possible combined toxic effects of azaspiracid-1 and okadaic acid in mice via the oral route. *Toxicon* 60, 895–906.

Ayres P. (1975) Mussel poisoning in Britain with special reference to paralytic shellfish poisoning: Review of cases reported 1814–1968. *Environmental Health* 83, 261–265.

Backer L.C., Kirkpatrick B., Fleming L.E., Cheng Y.S., Pierce R., Bean J.A., Clark R., Johnson D., Wanner A., Tamer R. and Baden D. (2005) Occupational exposure to aerosolized brevetoxins during Florida red tide events: Impacts on a healthy worker population. *Environmental Health Perspectives* 113, 644–649.

Baden D.G. and Trainer V.L. (1993) Mode of action of toxins of seafood poisoning. In Falconer I. (ed.) *Algal toxins in seafood and drinking water*. New York, NY: Academic Press, pp. 49–74.

Baron A.W., Steeg R., Morris C.M., Blain P.G. and Judge S.J. (2011) Motor activity is a sensitive behavioral biomarker of low-level exposure to the shellfish toxin, domoic acid, in male and female rats. *Toxicology* 290, 122.

Bates S.S., Bird C.J., de Freitas A.S.W., Foxall R., Gilgan M., Hanic L.A., Johnson G.R., McCulloch A.W., Odense P., Pocklingtonm R., Quilliam M.A., Sim P.G., Smith J.C., Subba Rao D.V., Todd E.C.D., Walter J.A. and Wright J.L.C. (1989) Pennate diatom Nitzschia pungens as the primary source of domoic acid, a toxin in shellfish from Eastern Prince Edward Island, Canada. *Canadian Journal of Fisheries and Aquatic Sciences* 46, 1203–1215.

Bauer M., Hoagland P., Leschine T.M., Blount B.G., Pomeroy C.M., Lampl L.L., Scherer C.W., Ayres D.L., Tester P.A., Sengco M.R., Sellner K.G. and Schumacker J. (2009) The importance of human dimensions research in managing harmful algal blooms. *Frontiers in Ecology and the Environment* 8, 75–83.

Bean J.A., Fleming L.E., Kirkpatrick B., Backer L.C., Nierenberg K., Reich A., Cheng Y.S., Wanner A., Benson J., Naar J., Pierce R., Abraham W.M., Kirkpatrick G., Hollenbeck J., Zaias J., Mendes E. and Baden D.G. (2011) Florida red tide toxins (brevetoxins) and longitudinal respiratory effects in asthmatics. *Harmful Algae* 10, 744–748.

Berdalet E., Vila M. and Abo's-Hernández R. (2015) *Expansion of the benthic dinoflagellate Ostreopsis with climate change: Health risks assessment and policy strategies for management*. Harmful Algal Blooms and Climate Change Scientific Symposium. Gothenburg, Sweden, 19–22 May. https://pices.int/meetings/international_symposia/2015/2015-HAB/scope.aspx.

Bernard S., Kudela R.M. and Velo-Suárez L. (2014) Developing global capabilities for the observation and prediction of harmful algal blooms. In Djavidnia S., Cheung V., Ott M. and Seeyave S. (eds.) *Oceans and society: Blue planet*. Cambridge: Cambridge Scholars Publishing, Chapter 6.

Blanco J., Correa J., Muñíz S., Mariño C., Martín H. and Arévalo F. (2013) Evaluación del impacto de los métodos y niveles utilizados para el control de toxinas en el mejillón. *Revista Galega dos Recursos Mariños* 3, 1–55.

Boni L., Mancini L., Milandri A., Poletti R., Pompei M. and Viviani R. (1992) First cases of diarrhetic shellfish poisoning in the Northern Adriatic Sea. In Vollenweider R.A., Marchetti R. and Viviani R. (eds.) *Marine coastal eutrophication*. Amsterdam: Elsevier, pp. 419–426.

Bradley W.G., Borenstein A.R., Nelson L.M., Codd G.A., Rosen B.H., Stommel E.W. and Cox P.A. (2013) Is exposure to cyanobacteria an environmental risk factor for amyotrophic lateral sclerosis and other neurodegenerative diseases? *Amyotrophic Lateral Sclerosis and Frontotemporal Degeneration* 14, 325–333.

Brand L.E., Pablo J., Compton A., Hammerschlag N. and Mash D.C. (2010) Cyanobacterial blooms and the occurrence of the neurotoxin, beta-N-methylamino-L-alanine (BMAA), in South Florida aquatic food webs. *Harmful Algae* 9, 620–635.

Bravo I., Vila M., Casabianca S., Rodriguez F., Rial P., Riobó P. and Penna A. (2012) Life cycle stages of the benthic palytoxin-producing dinoflagellate Ostreopsis cf. ovata (Dinophyceae). *Harmful Algae* 18, 24–34.

Brissard C., Herrenknecht C., Séchet V., Hervé, F., Pisapia, F., Harcouet, J., Lémée, R., Chomérat N., Hess P. and Amzil Z. (2014) Complex toxin profile of French Mediterranean Ostreopsis cf. ovata strains, seafood accumulation and ovatoxins pre purification. *Marine Drugs* 12, 2851–2876.

Brissard C., Hervé F., Sibat M., Séchet V., Hess P., Amzil Z. and Herrenknecht C. (2015) Characterization of ovatoxin-h, a new ovatoxin analog, and evaluation of chromatographic columns for ovatoxin analysis and purification. *Journal of Chromatography A* 1388, 87–101.

Brown C.W., Green D., Hickey B.M., Jacobs J.M., Lanerolle L.W.J., Moore S., Schwab D.J., Trainer V.L., Trtanj J., Turner E., Wood R.J. and Wynne T.T. (2012) Towards operational forecasts of algal blooms and pathogens. In Morain S.A. and Budge A.M. (eds.) *Environmental tracking for public health surveillance*. Leiden: CRC Press, 1st ed., pp. 345–368.

Campbell K., McNamee S.E., Huet A.C., Delahaut P., Vilarino N., Botana L.M., Poli M. and Elliott C.T. (2014) Evolving to the optoelectronic mouse for phycotoxin analysis in shellfish. *Analytical and Bioanalytical Chemistry* 406, 6867–6881.

Campbell L., Henrichs D.W., Olson R.J. and Sosik H.M. (2013) Continuous automated imaging-in-flow cytometry for detection and early warning of *Karenia brevis* blooms in the Gulf of Mexico. *Environmental Science and Pollution Research* 20, 6896–6902.

Casabianca S., Casabianca A., Riobó P., Franco J.M., Vila M. and Penna A. (2013) Quantification of the toxic dinoflagellate Ostreopsis spp. by qPCR assay in marine aerosol. *Environmental Science and Technology* 47, 3788–3795.

Centers for Disease Control and Prevention. (2002) Neurologic illness associated with eating Florida pufferfish, 2002. *Morbidity and Mortality Weekly Report* 51(16), 321–323.

Chateau-Degat M.L., Chinain M., Cerf N., Gingras S., Hubert B. and Dewailly E. (2005) Sea water temperature, Gambierdiscus spp. variability and incidence of ciguatera poisoning in French Polynesia. *Harmful Algae* 4, 1053–1062.

Chateau-Degat M.L., Chinain M., Darius H.T., Dewailly E. and Mallet H.P. (2009) Epidemiological surveillance of ciguatera in French Polynesia. *Bulletin Epidemiologique Hebdomadaire The'matique* 48–50, 522–525.

Chinain M., Darius H.T., Ung A., Fouc M.T., Revel T., Cruchet P., Pauillac S. and Laurent D. (2010b) Ciguatera risk management in French Polynesia: The case study of Raivavae Island (Australes Archipelago). *Toxicon* 56, 674–690.

Ciminiello P., Dell'Aversano C., Dello Iacovo E., Fattorusso E., Forino M. and Tartaglione L. (2014) First finding of Ostreopsis cf. ovata toxins in marine aerosols. *Environmental Science and Technology* 48, 3532–3540.

Ciminiello P., Dell'Aversano C. and Forino M. (2015) Chemistry of palytoxin and its analogues. In Botana L. and Alfonso A. (eds.) *Phycotoxins: Chemistry and biochemistry*. Hoboken, NJ: Wiley-Blackwell, pp. 85–111.

Daigo K. (1959) Constituents of Chondria armata. III: Constitution of domoic acid. *Journal of the Pharmaceutical Society of Japan. Yakugaku Zasshi* 79, 360–364. [In Japanese, with English abstract]

Davidson K. (2014) The challenges of incorporating realistic simulations of marine protists in biogeochemically based mathematical models. *Acta Protozoologica* 53, 129–138.

Davidson K. and Bresnan E. (2009) Shellfish toxicity in UK waters: A threat to human health? *Environmental Health* 8(Supplement 1), S12.

Davidson K., Gowen R.J., Harrison P.J., Fleming L., Hoagland P. and Moschonas G. (2014) Anthropogenic nutrients and harmful algae in coastal waters. *Journal of Environmental Management* 146, 206–216.

Deeds J.R., Landsberg J.H., Etheridge S.M., Pitcher G.C. and Longan S.W. (2008) Non-traditional vectors for paralytic shellfish poisoning. *Marine Drugs* 6, 308–348.
Deeds J.R. and Schwartz M.D. (2010) Human risk associated with palytoxin exposure. *Toxicon* 56, 150–162.
DeGrasse S.L. and Martinez-Diaz K. (2012) Biotoxin control programs in North, Central and South American countries. In Cabado A.G. and Vieites J.M. (eds.) *New trends in marine and freshwater toxins: Food safety concerns*. New York, NY: Nova Science Publishers.
Dewailly E., Chateau-Degat M.L. and Suhas E. (2008) Fish consumption and health in French Polynesia. *Asian Pacific Journal of Clinical Nutrition* 17, 86–93.
Epelboin L., Pérignon A., Hossen V., Vincent R., Krys S. and Caumes E. (2014) Two clusters of ciguatera fish poisoning in Paris, France, related to tropical fish imported from the French Caribbean by travelers. *Journal of Travel Medicine* 21, 397–402.
Epstein P. and Rapport D.J. (1996) Changing coastal marine environments and human health. *Ecosystem Health* 2, 166–176.
Estrada M., Sa'nchez F.J. and Fraga S. (1984) Gymnodinium catenatum (Graham) en las rı'as gallegas (NO de Espan˜a). *Investigación pesquera* 48, 31–40.
European Commission (2011) Commission Regulation (EU) No 15/2011 of 10 January 2011 amending Regulation (EC) No 2074/2005 as regards recognized testing methods for detecting marine biotoxins in live bivalve molluscs. *Official Journal* L6, 3–6. http://eur-lex. europa.eu/legal-content/EN/TXT/?uri=celex:32011R0015 (accessed 4 November 2015).
FAO (2006) *State of world aquaculture, 2006*. FAO Fisheries Technical Report Paper No. 500. Rome: Inland Water and Aquaculture Service. Fishery Resources Division, FAO Fisheries Department.
Ferrando R. (1984) *Alvar Núñez Cabeza de Vaca, Naufragios y Comentarios*. Madrid: Historia, vol. 16, p. 318.
Fleming L.E., Backer L. and Rowan A. (2002) The epidemiology of human illnesses associated with harmful algal blooms. In Baden D. and Adams D. (eds.) *Neurotoxicology handbook*. Totowa, NJ: Humana Press, vol. 1, pp. 363–381.
Fleming L.E., Kirkpatrick B., Backer L.C., Walsh C.J., Nierenberg K., Clark J., Reich A., Hollenbeck J., Benson J., Cheng Y.S., Naar J., Pierce R., Bourdelais A.J., Abraham W.M., Kirkpatrick G., Zaias J., Wanner A., Mendes E., Shalat S., Hoagland P., Stephan W., Bean J., Watkins S., Clarke T., Byrne M. and Baden D.G. (2011) Review of Florida red tide and human health effects. *Harmful Algae* 20, 224–233.
Friedman M.A., Fleming L.E., Fernandez M., Bienfang P., Schrank K., Dickey R., Bottein M.Y., Backer L., Ayyar R., Weisman R., Watkins S., Granade R. and Reich A. (2008) Ciguatera fish poisoning: Treatment, prevention and management. *Marine Drugs* 6, 456–479.
Fritz S., Scholes R.J., Obersteiner M., Bouma J. and Reyers B. (2008) A conceptual framework for assessing the benefits of a global earth observation system of systems. *IEEE Systems Journal* 2, 338–348.
Frolov S., Kudela R.M. and Bellingham J.G. (2013) Monitoring of harmful algal blooms in the era of diminishing resources: A case study of the US west coast. *Harmful Algae* 21–22, 1–12.
Fukuyo Y., Imai I., Kodama M. and Tamai K. (2002) Red tides and harmful algal blooms in Japan. In Taylor F.J. and Trainer V.L. (eds.) *Harmful algal blooms in the PICES region of the North Pacific*. PICES Scientific Report No. 23. Sidney, BC: North Pacific Marine Science Organization (PICES), pp. 7–20.

Fux E., Bire R. and Hess P. (2009) Comparative accumulation and composition of lipophilic marine biotoxins in passive samplers and mussels (M. edulis) on the West Coast of Ireland. *Harmful Algae* 8, 523–537.

Gaines G. and Taylor F.J.R. (1985) An exploratory analysis of PSP patterns in British Columbia. In Anderson D.M., White A.W. and Baden D.G. (eds.) *Toxic dinoflagellates. Proceedings of the third international conference on toxic dinoflagellates, New Brunswick, Canada*. New York, NY: Elsevier Science, pp. 439–444, 8–12 June.

GEOHAB (2011) *GEOHAB modeling: A workshop report*. McGillicuddy D.J. Jr., Glibert P.M., Berdalet E., Edwards C., Francks P., and Ross O. (eds.). Paris and Newark, DE: IOC and SCOR, p. 85.

GESAMP (2001) *Global environment outlook 3, EARTH SCAN, past, present and future perspectives: Protecting the oceans from land-based activities. Land-based sources and activities affecting the quality and uses of the marine, coastal, and associated freshwater environment*. GESAMP Reports and Studies No. 71. Nairobi: United Nations Environment Programme.

Golubic S., Abed R.M.M., Palin´ska K., Pauillac S., Chinain M. and Laurent D. (2010) Marine toxic cyanobacteria: Diversity, environmental responses and hazards. *Toxicon* 56, 836–841.

Gowen R.J., Tett P., Bresnan E., Davidson K., McKinney A., Harrison P.J., Milligan S., Mills D.K., Silke J. and Crooks A.-M. (2012) Anthropogenic nutrient enrichment and blooms of harmful microalgae. *Oceanography and Marine Biology: An Annual Review* 50, 65–126.

Hai D.-N., Lam N.-N. and Dippner J. (2010) Development of phaeocystis globosa blooms in the upwelling waters of the South Central coast of Viet Nam. *Journal of Marine Systems* 83, 253–261.

He R., McGillicuddy D.J., Keafer B.A. and Anderson D.M. (2008) Historic 2005 toxic bloom of Alexandrium fundyense in the Western Gulf of Maine: 2. *Coupled Biophysical Numerical Modeling. Journal of Geophysical Research-Oceans* 113, C07040.

Hess P. (2012) Phytoplankton and biotoxin monitoring programs for the safe exploitation of shellfish in Europe. In Cabado A.G. and Vieites J.M. (eds.) *New trends in marine and freshwater toxins: Food safety concerns*. New York, NY: Nova Science Publishers, pp. 305–314.

Hess P., Abadie E., Herve F., Berteaux T., Sechet V., Araoz R., Molgo J., Zakarian A., Sibat M., Rundberget T., Miles C.O. and Amzil Z. (2013) Pinnatoxin G is responsible for atypical toxicity in mussels (Mytilus galloprovincialis) and clams (Venerupis decussata) from Ingril, a French Mediterranean lagoon. *Toxicon* 75, 16–26.

Hess P., Amzil Z., Belin C., Compere C., Lassus P. and Menesguen A. (2012) Evolution of European monitoring systems for shellfish toxins—an increased need for the surveillance of phytoplankton. In Pagou K.A. and Hallegraeff G.M. (eds.) *Proceedings of the 14th international conference on harmful algae*. Hersonissos, Crete. Copenhagen: International Society for the Study of Harmful Algae and IOC of UNESCO, pp. 288–291, 1–5 November.

Hess P., Grune B., Anderson D.B., Aune T., Botana L.M., Caricato P., van Egmond H.P., Halder M., Hall S., Lawrence J.F., Moffat C., Poletti R., Richmond J., Rossini G.P., Seamer C. and Serratosa Vilageliu J. (2006) Three Rs approaches in marine biotoxin testing—the report and recommendations of a joint ECVAM/DG SANCO workshop (ECVAM Workshop 55). *Alternatives to Laboratory Animals (ATLA)* 34, 193–224.

Heymann D.L. (2004) *Control of communicable diseases manual*. Washington, DC: American Public Health Association, 18th ed.

Hiolski E.M., Preston S.K., Frame E.R., Myers M.S., Bammler T.K., Beyer R.P., Farin F.M., Wilkerson H.-W., Smith D.R., Marcinek D.J. and Lefebvre K.A. (2014) Chronic low-level domoic acid exposure alters gene transcription and impairs mitochondrial function in the CNS. *Aquatic Toxicology* 155, 151–159.

Hoagland P., Anderson D.M., Kaoru Y. and White A.W. (2002) The economic effects of harmful algal blooms in the United States: Estimates, assessment issues, and information needs. *Estuaries* 25, 677–695.

Hoagland P., Jin D., Beet A., Kirkpatrick B., Reich A., Ullman S., Fleming L.E. and Kirkpatrick G. (2014) The human health effects of Florida Red Tide (FRT) blooms: An expanded analysis. *Environment International* 68, 144–153.

Hoagland P. and Scatasta S. (2006) The economic effects of harmful algal blooms. In Grane'li E. and Turner J.T. (eds.) *Ecology of harmful algae*. New York, NY: Springer-Verlag, pp. 391–402.

ICES (2006) *Report of the ICES-IOC working group on harmful algal bloom dynamics (WGHABD)*. Gdynia, Poland: ICES CM, p. 47, 3–6 April.

ICES (2015) *Report of the international council for the exploration of the sea—IOC working group on harmful algal bloom dynamics (WGHABD), 28 April–2 May 2014*. Haarlem, The Netherlands: ICES CM/SSGHIE 12, p. 87.

Illoul H., Rodríguez F., Vila M., Adjas N., Aït Younes A., Bournissa M., Koroghli A., Marouf N., Rabia S. and Ameur F.L.K. (2012) The genus Ostreopsis along the Algerian coastal waters (SW Mediterranean Sea) associated with a human respiratory intoxication episode. *Cryptogamie, Algologie* 33, 209–216.

Imai I., Shimada H., Shinada A., Baba K., Kanamori M., Sato M., Kuwahara Y., Miyoshi K., Tada M., Hirano K., Miyazono A. and Itakura S. (2014) Prediction of toxic algal bloom occurrences and adaptation to toxic blooms to minimize economic loss to the scallop aquaculture industry in Hokkaido, Japan. In Trainer V.L. and Yoshida T. (eds.) *Proceedings of the workshop on economic impacts of harmful algal blooms on fisheries and aquaculture*. PICES Scientific Report No. 47. Sidney, BC: North Pacific Marine Science Organization (PICES), p. 85.

Jackson J.J., Stivala C.E., Iorga B.I., Molgo J. and Zakarian A. (2012) Stability of cyclic imine toxins: Interconversion of pinnatoxin amino ketone and pinnatoxin A in aqueous media. *Journal of Organic Chemistry* 77, 10435–10440.

Jiang L., Eriksson J., Lage S., Jonasson S., Shams S., Mehine M., Ilag L.L. and Rasmussen U. (2014a) Diatoms: A novel source for the neurotoxin BMAA in aquatic environments. *PLOS One* 9, e84578.

Jiang S.S., Kuwano K., Ishikawa N., Yano M., Takatani T. and Arakawa O. (2014b) Production of domoic acid by laboratory culture of the red alga Chondria armata. *Toxicon* 92, 1–5.

Jin D., Thunberg E. and Hoagland P. (2008) Economic impact of the 2005 red tide event on commercial shellfish fisheries in New England. *Ocean and Coastal Management* 51, 420–429.

Kat M. (1983) Diarrhetic mussel poisoning in the Netherlands related to the dinoflagellate Dinophysis acuminata. *Antonie van Leeuwenhoek* 49, 417–427.

Kibler S.R., Tester P.A., Kunkel K., Moore S.K. and Litaker R.W. (2015) Effects of ocean warming on growth and distribution of dinoflagellates associated with ciguatera fish poisoning in the Caribbean. *Ecological Modelling* 316, 194–210.

Kilcoyne J., Jauffrais T., Twiner M.J., Doucette G.J., Aasen J.A.B., Sosa S., Krock B., Se´chet V., Nulty C., Salas R., Clarke D., Geraghty J., Duffy C., Foley B., John U., Quilliam M.A., McCarron P., Miles C.O., Silke J., Cembella A., Tillmann U. and Hess P. (2014) *Azaspiracids—toxicological evaluation, test methods and the source organisms (ASTOX II)*. Final Project Report. Galway: Marine Institute.

Kilcoyne J., Keogh A., Clancy G., LeBlanc P., Burton I.W., Quilliam M.A., Hess P. and Miles C.O. (2012) Improved isolation procedure for Azaspiracids from shellfish, structural elucidation of azaspiracid-6, and stability studies. *Journal of Agricultural and Food Chemistry* 60, 2447–2455.

Kim H.G. (2006) Mitigation and controls of HABs. In Grane'li E. and Turner J.T. (eds.) *Ecology of harmful algae: Ecological studies*. Berlin: Springer-Verlag, vol. 189, pp. 327–338.

Kirkpatrick B., Fleming L.E., Squicciarini D., Backer L.C., Clark R.C., Abraham W., Benson J., Cheng Y.S., Johnson D., Pierce R., Zaias J., Bossart G.D. and Baden D.G. (2004) Literature review of Florida red tide: Implications for human health effects. *Harmful Algae* 3, 99–115.

Koike K., Sato S., Yamaji M., Nagahama Y., Kotaki Y., Ogata T. and Kodama M. (1998) Occurrence of okadaic acid-producing Prorocentrum lima on the Sanriku coast, Northern Japan. *Toxicon* 36, 2039–2042.

Landsberg J.H., Hall S., Johannessen J.N., White K.D., Conrad S.M., Abbott J.P., Felwelling L.J., Richardson R.W., Dickey R.W., Jester E.L.E., Etheridge S.M., Deeds J.R., Van Dolah F.M., Leighfield T.A., Zou Y., Beaudry C.G., Benner R.A., Rogers P.L., Scott P.S., Kawabata K., Wolny J.L. and Steidinger K.A. (2006) Saxitoxin puffer fish poisoning in the United States, with the first report of Pyrodinium bahamense as the putative toxin source. *Environmental Health Perspective* 114, 1502–1507.

Lane J.Q., Raimondi P.T. and Kudela R.M. (2009) Development of a logistic regression model for the prediction of toxigenic Pseudo-nitzschia blooms in Monterey Bay, California. *Marine Ecology Progress Series* 383, 37–51.

Larkin S. and Adams C. (2007) Harmful algal blooms and coastal business: Economic consequences in Florida. *Society and Natural Resources* 20, 849–859.

Lawrence J., Loreal H., Toyufuku H., Hess P., Karunasagar I. and Ababouch L. (2011) *Assessment and management of biotoxin risks in bivalve molluscs*. FAO Fisheries Technical Paper 551. Rome: FAO Fisheries Department.

Laycock M.V., Anderson D.M., Naar J., Goodman A., Easy D.J., Donovan M.A., Li A., Quilliam M.A., Al Jamali E. and Alshihi R. (2012) Removal of four algal toxins from seawater during desalination using reverse osmosis and distillation. *Desalination* 293, 1.

Lefebvre K.A., Frame E.R., Gulland F., Hansen J.D., Kendrick P.S., Beyer R.P., Bammler T.K., Farin F.M., Hiolski E.M., Smith D.R. and Marcinek D.J. (2012) A novel antibody-based biomarker for chronic algal toxin exposure and sub-acute neurotoxicity. *PLOS One* 7, e36213. doi: 10.1371/journal.pone.0036213.

Levin E.D., Pizarro P., Pang W.G., Harrison J. and Ramsdell J.S. (2005) Persisting behavioral consequences of prenatal domoic acid exposure in rats. *Neurotoxicology and Teratology* 27, 719–725.

Lewis R. and Ruff T.A. (1993) Ciguatera: Ecological, clinical and socioeconomic perspectives. *Critical Reviews in Environmental Science and Technology* 23, 137–156.

Louzao M.C., Vilarin˜o N. and Yotsu-Yamashita M. (2014) Polycavernosides and other scarce new toxins. In Botana L.M. (ed.) *Seafood and freshwater toxins*. Boca Raton, FL: CRC Press, pp. 857–872.

MacKenzie L., Beuzenberg V., Holland P., McNabb P. and Selwood A. (2004) Solid phase adsorption toxin tracking (SPATT): A new monitoring tool that simulates the biotoxin contamination of filter-feeding bivalves. *Toxicon* 44, 901–918.

Magnien R.E. (2001) The dynamics of science, perception, and policy during the outbreak of Pfiesteria in the Chesapeake Bay. *BioScience* 51, 843–852.

Mangialajo L., Ganzin N., Accoroni S., Asnaghi V., Blanfune A., Cabrini M., Cattaneo-Vietti R., Chavanon F., Chiantore M., Cohu S., Costa E., Fornasaro D., Grossel H., Marco-Miralles F., Maso´ M., Ren˜e´ A., Rossi A.M., Sala M.M., Thibaut T., Totti C., Vila M. and Leme´e R. (2011) Trends in Ostreopsis proliferation along the Northern Mediterranean coasts. *Toxicon* 57, 408–420.

Mattei C., Vetter I., Eisenbla¨tter A., Krock B., Ebbecke M., Desel H. and Zimmermann K. (2014) Ciguatera fish poisoning: A first epidemic in Germany highlights an increasing risk for European countries. *Toxicon* 91, 76–83.

McGillicuddy D.J., Jr., Anderson D.M., Lynch D.R. and Townsend D.W. (2005) Mechanisms regulating large-scale seasonal fluctuations in Alexandrium fundyense populations in the Gulf of Maine: Results from a physical-biological model. *Deep-Sea Research Part II* 52, 2698–2714.

Medcof J.F.R. (1985) Life and death with Gonyaulax: An historical perspective. In Anderson D.M., White A.W. and Baden D.G. (eds.) *Toxic dinoflagellates. Proceedings of the Third International Conference on Toxic Dinoflagellates, New Brunswick, Canada*. New York, NY: Elsevier Science, pp. 1–10, 8–12 June 1985.

Moestrup Ø., Akselman R., Cronberg G., Elbraechter M., Fraga S., Halim Y., Hansen G., Hoppenrath M., Larsen J., Lundholm N., Nguyen L.N. and Zingone A. (2009) *IOC-UNESCO taxonomic reference list of harmful microalgae*. http://www.marinespecies.org/hab (accessed 20 April 2015).

Molgo´ J., Ara´oz R., Benoit E. and Iorga B.I. (2014) Cyclic imine toxins. In Botana L.M. (ed.) *Seafood and freshwater toxins*. Boca Raton, FL: CRC Press, 3rd ed., pp. 951–990.

Morgan K., Larkin S.L. and Adams C.M. (2010) Red tides and participation in marine-based activities: Estimating the response of Southwest Florida residents. *Harmful Algae* 9, 333–341.

Mudie P.J., Rochon A. and Levac E. (2002) Palynological records of red tide-producing species in Canada: Past trends and implications for the future. *Paleogeography, Palaeoclimatology, Palaeoecology* 180, 159–186.

O'Connor A. (2008) The claim: Never eat shellfish in a month without an r. *The New York Times*. http://www.nytimes.com/2008/07/22/health/nutrition/22real.html?_r=0 (accessed 4 November 2015).

Olson R.J. and Sosik H.M. (2007) A submersible imaging-in-flow instrument to analyze nano- and microplankton: Imaging FlowCytobot. *Limnology and Oceanography: Methods* 5, 195–203.

Parsons G., Morgan A., Whitehead J.C. and Haab T.C. (2006) The welfare effects of Pfiesteria-related fish kills in seafood markets: A contingent behavior analysis. *Agricultural and Resource Economic Review* 35, 348–356.

Paz B., Riobo´ P., Fernandez M.L., Fraga S. and Franco J.M. (2004) Production and release of yessotoxins by the dinoflagellates Protoceratium reticulatum and Lingulodinium polyedrum in culture. *Toxicon* 44, 251–258.

Pennotti R., Scallan E., Backer L., Thomas J. and Angulo F.J. (2013) Ciguatera and scombroid fish poisoning in the United States. *Foodborne Pathogens and Disease* 10, 1059–1066.

Pottier I., Vernoux J.P. and Lewis R.J. (2001) Ciguatera fish poisoning in the Caribbean Islands and Western Atlantic. *Reviews of Environmental Contamination and Toxicology* 168, 99–141.

Proenc¸a L.A.O., Boemer G.L., Dias J.P., Hatherly M.M., Mendes I.L., Mendes L.A.M., Mendes M.C.Q., Rossi W.C., Tamanaha M.S., Tenenbaum D.R. and Schramm M.A. (2010) *Can the cases of airborne intoxication of beach users in south coast of Bahia (16824' S– 39802' W) be related to microalgae?* GEOHAB Open Science Meeting: HABs in Benthic Systems, Honolulu, Hawai' i, 21–23 June.

Radke E.G., Reich A. and Morris J.G. Jr (2015) Epidemiology of ciguatera in Florida. *American Journal of Tropical Medicine and Hygiene* 93, 425–432.

Ramos P.B., Dieh F., dos Santos J.M., Monserrat J.M. and Yunes J.S. (2014) Oxidative stress in rats induced by consumption of saxitoxin contaminated drink water. *Harmful Algae* 37, 68–74.

Reguera B., Riobo´ P., Rodrı´guez F., Dı´az P.A., Pizarro G., Paz B., Franco J.M. and Blanco J. (2014) Causative organisms, distributions and fate in shellfish. *Marine Drugs* 12, 394–461.

Reguera B., Velo-Sua´rez L., Raine R. and Park M.G. (2012) Harmful Dinophysis species: A review. *Harmful Algae* 14, 87–106.

Reich A., Lazensky R., Faris J., Fleming L.E., Kirkpatrick B., Watkins S., Ullman S., Kohler K. and Hoagland P. (2015) Assessing the impact of shellfish harvesting area closures on neurotoxic shellfish poisoning (NSP) incidence during red tide (*Karenia brevis*) blooms. *Harmful Algae* 43, 13–19.

Reiss C.R., Robert C., Owen C. and Taylor J.S. (2006) Control of MIB, geosmin and TON by membrane systems. *Journal of Water Supply: Research and Technology—AQUA* 55, 95–108.

Re´veillon D., Abadie E., Se´chet V., Masseret E., Hess P. and Amzil Z. (2015) B-methylamino-L-alanine (BMAA) and isomers: Distribution in different food web compartments of Thau Lagoon, French Mediterranean sea. *Marine Environmental Research* 110, 8–18.

Rhodes L. (2011) World-wide occurrence of the toxic dinoflagellate genus Ostreopsis Schmidt. *Toxicon* 57, 400–407.

Richlen M.L., Morton S.L., Jamali E.A., Rajan A. and Anderson D.M. (2010) The catastrophic 2008–2009 red tide in the Arabian Gulf region, with observations on the identification and phylogeny of the fish-killing dinoflagellate Cochlodinium polykrikoides. *Harmful Algae* 9, 163–172.

Rongo T. and van Woesik R. (2012) Socioeconomic consequences of ciguatera poisoning in Rarotonga, Southern Cook Islands. *Harmful Algae* 20, 92–100.

Roue´ M., Gugger M., Golubic S., Amzil Z., Ara´oz R., Turquet J., Chinain M. and Laurent D. (2014) Marine cyanotoxins potentially harmful to human health. In La Barre S. and Kornprobst J.-M. (eds.) *Outstanding marine molecules*. Weinheim: Wiley-VCH Verlag GmbH and Co. KGaA, pp. 1–22.

Ruiz N., Petit K., Vansteelandt M., Kerzaon I., Baudet J., Amzil Z., Biard J.F., Grovel O. and Pouchus Y.F. (2010) Enhancement of domoic acid neurotoxicity on Diptera larvae bioassay by marine fungal metabolites. *Toxicon* 55, 805–810.

Ryan J.P., Greenfield D., Marin III R., Preston C., Roman B., Jensen S., Pargett D., Birch J., Mikulski C., Doucette G. and Scholin C. (2011) Harmful phytoplankton ecology studies using an autonomous molecular analytical and ocean observing network. *Limnology and Oceanography* 56, 1255–1272.

Satake M., Ofuji K., Naoki H., James K.J., Furey A., McMahon T., Silke J. and Yasumoto T. (1998) Azaspiracid, a new marine toxin having unique spiro ring assemblies, isolated from Irish mussels, Mytilus edulis. *Journal of the American Chemical Society* 120, 9967–9968.

Scatasta S., Stolte W., Grane´li E. and van Ierland E. (2003) *The socio-economic impact of harmful algal blooms in European marine waters and description of future risks.* Fifth Deliverable for the EU-funded project ECOHARM.

Seki T., Satake M., MacKenzie A.L., Kaspar H.F. and Yasumoto T. (1995) Gymnodimine, a new marine toxin of unprecedented structure isolated from New Zealand oysters and the dinoflagellate, Gymnodinium sp. *Tetrahedron Letters* 36, 7093–7096.

Seubert E.L., Trussell S., Eagleton J., Schnetzer A., Cetinic I., Lauri P., Jones B.H. and Caron D.A. (2012) Algal toxins and reverse osmosis desalination operations: Laboratory bench testing and field monitoring of domoic acid, saxitoxin, brevetoxin, and okadaic acid. *Water Research* 46, 6563–6573.

Silva C.A., Morais E.C.P., Costa M.D.M., Ribas J.L.C., Guiloski I.C., Ramsdorf W.A., Zanata S.M., Cestari M.M., Oliveira Ribeiro C.A., Magalhaes V.F., Trudeau V.L. and Silva de Assis H.C. (2014) Saxitoxins induce cytotoxicity, genotoxicity and oxidative stress in teleost neurons in vitro. *Toxicon* 86, 8–15.

Skinner M.P., Brewer T.D., Johnstone R., Fleming L.E. and Lewis R.J. (2011) Ciguatera fish poisoning in the Pacific Islands (1998 to 2008). *PLOS Neglected Tropical Diseases* 5, e1416. doi: 10.1371/journal.pntd.0001416.

Sosa S., Ardizzone M., Beltramo D., Vita F., Dell'Ovo V., Barreras A., Yasumoto T. and Tubaro A. (2013) Repeated oral co-exposure to yessotoxin and okadaic acid: A short term toxicity study in mice. *Toxicon* 76, 94–102.

Stewart I., Seawright A.A. and Shaw G.R. (2008) Cyanobacterial poisoning in livestock, wild mammals and birds—an overview. *Advances in Experimental Medicine and Biology* 6, 613–637.

Stumpf R.P., Litaker R.W., Lanerolle L. and Tester P.A. (2008) Hydrodynamic accumulation of Karenia off the west coast of Florida. *Continental Shelf Research* 28, 189–213.

Suikkanen S., Kremp A., Hautala H. and Krock B. (2013) Paralytic shellfish toxins or spirolides? The role of environmental and genetic factors in toxin production of the Alexandrium ostenfeldii complex. *Harmful Algae* 26, 52–59.

Suzuki T. and Watanabe R. (2012) Shellfish toxin monitoring system in Japan and some Asian countries. In Cabado A.G. and Vieites J.M. (eds.) *New trends in marine and freshwater toxins: Food safety concerns.* New York, NY: Nova Science Publishers, pp. 347–377.

Tester P.A., Feldman R.L., Nau A.W., Kibler S. and Litaker R.W. (2010) Ciguatera fish poisoning and sea surface temperatures in the Caribbean Sea and the West Indies. *Harmful Algae* 56, 698–710.

Tester P.A., Kibler S.R., Holland W.C., Usup G., Vandersea M.W., Leaw C.P., Lim P.T., Jacob Larsen J., Mohammad-Noor N., Faust M.A. and Litaker R.W. (2014) Sampling harmful benthic dinoflagellates: Comparison of artificial and natural substrate methods. *Harmful Algae* 39, 8–25.

Tillmann U., Elbra¨chter M., Krock B., John U. and Cembella A.D. (2009) Azadinium spinosum gen. et sp. nov. (Dinophyceae) identified as a primary producer of azaspiracid toxins. *European Journal of Phycology* 44, 63–79.

Touzet N., Davidson K., Pete R., Flanagan K., McCoy G.R., Amzil Z., Maher M., Chapelle A. and Raine R. (2010) Co-occurrence of the West European (Gr. III) and North American (Gr. I) ribotypes of Alexandrium tamarense (Dinophyceae) in Shetland, Scotland. *Protist* 161, 370–384.

Touzet N., Franco J.M. and Raine R. (2007) Characterization of nontoxic and toxin-producing strains of Alexandrium minutum (Dinophyceae) in Irish coastal waters. *Applied Environmental Microbiology* 73, 3333–3342.

Trainer V.L. and Suddleson M. (2005) Monitoring approaches for early warning of domoic acid events in Washington state. *Oceanography* 18, 228–237.

Trainer V.L. and Yoshida T. (eds.) (2014) Proceedings of the workshop on economic impacts of harmful algal blooms on fisheries and aquaculture. *PICES Scientific Reports* 47, 85.

Trainer V.L., Moore L., Bill B.D., Adams N.G., Harrington N., Borchert J., Silva D.A.M. and Eberhart B.-T.L. (2013) Diarrhetic shellfish toxins and other lipophilic toxins of human health concern in Washington State. *Marine Drugs* 11, 1815–1835.

Turner A., Higgins C., Veszelovski A., Payne D., Davidson K., Hungerford J. and Higman W. (2015) Monitoring of new or emerging marine biotoxins in UK waters: Brevetoxins. *Marine Drugs* 13, 1224–1254.

Twiner M.J., Rehmann N., Hess P. and Doucette G.J. (2008) Azaspiracid shellfish poisoning: A review on the chemistry, ecology, and toxicology with an emphasis on human health impacts. *Marine Drugs* 6, 39–72.

Uemura D., Chou T., Haino T., Nagatsu A., Fukuzawa S., Zheng S., and Chen H. (1995) Pinnatoxin A: A toxic amphoteric macrocycle from the Okinawan bivalve Pinna muricata. *Journal of the American Chemical Society* 117, 1155–1156.

Van Dolah F.M. (2000) Marine algal toxins: Origins, health effects, and their increased occurrence. *Environmental Health Perspectives* 108(Supplement 1), 133–141.

Van Dolah F.M., Fire S.E., Leighfield T.A., Mikulski T.A. and Doucette G.L. (2012) Determination of paralytic shellfish toxins in shellfish by receptor binding assay: A collaborative study. *Journal of AOAC International* 95, 795–812.

Velo-Sua´rez L., Gonza´lez-Gil S., Pazos Y. and Reguera B. (2014) The growth season of Dinophysis acuminata in an upwelling system embayment: A conceptual model based on in situ measurements. *Deep Sea Research Part II* 101, 141–151.

Vila M., Riobo´ P., Bravo I., Maso´ M., Penna A. and Ren˜e´ A. (2014) A Three-year time series of toxic Ostreopsis blooming in a NW Mediterranean coastal site: Preliminary results. In Pagou P. and Hallegraeff G. (eds.) *Proceedings of the 14th international conference on harmful algae.* Copenhagen: ISSHA and IOC of UNESCO, pp. 111–113.

Villareal T.A., Hanson S., Qualia S., Jester E.L.E., Granade H.R., and Dickey R.W. (2007) Petroleum production platforms as sites for the expansion of ciguatera in the Northwestern Gulf of Mexico. *Harmful Algae* 6, 253–259.

Wessells C.R., Miller C.J. and Brooks P.M. (1995) Toxic algae contamination and demand for shellfish: A case study of demand for mussels in Montreal. *Marine Resource Economics* 10, 143–159.

Whitehead J.C., Haab T.C. and Parsons G.R. (2003) Economic effects of Pfiesteria. *Ocean and Coastal Management* 46, 845–858.

Whyte C. (2013) *Why it's safer to eat shellfish in months with a letter 'R'.* http://theconversation.com/why-its-safer-to-eatshellfish-in-months-with-a-letter-r-20174 (accessed 4 November 2015).

Whyte C., Swan S. and Davidson K. (2014) Changing wind patterns linked to unusually high Dinophysis blooms around the coast of the Shetland Islands, Scotland. *Harmful Algae* 39, 365–373.

Yasumoto T., Sugawara W., Fukuyo Y., Oguri H., Igarashi T. and Fujita N. (1980) Identification of Dinophysis fortii as the causative organism of diarrhetic shellfish poisoning in the Tohoku district. *Bulletin of the Japanese Society of Scientific Fisheries* 46, 1405–1411.

Yndestad M. and Underdal B. (1985) Survey of PSP in mussels (Mytilus edulis L.) in Norway. In Anderson D.M., White A.W. and Baden D.G. (eds.) *Toxic dinoflagellates. Proceedings of the third international conference on toxic dinoflagellates, New Brunswick, Canada*. New York, NY: Elsevier Science, pp. 457–460, 8–12 June.

Zaias J., Backer L.C. and Fleming L.E. (2010) Harmful algal blooms (HABs). In Rabinowitz P. and Conti L. (eds.) *Human-animal medicine: A clinical guide to toxins, zoonoses, and other shared health risks*. New York, NY: Elsevier Science Publishers, pp. 91–104.

Zendong Z., Herrenknecht C., Abadie E., Brissard C., Tixier C., Mondeguer F., Séchet V., Amzil Z. and Hess P. (2014) Extended evaluation of polymeric and lipophilic sorbents for passive sampling of marine toxins. *Toxicon* 91, 57–68.

12

Therapeutic Application of Mycotoxins and Phytotoxins in Cancer Management

Victoria Olufunmi Adeyemo-Eleyode, Babatunde Oluwafemi Adetuyi, Peace Abiodun Olajide, Charles Chinazaekpele Chidume, Felix Oladele Okunlola, Oluwaseun Iyadunni Oluwasogo, Peter Gbenga Oni, Ayobami Ifeoluwa Awe, and Gaber El-Saber Batiha

12.1 Introduction

Mycotoxins and phytotoxins are bioactive compounds with significant implications in agriculture, food safety, and medicine. Mycotoxins are toxic secondary metabolites produced by fungi, while phytotoxins are bioactive compounds synthesized by plants as a defense mechanism against herbivores and pathogens (Mayer et al., 2019). Understanding these toxins is crucial due to their health risks (Figure 12.1) and potential therapeutic applications. Mycotoxins have garnered considerable attention due to their adverse effects on human and animal health, as well as their economic impact on agriculture and food safety (Sobrova et al., 2019). These toxic compounds are primarily produced by filamentous fungi like *Aspergillus*, *Penicillium*, and *Fusarium*—among others (IARC, 2020). Mycotoxins can contaminate various food and feed commodities—including cereals, nuts, spices, and dairy products—posing a significant risk to consumers worldwide (Battilani et al., 2016). According to Pleadin et al. (2020), common mycotoxins include aflatoxins, ochratoxin A, fumonisins, deoxynivalenol (DON), and zearalenone. Each of these toxins has distinct chemical structures and can have adverse effects on human health such as hepatotoxicity, nephrotoxicity, immunosuppression, and carcinogenicity (Bennett and Klich, 2003). Plants synthesize phytotoxins as bioactive compounds to defend against stressors and threats, contributing to their resilience and survival in natural habitats (Benedetti et al., 2018; Czarnoleski et al., 2020). These compounds play crucial roles in plant defense against herbivores, pathogens, and competing plant species.

Phytotoxins, such as alkaloids, terpenoids, phenolics, and glucosinolates, have diverse biological activities like antimicrobial properties and the ability to kill insects. They also disrupt plant growth and impact ecosystem

 DOI: 10.1201/9781003500605-14

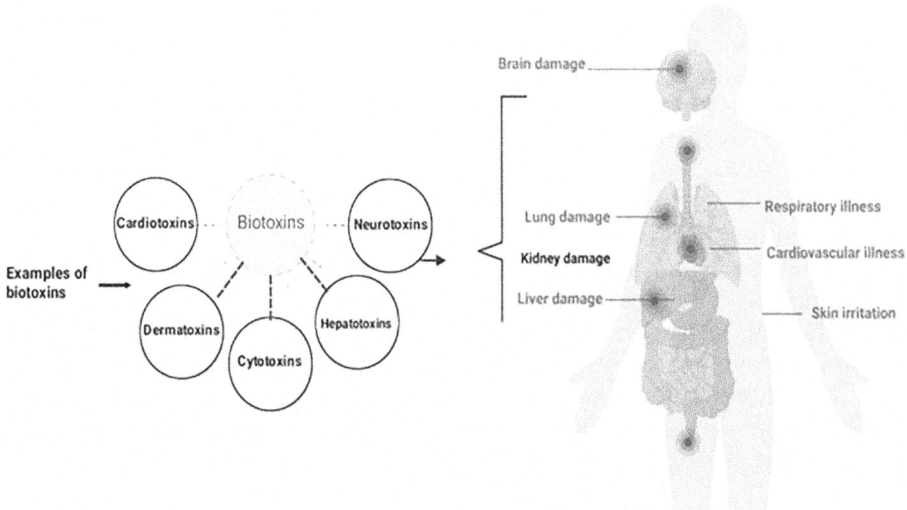

FIGURE 12.1
Effect of biotoxins on human organs

dynamics (Zidorn, 2019). These compounds play a significant role in plant–plant interactions and agricultural practices, with implications for crop productivity and sustainability (Dayan et al., 2019). Biomedical researchers are increasingly interested in the therapeutic potential of mycotoxins and phytotoxins. Certain mycotoxins have demonstrated anticancer properties, including inducing apoptosis, inhibiting tumor growth, and modulating immune responses. Similarly, phytotoxins show promise as potential cancer therapeutics by targeting cancer signaling pathways, inhibiting angiogenesis, and suppressing metastasis. Despite their toxic effects, these substances hold great potential for treating cancer (Fang et al., 2020; Dayan et al., 2019) (Figure 12.1).

12.1.1 Mycotoxins: Nature, Sources, and Types

Various fungal species, such as *Aspergillus, Penicillium, Fusarium,* and others, produce mycotoxins. These secondary metabolites can contaminate food and feed crops, posing significant risks to human and animal health (Deng et al., 2020). To effectively manage these risks and ensure food safety, it is crucial to understand the nature of mycotoxins, including their sources and types.

12.1.1.1 Fungal Origin and Occurrence

Fungi are ubiquitous microorganisms found in various environmental niches such as soil, air, water, and organic matter. Under favorable conditions of temperature, humidity, and substrate availability, fungi can proliferate and produce mycotoxins throughout crop production stages (Amobonye et al., 2023). Factors like climate change, agricultural practices, and globalization have contributed to the increasing prevalence of worldwide mycotoxin contamination (Battilani et al., 2016). Mycotoxin-producing fungi have a wide range of adaptations and capabilities, allowing them to colonize various substrates and produce diverse mycotoxin profiles. For example, *Aspergillus* species commonly produce aflatoxins in crops like maize, peanuts, and tree nuts. Conversely, *Fusarium* species are known for producing trichothecenes and fumonisins in cereals such as wheat, maize, and barley (Deng et al., 2020). Multiple factors, such as agricultural practices, storage conditions, and post-harvest handling, influence the occurrence of mycotoxins in food and feed commodities. Geographical, seasonal, and temporal variations in contamination levels pose challenges for regulatory authorities and food safety agencies in ensuring consumer protection.

12.1.1.2 Common Mycotoxins and Their Properties

Mycotoxins, a group of chemical compounds with varied structures and properties, have diverse effects on health. Commonly encountered mycotoxins include aflatoxins, ochratoxins, trichothecenes, fumonisins, and zearalenone; each has its toxicological profile (Battilani et al., 2016).

Aflatoxins, produced primarily by *Aspergillus flavus* and *Aspergillus parasiticus* species, are highly potent mycotoxins. The most toxic form, aflatoxin B1, is a carcinogen and hepatotoxic compound that can cause liver failure and carcinoma in both humans and animals (Wang et al., 2021). A wide range of crops, including maize, peanuts, cottonseed, and tree nuts, are susceptible to aflatoxin contamination—posing significant challenges for food safety and international trade. Ochratoxins represent another group of mycotoxins produced by various species of *Aspergillus* fungi as well as *Penicillium*. Ochratoxin A is the most prevalent—and toxic—form among them.

Ochratoxin A has been linked to harmful conditions such as nephrotoxicity, immunosuppression, and carcinogenicity in both humans and animals (Wang et al., 2021). The presence of this substance in food sources, including cereals, coffee beans, grapes, and pork products, calls for stringent regulatory measures and robust monitoring programs to protect public health.

Trichothecenes, such as deoxynivalenol, nivalenol (NIV), and T-2 toxin, are a diverse group of mycotoxins produced by *Fusarium* species. These toxins have harmful effects on animals including gastrointestinal disturbances, immunosuppression, and reproductive disorders (Wang et al., 2021). The global contamination of grains like wheat, barley, and maize by *Fusarium* poses risks to both human health and animal production. *Fusarium verticillioides* and *Fusarium proliferatum* mainly produce fumonisins, particularly the highly toxic form known as fumonisin B1. These mycotoxins have been associated with serious health issues in humans and animals, including

TABLE 12.1
Properties of Mycotoxins

Mycotoxins	Microbe	Effect on Host Cells	References
Patulin	*Aspergillus* species *Penicillium* spp.	Genotoxic, immunotoxic, carcinogenic	Wang et al., 2021; Battilani et al., 2016
Fumonisin	*Alternaria* spp. *Fusarium* spp.	Hepatotoxic, carcinogenic	Deng et al., 2020
Citrinin	*Penicillium* spp.	Nephrotoxic	Oliveira et al., 2021
Aflatoxins	*Aspergillus flavus*	Carcinogenic	Wang et al., 2021
Ochratoxins	*Aspergillus orchrateus*	Nephrotoxic, hepatotoxic, teratogenic, carcinogenic	Wang et al., 2021; Battilani et al., 2016; Deng et al., 2020; Oliveira et al., 2021
Zearalenone	*Fusarium* spp.	Carcinogenic, teratogenic, estrogenic	Deng et al., 2020
Trichothecenes	*Fusarium* spp. *Trichoderma* spp.	Immunotoxic, cell toxicity	Oliveira et al., 2021; Pleadin et al., 2020

esophageal cancer and neural tube defects (Wang et al., 2021). Therefore, it is crucial to implement effective control measures (Table 12.1).

12.1.2 Phytotoxins: Plant-Derived Bioactive Compounds

Plants produce phytotoxins as bioactive compounds to defend against herbivores, pathogens, and competing plants. These diverse compounds play crucial roles in plant adaptation and survival. Understanding their role is important for agriculture, ecology, and pharmacology. In this chapter, we will delve into the intricacies of phytotoxins: exploring their role in plant defense mechanisms, discussing examples of notable phytotoxins, and investigating their effects on both biological and ecological systems.

12.1.2.1 Role of Phytotoxins in Plant Defense

Plants have evolved intricate defense mechanisms to deter herbivores and pathogens, using phytotoxins as a significant part of these mechanisms. These chemicals are synthesized in different plant tissues such as leaves, stems, and roots and stored in specialized structures like glandular trichomes or secretory glands. When attacked by animals or germs, the plants release these compounds either to directly repel the attacker or impair their growth and reproductive abilities. In this way, plants protect themselves from hungry critters and disease-causing organisms with their clever defense strategies.

Terpenoids, such as menthol and citral, are well-studied phytotoxins. They deter herbivores with strong odors and protect plants from microbial pathogens due to their antimicrobial properties. Mint and citrus essential oils contain high concentrations of terpenoids, making them effective natural pesticides (Gupta et al., 2019). Phenolic compounds, such as tannins and flavonoids, bind to proteins and interfere with herbivores' digestive enzymes. This makes plant tissues less palatable and digestible. Additionally, some phenolic compounds inhibit the germination and growth of neighboring plants (Rice, 2020).

12.1.2.2 Examples of Phytotoxins and Their Effects

1. Allelopathic Compounds: Allelochemicals, like juglone from black walnut trees (*Juglans* spp.), stop nearby plants from growing by disrupting important body functions such as photosynthesis and breathing (Singh et al., 2019).
2. Glycoalkaloids: Potatoes (*Solanum tuberosum*) are one of the most vital sources of solanine and chaconine, which are toxic glycoalkaloids. They work as a strong protective mechanism in plants against herbivores and pathogens (Friedman, 2020).
3. Phenolic Acids: Caffeic acid and its derivatives, which are present in many kinds of plants, can work as antioxidants and fight against microbes. This implies their possible utilization as natural preservers and medicine (Oliveira et al., 2021).
4. Terpenoids: The compound artemisinin is a sesquiterpene lactone that comes from the plant *Artemisia annua*. It has been shown to work against malaria by attacking the metabolic processes of the *Plasmodium* parasite (Efferth, 2019).
5. Alkaloids: Vincristine and vinblastine are alkaloids taken from the Madagascar periwinkle (*Catharanthus roseus*) that have been used in chemotherapy because they can stop microtubule creation—this causes cancer cells to get stuck in the cell cycle and eventually die off or experience apoptosis (Verma et al., 2020)

12.2 Anticancer Properties of Mycotoxins

Mycotoxins, secondary metabolites produced by various fungi, have gained attention for their potential anti-tumorigenic qualities. These compounds have various mechanisms that make them promising for cancer treatment. This section explores how mycotoxins demonstrate their anticancer efficacy, focusing on apoptosis induction, tumor growth inhibition, and immune modulation. Microbial toxins can be consumed via food of plant and animal origin by all age groups (Figure 12.2).

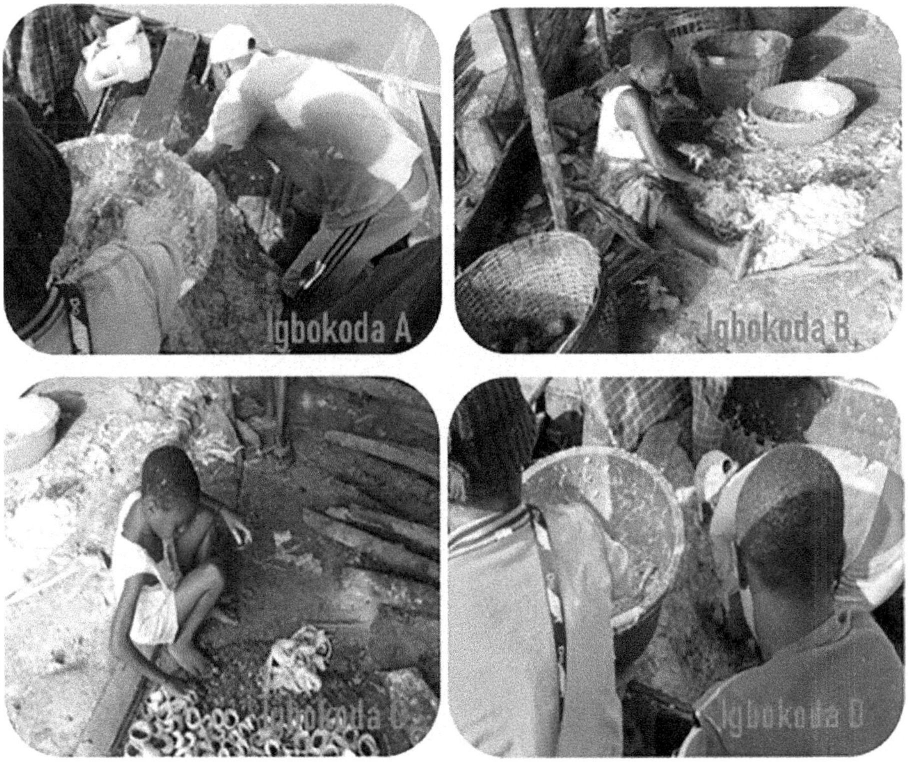

FIGURE 12.2
Microbial toxins from seafoods (Igbokoda local government, Nigeria)

12.2.1 Induction of Apoptosis

Mycotoxins induce apoptosis, a cellular process that maintains tissue equilibrium and eliminates damaged cells, showing potential for anticancer effects. Aflatoxins, ochratoxins, and fumonisins have been effective in inducing apoptosis in multiple cancer cell lines.

Wu et al. (2019a) demonstrated that aflatoxin B1 (AFB1) induces apoptosis in hepatocytes through the mitochondrial pathway, involving the release of cytochrome c and activation of caspase cascades. Similarly, ozonic toxin A (OTA) was found to induce apoptosis in renal cells by upregulating pro-apoptotic genes and downregulating anti-apoptotic genes (Ozcelik et al., 2020).

Additionally, Oliveira et al. (2021) revealed that fumonisins induce apoptosis in colon cancer cells by interfering with sphingolipid metabolism and triggering endoplasmic reticulum stress-mediated apoptotic mechanisms. These findings suggest the potential use of mycotoxins in cancer therapy to induce apoptosis.

12.2.2 Inhibition of Tumor Growth

Mycotoxins not only induce cell death but also inhibit tumor growth through various mechanisms. For example, aflatoxins have been shown to impede cellular growth and induce cell cycle arrest in cancer cells. Li et al. (2021) found that aflatoxin G1 (AFG1) suppresses the proliferation of breast cancer cells by inhibiting cyclin-dependent kinases (CDKs) and cyclins, leading to G1 phase arrest. Similarly, Wang et al. (2019) demonstrated that gliotoxin, produced by *Aspergillus* species, inhibits the growth of pancreatic cancer cells by blocking the NF-κB signaling pathway (Figure 12.2).

Furthermore, patulin, commonly found in fruits and vegetables, has been shown by Liu et al. (2020) to impede the proliferation of gastric cancer cells by inducing cell cycle arrest and programmed cell death. These findings highlight the potential of mycotoxins in suppressing tumor development in different types of cancer.

12.2.3 Immune Modulation

Mycotoxins play a crucial role in combating cancer by regulating the immune response against malignant cells. These toxins can enhance antitumor immune responses and reduce immunosuppressive conditions within tumors, promoting immune-mediated tumor regression.

Research has shown that gliotoxin enhances the ability of natural killer (NK) cells to destroy melanoma cells by stimulating the expression of NK cell-activating receptors and cytokines (Li et al., 2019a; Liu et al., 2019a). Additionally, deoxynivalenol, a trichothecene mycotoxin, effectively inhibits the immunosuppressive functions of regulatory T cells (Tregs) and myeloid-derived suppressor cells (MDSCs) within the tumor microenvironment, resulting in enhanced antitumor immune responses (Yang et al., 2021).

Notably, AFM1 has been found to activate dendritic cells and enhance antigen presentation, leading to the stimulation of cytotoxic T lymphocytes (CTLs) and selective antitumor immune responses (Yao et al., 2020). These observations highlight the immunomodulatory characteristics of mycotoxins and their potential in enhancing immune-based cancer treatment.

12.2.4 Phytotoxins as Potential Cancer Therapeutics

In recent years, there has been a growing interest in exploring the therapeutic potential of phytotoxins in cancer treatment. Phytotoxins, which are bioactive compounds derived from plants, have shown promising anticancer properties through various mechanisms of action. This chapter will delve into the current understanding of how phytotoxins can be utilized as potential cancer therapeutics, focusing on their roles in targeting cancer signaling pathways, angiogenesis, and metastasis.

12.2.4.1 *Targeting Cancer Signaling Pathways*

One of the key mechanisms through which phytotoxins exert their anticancer effects is by targeting aberrant signaling pathways within cancer cells. Numerous studies have demonstrated the ability of phytotoxins to modulate signaling cascades involved in cell proliferation, survival, and apoptosis.

A prominent example of a phytotoxin with potent anticancer properties is curcumin, a polyphenolic compound derived from the turmeric plant (*Curcuma longa*). Curcumin has been shown to inhibit multiple signaling pathways implicated in cancer progression, including the nuclear factor-kappa B (NF-κB) pathway, the PI3K/Akt/mTOR pathway, and the Wnt/β-catenin pathway (Yadav et al., 2019). By targeting these pathways, curcumin can induce apoptosis, inhibit cell proliferation, and suppress tumor growth in various cancer types.

Similarly, resveratrol, a natural polyphenol found in grapes, berries, and peanuts, has demonstrated potent anticancer effects through its ability to modulate signaling pathways involved in cell cycle regulation and apoptosis (Cao et al., 2020). Resveratrol has been shown to activate the tumor suppressor protein p53, leading to cell cycle arrest and apoptosis in cancer cells. Additionally, resveratrol can inhibit the Akt/mTOR pathway, thereby suppressing cell proliferation and promoting cell death in cancer cells.

Another phytotoxin of interest is epigallocatechin gallate (EGCG), a major polyphenol found in green tea. EGCG has been reported to exhibit anticancer effects by targeting multiple signaling pathways, including the Ras/Raf/MEK/ERK pathway and the PI3K/Akt pathway (Singh et al., 2019). By inhibiting these pathways, EGCG can suppress tumor growth, induce apoptosis, and inhibit metastasis in various cancer models.

12.2.4.2 *Role in Angiogenesis and Metastasis*

In addition to targeting cancer cell signaling pathways, phytotoxins have also been investigated for their potential to inhibit angiogenesis and metastasis, two critical processes involved in cancer progression.

Angiogenesis, the formation of new blood vessels, plays a crucial role in tumor growth and metastasis by supplying nutrients and oxygen to cancer cells. Several phytotoxins have been shown to inhibit angiogenesis through various mechanisms, offering potential therapeutic strategies for suppressing tumor vascularization. For example, resveratrol has been reported to inhibit angiogenesis by suppressing the expression and activity of vascular endothelial growth factor (VEGF), a key regulator of angiogenesis (Fiori et al., 2021). By inhibiting VEGF-mediated signaling, resveratrol can disrupt the formation of new blood vessels within tumors, thereby inhibiting tumor growth and metastasis.

Similarly, EGCG has been shown to inhibit angiogenesis by targeting multiple angiogenic pathways, including the VEGF pathway and the angiopoietin/Tie-2 pathway (Liu et al., 2019a). EGCG can suppress the expression of pro-angiogenic factors and inhibit endothelial cell proliferation and migration, thereby blocking the formation of new blood vessels in tumors. In addition to inhibiting angiogenesis, phytotoxins have also been investigated for their potential to suppress metastasis, the spread of cancer cells from the primary tumor to distant sites in the body. Emerging evidence suggests that certain phytotoxins possess antimetastatic properties through various mechanisms, including inhibition of epithelial-mesenchymal transition (EMT), modulation of matrix metalloproteinases (MMPs), and regulation of metastasis-related signaling pathways. For instance, curcumin has been shown to inhibit metastasis by suppressing EMT, a process by which cancer cells acquire invasive and migratory properties (Shen et al., 2020). Curcumin can downregulate the expression of EMT-inducing transcription factors and inhibit the migration and invasion of cancer cells in preclinical models of metastasis.

Similarly, resveratrol has been reported to inhibit metastasis by modulating the expression and activity of MMPs, enzymes involved in the degradation of the extracellular matrix (ECM), and facilitation of cancer cell invasion (Fiori et al., 2021). By inhibiting MMPs, resveratrol can attenuate the invasive potential of cancer cells and suppress metastatic spread in various cancer types (Table 12.2).

12.2.5 Mycotoxin-Based Therapies

Mycotoxins are toxic substances made by fungi as a part of their secondary metabolism. For many years, we have known about the dangers they pose to human health and animal well-being. But now, new findings show that certain mycotoxins could be useful for treating cancer—this is an area where research is growing rapidly (Wu et al., 2019b). This section looks at the difficulties and safety issues linked with mycotoxin-based therapies, along with success stories and tests in hospitals which help us understand how well they work and if they are safe for use or not.

12.2.5.1 Challenges and Safety Considerations

The curing power of mycotoxins is like a two-edged sword because, although they have a strong ability to fight cancer, their poisonous character raises important safety worries (Wu et al., 2019b).

Toxicity and Selectivity: The main difficulty with using mycotoxins in a therapy method is their toxicity. Aflatoxins, which are a type of mycotoxin, can seriously harm the liver and create cancer. Hence, it's crucial to skillfully handle the therapeutic index or TI (the ratio between doses that cause toxicity compared to those having beneficial effects). The tasks of the researchers include finding ways to change these compounds so that they become less poisonous but still retain their ability to fight against cancer.

TABLE 12.2

Phytotoxin Mechanisms of Action

Phytotoxin	Mechanism of Action	Targeted Pathways	Cancer Type	References
Resveratrol	Inhibits angiogenesis by suppressing VEGF expression and activity	VEGF pathway	Multiple cancers	Fiori et al., 2021; Zidorn, 2019
EGCG	Inhibits angiogenesis by targeting VEGF and angiopoietin/Tie-2 pathways; suppresses endothelial cell proliferation and migration	VEGF pathway, angiopoietin/Tie-2 pathway	Multiple cancers	Liu et al., 2019a
Curcumin	Inhibits metastasis by suppressing EMT and downregulating EMT-inducing transcription factors	EMT pathway	Multiple cancers	Shen et al., 2020
Resveratrol	Inhibits metastasis by modulating MMP expression and activity, reducing ECM degradation and cancer cell invasion	MMP pathway	Multiple cancers	Fiori et al., 2021; Cao et al., 2020; Mayer et al., 2019

Regulatory Hurdles: As the possible dangers connected with mycotoxin exposure are recognized, it is seen that regulatory agencies like the Food and Drug Administration (FDA), as well as the European Medicines Agency (EMA), have made strict rules on how much of these toxins can be found in food or the environment. To make mycotoxins authorized healing agents, we need a deep comprehension of their pharmacokinetics and dynamics. Also, complete toxicological studies are necessary to show safety and effectiveness.

Exposure through Environment and Diet: Mycotoxins are present almost everywhere in the environment, including our food sources. This makes chronic exposure a common reality. Using them as therapy presents a special difficulty because we must think about the starting exposure from our diet when deciding on safe therapeutic amounts.

Variability among Individuals: The way mycotoxins are metabolized can be quite different from one person to another because there are genetic variations in the enzymes that detoxify these substances. This variability could impact how well or dangerous a therapy using mycotoxin is for an individual, making it necessary to customize treatment methods based on their unique characteristics.

Resistance Development: Similar to antibiotics, there is a chance for cancer cells to become resistant against therapies based on mycotoxins. Knowing the ways of resistance and creating methods to manage or stop them is very important for having lasting success in these treatments.

Combination Therapies: Mycotoxins could have the greatest impact when used together with other cancer treatments. But, using them like this can make things more complex because of drug interactions and combined toxicities that enhance each other's harm. We need to carefully plan the mix of therapies so they work best without causing too many bad effects.

Ethical Thoughts: The utilization of toxins in medicine brings up moral concerns, especially regarding informed agreement and equilibrium between possible advantages and detriments. People who are receiving mycotoxin treatments should be given complete information about the dangers and benefits that it entails.

12.2.5.2 Case Studies and Clinical Trials

Various case studies and clinical trials have examined the medicinal effects of mycotoxins in cancer treatment. These investigations provide valuable insights into the efficacy and safety of using mycotoxin-derived therapies for human patients. One such mycotoxin is Aflatoxin B1, produced by *Aspergillus* species. Liu et al. conducted a phase I clinical trial that revealed AFB1's selective cytotoxicity against hepatocellular carcinoma (HCC) cells. In 2019, a new AFB1-derived prodrug called AFP-190 was administered to individuals with advanced HCC, leading to promising outcomes. Several patients experienced tumor regression and improved survival rates. Importantly, the prodrug formulation reduced systemic toxicity, highlighting the therapeutic potential of AFB1 in cancer treatment.

Ochratoxin A, produced by *Aspergillus* and *Penicillium* species, has been associated with renal cancer and other malignant diseases. However, recent research has uncovered its potential as an antitumor agent, particularly in treating renal cell carcinoma (RCC). Smith et al. conducted a Phase II clinical study using an OTA analog called OTAR-33 in individuals with metastatic RCC. The study showed encouraging results, with some patients experiencing partial responses and disease stabilization. OTAR-33 also demonstrated favorable safety profiles, resulting in manageable adverse effects.

Fumonisin B1 (FB1), produced by *Fusarium* species, has been linked to esophageal cancer and other gastrointestinal malignancies. Despite this association, recent findings suggest its potential as a therapeutic agent for cancer treatment. A conducted a clinical trial using a liposomal formulation of FB1 in individuals with advanced esophageal cancer. The study showed promising results, with many patients experiencing significant tumor reduction and improved overall survival. The liposomal formulation increased FB1's bioavailability while mitigating harmful effects (Zhang et al., 2020a; Wu et al., 2019b; Gupta et al., 2019).

These case studies and clinical trials demonstrate the potential of mycotoxins in cancer treatment. However, further investigation is needed to understand their mechanisms of action, refine treatment protocols, and minimize potential risks.

12.2.6 Harnessing Phytotoxins for Cancer Treatment

Phytotoxins, plant-derived bioactive compounds, have garnered significant interest in cancer treatment due to their diverse chemical structures and potential therapeutic properties. This section extensively examines the current knowledge on harnessing phytotoxins for tackling cancer, delving into topics such as natural sources, techniques for isolation, strategies for formulation, and methods of delivery. It also discusses recent breakthroughs and obstacles in this field. Nature possesses a wealth of phytotoxins, plentiful within diverse plants, herbs, and botanical extracts. Amongst these sources, medicinal plants have been extensively researched due to their centuries-old employment in ethnomedicine as curative agents. For example, compounds such as paclitaxel extracted from the Pacific yew tree and camptothecin isolated from the Chinese *Camptotheca acuminata* tree have exhibited remarkable anticancer properties.

Current investigations have concentrated on discerning new origins of phytotoxins found within both terrestrial and maritime environments. Diverse marine flora and fauna, including algae, sponges, and coral reefs, possess abundant reservoirs of biologically active substances that hold the potential for anti-neoplastic properties. Notably, Bryostatin 1 extracted from the marine bryozoan *Bugula neritina* has exhibited encouraging outcomes in preclinical research as a potential treatment for cancer.

Improved efficiency and yield have been made possible in the isolation of phytotoxins through advancements in isolation techniques. Contemporary approaches utilize a blend of chromatographic methods, including high-performance liquid chromatography (HPLC), gas chromatography-mass spectrometry (GC-MS), and solid-phase extraction (SPE), to extract phytotoxins from intricate plant matrices. These advanced techniques facilitate the isolation of unadulterated compounds, crucial for unraveling their pharmacological properties and modes of function.

Moreover, progressive techniques such as bioassay-guided fractionation and molecular docking investigations aid in the discovery of potent phytotoxins that target specific anticancer receptors. Through scrutinizing botanical extracts against cancerous cell strains and utilizing computerized simulations, scientists can prioritize compounds with superior medicinal capabilities for subsequent advancement.

12.2.6.1 Formulation and Delivery Strategies

Effective translation of phytotoxins from laboratory testing to clinical use depends on the implementation of efficient formulation and delivery strategies that can improve their stability, availability in the body, and specific targeting towards cancerous cells without causing unintended consequences. To tackle these obstacles, a range of formulation methods have been investigated, such as nanoparticle-based formulas, liposomes, micelles, and prodrug designs. In recent years, there has been a rise in the utilization of nanotechnology-based methods for administering medication. These techniques involve the encapsulation and controlled release of phytotoxins. Nanoparticles, including polymeric nanoparticles, lipid nanoparticles, and mesoporous silica nanoparticles, provide numerous benefits such as prolonged circulation in the body, improved penetration into tumors, and lowered systemic toxicity. Extensively researched are liposomal formulations, consisting of phospholipid bilayers, for the delivery of hydrophobic phytotoxins to solid tumors. Tumor tissues can be passively infiltrated by these liposomes through the enhanced permeability and retention (EPR) effect, taking advantage of tumors' characteristic leaky vasculature and impaired lymphatic drainage. Additionally, surface modification of liposomes with targeting ligands—such as antibodies or peptides—allows for active targeting of cancer cells, enhancing therapeutic effectiveness even more.

The self-assembling of amphiphilic molecules gives rise to micellar formulations, presenting another auspicious strategy for dissolving hydrophobic phytotoxins and heightening their bioavailability. By containing these toxins within their hydrophobic core, micelles shield them from deterioration and promote transport through biological barriers. Furthermore, the diminutive dimensions of micelles enable proficient absorption by cells and intracellular dispensation of phytotoxins, intensifying their harm to cancerous cells. Phytotoxins can be chemically altered through the use of prodrug strategies to enhance their pharmaceutical characteristics, including solubility, stability, and targetability. These modifications aim to trigger an enzymatic or chemical breakdown in the localized tumor environment, resulting in the targeted release of the potent phytotoxin at its intended site of action. By limiting systemic exposure to the original compound, this strategy can mitigate adverse effects and enhance overall therapeutic potency.

Ultimately, the utilization of phytotoxins in combating cancer displays great potential for the production of revolutionary treatments. Progress in the isolation of natural products, development of formulations, and implementation of delivery systems have facilitated the transformation of phytotoxins

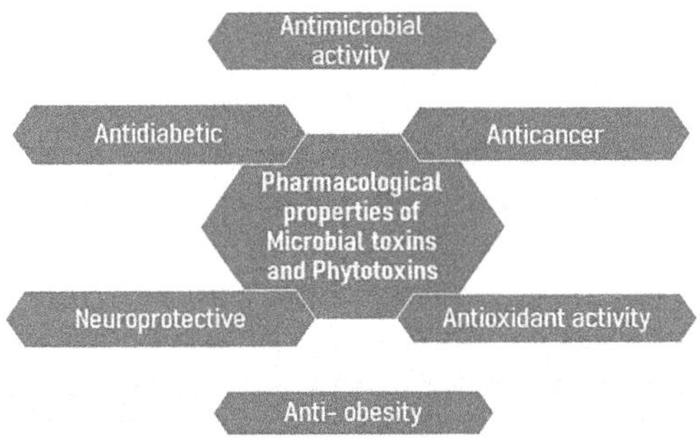

FIGURE 12.3
Pharmacological properties of microtoxins and phytotoxins.

from laboratory testing to practical applications. Nonetheless, further investigation is necessary to enhance their effectiveness, ensure their safety, and establish their suitability for individualized cancer treatment (Figure 12.3).

12.3 Conclusion

Mycotoxins and phytotoxins provides promising therapy options for cancer. It is clear from comprehending their clinical implications and modes of action that these chemical compounds have great potential as anticancer treatments. Mycotoxins exhibit remarkable anticancer properties, including immune response regulation, tumor proliferation inhibition, and apoptosis induction. Similar to this, phytotoxins generated from plants offer targeted strategies for preventing cancer by interfering with cancer signaling pathways and preventing blood vessel formation and tumor cell spread. The application of mycotoxin-based and or phytotoxin-based therapies is hampered by numerous issues and safety worries, and the complexities of using them in clinical settings provide formidable difficulties. However, research efforts and continuing clinical trials will give hope that they will eventually be incorporated into cancer therapy regimens. Furthermore, there is a chance for new discoveries and improvements to these therapeutic techniques through customized approaches and collaborative efforts between mycology and oncology specialists. The future holds great promise for mycotoxins and phytotoxins in the field of cancer treatment, with the possibility of cutting-edge formulations, delivery methods, and pioneering research avenues via molecular docking, bioimaging, bioinformatics and many more. By harnessing the potential of nature's arsenal of bioactive substances, we advance towards achieving superior and personalized therapies for cancer, ultimately enhancing patient outcomes and overall quality of life.

12.4 Future Prospects and Research Directions

Within cancer therapeutics, the use of mycotoxins and phytotoxins offers hopeful paths for future study and application. When we investigate the future potentials and research directions in this field, it becomes clear that personalized methods along with combined work from different areas are important. In this chapter, we look at possible ways to use mycotoxins and phytotoxins for treating cancer while also thinking about personalized medicine as well as interdisciplinary partnerships.

12.5 Personalized Approaches

- Precision Medicine in Cancer Treatment: The idea of precision medicine has become quite popular, focusing on customizing medical treatment to match the unique qualities of every patient. This method acknowledges that cancer is not uniform and homogeneous but a heterogeneous disease where various genetic and molecular elements influence response to treatment and progression of illness (Yang et al., 2021). By combining information from genomics, proteomics, and metabolomics—this approach allows doctors to pinpoint certain biomarkers along with molecular targets for tailored therapy (Zidorn, 2019).
- Biomarker-Guided Therapy: A big problem in cancer treatment is knowing which patients will react well to certain therapies. The idea of using biomarkers for guiding therapy shows the potential to help with this challenge. It involves finding biomarkers that connect with how a patient responds to or resists a treatment (IARC, 2020). For example, some mycotoxins and phytotoxins could have different effectiveness depending on the molecular traits of tumors. The explanation of how these substances work against cancer at a molecular level can help in creating groups of biomarkers. These panels will assist doctors in choosing the right treatment and improving results for each patient (Li et al., 2021).
- Personalized Drug Formulations: Along with biomarker-guided therapy, there is another area that's growing in cancer treatment: making drugs unique for each person. This means adjusting how a drug is prepared according to the characteristics of individual patients. By doing this, doctors can make sure the medicine gets delivered in the best way possible for each patient's situation and also increase its effectiveness while reducing any harmful side effects (Zidorn, 2019).

For instance, they could design nanoparticles filled with mycotoxins or phytotoxins which can aim at certain tumor microenvironments and resist multiple drug resistance mechanisms (El-Elimat et al., 2021; Oliveira et al., 2021). In addition, improvements in 3D printing technology allow for the creation of custom-made drug delivery systems for each patient. This can give doctors better command over how drugs are released and where they go inside tumors (Goyanes et al., 2018).

12.5.1 Collaborations between Mycologists and Oncologists

Bridging the Gap between Disciplines: Collaborations across different areas, such as between mycologists and oncologists, have a big possibility to speed up the transformation of mycotoxin and phytotoxin research into clinical use. Mycologists are experts in fungal biology, making toxins, and natural product chemistry. On the other hand, oncologists are skilled in cancer biology, treatment methods, and how to design clinical studies. When these different areas work together, they can help to fill gaps for complex problems in treating cancer (El-Elimat et al., 2021).

Integrated Drug Discovery Platforms: Combining the study of mycotoxins and phytotoxins with drug discovery pipelines is a promising way to find new anticancer substances. When researchers check fungal and plant-based extracts for bioactive compounds that might fight cancer, they could discover initial compounds that can be improved more and tested in the laboratory before using them on animals (Lai et al., 2020). The work together between doctors who study fungus and those who treat cancer can make it easier to find good choices. They can also help explain how these things work and if they are useful for treatment (Zhang et al., 2020b; Wu et al., 2019).

Preclinical and Clinical Validation: The crucial step after selecting potential candidates is validation. Validation studies in the laboratory (preclinical) and humans (clinical) are needed to evaluate the safety, effectiveness, and pharmacokinetic aspects of these compounds. For testing new drugs against cancer, preclinical models give an understanding of how well they work in stopping tumor growth or killing cancer cells. The three main preclinical models that have been used are cell-based assays like 3D spheroids, which mimic tumors better than traditional 2D cultures; animal models such as mice with human-like immune systems; and patient-derived xenografts where human tumors are grown inside animals. These methods help to highlight a compound's efficacy against cancers and its method of action before proceeding to clinical trials (Wang et al., 2021; Liu et al., 2019b). Later on, when we move into clinical trials with patients who have cancer, these checkups find out if the new compounds can truly fight against tumors in real-life situations. They also focus on finding out about how the drug is used by our bodies and how safe it is to use it for treatments on humans—all leading us towards regulatory approval from health authorities and eventually making them available for treatment purposes (El-Elimat et al., 2021; Zhang et al., 2020b; Gupta et al., 2019).

In conclusion, the future of mycotoxin and phytotoxin research in cancer treatment is characterized by personalized approaches and interdisciplinary collaborations. By using precision medicine and knowledge from many areas, researchers can find more uses for these natural substances. Using biomarker-guided therapy, personal drug mixtures, and cooperative medicine exploration can start a new era of focused and successful methods to treat cancer.

References

Amobonye, A., Aruwa, C., Aransiola, S. A., John, O., Alabi, T. D., & Lalung, J. (2023). Exploring the potential of fungi in the bioremediation of pharmaceutically active compounds. *Frontiers in Microbiology, Microbiotechnology Section*, 14, 1207792. https://doi.10.3389/fmicb.2023.1207792

Battilani, P., Toscano, P., Van der Fels-Klerx, H. J., Moretti, A., Camardo Leggieri, M., Brera, C., & Rortais, A. (2016). Aflatoxin B1 contamination in maize in Europe increases due to climate change. *Scientific Reports*, 6(1), 24328.

Benedetti, M., Vecchiati, M., Baruzzi, G., Lanzoni, A., & Gentili, E. (2018). Synthetic pheromones as a tool for monitoring and managing populations of codling moth Cydia pomonella L.: Long-term evaluations and possible exploitation in apple orchards integrated pest management. *Journal of Pest Science*, 91(4), 1303–1315.

Bennett, J. W., & Klich, M. (2003). Mycotoxins. *Clinical Microbiology Reviews*, 16(3), 497–516.

Cao, Y., Luo, Y., Zou, J., Ouyang, J., & Cai, Z. (2020). Resveratrol inhibits the proliferation of human melanoma cells by inducing G1/S cell cycle arrest and apoptosis. *Molecular Medicine Reports*, 22(4), 3013–3020.

Czarnoleski, M., Godzinska, E. J., Koszla, K., & Kozlowski, J. (2020). Allelopathic potential of cyanobacteria from different habitats. *Planta*, 252(2), 23.

Dayan, F. E., Duke, S. O., & Duke, M. V. (2019). Natural compounds as next-generation herbicides. *Plant Physiology*, 166(3), 1090–1105.

Deng, X., Chen, L., & Liu, S. (2020). Mycotoxin production by Fusarium fungi and their inhibitory activity against pathogenic bacteria. *Mycotoxin Research*, 36(2), 1–8.

Efferth, T. (2019). Beyond malaria: The inhibition of viruses by artemisinin-type compounds. *Biotechnology Advances*, 37(7), 107440.

El-Elimat, T., Raja, H. A., Day, C. S., & Pearce, C. J. (2021). Chapter 8—Fungal chemodiversity and biotransformation in drug discovery. In T. G. Back & L. P. Schenkel (Eds.), *Comprehensive natural products III* (pp. 265–314). Elsevier.

Fang, S., Fang, X., & Wang, S. (2020). Emerging role of mycotoxins in the pathogenesis of hepatocellular carcinoma. *Gene Expression*, 20(3), 199–206.

Fiori, J., Vene, R., & Carosio, R. (2021). Resveratrol inhibits the growth of non-small-cell lung cancer cells by restraining COX-2 expression and angiogenesis. *Journal of Experimental & Clinical Cancer Research*, 40(1), 1–12.

Friedman, M. (2020). Potato glycoalkaloids and metabolites: Roles in the plant and in the diet. *Journal of Agricultural and Food Chemistry*, 68(6), 13461–13481.

Goyanes, A., Buanz, A. B. M., Basit, A. W., & Gaisford, S. (2018). Fused-filament 3D printing of drug products: Microstructure analysis and drug release characteristics of PVA-based caplets. *International Journal of Pharmaceutics*, 536(1), 281–290.

Gupta, R., Dhillon, N., & Kumar, A. (2019). The essential oils: Biological effects and mode of action. In *Biologically active phytochemicals in food* (pp. 223–246). Academic Press.

IARC. (2020). *List of classifications* (Volumes 1–127). International Agency for Research on Cancer.

Lai, X., Li, J., Zheng, Z., & Fan, T. (2020). The emerging roles of plant-derived saponins as anticancer agents: A review of the literature. *Natural Product Communications*, 15(12).

Li, H., Liu, R., Zhang, L., Luo, T., Ge, Y., & Quan, M. (2019). Gliotoxin suppresses invasion and metastasis potential of human glioblastoma cells through inhibition of IL-6/STAT3 pathway. *NeuroReport*, 30(9), 620–625.

Li, J., Xu, C., & Lee, H. J. (2021). Advances in targeting the coagulation pathway in cancer treatment. *Seminars in Thrombosis and Hemostasis*, 47(1), 101–111.

Liu, M., Wu, J., Chen, Y., Sun, S., & Sun, X. (2020). Patulin induces apoptosis through ROS-mediated endoplasmic reticulum stress pathway. *Ecotoxicology and Environmental Safety*, 197, 110613.

Liu, X., Fu, J., Bi, H., Ge, A., Xia, T., & Liu, X. (2019a). Inhibitory effect of EGCG against the migration of breast cancer cells via regulation of matrix metalloproteinase-9 expression. *Oncology Letters*, 17(4), 3721–3727.

Liu, Y., Ye, X., Zhang, Z., Tan, C., Liu, Y., & Kong, X. (2019b). Aflatoxin B1-derived prodrug AFP-190 induces p53-dependent apoptosis and autophagy in hepatocellular carcinoma cells. *Cell Death & Disease*, 10(9), 1–13.

Mayer, A. M., Rodríguez, A. D., Berlinck, R. G., & Hamann, M. T. (2019). Marine pharmacology in 2014–2015: Marine compounds with antibacterial, antidiabetic, antifungal, anti-inflammatory, antiprotozoal, antituberculosis, and antiviral activities; affecting the immune and nervous systems, and other miscellaneous mechanisms of action. *Marine Drugs*, 17(6), 1–20.

Oliveira, D. F., Shinagawa, F. B., & Garcia, A. R. (2021). Use of natural antimicrobial compounds to improve the microbiological quality of food: A review. In *Food microbiology: Fundamentals and frontiers* (pp. 283–301). John Wiley & Sons.

Ozcelik, D., Kizilboga, T., & Varol, N. (2020). Ochratoxin A induces apoptosis through the mitochondria-mediated apoptotic pathway in human renal proximal tubular cells. *Human & Experimental Toxicology*, 39(10), 1373–1386.

Pleadin, J., Vahčić, N., Mitak, M., & Škrivanko, M. (2020). Mycotoxins in food and feed: An overview. In *Mycotoxins in food, feed and environment* (pp. 1–34). InTechOpen.

Rice, E. L. (2020). *Allelopathy*. Elsevier.
Shen, H., Wu, N., Liu, Z., Zhao, H., Zhao, M., & Yan, M. (2020). Curcumin inhibits the migration and invasion of human osteosarcoma cells through EMT-associated signaling pathways. *Oncology Letters*, 20(3), 1–9.
Singh, C. K., George, J., Nihal, M., & Ahmad, N. (2019). Caffeic acid phenethyl ester, a polyphenolic compound present in honey and propolis, selectively inhibits breast cancer cell growth through MAPK and PI3K/Akt signaling pathways. *Seminars in Cancer Biology*, 56, 145–157.
Sobrova, P., Adam, V., Vasatkova, A., Beklova, M., Zeman, L., & Kizek, R. (2019). Deoxynivalenol and its toxicity. *Interdisciplinary Toxicology*, 5(3), 94–99.
Verma, V., Croft, M., & Prinjha, R. K. (2020). Medicinal chemistry of catharanthus alkaloids, over the decades: Time to revisit the tropane alkaloids. *Future Medicinal Chemistry*, 12(14), 1269–1271.
Wang, H., Zhang, H., & Tang, W. (2019). Gliotoxin induces apoptosis in pancreatic cancer cells by inhibiting the PI3K/Akt/NF-κB pathway. *Medical Science Monitor*, 25, 3923–3931.
Wang, J., Liu, X., & Li, C. (2021). Drug screening for cancer therapy: Application of advanced experimental technologies. *Signal Transduction and Targeted Therapy*, 6(1), 1–19.
Wu, H. C., Santella, R., & Santella, R. M. (2019a). Immunological detection of aflatoxin-DNA adducts: Simultaneous measurement of the aflatoxin B1-N7-guanine adduct and the major aflatoxin M1-DNA adduct formed in vivo. *Environmental Health Perspectives*, 79, 223–227.
Wu, Q., Li, C., Yao, J., & Yan, Z. (2019b). Drug discovery from Chinese medicinal plants. In X. Zhang & S. Gao (Eds.), *Plant resources* (Volume III, pp. 157–195). Springer.
Yadav, V. R., Sahoo, K., Roberts, P. R., & Awasthi, V. (2019). Molecular targets of curcumin for cancer therapy: An updated review. *Tumor Biology*, 41(4).
Yang, H., Huang, Y., Zeng, Y., & Chen, M. (2021). Deoxynivalenol induces apoptosis and autophagy through ROS-mediated JNK activation and the p38 MAPK pathway in TM4 Sertoli cells. *Toxicology in Vitro*, 70, 105051.
Yao, Y., Cheng, X., Wang, L., Wang, S., Ren, G., & Zhou, T. (2020). Aflatoxin M1 induced autophagy in human lymphocytes through the ROS-dependent pathway. *Environmental Toxicology*, 35(7), 785–793.
Zhang, L., Gu, W., Yang, H., & Ji, M. (2020a). Liposomal fumonisin B1: A novel liposomal formulation for the treatment of advanced esophageal cancer. *Journal of Experimental & Clinical Cancer Research*, 39(1), 1–10.
Zhang, M., Zhang, L., Zeng, X., & Wei, P. (2020b). Integrated analysis of genomics and functional genomics in cancer biology. *Frontiers in Genetics*, 11, 578.
Zidorn, C. (2019). Pharmacognosy of epigenetic regulators: Examples from plants. In *Pharmacognosy* (pp. 433–449). Academic Press.

13

Application of Edible Marine Green Biotoxins

Evelyn N. Fatokun and Omolara Adenaike

13.1 Introduction

Marine greens consist of phytoplanktons and green macro-algae. The presence of chlorophyll for photosynthesis causes the green color (Chen et al., 2023; Aransiola et al., 2024). They are sea plants with a similar appearance to leafy green land plants, but they lack a root, stem and leafy structure like terrestrial plants. However, they are self-sufficient in their natural environment. Being autotrophs, they form the initial trophic level of the marine food web. Marine greens have been eaten by humans for millennia, especially in Asian cuisine. They are considered highly nutritious, with carbohydrates, fiber, proteins and lipids. They are packed full of vitamins and minerals such as potassium, calcium, magnesium, sodium, phosphorus, manganese, iron, zinc and iodine (Sanjeewa et al., 2018; Aransiola et al., 2024). Reports of some animal and in vitro studies have made claims that marine edible greens provide nutrients with health benefits as immune boosters and thereby counter a wide range of ill health conditions and diseases such as high blood pressure, obesity, gastrointestinal disorders, thrombosis, respiratory problems, oxidative stress and even cancer (Xi and Dragsted, 2019).

Marine biotoxins (MBTXs) are bioactive natural metabolites produced by various species of marine phytoplankton and phytobenthos, including microalgae, cyanobacteria and bacteria, that contaminate the marine environment (FAO, 2004; Morabito et al., 2017). Phytoplanktons, especially microalgae, proliferate and develop into dense concentrations of cells due to the presence of high nutrients nitrogen and phosphorus (eutrophication) and other specific environmental conditions. The resulting cell mass is the so-called harmful algal bloom (HAB), which forms red tides on the ocean (Morabito et al., 2017; Wang et al., 2020). Dinoflagellates account for up to 75% of HAB species (Wang et al., 2020). The associated MBTXs may bio-accumulate in plankton-feeding marine animals through feeding and other physiological

DOI: 10.1201/9781003500605-15

activity during their growth (O'Mahony, 2018). The direct effects of HABs in marine waters on human health are due to ingestion, skin contact and inhalation of contaminated seafood, water and aerosolized biotoxins, respectively. However, intoxication through various steps of the food chain by eating contaminated seafood is the most common documented consequence (Morabito et al., 2017). Consumption of toxin-contaminated seafood is associated with intoxication, such as neurologic, diarrheic, paralytic, azaspiracid and amnesic (demoic) shellfish poisoning in humans (Mafra et al., 2023; Oshiro et al., 2024). These poisonings are mostly caused by neurotoxins, with very specific effects upon the nervous system in animals or even humans (Wang, 2008). Some of these toxins are lethal, even at levels as low as a microgram per kilogram dose, hence constituting a specific concern as environmental contaminants (Ciminiello and Fattorusso, 2006). Vectors of HAB-related toxins include bivalve mollusks, fish, tunicates, echinoderms and gastropods (Murk et al., 2019).

Ecologically, the deleterious effects of MBTXs can impact an entire ecosystem. Chronic impacts from sublethal toxic HABs can affect the structure and function of ecosystems and wildlife health, including massive mortality of fish, larval or juvenile stages of fish, seabirds, dolphins, whales and other marine animals, in a single outbreak, with resultant long- and short-term ecosystem impacts critical to the sustainability and/or recovery of natural populations at higher trophic levels (Suresh et al., 2014).

However, despite the hazardous effects of HAB-associated biotoxins, their unique structure and varying chemical compositions make them valuable and quite interesting compounds with pharmacological and biotechnological potential (Assunção et al., 2017; Mafra et al., 2023). This chapter focuses on edible marine green biotoxins, with an emphasis on those associated with harmful algal blooms and their types, distribution, monitoring and possible applications of marine microbial toxins.

13.2 Marine Biotoxins

Marine biotoxins can be grouped according to their chemical structure as polyether, polypeptide or alkaloid toxins; according to their molecular size as low molecular weight and large molecular weight; as a function of their solubility in solvents; or on the basis of the effects produced (Morabito et al., 2017). Several classes of biotoxins based on their chemical structure have been recognized, including okadaic acid (OA), brevetoxin (BTX), domoic acid (DA), cyclic imines (CI) group, saxitoxin (STX), yessotoxin (YTX), tetrodotoxin (TTX), pectenotoxin (PTX), azaspiracid (AZA), palytoxin (PlTX) and ciguatoxin (CTX) (Visciano et al., 2016; Morabito et al., 2017; Ettoubi et al., 2020).

These toxins elicit varying symptoms in humans (Visciano et al., 2016). Therefore, classification based on effects produced includes paralytic (PSP), diarrheic (DSP), amnesic (ASP) or domoic acid poisoning (DAP); neurotoxic (NSP) and azaspiracid (AZP) shellfish poisonings; and ciguatera fish poisoning (CFP) (Morabito et al., 2017; Zhao et al., 2018). They are classified according to their solubility in solvents into fat- and water-soluble marine biotoxins. The lipophilic marine toxins consist of five distinct chemical groups: okadaic acid, pectenotoxins, yessotoxins, brevetoxins and azaspiracids, while the hydrophilic toxins are made up of different groups including domoic acid, saxitoxin and tetrodotoxin (Bacchiocchi et al., 2015; Otero and Silva, 2022). Also, there is the amphipathic type of marine toxin, such as palytoxins, which shows both hydrophilic and lipophilic properties (Louzao et al., 2022). However, new compounds are continuously being discovered and added to the list of these toxins and their analogues (Murk et al., 2019).

13.2.1 Health Impact of Marine Biotoxins

Marine biotoxins are a heterogeneous group of naturally occurring metabolites from marine microorganisms and enter the food chain as they are fed upon by filter-feeding shellfish and mollusks and passed to higher trophic levels to the tissues of the consumers, where they bio-accumulate (Figure 13.1). They pose a danger and threat to public health, as they are highly potent and poisonous to humans and animals, being able to trigger toxicological responses in the body even at low concentrations (Ferrara, 2020; Würger et al., 2024). Harmful algae blooms have been identified as the major source of introduction of various toxins (Kasheverov et al., 2022).

Most MBTXs cannot be destroyed by cooking or freezing; the toxicity is acute and short term, with symptoms manifesting in some cases 5 to 60 minutes after consuming contaminated mollusks (Nicolas et al., 2017; Ettoubi et al., 2020). The highest concentration of the toxins occurs mostly in the digestive tract of vector species, for instance, in shellfish, fish, snails and crabs. Therefore, the risk of intoxication is mostly from seafood such as clams and mussels that can be consumed without first removing the digestive tract (Murk et al., 2019). However, there are insufficient purified forms of most toxins for toxicity trials, which makes the toxicity mechanism of some of them unknown (Louzao et al., 2022). MBTXs elicit varying symptoms ranging

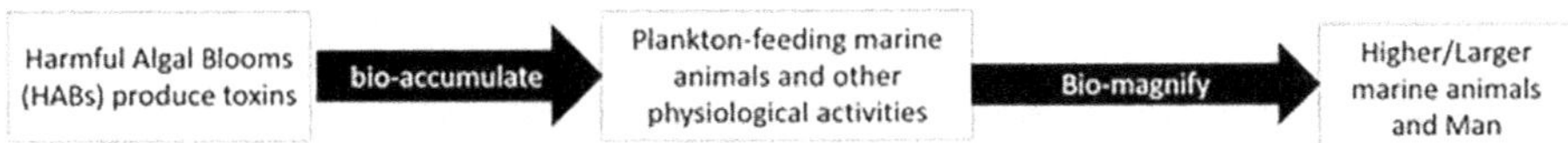

FIGURE 13.1
Marine biotoxin transmission pathway.

from severe gastrointestinal (GI) intoxication with abdominal cramps, diarrhea, nausea and vomiting to neurological disorders, including respiratory distress, dizziness, ataxia and partial paralysis toxic shock and even death (Visciano et al., 2016; Zhao et al., 2018). Some intoxication may be acute, requiring the hospitalization of victims, or chronic, especially at sublethal doses (Suresh et al., 2014; Abraham et al., 2021).

13.2.2 Environmental Impact of Marine Biotoxins

Exposure to MBTXs is mostly through accidental ingestion or nasal uptake of toxin-contaminated water during recreational activities (WHO, 2021). Aerosolized brevetoxin was implicated in intoxication of humans which elicited non-fatal symptoms such as skin irritation, shortness of breath and non-productive cough (Louzao et al., 2022). Several MBTXs have also been associated with the morbidity and mortality of large numbers of fish, marine mammals and wildlife (Suresh et al., 2014).

13.3 Types and Distribution of Marine Biotoxins

Marine food intoxications initially considered endemic have become a global phenomenon, with the proliferation of HABs producing MBTXs occurring in different regions of the world, especially along coastal areas (Ettoubi et al., 2020). This has been attributed to increase in diverse anthropogenic activities such as higher exports and consumption of seafood, nutrient contamination, tourism and global climate change such as ocean acidification and global warming (Faggio et al., 2016; Morabito et al., 2017).

Regions that were formerly free of or with low incidences of marine food intoxications have witnessed not just new but increased episodes of MBTX poisonings (Díaz-Marrero et al., 2023). For instance, a cyclic imine group of toxins, pinnatoxins, has been reported in different vectors from coasts across several countries, including Canada, Spain, France and Cuba (Otero and Silva, 2022). Nevertheless, incidences of marine biointoxication have been under-recognized, especially in the tropic and subtropic regions, including most African countries (Zendong et al., 2016; Ansdell, 2024).

13.3.1 Okadaic Acid

Okadaic acid is a lipophilic polyether toxin that was initially isolated from *Halichondria* spp. and other sea sponges, including *H. okadai*, from which the name was derived, and from some dinoflagellate genera such as the *Prorocentrum* spp. and *Dinophysis* spp. (Reguera et al., 2014; Fu et al., 2019). Studies have shown that chronic exposure to low levels of OA toxin can cause neurological damage, can impact several metabolic pathways and may result in apoptosis (Murk et al., 2019). Okadaic acid and its derivatives, dinophysistoxins (DTXs), elicit acute GI symptoms of diarrhetic shellfish poisoning, characterized by nausea, vomiting, abdominal cramps, diarrhea and chills that resolve within three days (Vale and Botana, 2008) and in the most severe cases, dizziness, seizures, hallucinations and short-term memory loss (Ettoubi et al., 2020). Incidences of OA poisoning have occurred over the years at different times globally, with reported cases across the continents of Europe, North and South America, Asia and Africa (Zendong et al, 2016; Ettoubi et al., 2020).

13.3.2 Pectenotoxins

Pectenotoxins are heat-stable lipophilic cyclic polyether compounds originally isolated from the phytoplankton dinoflagellate *Dinophysis fortii* in Japan and Europe (Visciano et al., 2016). They produce symptoms similar to those induced by OA and its derivatives, such as diarrhea. They disrupt actin cytoskeleton and may cause cell cycle arrest and apoptosis (Espiña et al., 2008).

13.3.3 Brevetoxins

Brevetoxins are heat-stable lipophilic cyclic polyether toxins, grouped based on their backbone structure into A type and B type, with the former having 10 transfused ether rings and the latter 11 (Shimizu et al., 1986). BTXs are synthesized by some species of dinoflagellates of the genus *Karenia*, specifically *K. brevis*. Vectors of BTXs are clams, gastropods, oysters and greenshell mussels (Abraham et al., 2021). These toxins elicit neurologic shellfish poisoning, characterized by a wide range of neurological and GI symptoms, which manifest within 30 min to a few hours after ingestion. The symptoms include diarrhea, nausea and vomiting, paresthesias around the mouth and extremities, hot/cold temperature reversal, vertigo, loss of coordination and seizures and in severe cases may result in coma (Morabito et al., 2017; Abraham et al., 2021). BTXs have been associated with the morbidity and mortality of marine mammals and great numbers of fish (Gebhard et al., 2015). Brevetoxins, although endemic in some places such as Florida (USA), New Zealand and the West Indies, have been detected in seafoods across many regions, including the Gulf of Guinea (Nigeria) and Japan, although with no intoxication recorded in some cases (Murk et al., 2019; Otero and Silva, 2022).

13.3.4 Yessotoxins

Yessotoxins and their derivatives are lipophilic sulphate-polyether toxins synthesized by dinoflagellates, including *Gonyaulax spinifera* and *Protoceratium reticulatum* (Visciano et al., 2016). The structural composition makes YTX a polar lipophilic compound, conferring an amphoteric characteristic to the molecule (Paz et al., 2008). Human intoxication has so far not been reported (Visciano et al., 2016; Louzao et al., 2022).

13.3.5 Tetrodotoxins

Tetrodotoxins were initially isolated from pufferfish but are produced by enteric marine bacteria of the genera *Vibrio, Pseudomonas, Actinomycetes* and *Pseudoalteromonas* present in other marine animals, including octopuses, crabs, some species of gobies, sea stars, bivalves and gastropods, either as part of the animals' microbiomes or acquired through the food chain (Mackieh et al., 2021). TTXs are hydrophilic low molecular weight neurotoxins, adjudged to be over a thousand times more toxic to humans than cyanide (Lago et al., 2015). Intoxication with TTX is by consumption of contaminated seafoods, especially fish, and is characterized by paresthesia of the mouth, lack of muscular coordination, respiratory distress and death (Louzao et al., 2022). TTXs were initially thought to be endemic in Asia, especially Japan, but incidences of the toxin have been reported across Europe, the USA, Mexico, Oceania and Morocco (Lago et al., 2015; Ettoubi et al., 2020).

13.3.6 Ciguatoxins

Ciguatoxins are large thermostable fat-soluble molecules synthesized by benthic dinoflagellates of the species *Gambierdiscus toxicus* that are prevalent in dying or dead coral reefs (Otero and Silva, 2022). Ciguatera poisoning is the most significant and severe type of MBTX-related poisoning globally, associated with fish consumption (Visciano et al., 2016; Murk et al., 2019; Mafra et al., 2023). CTX is the most common illness that is not bacteria related with consumption of seafood worldwide, affecting from 50,000 to 500,000 people annually, including occasional mortality cases (Louzao et al., 2022). The geographical distribution of ciguatera poisoning was initially limited to tropical regions with extended coral reefs, mostly the Caribbean and various island regions in the Pacific and Indian Oceans (Oshiro et al., 2024). However, ciguatera fish poisoning cases have been recorded in non-tropical areas due to seafood trade. Moreover, the emergence of remote tourism and increasing reef fish imports have led to incidence of the illness in other continents, such as North America and Europe (Friedman et al., 2017; Murk et al., 2019; Otero and Silva, 2022; Oshiro et al., 2024). CTX intoxication syndrome is characterized by over 100 symptoms, encompassing several neurological disturbances such as paresthesia, myalgia and cold allodynia, cardiovascular derangement including bradycardia and hypotension and GI distress (Otero and Silva, 2022).

13.3.7 Azaspiracids

This group of marine toxins has worldwide distribution but was initially identified following an outbreak of food poisoning in the Netherlands and subsequently in other countries after the consumption of exported contaminated Irish mussels (FAO and WHO, 2016). Azaspiracid toxins are produced by the dinoflagellate genera *Azadinium* and *Amphidoma* (Tillmann et al., 2009). AZA was so named because of its chemical structure, which is a cyclic amine or aza group, containing a tri-spiro-assembly assembly and carboxylic acid group (FAO and WHO, 2016). Incidences of AZA toxins in shellfish have also been reported from several coastal regions of North and South America, Europe and North Africa (Amzil et al., 2008; Elgarch et al., 2008; Alvarez et al., 2010; Hess et al., 2014). In the Asian countries of Korea and China, AZAs were isolated from the dinoflagellate *Azadinium poporum*, which was previously recognized as non-toxigenic (FAO and WHO, 2016). AZAs have also been detected in oysters and clams and in crabs and sponges from Scandinavia and Japan, respectively (FAO and WHO, 2016). The symptoms of intoxication in humans are vomiting, nausea, diarrhea and stomach cramps, which appear after a few hours and last for up to two days (Klontz et al., 2009).

13.3.8 Domoic Acid

This toxin is a hydrophilic small molecule neurotoxic amino acid derivate consisting of a cyclic amino acid with three carboxylic acid groups (FAO and WHO, 2016). DA was originally detected in *Chondria armata*, a red algae species, but outbreaks of poisoning from toxins produced by diatoms, especially in the genus *Pseudo-nitzschia*, have been reported (Trainer et al., 2012). DA is responsible for amnesic shellfish poisoning, the only shellfish poison produced by a diatom (Smida et al., 2014). However, DA-producing *Pseudo-nitzschia* and *Nitzschia* diatom species are prevalent globally in many regions and climatic zones, including Southeast Asia, Japan, France, North and Central America, Portugal and Ireland. The assumed minimum infectious dose for human ranges from 0.2 to 0.9 mg/kg body weight (Murk et al., 2019). Vectors include bivalves and other species that have accumulated the toxin either through grazing on benthic algae or by filtration of phytoplankton (FAO and WHO, 2016). Domoic acid is regarded as an excitatory amino acid, capable of neurotransmission and neurotoxic activities to the central nervous system (Morabito et al., 2017). DA toxin is responsible for amnesic shellfish poisoning or domoic acid poisoning, since amnesia does not always occur. This intoxication is characterized by initial GI signs such as nausea, vomiting and diarrhea, followed by neurological complications, including headache, disorientation, confusion, seizures, memory loss, difficulty in breathing, coma and in some cases death (Louzao et al., 2022).

13.3.9 Saxitoxins

Saxitoxin and its analogues are produced mostly by dinoflagellates of the genera *Alexandrium*, *Gymnodinium* and *Pyrodinium* and by planktonic and benthic marine and freshwater cyanobacteria, including *Anabaena* spp.,

Aphanizomenon spp. and *Planktothrix* (Vilariño et al., 2018). Saxitoxins are widely distributed around the world, with reports of toxin-related symptoms in coastal regions of temperate and tropical areas, including North and South America, Japan, Europe, Australia, Canada, Southeast Asia, China, the Indo-Pacific region and on the coasts of Morocco (Silva et al., 2018; Ettoubi et al., 2020). This has been attributed to climate change rather than the introduction of dinoflagellates by sea transport (FAO and WHO, 2016; Silva et al., 2018; Ettoubi et al., 2020). Vectors of STX include mussels, oysters and clams, marine snails and pufferfish (FAO and WHO, 2016). Saxitoxin and its derivatives are hydrophilic tetrahydropurine neurotoxins which cause PSP in humans, with the primary site of action being the peripheral nervous system, where its link causes a rapid initiation of symptoms under an hour (Morabito et al., 2017; Otero and Silva, 2022). Symptoms are characterized by numbness and tingling sensations starting from the lips, then the face, neck, arms and fingertips, legs and toes, occasionally with dizziness, headache, nausea and sometimes transitory blindness, under mild intoxication (Vilariño et al., 2018; Morabito et al., 2017; Otero and Silva, 2022). Severe PSP symptoms include progression of tingling sensation in the extremities to stiffness and incoordination, incoherent speech, ataxia and a feeling of lightness. These symptoms may be accompanied by weakness, myalgia and respiratory difficulty, and in very severe cases, muscular paralysis and difficulty in breathing may progress to respiratory arrest and death within 24 h unless respiratory support is administered (Morabito et al., 2017; Otero and Silva, 2022).

13.4 Monitoring and Prevention

The last decade has witnessed increased episodes of marine biotoxin intoxication due to worldwide higher incidences of HABs (Louzao et al., 2022). This has necessitated the requirement for risk assessment and collation of data on the safety monitoring of MBTXs. However, monitoring the presence of toxigenic microbes in aquatic environments and toxic compounds in seafood is insufficient or still lacking in several places (Mafra et al., 2023).

Risk assessment can be approached at various levels, including hazard monitoring of the marine environment for incidence of higher concentrations of harmful algal species, risk assessment and management of seafoods and non-foods and registration of intoxications in humans that have been analytically verified (Daneshian et al., 2013).

The gold standard for biotoxin assessment in aquatic food is the mouse bioassay (MBA). This involves injecting seafood extract into the peritoneum of a group of mice and recording the duration for lethality of the mice, which is then correlated with the toxin content of the sample. The test estimates the total toxicity of the extract, that is, the sum of the toxicities of the many congeners (related substances) present in the sample (FAO and WHO, 2016).

However, besides the ethical issues with this bioassay, there are some insufficient specificities such as different exposure routes (intraperitoneal versus oral), high intra-species and low inter-species variability and comparability and doubtful extrapolation of quantitative risk to humans (Daneshian et al., 2013; FAO and WHO, 2016). Although for practical reasons the MBA is still being used in various countries (FAO and WHO, 2016), the use of an analytical method by liquid chromatography with mass spectrometry (LC-MS) has been advocated by the European Food Safety Authority (EFSA) as a substitute for almost all classes of marine toxins (Daneshian et al., 2013; Visciano et al., 2016). Nevertheless, the use of LC-MS is limited by its difficulty in detecting new toxins, and quantitative analysis is highly dependent on the availability of calibration standards for the biotoxin analogues and metabolites (FAO and WHO, 2016). Consequently, when new toxin analogues are detected but accurate standards are not yet available, only an approximate quantitation is possible using estimated response factors (Daneshian et al., 2013).

For the purpose of risk assessment of food, however, it is vital to focus on the possible adverse effects, either from one toxin or a combination of toxins (Daneshian et al., 2013). In that case, total toxicity of the material in the extract can be estimated by determining the toxicity equivalency factors (TEFs), which is the toxicity ratio of a compound from a chemical group that shares the same mode of action of a reference compound in the same group (FAO and WHO, 2016). However, an appropriate definition of the toxicity of each compound is necessary for adequate TEF estimation (Louzao et al., 2022).

European Union (EU) food legislation focuses on monitoring of biotoxins in bivalve mollusks, and the EU has enacted Regulation 854/2004/EC, which establishes periodic sampling and monitoring of live bivalve mollusk production areas in order to check the incidence and occurrence of toxin-producing plankton in live bivalve mollusks (Visciano et al., 2016). Monitoring is usually performed weekly during the harvesting period but may be reduced if a low risk of intoxication is established during the risk assessment. However, production areas shall be closed by the competent authority if the results of monitoring exceed the regulatory limits and reopened when at least two consecutive results of biotoxin levels in mollusks meet the limits (Berdalet et al., 2015; Visciano et al., 2016; Louzao et al., 2022).

The Codex Committee on Fish and Fishery Products (CCFFP) set the limits for marine biotoxins for international trade some years ago and has developed the standard for live and raw bivalve mollusks (CODEX STAN 292–2008), which was revised a decade ago (Louzao et al., 2022). However, there has been a lack of updates and harmonization in the regulatory criteria about the marine biotoxins. Hence, the most frequently given advice in some instances, such as ciguatoxigenesis, is to avoid consuming fish weighing more than 2 kg and fish parts such as the viscera, brain, and gonads, where ciguatoxins are mostly accumulated (Louzao et al., 2022).

However, monitoring and management programs for marine biotoxins should be designed in such a manner as to guarantee public health and minimal impacts to fishing and aquaculture operations (Free et al., 2022).

13.5 Applications of Marine Biotoxins

Natural environment like soils, water and plants have been found to be reservoirs of enormous bioactive compounds of immense beneficial value to humans and other living things. Worthy of note is that several of these compounds of marine origin have been found to be more abundant than those of terrestrial origin (Kraus, 2021). Marine biotoxins, also known as phycotoxins, have attracted the attention of researchers because of their features and properties, which can be classified into three major classes (Figure 13.2): their complex chemical structures, pharmacological activity and ability to carry out modification and activation of vital metabolic pathways (Louzao et al., 2022; Flores-Holguín et al., 2024).

The unique structure and varying chemical compositions and their mechanisms of action make MBTXs valuable and quite interesting compounds with pharmacological and biotechnological potential (Assunção et al., 2017; Mafra et al., 2023).

Accordingly, MBTXs of the classes tetrodotoxin and saxitoxin, brevetoxins and ciguatoxins all bind on the voltage gated sodium channels (VGSCs) at different sites, which results in either the activation or inhibition of the Na^+ flux through the channel. While TTX and STX both bind to VGSCs at site 1, BTX and CTX both bind at site 5. The activity of TTX and STX inhibits the action potential in the muscles and neurons, thereby immobilizing the tissues, which leads to physiological conditions associated with tetrodotoxin poisoning and paralytic shellfish poisoning, respectively (Pratheepa and Vasconcelos, 2017; Louzao et al., 2022). These properties are being harnessed in the exploration of novel pharmaceuticals.

For instance, the ability of TTX to block VGSCs is being harnessed by researchers in the production of analgesics for relieving severe cancer pains and treatment of drug withdrawal craving and anxiety (Lago et al., 2015).

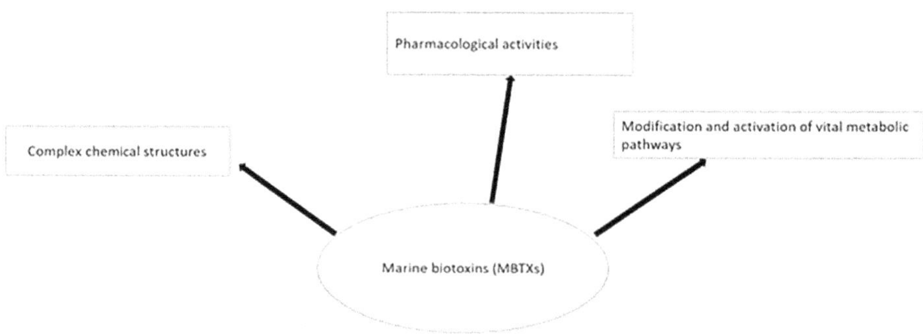

FIGURE 13.2
Features and properties of marine biotoxins.

Several studies have documented the effectiveness of TTX in neuropathic pains and demonstrated the absence of clinically significant toxicity on administration (Mackieh et al., 2021).

Flores-Holguín et al. (2024) were able to elucidate the chemical reactivity and estimated pharmacokinetic properties of saxitoxin derivatives using computational tools and concluded that there is a need to consider the potential of the toxins as new pharmaceutical candidates. Furthermore, active compounds of TTX and STX and their derivatives and analogues can be administered by needles or as tablets and patches as an established method to control musculoskeletal pain (Mackieh et al., 2021).

Yessotoxin and its derivatives have been reported as fascinating tools for biological probes and pharmacological mechanisms (Korsnes et al., 2014; Assunção et al., 2017). They can interfere with certain cellular pathways such as apoptotic and non-apoptotic cell death. The potential of yessotoxin to induce cellular death (apoptosis) in some types of tumor cells and produce a cytotoxic effect in neuronal cortical neurons has been reported (Alonso et al., 2013; Tobio et al., 2016). Although lethality has been reported on mice after intraperitoneal injection, poisoning symptoms did not develop when YTX was administered orally; interestingly, human intoxication events have not been recorded (Louzao et al., 2022). Moreover, YTX could be useful in the prevention and treatment of cholesterol level and glucose metabolism-associated diseases (Alfonso et al., 2016).

Ciguatoxin has been suggested as an important tool in the investigation of the biological function and structure of voltage gated sodium channels due to its discriminatory affinity for the various VGSC subtypes (Assunção et al., 2017; Mackieh et al., 2021). Azaspiracid, with its distinctive cyclic amine structure, offers great biotechnological importance, including its ability to alter cell morphology, gene expression and cytoskeleton structure and activate apoptosis, cell damage and cytoskeleton regulation, among others (Twiner et al., 2012).

Although the potential of marine biotoxins in pharmacological and biotechnological applications is enormous, with several patent applications already existing, progress in this direction has been hampered mostly due to the scarcity of purified forms of most of the toxins for preclinical testing, and cultivation of dinoflagellates for biotoxin synthesis under controlled conditions has been challenging (Assunção et al., 2017; Louzao et al., 2022).

13.6 Conclusion

Marine biotoxins are a plethora of complex biomolecules with particular characteristics. Although progress has been made in the identification and elaboration of their mechanisms of action and effect on marine wildlife and human health, there are still some information gaps regarding the recognition and recording of emerging cases of intoxication. On the other hand, despite the immense possibilities in harnessing marine biotoxins in the advancement of drug discovery and as biotechnological tools, a lack of availability of requisite quantities of these toxins for further investigations has limited these possibilities.

References

Abraham, A., Flewelling, L.J., El Said, K.R., Odom, W., Geiger, S.P., Granholm, A.A., et al. (2021). An Occurrence of Neurotoxic Shellfish Poisoning by Consumption of Gastropods Contaminated with Brevetoxins. *Toxicon*. 191:9–17. https://doi.org/10.1016/j.toxicon.2020.12.010.

Alfonso, A., Vieytes, M. and Botana, L. (2016). Yessotoxin, a Promising Therapeutic Tool. *Mar. Drugs*. 14:30.

Alonso, E., Vale, C., Vieytes, M.R. and Botana, L.M. (2013). Translocation of PKC by Yessotoxin in an In Vitro Model of Alzheimer's Disease with Improvement of Tau and Beta-Amyloid Pathology. *ACS Chem. Neurosci*. 4:1062–1070.

Alvarez, G., Uribe, E., Avalos, P., Marino, C. and Blanco, J. (2010). First Identification of Azaspiracid and Spirolides in *Mesodesma donacium* and *Mulinia edulis* from Northern Chile. *Toxicon*. 55(2–3):638–641.

Amzil, Z., Sibat, M., Royer, F. and Savar, V. (2008). First Report on Azaspiracid and Yessotoxin Groups Detection in French Shellfish. *Toxicon*. 52(1):39–48.

Ansdell, V.E. (2024). Food Poisoning from Marine Toxins. *Environmental Hazards & Risks: CDC Yellow Book 2024*. https://wwwnc.cdc.gov/travel/yellowbook/2024/environmental-hazards-risks/food-poisoning-from-marine-toxins (Accessed 4/7/2024).

Aransiola, S.A., Oyewole, O.A., Maddela, N.R., Ijah, U.J.J. and Manjunatha, B. (Eds.). (2024). *Marine Greens: Environmental, Agricultural, Industrial and Biomedical Applications* (1st ed.). Boca Raton, FL: CRC Press, Taylor and Francis Group. https://doi.org/10.1201/9781003369738.

Assunção, J., Guedes, A.C. and Malcata, F.X. (2017). Biotechnological and Pharmacological Applications of Biotoxins and Other Bioactive Molecules from Dinoflagellates. *Mar. Drugs*. 15:393. https://doi.org/10.3390/md15120393.

Bacchiocchi, S., Siracusa, M., Ruzzi, A., Gorbi, S., Ercolessi, M., Cosentino, M.A., et al. (2015). Two-Year Study of Lipophilic Marine Toxin Profile in Mussels of the North-Central Adriatic Sea: First Report of Azaspiracids in Mediterranean Seafood. *Toxicon*, 108:115–125. http://doi.org/10.1016/j.toxicon.2015.10.002.

Berdalet, E., Fleming, L., Gowen, R., Davidson, K., Hess, P., Backer, L., et al. (2015). Marine Harmful Algal Blooms, Human Health and Wellbeing: Challenges and Opportunities in the 21st Century. *J. Mar. Biol. Assoc. U.K*. 96:61–91. https://doi.org/10.1017/S0025315415001733.

Chen, Z., Wu, W., Wen, Y., Zhang, L., Wu, Y., Farid, M.S., et al. (2023). Recent advances of natural pigments from algae. *Food Prod. Process Nutr.* 5:39. https://doi.org/10.1186/s43014-023-00155-y.

Ciminiello, P. and Fattorusso, E. (2006). Bivalve Molluscs as Vectors of Marine Biotoxins Involved in Seafood Poisoning. In *Molluscs: Progress in Molecular and Subcellular Biology*, Cimino, G. and Gavagnin, M., Eds. Berlin, Heidelberg, Germany: Springer, pp. 53–82.

Daneshian, M., Botana, L.M., Dechraoui Bottein, M.Y., Buckland, G., Campàs, M., Dennison, N., et al. (2013). A roadmap for hazard monitoring and risk assessment of marine biotoxins on the basis of chemical and biological test systems. *ALTEX*. 30(4)-S:487–545.

Díaz-Marrero, A.R., Fernandez, J.J., Rodríguez, F., Band-Schmidt, C.J., Diogène, J. and Novelli, A. (2023). Editorial: Marine Microalgae and Biotoxins. *Front. Mar. Sci.* 10:1172371. https://doi.org/10.3389/fmars.2023.1172371.

Elgarch, A., Vale, P., Rifai, S. and Fassouane, A. (2008). Detection of Diarrheic Shellfish Poisoning and Azaspiracid Toxins in Moroccan Mussels: Comparison of the LC-MS Method with the Commercial Immunoassay Kit. *Mar. Drugs*. 6(4):587–594.

Espiña, B., Louzao, M.C., Ares, I.R., Cagide, E., Vieytes, M.R., Vega, F.V., et al. (2008). Cytoskeletal Toxicity of Pectenotoxins in Hepatic Cells. *Br. J. Pharmacol*. 155:934–944. https://doi.org/10.1038/bjp.2008.323.

Ettoubi, E., Akif, F., Genten, F. and Blaghen, M. (2020). Marine Biotoxins: Origins, Effects, Distribution, Prevention and Treatment. *Int. J. Innov. Sci. Res. Technol.* 5:11. ISSN No:2456-2165.

Faggio, C., Pagano, M., Dottore, A., Genovese, G. and Morabito, M. (2016). Evaluation of Anticoagulant Activity of Two Algal Polysaccharides. *Nat. Prod. Res.* 30:1934–1937.

FAO. (2004). *Marine Biotoxins; Food and Agriculture Organization of the United Nations.* Food and Nutrition Paper 80. Rome, Italy: FAO. https://www.fao.org/4/y5486e/y5486e00.htm (Accessed 24/5/2024).

FAO and WHO. (2016). *Toxicity Equivalency Factors for Marine Biotoxins Associated with Bivalve Molluscs*. Joint FAO/WHO Technical Paper. www.fao.org/publications (Accessed 29/6/2024).

Ferrara, L. (2020). Dinoflagellates important marine producers of natural bio-compounds with high biotechnological and pharmacological potential. *J. Food Chem. Nanotechnol*. 6:138–149.

Flores-Holguín, N., Salas-Leiva, J.S., Núñez-Vázquez, E.J., Tovar-Ramírez, D. and Glossman-Mitnik, D. (2024). Marine Toxins as Pharmaceutical Treasure Troves: A Focus on Saxitoxin Derivatives from a Computational Point of View. *Molecules*. 29:275. https://doi.org/10.3390/molecules29010275.

Free, C.M., Moore, S.K. and Trainer, V.L. (2022). The value of monitoring in efficiently and adaptively managing biotoxin contamination in marine fisheries. *Harmful Algae* 114:102226. https://doi.org/10.1016/j.hal.2022.102226.

Friedman, M.A., Fernandez, M., Backer, L.C., Dickey, R.W., Bernstein, J., Schrank, K., et al. (2017). An Updated Review of Ciguatera Fish Poisoning: Clinical, Epidemiological, Environmental, and Public Health Management. *Mar. Drugs*. 15:72.

Fu, L.L., Zhao, X.Y., Ji, L.D. and Xu, J. (2019). Okadaic Acid (OA): Toxicity, Detection and Detoxification. *Toxicon*. 160:1–7.

Gebhard, E., Levin, M., Bogomolni, A. and De Guise, S. (2015). Immunomodulatory Effects of Brevetoxin (PbTx-3) upon In Vitro Exposure in Bottlenose Dolphins (*Tursiops truncatus*). *Harmful Algae*. 44:54–62. https://doi.org/10.1016/j.hal.2015.02.010.

Hess, P., McCarron, P., Krock, B., Kilcoyne, J. and Miles, C.O. (2014). *Azaspiracids: Chemistry, Biosynthesis, Metabolism, and Detection, Seafood and Freshwater Toxins*. Boca Raton: CRC Press, pp. 799–822. https://doi.org/10.3390/md20030199.

Kasheverov, I., Kudryavtsev, D., Shelukhina, I., Nikolaev, G., Utkin, Y. and Tsetlin, V. (2022). Marine Origin Ligands of Nicotinic Receptors: Low Molecular Compounds, Peptides and Proteins for Fundamental Research and Practical Applications. *Biomolecules*. 12:189. https://doi.org/10.3390/biom12020189.

Klontz, K.C., Abraham, A., Plakas, S.M. and Dickey, R.W. (2009). Mussel-Associated Azaspiracid Intoxication in the United States. *Annals Intern. Med*. 150(4):361–361.

Korsnes, M.S., Røed, S.S., Tranulis, M.A., Espenes, A. and Christophersen, B. (2014). Yessotoxin Triggers Ribotoxic Stress. *Toxicol. In Vitro*. 28:975–981.

Kraus, J.-L. (2021). Natural Products as Potential Antiviral Drugs: The Specific Case of Marine Biotoxins. *Russian J. Bioorganic Chem*. 47(6):1127–1132.

Lago, J., Rodríguez, L.P., Blanco, L., Vieites, J.M. and Cabado, A.G. (2015). Tetrodotoxin, an Extremely Potent Marine Neurotoxin: Distribution, Toxicity, Origin and Therapeutical Uses. *Mar. Drugs*. 13:6384–6406. https://doi.org/10.3390/md13106384.

Louzao, M.C., Vilariño, N., Vale, C., Costas, C., Cao, A., Raposo-Garcia, S., et al. (2022). Current Trends and New Challenges in Marine Phycotoxins. *Mar Drugs*. 8;20(3):198. https://doi.org/10.3390/md20030198.

Mackieh, R., Abou-Nader, R., Wehbe, R., Mattei, C., Legros, C., Fajloun, Z., et al. (2021). Voltage-Gated Sodium Channels: A Prominent Target of Marine Toxins. *Mar. Drugs*. 19(10):562. https://doi.org/10.3390/md19100562ff.

Mafra, L.L., de Souza, D.A., Menezes, M., Schramm, M.A. and Hoff, R. (2023). Marine Biotoxins: Latest Advances and Challenges Toward Seafood Safety, Using Brazil as a Case Study. *Curr. Opin. Food Sci*. 53:101078. https://doi.org/10.1016/j.cofs.2023.101078.

Morabito, S., Silvestro, S. and Faggio, C. (2017). How the marine biotoxins affect human health. *Nat. Prod. Res*. 32(6):621–631. https://doi.org/10.1080/14786419.2017.1329734.

Murk, A.J., Nicolas, J., Smulders, F.J., Bürk, C. and Gerssen, A. (2019). Marine Biotoxins: Types of Poisoning, Underlying Mechanisms of Action and Risk Management Programmes. In *Chemical Hazards in Foods of Animal Origin Food Safety Assurance and Veterinary Public Health No. 7*, Smulders, F.J.M., Rietjens, I.M.C.M. and Rose, M., Eds. © Wageningen Academic Publishers. https://doi.10.3920/978-90-8686-877-3_09.

Nicolas, J., Hoogenboom, R.L.A.P., Hendriksen, P.J.M., Bodero, M., Bovee, T.F.H., Rietjens, I.M.C.M. and Gerssen, A. (2017). Marine Biotoxins and Associated Outbreaks Following Seafood Consumption: Prevention and Surveillance in the 21st Century. *Glob. Food Secur*. 15:11–21. https://doi.org/10.1016/j.gfs.2017.03.002.

O'Mahony, M. (2018). EU Regulatory Risk Management of Marine Biotoxins in the Marine Bivalve Mollusc Food-Chain. *Toxins*. 10:118. https://doi.org/10.3390/toxins10030118.

Oshiro, N., Gago-Martínez, A. and Tubaro, A. (2024). Chemistry, Toxicology and Etiology of Marine Biotoxins. *J. Mar. Sci. Eng*. 12L:236. https://doi.org/10.3390/jmse12020236.

Otero, P. and Silva, M. (2022). Emerging Marine Biotoxins in European Waters: Potential Risks and Analytical Challenges. *Mar. Drugs*. 20:199.

Paz, B., Daranas, A.H., Norte, M., Riobó, P., Franco, J.M. and Fernández, J.J. (2008). Yessotoxins, a Group of Marine Polyether Toxins: An Overview. *Mar. Drugs*. 6:73–102.

Pratheepa, V. and Vasconcelos, V. (2017). Binding and Pharmacokinetics of the Sodium Channel Blocking Toxins (Saxitoxin and the Tetrodotoxins). *Mini Rev. Med Chem*. 17:320–327.

Reguera, B., Riobo, P., Rodriguez, F., Diaz, P.A., Pizarro, G., Paz, B., Franco, J.M. and Blanco, J. (2014). Dinophysis Toxins: Causative Organisms, Distribution and Fate in Shellfish. *Mar. Drugs*. 12:394–461.

Sanjeewa, K.K.A., Lee, W. and Jeon, Y.-J. (2018). Nutrients and Bioactive Potentials of Edible Green and Red Seaweed in Korea. *Fish Aquat. Sci*. 21:19. https://doi.org/10.1186/s41240-018-0095-y.

Shimizu, Y., Chou, H.N., Bando, H., Van Duyne, G. and Clardy, J. (1986). Structure of Brevetoxin A (GB-1 Toxin), the Most Potent Toxin in the Florida Red Tide Organism *Gymnodinium breve* (*Ptychodiscus brevis*). *J. Am. Chem. Soc*. 108(3):514–515.

Silva, M., Rey, V., Barreiro, A., Kaufmann, M., Neto, A.I., Hassouani, M., et al. (2018). Paralytic Shellfish Toxins Occurrence in Non-Traditional Invertebrate Vectors from North Atlantic Waters (Azores, Madeira, and Morocco). *Toxins*. 10(9):362.

Smida, D.B., Lundholm, N., Kooistra, W.H.C.F., Sahraoui, I., Ruggiero, M.V., Kotaki, Y., et al. (2014). Morphology and Molecular Phylogeny of *Nitzschia bizertensis* sp. nov.—A New Domoic Acid-Producer. *Harmful Algae*. 32:49–63.

Suresh, S.P., Gauri, S., Desai, S., Kavitha, M. and Padmavathy, P. (2014). Marine Biotoxins and Its Detection. *Afri. J. Environ. Sci. Technol*. 8(6):350–365. https://doi.org/10.5897/AJEST12.065.

Tillmann, U., Elbrächter, M., Krock, B., John, U. and Cembella, A. (2009). *Azadinium spinosum* gen. et sp. nov. (*Dinophyceae*) Identified as a Primary Producer of Azaspiracid Toxins. *Eur. J. Phycol*. 44(1):63–79.

Tobio, A., Alfonso, A., Madera-Salcedo, I., Botana, L.M. and Blank, U. (2016). Yessotoxin, a Marine Toxin, Exhibits Anti-Allergic and Anti-Tumoural Activities Inhibiting Melanoma Tumour Growth in a Preclinical Model. *PLOS One*. 11:e0167572.

Trainer, V.L., Bates, S.S., Lundholm, N., Thessen, A.E., Cochlan, W.P., Adams, N.G. et al. (2012). Pseudo-Nitzschia Physiological Ecology, Phylogeny, Toxicity, Monitoring and Impacts on Ecosystem Health. *Harmful Algae*. 14(Special issue):271–300.

Twiner, M.J., Hanagriff, J.C., Butler, S., Madhkoor, A.K. and Doucette, G.J. (2012). Induction of Apoptosis Pathways in Several Cell Lines Following Exposure to the Marine Algal Toxin Azaspiracid. *Chem. Res. Toxicol*. 25:1493–1501.

Vale, C. and Botana, L.M. (2008). Marine Toxins and the Cytoskeleton: Okadaic Acid and Dinophysistoxins. *FEBS J*. 275(24):6060–6066.

Vilariño, N., Louzao, M.C., Abal, P., Cagide, E., Carrera, C., Vieytes, M.R. et al. (2018). Human Poisoning from Marine Toxins: Unknowns for Optimal Consumer Protection. *Toxins*. 10:324. https://doi.org/10.3390/toxins10080324.

Visciano, P., Schirone, M., Berti, M., Milandri, A., Tofalo, R. and Suzzi, G. (2016). Marine Biotoxins: Occurrence, Toxicity, Regulatory Limits and Reference Methods. *Front. Microbiol*. 7:1051. https://doi.org/10.3389/fmicb.2016.01051.

Wang, D.-Z. (2008). Neurotoxins from Marine Dinoflagellates: A Brief Review. *Mar. Drugs*. 6:349–371.

Wang, H., Hu, Z., Chai, Z., Deng, Y., Zhan, Z. and Tang, Y.Z. (2020). Blooms of *Prorocentrum donghaiense* Reduced the Species Diversity of Dinoflagellate Community. *Acta Oceanol. Sin*. 39:110–119. https://doi.org/10.1007/s13131-020-1585-1.

WHO. (2021). *Guidelines on Recreational Water Quality: Volume 1 Coastal and Fresh Waters. Harmful Algal Blooms*. Geneva: World Health Organization, p. 5. https://www.ncbi.nlm.nih.gov/books/NBK572631/ (Accessed 29/6/2024).

Würger, L.T., Alarcan, J. and Braeuning, A. (2024). Effects of marine biotoxins on drug-metabolizing cytochrome P450 enzymes and their regulation in mammalian cells. *Arch. Toxicol*. 98(5):1311–1322.

Xi, M. and Dragsted, L.O. (2019). Biomarkers of Seaweed Intake. *Genes Nutri*. 14:24. https://doi.org/10.1186/s12263-019-0648-4.

Zendong, Z., Kadiri, M., Herrenknecht, C., Nézan, E., Mazzeo, A. and Hess, P. (2016). Algal Toxin Profiles in Nigerian Coastal Waters (Gulf of Guinea) Using Passive Sampling and Liquid Chromatography Coupled to Mass Spectrometry. *Toxicon*. 114:16–27. https://doi.org/10.1016/j.toxicon.2016.02.011.

Zhao, L., Huang, Y., Dong, Y., Han, X., Wang, S. and Liang, X. (2018). Aptamers and Aptasensors for Highly Specific Recognition and Sensitive Detection of Marine Biotoxins: Recent Advances and Perspectives. *Toxins*. 10:427. http://doi.org/10.3390/toxins10110427.

14

Exploring the Therapeutic Potential of Snake Venom Biotoxins

Edward Kwame Opata, Ayobami Ifeoluwa Awe, Peter Gbenga Oni, and Babatunde Oluwafemi Adetuyi

14.1 Introduction

Biotoxins are considered natural products obtained from plant, animal and microorganism sources which can induce pain and other deleterious effects, changing the physiology of the cell, tissue or organ affected, leading to death. These 'toxins' could elicit some toxicological, pharmacological or therapeutic effects due to their sources and constituent composition. These biotoxins could serve as ideal raw materials or novel compounds for drug design to tackle pathological problems such as atherothrombosis, atherosclerosis, cancers and neurological defects, among others (Liu et al., 2014).

Numerous bioactive natural compounds are obtained from diverse species of snakes, lizards, scorpions, spiders, bees, octopi and centipedes. Currently, there are over 11,000 reptile species recognized worldwide. Among these, snakes are one of the most scientifically studied, with many snake species known, yet a few of these are highly venomous, such as *Viperidae, Elapidea* and *Colubridea*. They have a wide degree of constituents which make up their poisonous glandular content, such as amino acids, lipids, carbohydrates, proteins, polypeptides, peptides, nucleic acids and more, which have been considered to have pharmacological benefits when they are isolated and characterized (Calderón-Celis et al., 2017; Simoes-Silva et al., 2018).

Their range of actions targets significant physiological pathways such as those associated with cytotoxic, neurotoxic, myotoxic, cardiotoxic and other enzymatic or non-enzymatic activities (Ciolek et al., 2022; Isbister et al., 2020; Yang et al., 2016). Hence, snake envenoming is considered a health risk in humans, as it has been reported to result in mortality ranging between 80,000 and 140,000 annually, as well as over half a million individuals being left with unfortunate outcomes such as amputation, blindness and other post-traumatic disorders on a global scale (Carey et al., 2012; Gutiérrez et al., 2017).

DOI: 10.1201/9781003500605-16

Nonetheless, several of these toxins have been exploited in the medical field to serve as beneficial final products, as they have been demonstrated in different studies to serve as promising diagnostic tools and pharmacological and therapeutic agents in many medical fields such as cardiovascular research, cancer chemotherapy, neurological sciences and antimicrobial and antiviral research fields (Offor & Piater, 2023; Oliveira et al., 2022; Teixeira et al., 2022).

This chapter aims to elucidate the general outlook of the snake venom, their constituents, and applications as therapeutic candidates in the medical field, covering disease conditions such as cardiovascular dysfunction, neurological disorders and the risk of cancer.

14.2 Snake Venom

Snake venoms are secretions of complex stores of proteins, peptides and enzymes present in the venomous gland of the parotid salivary gland, situated on either side of the head within encapsulated membranes (Kantivan Goswami et al., 2014). These enzymatic and non-enzymatic components consist of metalloproteinases, proteolytic enzymes, phospholipases, coagulating proteins, cytotoxins and neurotoxins. Venomous enzymes are responsible for the hydrolysis and degradation of the membrane components, which emanates into tissue necrosis, apoptosis and blood clotting or fibrinolysis (Jin & Varner, 2004). The proinflammatory effects of snake venoms are ascribed to the presence of metalloproteinases and phospholipases (Chan et al., 2016). However, the non-enzymatic constituents potentiate the gravity of the envenomation from the snake bites.

14.3 Types and Sources of Snake Biotoxins

The types of snake venom or biotoxins are dependent upon their species, geographical locations and habitats where they are found; their associated climates; and their ages. These are classified into the following main categories:

> Hemotoxic venom affects the cardiovascular system, especially as it relates with the hemostatic system. They are characterized by onset of hypotension, increasing vasodilation and permeability via the degradation of the basement membranes leading to systemic hypotensive shock.
>
> **(Gutiérrez et al., 2016)**

Cytotoxic venoms target specific cellular sites and components, which could induce necrosis; apoptosis; and cell proliferation, migration and growth. Victims express or show characteristic inflammation, blistering, bruises and systemic effects. If these are not attended to promptly, they result in detrimental states requiring surgery or amputation of the affected areas. They are known to produce neutrophil extracellular traps (NETS), block blood vessels, promote coagulopathy and in some incidences enhance fibrin formation, leading to either hypoxia or hemorrhagic shock (Kalita et al., 2022; Rivel et al., 2016).

Neurotoxic venom, on the other hand, can harm the nervous system, inducing possible hemorrhagic shock. It is characterized by paralysis of the neuronal muscles, ptosis of the eyes and intermittent vasodilation and vasoconstriction of the cranial nerves, which proceeds to the respiratory tract and eventual flaccid paralysis (Slagboom et al., 2017). Most of these toxins are present in most snakes and are members of the phospholipase A_2 (PLA_2) and three finger toxin (3FTX) groups, which have the potential to alter chemical signaling at synaptic junctions, thereby inducing paralysis as a result (Casewell et al., 2013).

14.4 Composition of Snake Venom

Their composition varies mainly by their families and species to contain hundreds of bioactive compounds (Calvete et al., 2009). They have all been reported to consist of proteins, peptides, enzymes, phospholipase A2, three-finger toxin defensins, disintegrins, serine protease and metalloproteinase inhibitors. Others are cytotoxins, neurotoxins, coagulants, fibrinolytics and cysteine-rich secretory proteins, among others (Dennis et al., 2011). They are mostly considered hydrophilic compounds, having a pH of 4.5 for acidic phosphatases and 9–10 for alkaline phosphatases. They have a large range of enzymes serving dynamic functions in their victims. For instance, the phosphodiesterase A2 (PLA_2) causes cell lysis, oxidases and proteases enhance membrane hydrolysis and digestion and inorganic moieties act as cofactors/coenzymes (Oliveira et al., 2022). Table 14.1 shows the prominent features of snake venoms and their biological and therapeutic targets.

14.5 Snake Toxins, Disease Conditions and Therapeutic Potentials

14.5.1 Phospholipase A_2 and Neurotoxicity

The complexity of snake venom gives it the much-needed diversity it requires to have different medicinal possibilities. Their capacity to bind to several membrane bound and cytosolic receptors in a selective dimension has been

TABLE 14.1

Features of Snake Families and Their Toxins

Snake Family	Toxins	Pathology	Biological Target	Therapeutic Targets	Reference
Elapidea, Viperidae	PLA_2	Skeletal muscle necrosis, paralysis, local inflammatory reactions	Plasma membrane, synaptic nerve	Anti-neuromuscular paralysis., anti-bacterial, anti-fungi	(Ferraz et al., 2019; Gutiérrez et al., 2017)
Elapidea, Viperidae	SVSPs	Coagulopathy, fibrinolytics.	Coagulating and fibrinolysis proteins	Inhibits thrombus formation, and fibrinogen activation	(Serrano, 2013; Ullah et al., 2018)
Elapidea, Viperidae	SVSPs	Coagulating proteins and platelets adhesion, activation and aggregation factors	Platelets hypo and hyper-aggregation, fibrin degradation, membrane protein digestion, apoptosis	Regulates platelet aggregation, coagulation and fibrinolysis	(Ferraz et al., 2019; Olaoba et al., 2020; Ullah et al., 2018)
Elapidea, Colubridea	3FTX	Synaptic nerve degradation and demyelination leading to paralysis; cardiac arrest through lysis of cardiomyocytes	Neuromuscular acetylcholine receptors, acetylcholinesterase and cardiotoxin cardiomyocytes	Regulates blood pressure; coagulation disorders and analgesic action	(Kini & Doley, 2010; Kini & Koh, 2020)
Elapidea, Viperidae, Colubridea	Disintegrins	Cell migration, apoptosis and angiogenesis	Cell adhesion molecules, selectins, growth factors	Regulates cell cytotoxicity, migration and proliferation	(Carey et al., 2012; Jakubowski et al., 2013; Thangam et al., 2012)

reported to serve as selective therapeutic neurotoxins, having specific mechanisms of action (Chan et al., 2016; Osipov & Utkin, 2023).

The snakes of the families of Elapidea and Viperidae are considered to have the most abundant sources of neurotoxins with life-threatening effects.

Having two types of neurotoxins, the α and β-neurotoxins, the most active of these being the β-neurotoxin, which is typically composed of phospholipase A2. PLA_2 is regarded as one of the most important and abundant esterases and acts at the presynaptic nerve of neuro-transmuscular junctions. This is ensued by the hydrolytic action of PLA_2 on membrane bound phospholipids around the terminal junctions of nerve cells. The release of lysophospholipids, fatty acids and eventual exocytosis of vesicle-bound components from cytosolic membrane organelles enhances the permeability of ionic moieties, consequent depolarization and hyperpolarization of mitochondrial pores and eventually destruction of synaptic vesicles (Rossetto & Montecucco, 2008). In a nutshell, the uncontrolled influx of extracellular molecules such as Ca^{2+} and Na^{+} ions results in cell death arising from neuromuscular terminal paralysis (Barber et al., 2013; Rossetto & Montecucco, 2008). They are of two groups, with the pancreatic PLA_2 found in Elapids considered group I, while those of synovial PLA_2 are termed group II (Tasoulis & Isbister, 2022).

The active site of group II viper toxins is located at the 49th amino acid residue (Aspartate, Asp49), which is responsible for their catalytic activity (Tasoulis & Isbister, 2022). It should be noted that these PLA_2 are so therapeutically essential as their concentrations within the serum of victims/patients of snake bites can be highly elevated and useful in the detection of individuals who are undergoing systemic envenoming (Isbister et al., 2020).

Elapidea, having the most abundant PLA_2, has a diverse pharmacological profile, has been reported to have pre-synaptic neurotoxicity, cytotoxicity, myotoxicity, serve as anticoagulants and present immune-inflammatory tendencies (Johnston et al., 2013, 2017; Lane et al., 2011). Most importantly, the release of inflammatory cytokines is induced by the conversion of membrane-bound arachidonic acids into prostaglandins and leukotrienes, thereby enhancing the associated inflammation within the affected tissues, as it may relate to the pre- and post-synaptic cleft (Murakami et al., 2020).

In the nervous system, the peripheral axis is not protected by the blood–brain barrier (BBB); thus, its terminal ends are highly susceptible to neurotoxin attacks. These PLA_2-associated venoms cause neuromuscular flaccid paralysis, which is related to blocked nasal and oral muscles. This is because of the inadequacy of the neuromuscular tight junction transmission mechanism. The transmission mechanism consists of the nerve terminals, muscle fibers, Schwann cells, axon terminal and neurotransmitter acetylcholine's (Ach) synaptic cleft. The entry of soluble ions, such as Ca, K and Na, triggers the buildup of flux within voltage-gated channels, which mediates the induction of synaptic toxicity (Jimsheleishvili et al., 2023; Zambelli & Hösch, 2023).

They act by complex covalent interactions, producing toxicity by the depletion of synaptic vesicle degeneration of the motor nerve. Once PLA_2 is within the nerve terminal, it binds to the active site and induces conformational changes involving enzymatic hydrolysis of phospholipids and release of prostaglandins and leukotrienes, which are signals of neurotoxicity induced by inflammatory cytokines (Oliveira et al., 2022). These changes are also associated with membrane polarization via increased permeability and the influx of Ca^{2+} ions in exocytosis, which promotes the depletion of the reserved pool of the synaptic vesicles. They also induce the release of nucleotides (ADP, ATP, UTP), which have an affinity for binding to purinergic receptors and enhance the release of K^+ and Ca^{2+} ions, promoting sustained membrane polarization (Cintra-Francischinelli et al., 2010). This depletion and its associated intracellular events lead to possible sustained degenerative events with the onset of disease conditions (Gutiérrez et al., 2017).

These events all lead to prolonged and severe paralysis, characterized by pain and the release of neurotoxins. PLA_2 induces pain either directly through several inflammatory cytokines or mediators (such as interleukins, tumor necrosis factors, interferon gamma, prostaglandins, thromboxane, leukotrienes, etc.) or indirectly through nociceptors. However, these nociceptors have some receptors which recognize these inflammatory proteins earlier highlighted earlier, thereby increasing the nerve cell sensitivity to these membrane changes.

14.6 Snake Venom Metalloproteinases and Serine Proteinases in Cardiovascular Diseases

According to the WHO, cardiovascular diseases (CVDs) are the first leading cause of death globally, with a death rate of approximately 18 million annually. These include incidences of ischemic heart diseases, stroke/myocadiac infarction, atherosclerosis, atherothrombosis and arrhythmia, among others. The challenges associated with most CVDs are related to the development of thrombi or clots within blood vessels, which, if not resolved, mature, rupture and break out in the form of thrombosis.

Under physiological conditions, the endothelium is under a hemostatic state, evidenced by the existence of resting platelets; however, under pathological conditions, such as injuries, platelets need to be recruited and undergo adhesion, activation and aggregation to ensure the cessation of bleeding by the formation of a thrombus mesh link. Damaged blood vessels expose collagen fires, which have an affinity for the van Willebrand factor (vWF), which enhances the interaction with GP-Ib-IX in the platelet membrane. The adhered platelets undergo degranulation, enabling the release of the platelet's cytoplasmic contents or soluble mediators such as ADP, serotonin, thrombin, thromboxane and platelet activating factors, which induce the activation phase. Platelet aggregation begins once the platelets become activated, triggering the release of integrins, selectins and cadherins such as $\alpha IIb\beta 3$, glycoprotein VI (GPVI), P-selectin and E-cadherins. Aggregation and clot plug are further enhanced by the interaction of the released soluble mediators binding to their specific receptors.

In the management of CVD-related incidences, a high percentage of toxins from snake venom obtained from various families affect the hemostatic system, inhibiting platelet-related proteins and clotting factors and inducing fibrinolysis and hemorrhage, which enhances the endothelium function. These toxins are obtained from varieties of snake families, such as Viperidae, Crotalidae, Elapidea and Colubridea, among others. They produce specific toxins or, better still, venoms with a specific affinity for coagulation proteins. They serve as either procoagulants or anticoagulants, having either or both enzymatic or nonenzymatic effects on the coagulation hemostatic system (C. Xie et al., 2020). Several of these toxins affecting the coagulation system, classified based on their structure-function relations, are either metalloproteinases, serine proteinases or PLA_2 (Fox & Serrano, 2008; Serrano, 2013).

14.7 Snake Venom Serine Proteinases

These are mainly found in about 6%–26% of viper snakes' whole venom but also in Colubridea and Flapidea snakes and affect the hemostatic system. They impact hemostatic sub-functions in their physiological states, such as those implicated in platelet adhesion, activation and aggregation, influencing the coagulating zymogens, fibrinolytic proteins and complement system and the induction of inflammation during dysfunctional states, which result in endothelial damage. An interesting fact about snake venom serine proteinases (SVSPs) is their structural sequence identity, having a catalytic triad (His57, Asp102 and Ser 195) but different specificity to substrates, irrespective of their sources (Sanchez et al., 2017; Serrano, 2013). It should also be noted that SVSPs are associated with the pathologies and eventual side effects of snake envenoming, such as in incidences of coagulopathies. Aside from inducing hemorrhagic efficacy, these SVSPs are known to also serve other biological effects, such as procoagulants (due to the presence of the Stuart-Prower factor—FX—and prothrombin activators) and antiplatelets (White, 2005).

14.8 Snake Venom Metalloproteinases

Most toxins of this class are obtained from Viperidae and Crotalidea, which range from about 6%–72% of all snakes. A large percentage of these venoms of viper and crotalid origin affect the bulk of the hemostatic system. They have the tendency to induce coagulation and fibrinolytic processes simultaneously. They have been reported to induce the activation of platelets and tissue factors and enhance the conversion of prothrombin to thrombin, which are central to clot formation via the extrinsic coagulation pathway, and induce the fibrinolytic circuit (Calvete, 2013; Offor et al., 2022; Tan, 2022).

These processes are dependent on their enzymatic and non-enzymatic proteins present in these toxins, altering the integrity of the membrane by degrading the components of the extracellular matrix and endothelium, influencing coagulation cascade activity and causing hemorrhage in affected individuals (Dingwoke et al., 2024; Takeda et al., 2012; White, 2005). In clinical settings, coagulopathy is one of the main causes of mortality. However, in incidences of snake bite, traditional treatment regimens such as the use of heparin, antithrombin compounds, platelet inhibitors and other antagonists of coagulating enzymes are not applied due to their strong manifestation of thrombin-like enzymatic properties. This feature enhances the ability to use these enzymes to assay for the existence of hemostatic proteins (Gamulin et al., 2023; Lee et al., 2022; Maduwage et al., 2015). It is also important to understand that some snake toxins have the capability to disrupt the coagulation system but inhibit the proteins and/or receptors associated with platelet aggregation (such as collagen fibers, GPVI, vWF, αIIbβ3 integrin) and coagulation systems (such as FX, II, I, V and VII). The presence of some of the viperous constituents within a system aids in determining the toxicological dynamics of that condition. A classic example is seen in high incidences of hemophilia, in which metalloproteinases have been reported to be very highly expressed (Kolvekar et al., 2023).

With respect to their hemorrhagic activities, causing a high degree of bleeding, there is degradation of the basement membrane proteins (such as the collagen subtypes, laminin, selectins and cadherins) which are found within the endothelia of the blood vessels, causing systemic damage because of endothelial dysfunction (Olaoba et al., 2020). They are also implicated in non-hemorrhagic incidences, such as reported by Baldo et al. (2010), who showed that snake venom metalloproteinases (SVMPs) could use apoptotic mechanisms to degrade the basement membrane, such as with fibrinolytic activities, thereby causing sustained bleeding. Changes in the membrane assemblage, such as the cell adhesion-extracellular matrix, enhance the fibrinolytic process with an intact assembly, leading to the apoptotic course being sustained (Araki, 2016).

14.9 Disintegrins and Cancers

Cancers including hepatocarcinoma, melanoma, leukemia, lung, kidney, ovarian and testicular cancers, to mention just a few, all combine to give an estimated incidence of approximately 18.1 million as of 2020 globally (Sung et al., 2021). These rates affect both sexes and all age groups across all continents of the world; therefore, it is considered a global problem. It is therefore important to understand details about the epidemiology of cancers and how they affect population trends. This enhances the timely interventions and management of conditions associated with its incidences and mortality (Mattiuzzi & Lippi, 2019).

Disintegrins, as described earlier, consist of a plethora of polypeptides and many active proteins, which amount to approximately 90% of the dry mass of snake venom. These serve as pharmacologically active constituents which may be noxious or beneficial compounds in tackling tumors and associated cancers (White, 2005). They have been described to have highly potent and efficient actions against cancer related cases in various experimental models.

Specifically, disintegrins act against transmembrane receptors, integrins, which are predominantly found in the cell membranes of living organisms (mostly vertebrates and humans). These integrins consist of two major subunits, the α and β chains, from which the protein moiety is structurally built, giving various forms that act in hemostasis, cell adhesion and migration, coagulation and proliferation (Barczyk et al., 2010; Park et al., 2020). Examples of these heterodimeric proteins include αIIbβ3, α5β1, αvβ5 and α6β1 (Takada et al., 2007).

As a general description, disintegrins are considered small, non-toxic, non-enzymatic cysteine-rich peptides, having numerous sequences based on their amino acid residues (Saviola et al., 2015). They are a group of low molecular weight, cysteine-rich polypeptide units consisting of 45–84 amino acid residues found in snakes such as Elapidea, Colubridea, Viperidae and Crotalidea (Kele et al., 2015). The major classes of these disintegrins are the short sequence disintegrins, consisting of 41–51 amino acid residues with a secondary structure containing four cysteine bridges (found in echistatin-RGD and obtustatin-KTS). The second group of higher molecular weight contains approximately 70 amino acid residues linked by six cysteine residues such as barbourin-KGD and flavoviridin-RGD. The other groups contain approximately 84 amino acid residues linked by seven cysteine bridges (bitistatin-RGD), with the final group being those with either homodimers or heterodimer protein monomeric units, with about 67 amino acid residues which are not covalently bound. They consist of four cysteine-linked bridges within intra- or interchain formations (Kele et al., 2015; Lazarovici et al., 2019). The presence of these cysteine-linked groups enacts functionality on the disintegrins, giving them the necessary conformational exposures or changes they demand for effectiveness. They act by inhibiting the activities of integrins in physiological processes such as platelet adhesion, activation and aggregation, thereby inducing loss of blood and hemorrhagic shock (Kuo et al., 2019). They are inhibitors of cell adhesion molecules such as the intercellular adhesion molecule-1 (ICAM-1), P-selectins and E-cadherins implicated in cell migration, apoptosis and angiogenesis (Jakubowski et al., 2013). They are in themselves responsible for leukocyte recruitment and

TABLE 14.2
Snake Venoms and Their Mechanism of Action in Different Study Models

Snake Family	Species	Specific Disintegrin Toxins	Study Model	Mechanism of Action	Ref
Elapidea	*Naja naja*	Disintegrin protein	Breast cancer, MCF-7 Lung cancer, A549 Liver cancer, HepG2	Induces cytotoxicity and apoptosis	(Thangam et al., 2012)
Elapidea	*Naja oxiana* and *Naja haje*	Cytotoxin 1 Cytotoxin 2 Cytotoxin 3	Lung epithelia cells, A549 Human leukemia cells, HL60 Breast cancer, MCF-7	Induces cytotoxicity, apoptosis	(Ebrahim et al., 2016; Feofanov et al., 2005)
Elapidea	*Naja naja atra*	Cystatin	Skin melanoma, B16F10	Inhibit invasion, proliferation and metastasis	(Q. Xie et al., 2013)
Viperidae	*A. hays brevicaudus*	Salmosin	Skin melanoma, B16F10	Inhibits metastasis, cell proliferation	(Kim et al., 2003; Offor & Piater, 2023)
Viperidae	*Vipera lebetina obtuse*	Obtustatin	Lung carcinoma, LLC cells	Inhibits angiogenesis	(Marcinkiewicz & Kisiel, 2003)
Viperidae	*Crotalus ruber ruber*	Recombinant rubistatin	Malignant skin melanoma, SK-Mel-28	Inhibits cell proliferation, migration and apoptosis	(Carey et al., 2012)
Viperidae	*Bothrops alternatus*	Alternagin-C	Endothelial cells, HUVEC; triple negative breast cancer, MDA-MB-231	Inhibits angiogenesis	(dos Santos et al., 2020)
Elapidea	*Walterinnesia aegyptia*	*Walterinnesia aegyptia* venom (WEV)	Negative breast cancer, MDA-MB-231; breast cancer, MCF-7	Inhibits angiogenesis, cell proliferation and apoptosis and induces cell cycle arrest	(Badr et al., 2013)

serve as antagonists against integrins (such as αIIbβ3—the fibrinogen receptor, αvβ3—the vitronectin receptor and α5β1—the fibronectin receptor) in the pathogenesis of specific cancers (Lazarovici et al., 2019).

Table 14.2 shows the efficacy of diverse snake venoms serving as therapeutic agents against related tumorigenic onsets.

The history of the use of snake venom in the treatment of cancer-related conditions dates to the year 1993, when Calmette and colleagues reported the antitumor efficacy of the venom of *Naja* sp. on adenocarcinoma cells (Da Silva et al., 1996). The venom or *Vipera lebentina* has been shown to induce cell death via apoptosis in cancerous ovarian cells. In the place of the *Walterinnesia aegyptia* venom (WEV), it was reported to cause cell cycle arrest in prostate cancer cells and enhanced antitumor potency in breast cancer cell lines, either when administered singly or in combination with silica nanoparticles, which served as a delivery vehicle of the toxin (Al-Sadoon et al., 2013; Badr et al., 2013). At very low doses or concentrations, they could be useful as chemotherapeutic agents, as they have been shown to inhibit tumor growth by inducing cell cycle arrest and apoptosis without any significant effect on normal cells (Kele et al., 2015; Macêdo et al., 2015). Aggretin (purified from *Calloselasma rhodostoma*), a collagen-like agonist, has been found to target platelets, their associated integrins (α2β1) and growth factors, thereby exerting anti-tumor effects on affected cells during metastatic cancer progression (Cañas et al., 2021; Oliveira et al., 2022).

14.10 Three-Finger Toxins and Multi-Therapy in Diseases

Three-finger toxins are one of the most prominent venoms, found in different snakes such as vipers, elapids and colubrids. They are one of the most useful non-enzymatic snake toxins. Structurally, they differ in the length of amino acid residues, as they have been identified to range between 58 and 81 amino acid residues linked by different numbers of disulfide bridges (Kessler et al., 2017). For instance, based on the source species, the short variants, α-neurotoxins, β-cardiotoxins and cytotoxins, have been reported to consist of between 55 and 65 amino acid residues, linked by four disulfide bridges. On the other hand, the long-chain variants consist of between 66 and 75 amino acid residues with five disulfide bridges (Kini & Doley, 2010). As described, they are highly diverse, and this could be due to their evolutionary genetic duplication and deletions, clonal selection and differential genetic accumulation occurring within their molecular genetic skeleton (Junqueira-De-Azevedo et al., 2015; Kini & Doley, 2010; Pawlak et al., 2006). The result of these evolutionary changes is shown in the various isoforms of the 3FTX having diverse structural and functional differences. These variabilities are mostly expressed in their functions and activities, such as being neurotoxins, cytotoxins and cardiotoxins, as represented in Table 14.3 (Laustsen et al., 2018). To this end, the 3FTX is highly multi-functional. However, in some species, there is conservational functionality, and the reason for this remains to be seen, such as with the Elapidea cobra (*Naja naja* species) being rich in cytotoxins, while the mamba (genus *Dendroaspis*) is rich in neurotoxins and anticoagulants (Laustsen et al., 2018; Pawlak et al., 2006).

One interesting fact about the 3FTXs is that they are not involved in inflammation or tissue hyperplasia. The unique multifactorial functionality of these snake venom toxins is in their conserved regions with structo-functional loops with a Tyr25 or Phe27 amino acid residue responsible for their folding (Kini & Koh, 2020; Pawlak et al., 2006). These create diverse loops, such as loops I, II and III, based on the degree of folding and the nature of amino acid residues present in their active sites. Their β-pleated sheets enhance their native structural conformational stability and integrity due to the interaction

TABLE 14.3

3FTX Snake Venom Functions in Diverse Species

Snake Family	Species	Functionality	Therapeutic Mechanism of Action	References
Elapidea	*Bungarus multicinctus*	Neurotoxins	α-neurotoxin inhibits muscle and neuronal acetylcholinesterase receptor (AChR)	(Changeux, 1990; Nirthanan & Gwee, 2004)
Elapidea	*Dendroaspis polylepis*	Neurotoxins	Inhibits muscarinic receptors	(Marchot et al., 1998; Miwa et al., 2011)
Elapidea	*Naja oxiana, Naja kaouthia*	Cardiotoxins	Non-specific action on phospholipids and insulin receptors	(Averin et al., 2022; Nguyen et al., 2012)
Viperidae	*Bothrops jararaca*	Cardiotoxins (mambins and exactin)	Regulates platelets activities; inhibits factor X action, which alters the stability of hemostatic proteins	(Girish & Kini, 2016; Messadi, 2023)
Elapidea	*Dendroaspis* spp. (African mamba)	Cardiotoxins (fasciculi, muscarinic toxin)	α- and β-adrenoreceptor regulation, which alters cardiac rates	(Fruchart-Gaillard et al., 2008; Näreoja et al., 2011)
Elapidea	*Calliophis bivirgatus*	Cytotoxins	Activates voltage-gated channels (Na^+, K^+, Ca^{2+})	(Vidya et al., 2021; Yang et al., 2016)

of van der Waals, hydrogen and ionic forces. Other toxins such as fasciculi, a cardiotoxin, have about six to eight amino acid residues in active sight, which facilitates hydrophobic interactions (Averin et al., 2022; Messadi, 2023). Another toxin, the beta muscarinic toxin (MTβ) from the mamba, the elapid family, has affinity for the muscarinic receptor. However, upon structural changes via the substitution reaction in the amino acid residue from Ile/Ser38 to Ala/Val 43, it increases the affinity of the MTβ for adrenoreceptors but has little or no affinity for the muscarinic receptor (Ciolek et al., 2022; Fruchart-Gaillard et al., 2008).

In the same vein, the short chain α-neurotoxin, a potent neuronal AChR blocker, is formed by a rearrangement reaction within its binding pocket. The loop II insertion into this pocket induces its functionality as an α-neurotoxin with affinity for the nAChR, while loop I and III interactions, occurring from charged residue (van der Waals and hydrogen bond) interactions, determine their immunogenicity (Nys et al., 2022; Pruksaphon et al., 2022).

14.11 Common Drugs Used against Snake Envenomation

The treatment regimen against snakebites and envenomation involves the use of antivenoms. They remain the only specific mode which can potentially prevent, reverse, mitigate and abrogate most of the effects of envenoming upon administration at therapeutic doses. However, aside from antivenoms, other medical and paramedic measures are taken to effectively treat snakebite victims. They include administration of synthetic or pharmaceutical drugs, wound care, reconstructive surgery and prosthesis (Oliveira et al., 2022). Several synthetic drugs are also being explored for their potential as anticoagulants, antifibrinolytics, antiplatelets and anti-necrotic compounds. For example, a class of drugs known as anticholinesterases can be beneficial in restoring paralysis due to neuromuscular dysfunction after bites from neurotoxic venomous snakes (Gutiérrez et al., 2021; Morais, 2018). Also, drugs with anti-apoptotic/necrotic potential can reduce tissue damage around the affected local areas where the bite occurred by reducing local tissue damage, which can lead to severe disability and future amputation (Silva, Maduwage, et al., 2017). Therefore, early access to safe and effective antivenoms and other recommended or approved drugs is highly critical in reducing the morbidity and mortality arising from snake bites.

There are three major therapeutic applications of snake venom: toxin-based diagnostic markers, biological markers and pharmaceutical markers (Estevão-Costa et al., 2018; Herzig et al., 2020; Oliveira et al., 2022). Our focus will be on the US-based Food and Drug Administration's (FDA) approved pharmaceutical drugs. These drugs are typically considered neurotoxic, cytotoxic, cardiotoxic or hemotoxic. We understand, as earlier explained, that they function in tandem with their prefixes, such as neurotoxic, being responsible for treating neurological disorders; cytotoxins act against cancer related abnormalities; and cardiotoxins are related therapeutics against cardiovascular and hematological diseases (Oliveira et al., 2022).

14.12 Cardiotoxic Drugs

Captopril: It is a small, synthetic, orally administered bioactive antihypertensive drug obtained from snake venom, used to stimulate vasodilation of the bradykinin peptide after a snake bite. It was one of the first drugs produced to target angiotensin-converting enzyme (ACE). Snakes such as *Bothrops jararaca* produce this biotoxin, which potentiates the bradykinin potentiating factor (BPF), which inhibits ACE and increases the hypotensive capability of the bradykinins. The ACE converts angiotensin I (AC I) to angiotensin II (AC II), which results in an increase in blood pressure and subsequent degradation of bradykinin peptides, which are vasodilators. BPF is the principal component of the drug captopril (Cushman & Ondetti, 1991; Ferreira et al., 1970).

Mechanistically, BPF exerts its action on the extracellular matrix; binds to G-proteins; and degrades the phospholipid bilayer to release prostaglandins, phospholipases and protein kinases, leading to changes in intracellular Ca^{2+} concentrations. Onward synthesis of nitric oxide (NO), prostacyclin and proteins C and S, which are prominent inhibitors of platelet aggregation and onward coagulopathy, thus destroying the possibility of blood clot formation when bitten by thrombosis inducing venomous snakes (Camargo et al., 2012; Golias et al., 2007).

Captopril is, however, associated with certain physiologic and non-physiologic side effects when administered. These include hypotension, hyperkalemia, renal dysfunction, anemia and incessant cough (especially in excessive usage) (Sica, 2005). To circumvent these challenges, a modification was made in the structural conformation of this drug to produce an alternative product called Enalapril. However, both drugs are still in use in the management of cardiotoxic-related snake bites. Other examples of drug candidates used as alternatives to these principal compounds include ramipril, moexipril and lisinopril, among others (Acharya et al., 2003).

14.13 αIIbβ3 Integrin Inhibitors

Eptifibatide: This is a potent antiplatelet drug, used principally in the treatment of CVD-related coagulopathy associated with hypercoagulation due to intensive platelet reactivity. It was synthesized from the venom of the rattlesnake, *Sistrurus miliarius* barbourin, being a disintegrin that is antagonist of integrins (Jakubowski et al., 2013). They have strong affinity for the dimeric αIIbβ3 integrin, a known receptor for the coagulating zymogen fibrinogen. At its active site, it interacts with the amino acid residues within the KDG and RGD hybridized domain. The motif non-specificity of the active compound in the drug is currently a source of concern to clinicians (Lazarovici et al., 2019; Roffi & Mukherjee, 2008).

Tirofiban: This is another drug approved by the FDA, used as a prominent target of αIIbβ3 integrin, which aids in the management of coronary ischemic conditions arising from malaggregation of platelets (Nasrabadi et al., 2022). The active compound of this drug is obtained by synthetic crystallization from echistatin toxin, a prominent disintegrin obtained from the *Echis carinatus* viper snake. It is one of the first synthesized pharmacophore-based drugs, which has been considered more specific than eptifibatides due to its higher affinity for the RGD motif due to its structural resemblance. It binds other integrins with nanomolar affinity but with higher specificity for αIIbβ3 (Estevão-Costa et al., 2018; Hartman et al., 1992).

14.14 Neurotoxic Drugs

Cobrotoxin: This is a short-chain post-synaptic neurotoxin, which is a subtype of 3FTX. It is purified from the venom of *Naja atra.* It binds to nAChRs at the neuromuscular junction of the synaptic nerve. Its binding has been reported to increase the acetylcholine levels in the body by its inhibitory potency of the enzyme responsible for the hydrolysis of acetylcholine, acetylcholinesterase (Bedraoui et al., 2024; Chang et al., 1999).

Cobratoxin: Another 3FTX subtype is a long-chain post-synaptic cleft neurotoxin, which is isolated from *Naja naja kaouthi* (Huynh et al., 2022). A unique characteristic is how it works by blocking or opening ion channels on neuromuscular nerves by inhibiting synaptobrevin protein (responsible for the exocytosis of Ca^{2+} into synaptic vesicles), which aids in the release of modular neurotransmitters across the synaptic nerves. The inhibition confers an analgesic effect due to its suppression of inflammatory proteins arising from the CA^{2+} efflux (Gazerani & Cairns, 2014; Silva, Hodgson, et al., 2017).

14.15 Antineoplastic/Cytotoxic Drugs

Crotamine: A small molecular weight therapeutic defensin, isolated from the venom of the rattlesnake *Crotalus durissus.* Its structure is like human defensin subtypes (α and β), with about 42 peptide residues linked by disulfide bridges (Cañas, 2022; Tasima et al., 2020). It is very selective for proficiently proliferating cells, which are known with neoplastic and cytotoxic cells, thus making it a promising and effective antineoplastic compound. Due to its high oral bioavailability, it has been postulated to have excellent proteolytic resistance and penetrative potency, especially with tumorigenic cells. Aside from its antitumor feature, it has shown to be an anti-inflammatory agent as well (de Carvalho Porta et al., 2020; Kerkis et al., 2004).

14.16 Conclusion

At the mention of snakes in our world today, we are gripped with fear, yet, in ancient times, we had a vast interest in them due to their medicinal bioactive composition. It has been established that the complexity of snake venom is beyond doubt. It is a mixture of different biologically active proteins, peptides, enzymes and non-enzymic organic and inorganic compounds. This chapter has shown that snake venom is not new to the clinical world, as it has been a useful therapeutic agent in the treatment and management of many disease conditions such as cancers, neurological defects and cardiovascular dysfunction, among others. Their mechanism of action involves but is not limited to inhibition of cell proliferation, apoptosis and necrosis. Others, such as regulation of ion-gated channels along the synaptic cleft, regulation of cell adhesion and binding potency, cell cycle, selective destruction of membrane bound proteins with enhanced permeability and so many others. Based on these mechanisms, snake venoms have been modeled based on their structures into potent drugs used in clinical settings to tackle a host of diseases, as earlier mentioned. Most of these drugs have been approved by regulatory agencies such as the US FDA, yet they are associated with some challenges in their usage. Therefore, for future interest in the study of snake toxins, it is important to delve into their impact at the molecular level and how they can affect individualized medicine.

References

Acharya, K. R., Sturrock, E. D., Riordan, J. F., & Ehlers, M. R. W. (2003). Ace revisited: A new target for structure-based drug design. *Nature Reviews Drug Discovery*, 2(11), 891–902. https://doi.org/10.1038/nrd1227

Al-Sadoon, M. K., Rabah, D. M., & Badr, G. (2013). Enhanced anticancer efficacy of snake venom combined with silica nanoparticles in a murine model of human multiple myeloma: Molecular targets for cell cycle arrest and apoptosis induction. *Cellular Immunology*. https://doi.org/10.1016/j.cellimm.2013.07.016

Araki, S. (2016). Endothelial cell toxicity of vascular apoptosis-inducing proteins from hemorrhagic snake venom. *Snake Venoms*, 1–15. https://doi.org/10.1007/978-94-007-6648-8_5-1

Averin, A. S., Nenov, M. N., Starkov, V. G., Tsetlin, V. I., & Utkin, Y. N. (2022). Effects of Cardiotoxins from naja oxiana cobra venom on rat heart muscle and aorta: a comparative study of toxin-induced contraction mechanisms. *Toxins*, *14*(2), 88. https://doi.org/10.3390/TOXINS14020088/S1

Badr, G., Al-Sadoon, M. K., & Rabah, D. M. (2013). Therapeutic efficacy and molecular mechanisms of snake (Walterinnesia aegyptia) venom-loaded silica nanoparticles in the treatment of breast cancer- and prostate cancer-bearing experimental mouse models. *Free Radical Biology and Medicine*, *65*, 175–189. https://doi.org/10.1016/J.FREERADBIOMED.2013.06.018

Baldo, C., Jamora, C., Yamanouye, N., Zorn, T. M., & Moura-da-Silva, A. M. (2010). Mechanisms of vascular damage by hemorrhagic snake venom metalloproteinases: Tissue distribution and in situ hydrolysis. *PLOS Neglected Tropical Diseases*, *4*(6), e727. https://doi.org/10.1371/JOURNAL.PNTD.0000727

Barber, C. M., Isbister, G. K., & Hodgson, W. C. (2013). Alpha neurotoxins. *Toxicon: Official Journal of the International Society on Toxinology*, *66*, 47–58. https://doi.org/10.1016/J.TOXICON.2013.01.019

Barczyk, M., Carracedo, S., & Gullberg, D. (2010). Integrins. *Cell and Tissue Research*, *339*(1), 269. https://doi.org/10.1007/S00441-009-0834-6

Bedraoui, A., Suntravat, M., El Mejjad, S., Enezari, S., Oukkache, N., Sanchez, E. E., Galan, J. A., El Fatimy, R., & Daouda, T. (2024). Therapeutic potential of snake venom: Toxin distribution and opportunities in deep learning for novel drug discovery. *Medicine in Drug Discovery*, *21*, 100175. https://doi.org/10.1016/J.MEDIDD.2023.100175

Calderón-Celis, F., Cid-Barrio, L., Encinar, J. R., Sanz-Medel, A., & Calvete, J. J. (2017). Absolute venomics: Absolute quantification of intact venom proteins through elemental mass spectrometry. *Journal of Proteomics*, *164*, 33–42. https://doi.org/10.1016/J.JPROT.2017.06.001

Calvete, J. J. (2013). Snake venomics: From the inventory of toxins to biology. *Toxicon: Official Journal of the International Society on Toxinology*, *75*, 44–62. https://doi.org/10.1016/J.TOXICON.2013.03.020

Calvete, J. J., Sanz, L., Angulo, Y., Lomonte, B., & Gutiérrez, J. M. (2009). Venoms, venomics, antivenomics. *FEBS Letters*, *583*(11), 1736–1743. https://doi.org/10.1016/J.FEBSLET.2009.03.029

Camargo, A. C. M., Ianzer, D., Guerreiro, J. R., & Serrano, S. M. T. (2012). Bradykinin-potentiating peptides: Beyond captopril. *Toxicon: Official Journal of the International Society on Toxinology*, *59*(4), 516–523. https://doi.org/10.1016/J.TOXICON.2011.07.013

Cañas, C. A. (2022). Biological and medical aspects related to South American rattlesnake crotalus durissus (Linnaeus, 1758): A view from Colombia. *Toxins*, *14*(12). https://doi.org/10.3390/TOXINS14120875

Cañas, C. A., Castaño-Valencia, S., Castro-Herrera, F., Cañas, F., & Tobón, G. J. (2021). Biomedical applications of snake venom: From basic science to autoimmunity and rheumatology. *Journal of Translational Autoimmunity*, *4*. https://doi.org/10.1016/J.JTAUTO.2020.100076

Carey, C. M., Bueno, R., Gutierrez, D. A., Petro, C., Lucena, S. E., Sanchez, E. E., & Soto, J. G. (2012). Recombinant rubistatin (r-Rub), an MVD disintegrin, inhibits cell migration and proliferation, and is a strong apoptotic inducer of the human melanoma cell line SK-Mel-28. *Toxicon, 59*(2), 241. https://doi.org/10.1016/J.TOXICON.2011.12.002

Casewell, N. R., Wüster, W., Vonk, F. J., Harrison, R. A., & Fry, B. G. (2013). Complex cocktails: The evolutionary novelty of venoms. *Trends in Ecology & Evolution, 28*(4), 219–229. https://doi.org/10.1016/J.TREE.2012.10.020

Chan, Y. S., Cheung, R. C. F., Xia, L., Wong, J. H., Ng, T. B., & Chan, W. Y. (2016). Snake venom toxins: Toxicity and medicinal applications. *Applied Microbiology and Biotechnology, 100*(14), 6165–6181. https://doi.org/10.1007/S00253-016-7610-9

Chang, L. S., Chen, K. C., Wu, B. N., Lin, S. K., Wu, P. F., Hong, Y. R., & Yang, C. C. (1999). Expression and mutagenesis studies of cobrotoxin from Taiwan cobra. *Biochemical and Biophysical Research Communications, 263*(3), 652–656. https://doi.org/10.1006/bbrc.1999.1418

Changeux, J. P. (1990). The TiPS lecture the nicotinic acetylcholine receptor: An allosteric protein prototype of ligand-gated ion channels. *Trends in Pharmacological Sciences, 11*(12), 485–492. https://doi.org/10.1016/0165-6147(90)90049-E

Cintra-Francischinelli, M., Caccin, P., Chiavegato, A., Pizzo, P., Carmignoto, G., Angulo, Y., Lomonte, B., Gutiérrez, J. M., & Montecucco, C. (2010). Bothrops snake myotoxins induce a large efflux of ATP and potassium with spreading of cell damage and pain. *Proceedings of the National Academy of Sciences of the United States of America, 107*(32), 14140–14145. https://doi.org/10.1073/pnas.1009128107

Ciolek, J., Zoukimian, C., Dhot, J., Burban, M., Triquigneaux, M., Lauzier, B., Guimbert, C., Ferron, M., Ciccone, L., Tepshi, L., Boturyn, D., Stura, E., Legrand, P., Robin, P., Mourier, G., Schaack, B., Fellah, I., Blanchet, G., Gauthier-Erfanian, C., . . . Gilles, N. (2022). MT9, a natural peptide from black mamba venom antagonizes the muscarinic type 2 receptor and reverses the M2R-agonist-induced relaxation in rat and human arteries. *Biomedicine & Pharmacotherapy, 150*. https://doi.org/10.1016/j.biopha.2022.113094ï

Cushman, D. W., & Ondetti, M. A. (1991). History of the design of captopril and related inhibitors of angiotensin converting enzyme. *Hypertension, 17*(4), 589–592. https://doi.org/10.1161/01.HYP.17.4.589

Da Silva, R. J., Fecchio, D., & Barraviera, B. (1996). Antitumor effect of snake venoms. *Journal of Venomous Animals and Toxins, 2*(2), 79–90. https://doi.org/10.1590/S0104-79301996000200002

de Carvalho Porta, L., Fadel, V., D'Arc Campeiro, J., Oliveira, E. B., Godinho, R. O., & Hayashi, M. A. F. (2020). Biophysical and pharmacological characterization of a full-length synthetic analog of the antitumor polypeptide crotamine. *Journal of Molecular Medicine, 98*(11), 1561–1571. https://doi.org/10.1007/S00109-020-01975-Y/FIGURES/5

Dennis, E. A., Cao, J., Hsu, Y. H., Magrioti, V., & Kokotos, G. (2011). Phospholipase A2 enzymes: Physical structure, biological function, disease implication, chemical inhibition, and therapeutic intervention. *Chemical Reviews, 111*(10), 6130–6185. https://doi.org/10.1021/CR200085W

Dingwoke, E. J., Adamude, F. A., Salihu, A., Abubakar, M. S., & Sallau, A. B. (2024). Toxicological analyses of the venoms of Nigerian vipers Echis ocellatus and Bitis arietans. *Tropical Medicine and Health, 52*(1). https://doi.org/10.1186/S41182-024-00581-9

dos Santos, P. K., Altei, W. F., Danilucci, T. M., Lino, R. L. B., Pachane, B. C., Nunes, A. C. C., & Selistre-de-Araujo, H. S. (2020). Alternagin-C (ALT-C), a disintegrin-like protein, attenuates alpha2beta1 integrin and VEGF receptor 2 signaling resulting in angiogenesis inhibition. *Biochimie, 174*, 144–158. https://doi.org/10.1016/J.BIOCHI.2020.04.023

Ebrahim, K., Vatanpour, H., Zare, A., Shirazi, F. H., & Nakhjavani, M. (2016). Anticancer activity a of caspian cobra (Naja naja oxiana) snake venom in Anticancer activity a of caspian cobra (Naja naja oxiana) snake venom in human cancer cell lines via induction of apoptosis human cancer cell lines via induction of apoptosis. *Iranian Journal of Pharmaceutical Research: IJPR, 15.*

Estevão-Costa, M. I., Sanz-Soler, R., Johanningmeier, B., & Eble, J. A. (2018). Snake venom components in medicine: From the symbolic rod of Asclepius to tangible medical research and application. *The International Journal of Biochemistry & Cell Biology, 104*, 94–113. https://doi.org/10.1016/J.BIOCEL.2018.09.011

Feofanov, A. V., Sharonov, G. V., Astapova, M. V., Rodionov, D. I., Utkin, Y. N., & Arseniev, A. S. (2005). Cancer cell injury by cytotoxins from cobra venom is mediated through lysosomal damage. *Biochemical Journal, 390*(Pt 1), 11. https://doi.org/10.1042/BJ20041892

Ferraz, C. R., Arrahman, A., Xie, C., Casewell, N. R., Lewis, R. J., Kool, J., & Cardoso, F. C. (2019). Multifunctional toxins in snake venoms and therapeutic implications: From pain to hemorrhage and necrosis. *Frontiers in Ecology and Evolution, 7*(June), 463257. https://doi.org/10.3389/FEVO.2019.00218/BIBTEX

Ferreira, S. H., Greene, L. J., Alabaster, V. A., Bakhle, Y. S., & Vane, J. R. (1970). Activity of various fractions of bradykinin potentiating factor against angiotensin I converting enzyme. *Nature, 225*(5230), 379–380. https://doi.org/10.1038/225379a0

Fox, J. W., & Serrano, S. M. T. (2008). Insights into and speculations about snake venom metalloproteinase (SVMP) synthesis, folding and disulfide bond formation and their contribution to venom complexity. *The FEBS Journal, 275*(12), 3016–3030. https://doi.org/10.1111/J.1742-4658.2008.06466.X

Fruchart-Gaillard, C., Mourier, G., Marquer, C., Stura, E., Birdsall, N. J. M., & Servent, D. (2008). Different interactions between MT7 toxin and the human muscarinic M1 receptor in its free and N-methylscopolamine-occupied states. *Molecular Pharmacology, 74*(6), 1554–1563. https://doi.org/10.1124/MOL.108.050773

Gamulin, E., Mateljak Lukačević, S., Halassy, B., & Kurtović, T. (2023). Snake antivenoms—toward better understanding of the administration route. *Toxins, 15*(6), 398. https://doi.org/10.3390/TOXINS15060398

Gazerani, P., & Cairns, B. E. (2014). Venom-based biotoxins as potential analgesics. *Expert Review of Neurotherapeutics, 14*(11), 1261–1274. https://doi.org/10.1586/14737175.2014.962518

Girish, V. M., & Kini, R. M. R. (2016). Exactin: A specific inhibitor of factor X activation by extrinsic tenase complex from the venom of hemachatus haemachatus. *Scientific Reports, 6*(1), 1–13. https://doi.org/10.1038/srep32036

Golias, C., Charalabopoulos, A., Stagikas, D., Charalabopoulos, K. A., & Batistatou, A. (2007). The kinin system—bradykinin: Biological effects and clinical implications. Multiple role of the kinin system—bradykinin. *Hippokratia, 11*(3), 124. https://www.ncbi.nlm.nih.gov/pmc/articles/PMC2658795/

Gutiérrez, J. M., Albulescu, L. O., Clare, R. H., Casewell, N. R., Abd El-Aziz, T. M., Escalante, T., & Rucavado, A. (2021). The search for natural and synthetic inhibitors that would complement antivenoms as therapeutics for snakebite envenoming. *Toxins, 13*(7). https://doi.org/10.3390/TOXINS13070451

Gutiérrez, J. M., Calvete, J. J., Habib, A. G., Harrison, R. A., Williams, D. J., & Warrell, D. A. (2017). Snakebite envenoming. *Nature Reviews Disease Primers*, *3*(1), 1–21. https://doi.org/10.1038/nrdp.2017.63

Gutiérrez, J. M., Escalante, T., Rucavado, A., & Herrera, C. (2016). Hemorrhage caused by snake venom metalloproteinases: A journey of discovery and understanding. *Toxins*, *8*(4). https://doi.org/10.3390/TOXINS8040093

Hartman, G. D., Egbertson, M. S., Halczenko, W., Laswell, W. L., Duggan, M. E., Smith, R. L., Naylor, A. M., Manno, P. D., Lynch, R. J., Zhang, G., Chang, C. T. C., & Gould, R. J. (1992). Non-peptide fibrinogen receptor antagonists. 1: Discovery and design of exosite inhibitors. *Journal of Medicinal Chemistry*, *35*(24), 4640–4642. https://doi.org/10.1021/JM00102A020

Herzig, V., Cristofori-Armstrong, B., Israel, M. R., Nixon, S. A., Vetter, I., & King, G. F. (2020). Animal toxins—nature's evolutionary-refined toolkit for basic research and drug discovery. *Biochemical Pharmacology*, *181*. https://doi.org/10.1016/J.BCP.2020.114096

Huynh, T. M., Silva, A., Isbister, G. K., & Hodgson, W. C. (2022). Isolation and characterization of two postsynaptic neurotoxins from Indian cobra (naja naja) venom. *Frontiers in Pharmacology*, *13*. https://doi.org/10.3389/FPHAR.2022.815079

Isbister, G. K., Mirajkar, N., Fakes, K., Brown, S. G. A., & Veerati, P. C. (2020). Phospholipase A2 (PLA2) as an early indicator of envenomation in Australian elapid snakebites (ASP-27). *Biomedicines*, *8*(11), 1–9. https://doi.org/10.3390/BIOMEDICINES8110459

Jakubowski, P., Calvete, J. J., Eble, J. A., Lazarovici, P., & Marcinkiewicz, C. (2013). Identification of inhibitors of α2β1 integrin, members of C-lectin type proteins, in Echis sochureki venom. *Toxicology and Applied Pharmacology*, *269*(1), 34. https://doi.org/10.1016/J.TAAP.2013.03.002

Jimsheleishvili, S., Marwaha, K., & Sherman, A. L. (2023). *Physiology, neuromuscular transmission*. StatPearls. https://www.ncbi.nlm.nih.gov/books/NBK541133/

Jin, H., & Varner, J. (2004). Integrins: Roles in cancer development and as treatment targets. *British Journal of Cancer*, *90*(3), 561–565. https://doi.org/10.1038/sj.bjc.6601576

Johnston, C. I., Brown, S. G. A., O'Leary, M. A., Currie, B. J., Greenberg, R., Taylor, M., Barnes, C., White, J., & Isbister, G. K. (2013). Mulga snake (Pseudechis australis) envenoming: a spectrum of myotoxicity, anticoagulant coagulopathy, haemolysis and the role of early antivenom therapy—Australian snakebite project (ASP-19). *Clinical Toxicology*, *51*(5), 417–424. https://doi.org/10.3109/15563650.2013.787535

Johnston, C. I., Ryan, N. M., O'Leary, M. A., Brown, S. G. A., & Isbister, G. K. (2017). Australian taipan (Oxyuranus spp.) envenoming: Clinical effects and potential benefits of early antivenom therapy—Australian snakebite project (ASP-25). *Clinical Toxicology*, *55*(2), 115–122. https://doi.org/10.1080/15563650.2016.1250903

Junqueira-De-Azevedo, I. L. M., Bastos, C. M. V., Ho, P. L., Luna, M. S., Yamanouye, N., & Casewell, N. R. (2015). Venom-related transcripts from bothrops jararaca tissues provide novel molecular insights into the production and evolution of snake venom. *Molecular Biology and Evolution*, *32*(3), 754–766. https://doi.org/10.1093/MOLBEV/MSU337

Kalita, B., Utkin, Y. N., & Mukherjee, A. K. (2022). Current insights in the mechanisms of cobra venom cytotoxins and their complexes in inducing toxicity: Implications in antivenom therapy. *Toxins*, *14*(12). https://doi.org/10.3390/TOXINS14120839

Kantivan Goswami, P., Samant, M., & Srivastava, R. S. (2014). Snake venom, anti-snake venom & potential of snake venom. *International Journal of Pharmacy and Pharmaceutical Sciences, 6*(5).

Kele, J., Macêdo, A., Fox, J. W., & De Souza Castro, M. (2015). Disintegrins from snake venoms and their applications in cancer research and therapy. *Current Protein and Peptide Science, 16*, 532–548.

Kerkis, A., Kerkis, I., Rádis-Baptista, G., Oliveira, E. B., Vianna-Morgante, A. M., Pereira, L. V., & Yamane, T. (2004). Crotamine is a novel cell-penetrating protein from the venom of rattlesnake Crotalus durissus terrificus. *FASEB Journal: Official Publication of the Federation of American Societies for Experimental Biology, 18*(12), 1407–1409. https://doi.org/10.1096/FJ.03-1459FJE

Kessler, P., Marchot, P., Silva, M., & Servent, D. (2017). The three-finger toxin fold: A multifunctional structural scaffold able to modulate cholinergic functions. *Journal of Neurochemistry, 142*, 7–18. https://doi.org/10.1111/JNC.13975

Kim, S. I., Kim, H. S., & Jang, Y. (2003). *Inhibitory effect of the salmosin gene transferred by cationic liposomes on the progression of B16BL6 tumors*. https://www.researchgate.net/publication/242096015

Kini, R. M., & Doley, R. (2010). Structure, function and evolution of three-finger toxins: Mini proteins with multiple targets. *Toxicon: Official Journal of the International Society on Toxinology, 56*(6), 855–867. https://doi.org/10.1016/J.TOXICON.2010.07.010

Kini, R. M., & Koh, C. Y. (2020). Snake venom three-finger toxins and their potential in drug development targeting cardiovascular diseases. *Biochemical Pharmacology, 181*. https://doi.org/10.1016/J.BCP.2020.114105

Kolvekar, N., Bhattacharya, N., Sarkar, A., & Chakrabarty, D. (2023). How snake venom disintegrins affect platelet aggregation and cancer proliferation. *Toxicon, 221*, 106982. https://doi.org/10.1016/J.TOXICON.2022.106982

Kuo, Y. J., Chung, C. H., & Huang, T. F. (2019). From discovery of snake venom disintegrins to a safer therapeutic antithrombotic agent. *Toxins, 11*(7). https://doi.org/10.3390/TOXINS11070372

Lane, J., O'Leary, M. A., & Isbister, G. K. (2011). Coagulant effects of black snake (Pseudechis spp.) venoms and in vitro efficacy of commercial antivenom. *Toxicon, 58*(3), 239–246. https://doi.org/10.1016/J.TOXICON.2011.05.020

Laustsen, A. H., Karatt-Vellatt, A., Masters, E. W., Arias, A. S., Pus, U., Knudsen, C., Oscoz, S., Slavny, P., Griffiths, D. T., Luther, A. M., Leah, R. A., Lindholm, M., Lomonte, B., María Gutiérrez, J., & Mccafferty, J. (2018). In vivo neutralization of dendrotoxin-mediated neurotoxicity of black mamba venom by oligoclonal human IgG antibodies. *Nature, 9*(3928). https: / / doi.org / 10.1038 / s41467-018-06086-4

Lazarovici, P., Marcinkiewicz, C., & Lelkes, P. I. (2019). From snake venom's disintegrins and C-type lectins to anti-platelet drugs. *Toxins, 11*(303). https://doi.org/10.3390/toxins11050303

Lee, J. M., Song, J. H., & Song, K. H. (2022). A retrospective evaluation of snake envenomation in dogs in South Korea (2004–2021). *Toxins, 14*(8). https://doi.org/10.3390/TOXINS14080565

Liu, C. C., Yang, H., Zhang, L. L., Zhang, Q., Chen, B., & Wang, Y. (2014). Biotoxins for cancer therapy. *Asian Pacific Journal of Cancer Prevention, 15*(12), 4753–4758. https://journal.waocp.org/article_29331.html

Macêdo, J. K. A., Fox, J. W., & Castro, M. de S. (2015). Disintegrins from snake venoms and their applications in cancer research and therapy. *Current Protein & Peptide Science, 16*(6), 532. https://doi.org/10.2174/1389203716666150515125002

Maduwage, K., Buckley, N. A., de Silva, H. J., Lalloo, D. G., & Isbister, G. K. (2015). Snake antivenom for snake venom induced consumption coagulopathy. *The Cochrane Database of Systematic Reviews, 2015*(6). https://doi.org/10.1002/14651858.CD011428.PUB2

Marchot, P., Bourne, Y., Prowse, C. N., Kanter, J. R., Eads, J., Bougis, P. E., & Taylor, P. (1998). Fasciculin inhibition of mouse acetylcholinesterase. *Structure and Function of Cholinesterases and Related Proteins*, 331–338. https://doi.org/10.1007/978-1-4899-1540-5_94

Marcinkiewicz, C., & Kisiel, D. (2003). *Obtustatin: A potent selective inhibitor of 11 integrin in vitro and angiogenesis in vivo1*. https://www.researchgate.net/publication/7362783

Mattiuzzi, C., & Lippi, G. (2019). Current cancer epidemiology. *Journal of Epidemiology and Global Health, 9*(4), 217. https://doi.org/10.2991/JEGH.K.191008.001

Messadi, E. (2023). Snake venom components as therapeutic drugs in ischemic heart disease. *Biomolecules, 13*(10), 1539. https://doi.org/10.3390/BIOM13101539

Miwa, J. M., Freedman, R., & Lester, H. A. (2011). Neural systems governed by nicotinic acetylcholine receptors: Emerging hypotheses. *Neuron, 70*(1), 20–33. https://doi.org/10.1016/J.NEURON.2011.03.014

Morais, V. (2018). Antivenom therapy: Efficacy of premedication for the prevention of adverse reactions. *The Journal of Venomous Animals and Toxins Including Tropical Diseases, 24*(1). https://doi.org/10.1186/S40409-018-0144-0

Murakami, M., Sato, H., & Taketomi, Y. (2020). Updating phospholipase A2 biology. *Biomolecules, 10*(10), 1–33. https://doi.org/10.3390/BIOM10101457

Näreoja, K., Kukkonen, J. P., Rondinelli, S., Toivola, D. M., Meriluoto, J., & Näsman, J. (2011). Adrenoceptor activity of muscarinic toxins identified from mamba venoms. *British Journal of Pharmacology, 164*(2b), 538. https://doi.org/10.1111/J.1476-5381.2011.01468.X

Nasrabadi, N. N., Dounighi, N. M., Ahmadinejad, M., Rabiei, H., Tabarzad, M., Najafi, M., & Vatanpour, H. (2022). Isolation of the anticoagulant and procoagulant fractions of the venom of Iranian endemic echis carinatus. *Iranian Journal of Pharmaceutical Research: IJPR, 21*(1). https://doi.org/10.5812/IJPR-127240

Nguyen, T. T. N., Folch, B., Létourneau, M., Vaudry, D., Truong, N. H., Doucet, N., Chatenet, D., & Fournier, A. (2012). Cardiotoxin-I: An unexpectedly potent insulinotropic agent. *ChemBioChem, 13*(12), 1805–1812. https://doi.org/10.1002/CBIC.201200081

Nirthanan, S., & Gwee, M. C. E. (2004). Three-finger α-neurotoxins and the nicotinic acetylcholine receptor, forty years on. *Journal of Pharmacological Sciences, 94*(1), 1–17. https://doi.org/10.1254/JPHS.94.1

Nys, M., Zarkadas, E., Brams, M., Mehregan, A., Kambara, K., Kool, J., Casewell, N. R., Bertrand, D., Baenziger, J. E., Nury, H., & Ulens, C. (2022). The molecular mechanism of snake short-chain α-neurotoxin binding to muscle-type nicotinic acetylcholine receptors. *Nature Communications, 13*(1). https://doi.org/10.1038/S41467-022-32174-7

Offor, B. C., Muller, B., & Piater, L. A. (2022). A review of the proteomic profiling of African viperidae and elapidae snake venoms and their antivenom neutralisation. *Toxins, 14*(11). https://doi.org/10.3390/TOXINS14110723

Offor, B. C., & Piater, L. A. (2023). Snake venom toxins: Potential anticancer therapeutics. *Journal of Applied Toxicology*. John Wiley and Sons Ltd. https://doi.org/10.1002/JAT.4544

Olaoba, O. T., Karina dos Santos, P., Selistre-de-Araujo, H. S., & Ferreira de Souza, D. H. (2020). Snake venom metalloproteinases (SVMPs): A structure-function update. *Toxicon: X, 7*. https://doi.org/10.1016/J.TOXCX.2020.100052

Oliveira, A. L., Viegas, M. F., da Silva, S. L., Soares, A. M., Ramos, M. J., & Fernandes, P. A. (2022). The chemistry of snake venom and its medicinal potential. *Nature Reviews Chemistry, 6*(7), 451–469. https://doi.org/10.1038/s41570-022-00393-7

Osipov, A., & Utkin, Y. (2023). What are the neurotoxins in hemotoxic snake venoms? *International Journal of Molecular Sciences, 24*(3). https://doi.org/10.3390/IJMS24032919

Park, E. J., Myint, P. K., Ito, A., Appiah, M. G., Darkwah, S., Kawamoto, E., & Shimaoka, M. (2020). Integrin-ligand interactions in inflammation, cancer, and metabolic disease: Insights into the multifaceted roles of an emerging ligand irisin. *Frontiers in Cell and Developmental Biology, 8*, 588066. https://doi.org/10.3389/FCELL.2020.588066/BIBTEX

Pawlak, J., Mackessy, S. P., Fry, B. G., Bhatia, M., Mourier, G., Fruchart-Gaillard, C., Servent, D., Ménez, R., Stura, E., Ménez, A., & Kini, R. M. (2006). Denmotoxin, a three-finger toxin from the colubrid snake boiga dendrophila (Mangrove Catsnake) with bird-specific activity. *Journal of Biological Chemistry, 281*(39), 29030–29041. https://doi.org/10.1074/JBC.M605850200

Pruksaphon, K., Yuvaniyama, J., & Ratanabanangkoon, K. (2022). Immunogenicity of snake α-neurotoxins and the CD4 T cell epitopes. *Toxicon, 214*, 136–144. https://doi.org/10.1016/J.TOXICON.2022.05.009

Rivel, M., Solano, D., Herrera, M., Vargas, M., Villalta, M., Segura, Á., Arias, A. S., León, G., & Gutiérrez, J. M. (2016). Pathogenesis of dermonecrosis induced by venom of the spitting cobra, Naja nigricollis: An experimental study in mice. *Toxicon: Official Journal of the International Society on Toxinology, 119*, 171–179. https://doi.org/10.1016/J.TOXICON.2016.06.006

Roffi, M., & Mukherjee, D. (2008). Platelet glycoprotein IIb/IIIa receptor inhibitors—end of an era? *European Heart Journal, 29*(4), 429–431. https://doi.org/10.1093/EURHEARTJ/EHM624

Rossetto, O., & Montecucco, C. (2008). Presynaptic neurotoxins with enzymatic activities. *Handbook of Experimental Pharmacology, 184*(184), 129–170. https://doi.org/10.1007/978-3-540-74805-2_6

Sanchez, E. F., Flores-Ortiz, R. J., Alvarenga, V. G., & Eble, J. A. (2017). Direct fibrinolytic snake venom metalloproteinases affecting hemostasis: Structural, biochemical features and therapeutic potential. *Toxins, 9*(12). https://doi.org/10.3390/TOXINS9120392

Saviola, A. J., Modahl, C. M., & Mackessy, S. P. (2015). Disintegrins of Crotalus simus tzabcan venom: Isolation, characterization and evaluation of the cytotoxic and anti-adhesion activities of tzabcanin, a new RGD disintegrin. *Biochimie, 116*, 92–102. https://doi.org/10.1016/J.BIOCHI.2015.07.005

Serrano, S. M. T. (2013). The long road of research on snake venom serine proteinases. *Toxicon, 62*, 19–26. https://doi.org/10.1016/J.TOXICON.2012.09.003

Sica, D. A. (2005). Angiotensin-converting enzyme inhibitors' side effects—physiologic and non-physiologic considerations. *The Journal of Clinical Hypertension, 7*(Suppl 8), 17. https://doi.org/10.1111/J.1524-6175.2005.04556.X

Silva, A., Hodgson, W. C., & Isbister, G. K. (2017). Antivenom for neuromuscular paralysis resulting from snake envenoming. *Toxins, 9*(4). https://doi.org/10.3390/TOXINS9040143

Silva, A., Maduwage, K., Buckley, N. A., Lalloo, D. G., de Silva, H. J., & Isbister, G. K. (2017). Antivenom for snake venom-induced neuromuscular paralysis. *The Cochrane Database of Systematic Reviews*, *2017*(3). https://doi.org/10.1002/14651858.CD012604

Simoes-Silva, R., Alfonso, J., Gomez, A., Holanda, R. J., Sobrinho, J. C., Zaqueo, K. D., Moreira-Dill, L. S., Kayano, A. M., Grabner, F. P., da Silva, S. L., Almeida, J. R., Stabeli, R. G., Zuliani, J. P., & Soares, A. M. (2018). Snake venom, a natural library of new potential therapeutic molecules: Challenges and current perspectives. *Current Pharmaceutical Biotechnology*, *19*(4), 308–335. https://doi.org/10.2174/1389201019666180620111025

Slagboom, J., Kool, J., Harrison, R. A., & Casewell, N. R. (2017). Haemotoxic snake venoms: their functional activity, impact on snakebite victims and pharmaceutical promise. *British Journal of Haematology*, *177*(6), 947. https://doi.org/10.1111/BJH.14591

Sung, H., Ferlay, J., Siegel, R. L., Laversanne, M., Soerjomataram, I., Jemal, A., & Bray, F. (2021). Global cancer statistics 2020: GLOBOCAN estimates of incidence and mortality worldwide for 36 cancers in 185 countries. *CA: A Cancer Journal for Clinicians*, *71*(3), 209–249. https://doi.org/10.3322/CAAC.21660

Takada, Y., Ye, X., & Simon, S. (2007). The integrins. *Genome Biology*, *8*(5), 1–9. https://doi.org/10.1186/GB-2007-8-5-215/FIGURES/4

Takeda, S., Takeya, H., & Iwanaga, S. (2012). Snake venom metalloproteinases: Structure, function and relevance to the mammalian ADAM/ADAMTS family proteins. *Biochimica et Biophysica Acta*, *1824*(1), 164–176. https://doi.org/10.1016/J.BBAPAP.2011.04.009

Tan, C. H. (2022). Snake venomics: Fundamentals, recent updates, and a look to the next decade. *Toxins*, *14*(4). https://doi.org/10.3390/TOXINS14040247

Tasima, L. J., Serino-Silva, C., Hatakeyama, D. M., Nishiduka, E. S., Tashima, A. K., Sant'Anna, S. S., Grego, K. F., De Morais-Zani, K., & Tanaka-Azevedo, A. M. (2020). Crotamine in Crotalus durissus: Distribution according to subspecies and geographic origin, in captivity or nature. *The Journal of Venomous Animals and Toxins Including Tropical Diseases*, *26*. https://doi.org/10.1590/1678-9199-JVATITD-2019-0053

Tasoulis, T., & Isbister, G. K. (2022). A current perspective on snake venom composition and constituent protein families. *Archives of Toxicology*, *97*(1), 133–153. https://doi.org/10.1007/S00204-022-03420-0

Teixeira, S. C., da Silva, M. S., Gomes, A. A. S., Moretti, N. S., Lopes, D. S., Ferro, E. A. V., & Rodrigues, V. D. M. (2022). Panacea within a Pandora's box: The antiparasitic effects of phospholipases A2 (PLA2s) from snake venoms. *Trends in Parasitology*, *38*(1), 80–94. https://doi.org/10.1016/J.PT.2021.07.004

Thangam, R., Gunasekaran, P., Kaveri, K., Sridevi, G., Sundarraj, S., Paulpandi, M., & Kannan, S. (2012). A novel disintegrin protein from Naja naja venom induces cytotoxicity and apoptosis in human cancer cell lines in vitro. *Process Biochemistry*, *47*(8), 1243–1249. https://doi.org/10.1016/j.procbio.2012.04.020

Ullah, A., Masood, R., Ali, I., Ullah, K., Ali, H., Akbar, H., & Betzel, C. (2018). Thrombin-like enzymes from snake venom: Structural characterization and mechanism of action. *International Journal of Biological Macromolecules*, *114*, 788–811. https://doi.org/10.1016/J.IJBIOMAC.2018.03.164

Vidya, V., Achar, R. R., Himathi, M. U., Akshita, N., Kameshwar, V. H., Byrappa, K., & Ramadas, D. (2021). Venom peptides—a comprehensive translational perspective in pain management. *Current Research in Toxicology, 2*, 329. https://doi.org/10.1016/J.CRTOX.2021.09.001

White, J. (2005). Snake venoms and coagulopathy. *Toxicon: Official Journal of the International Society on Toxinology, 45*(8), 951–967. https://doi.org/10.1016/J.TOXICON.2005.02.030

Xie, C., Slagboom, J., Albulescu, L. O., Bruyneel, B., Still, K. B. M., Vonk, F. J., Somsen, G. W., Casewell, N. R., & Kool, J. (2020). Antivenom neutralization of coagulopathic snake venom toxins assessed by bioactivity profiling using nanofractionation analytics. *Toxins, 12*(1), 53. https://doi.org/10.3390/TOXINS12010053

Xie, Q., Tang, N., Lin, Y., Wang, X., Lin, X., & Lin, J. (2013). Recombinant adenovirus snake venom cystatin inhibits the growth, invasion, and metastasis of B16F10 cells in vitro and in vivo. *Melanoma Research, 23*(6), 444–451. https://doi.org/10.1097/CMR.0000000000000031

Yang, D. C., Deuis, J. R., Dashevsky, D., Dobson, J., Jackson, T. N. W., Brust, A., Xie, B., Koludarov, I., Debono, J., Hendrikx, I., Hodgson, W. C., Josh, P., Nouwens, A., Baillie, G. J., Bruxner, T. J. C., Alewood, P. F., Lim, K. K. P., Frank, N., Vetter, I., & Fry, B. G. (2016). The snake with the scorpion's sting: Novel three-finger toxin sodium channel activators from the venom of the long-glanded blue coral snake (Calliophis bivirgatus). *Toxins, 8*(10), 303. https://doi.org/10.3390/TOXINS8100303

Zambelli, V. O., & Hösch, N. G. (2023). Neurotoxicity and myotoxicity of snake venom-derived phospholipase A2. *Phospholipases in Physiology and Pathology, 7*, 153–166. https://doi.org/10.1016/B978-0-443-21800-2.00012-9

Section 3

Biotoxin Detection in Food

15

The Mode of Transmission of Biotoxins to Humans

Abraham Olufemi Asuku, Gbonjubola Oyinlola Ogungbanagbe, Asiat Na'Allah, Isaiah Woru Sabinari, and Salam Babatunde Saliu

15.1 Introduction

15.1.1 Definition of Biotoxins

Biotoxins can be referred to as natural materials produced by bacteria, plants, or animals and have been shown to have a pronounced effect on the human system following exposure. This exposure can be in various forms such through oral or nasal contact or contact with contaminated surfaces, which could result in multiple signs and symptoms. All these depend on the intensity and kind of toxins the individual has been exposed to (Parak et al., 2024). It should be known that these organisms produce biotoxins to defend (Janik et al., 2019).

Most of these biotoxins have detrimental effects, especially on the neurological system, such as preventing acetylcholine release or interrupting nerve impulse conduction. One major factor about these toxins is their inability to proliferate and their lack of contagiousness. This makes them stand out from similar infections (Zhang et al., 2014). They also have a substantial role to play in society, as some of these toxins are associated with natural intoxication, as well as being causative agents in many cases of food poisoning, such as botulinum neurotoxins (Dorner and Rummel, 2015). What makes them fatal is the amount absorbed into the human system, since a lethal dosage has been defined as the quantity needed to kill half of a set of experiment subjects (particularly rodents) (Janik et al., 2019).

DOI: 10.1201/9781003500605-18

15.2 Types of Biotoxins

15.2.1 Classification and Examples of Common Biotoxins

Biotoxins can be classified based on their sources, chemical nature, and mode of action. However, some biotoxins are more commonly discussed, and those will be focused on in this chapter.

15.2.1.1 Marine Biotoxins

Marine biotoxins are classified as natural toxins and are generated by marine species such as algae, dinoflagellates, bacteria, and aquatic creatures such as jellyfish and cone snails. They tend to build in sea animals such as shellfish, which humans regularly eat, and can pose a serious health concern (Costa et al., 2019). While seafood can serve as a great source of nutrients, it can also act as a breeding ground for the growth of diseases and germs, and the biotoxins formed can accumulate and be metabolized through the food chain. Additionally, they can lead to illnesses that are referred to as "bio intoxication" (Morabito et al., 2017). This intoxication can lead to a wide range of syndromes that include paralytic, diarrhetic, and even neurotoxic poisonings, with paralytic shellfish poisoning (PSP) being the most common (Morabito et al., 2017). Some of these biotoxins include saxitoxin and gonyautoxin (both found in clams), domoic acid, okadaic acid, pectenotoxin, yessotoxin, brevetoxin, and many more (Visciano et al., 2016).

15.2.1.2 Plant Toxins

These are toxins naturally produced by plants. Their main goal is as a form of protection for plants, deterring them from herbivores. Due to this, the ingestion of these toxins in humans could have harmful effects. A well-known toxin is ricin, which is a form of phytotoxin. This is commonly found in castor beans and is known for its biomedical uses and its toxic characteristics (Roxas Duncan, 2011). Its level of toxicity depends on the mode of exposure; for example, intravenous exposure can cause the formation of lesions in the spleen or kidney. For oral ingestion, the gastrointestinal tract (GIT) is severely damaged, and inhalation mostly affects the respiratory tract (Whitfield et al., 2017; Franke et al., 2019).

Cannabinoids can also have toxic attributes. Although they are known for their therapeutic effects as analgesics and appetite stimulants, a high dosage can lead to several neurological effects such as dizziness and drowsiness and can lead to seizures and comas. It can also affect the GIT and the cardiovascular system (CVS) (Malik et al., 2020; Breijyeh et al., 2021). These effects are, however, dose dependent and also depend on their mode of administration. A modest amount might result in temporary memory degradation or lack of focus, while a greater dosage can have more significant consequences. Thankfully most of these effects are short lived and may not cause lasting damage to the body (Boadu et al., 2018).

15.2.1.3 Viral Toxins

Certain viruses generate poisons or proteins, which may contribute to disease development. A good example is the toxin NS1, which is implicated in the dengue disease pathogenesis (Lebeau et al., 2021). Dengue fever is known as one of the most serious mosquito-borne illnesses, after malaria. It is a public health concern, with the dengue virus (DENV) and host factors playing important roles in its severity (Lebeau et al., 2021). This virus has a specific protein known as the DENV NS1 protein, which contributes to vascular leakage, a known sign of dengue severity. In this case, it disrupts the endothelium glycocalyx layer, which contributes to barrier failure and plasma leakage (Glasner et al., 2017). It also increases the production of cytokines, can lead to vascular problems (Beatty et al., 2015), and plays a role in complement blockage techniques of immune escape (Glasner et al., 2018), making it a deadly viral toxin.

Another example is the NSP4 from rotavirus, which is frequently the root of deadly intestinal inflammation, especially in younger people. (Troeger et al., 2018). It affects the epithelial cells by inhibiting their secretory pathway, changing their cytoskeleton architecture, and also activating the plasma membrane permeability, leading to diarrhea-induced complications (Tohmé and Delgui, 2021)

15.2.1.4 Animal Toxins

Animal toxins, more commonly known as their "venom", have been fine-tuned throughout many centuries of evolution by taking advantage of their victims' biological complexities to produce toxins that target specific systems of the latter, to produce varying results, like incapacitating, breaking down the defense, and even leading to more fatal outcomes (Chen et al., 2018; Herzig et al., 2020). This works by targeting various enzymes, receptors, and even ion channels of the neurological, circulatory, or musculoskeletal systems. Some of the animals known for their deadly venoms include snakes, spiders, snails, and scorpions (Fry et al., 2009). Some of these toxins include neurotoxins (Rossetto and Montecucco, 2019), dendrotoxins (Kularatne and Senanayake, 2014), cytotoxins (Tkachev et al., 2020), cardiotoxins (Averin et al., 2021), and more that can be found in these creatures.

15.3 Modes of Transmission

15.3.1 Direct Contact Transmission

This occurs when toxins are transferred from the host or source to humans through physical touch. This can be through skin contact, animal stings, or contact with contaminated objects. Botulinum toxin, generated by *Clostridium botulinum*, can be seen in contaminated edibles such as canned vegetables and fruits. It spreads through the circulation and subsequently inhibits the production of acetylcholine, which can be irreversible if not treated promptly. Botulinum can also be transmitted through contaminated objects and surfaces. Its exposure can cause paralysis ranging from the eyelids (ptosis) to the muscles that govern speech and damage other organs such as the bladder, resulting in urine retention (Anderson, 2012).

Most animals with venomous or toxins "inject" them into their victims by introducing the substance deep into the target tissues, using a structure specific for this purpose such as a bee stinger or a snake's fangs (Nelsen et al., 2013). Some animals such as the colubrid snakes "chew" the toxins with teeth that are grooved rather than hollow, and the toxins penetrate the skin via diffusion and surface tension (Rajabizadeh et al., 2020). Termites secrete toxins from their frontal glands with their mandibles (Oliveira Alves and Filho, 2017). Spitting cobras are known to subdue their prey and inflict damage by "spraying" their toxins, aiming at the victim's face and eyes (Jalink, 2020), and the *Lonomia* caterpillars have stiff hairs that can penetrate tissue and deliver their venom (González et al., 2023).

15.4 Ingestion

This is a common mode of transmission for biotoxins. This could be through contaminated food, improper food handling, or marine toxins. One of them is aflatoxins, which are extremely hazardous and have been linked to various foods, including fruits that are dried and groundnuts, as well as maize. These fungi are known to grow in tropical and subtropical regions and are unfortunately hard to eliminate from contaminated food due to their heat-resistant nature (Mahato et al., 2019). Repeated exposure results in chronic disorders such as primary liver cancer and other forms of cancer in other organs such as bone, blood, kidney, and more. They are also thought to have a role in illnesses such as micronutrient malabsorption, kwashiorkor, protein synthesis, and metabolic enzyme activity (Benkerroum, 2020).

Another toxin transferred by eating is saxitoxin, which is widely known due to being involved in paralytic shellfish poisoning (PSP). Large dosages are known to be lethal, but low dosages have the potential to impact neurodevelopment by acting voltage-gated sodium channels (VGSCs). This transmission mostly occurs in cultures that take a lot of seafood over long periods, as they may pick untested seafood (O'Neill et al., 2016). Victims of saxitoxin-contaminated shellfish have gastrointestinal pain or neurological manifestations within hours, varying from harmless circumoral paresthesias and limb tingling to dysphagia, ataxia, and mental abnormalities. A lot of patients describe the feeling of "suspension" or separation. Tachycardia and hypertension have been reported. Although the majority of people recover without treatment, weakness may swiftly result in respiratory failure and asphyxiation. Currently, there are no remedies for saxitoxin (Hurley et al., 2014).

15.5 Inhalation

Biotoxins can be aerosolized, forming small particles or droplets that become airborne. This can occur spontaneously, such as when fungus spores go airborne. When a person inhales polluted air, biotoxin particles accumulate in the respiratory system. Depending on their size, particles might become stuck in the upper respiratory tract or go further into the lungs. From there, they spread throughout the body, possibly reaching target organs (Janik et al., 2019). An excellent example is ricin, which is a type 2 ribosome-inactivating protein found in castor oil seeds (Falach et al., 2016). It enters cells via endocytosis, where it attaches to oligosaccharides or mannose receptors on the cell membrane. Inhaled ricin poisoning mostly causes pulmonary harm, which includes severe interstitial pneumonia, which occurs with local pro-inflammatory cytokine release, alveolar and perivascular edema, extensive neutrophil infiltration, bleeding, and widespread airway epithelial necrosis affecting all pulmonary lobes. Ultimately, inundation in the lungs causes trouble breathing and mortality. These modifications might be summarized as acute lung damage with medical symptoms comparable to symptoms of acute respiratory distress syndrome (Stoll et al., 2023).

Anthrax is a zoonotic occupational illness produced by *Bacillus anthracis*. It occurs in humans at random and with limited frequency, and no examples of direct transfer of the causative agent from human to human have been documented. However, infection is acquired by interaction with infected livestock or contaminated animal-derived products (Huang et al., 2015). Clinical manifestations of anthrax can be classified under three categories according to the mechanism of transmission: cutaneous, respiratory, and gastrointestinal. The respiratory variant of anthrax is regarded to be the most dangerous since it can induce fatal septicemia. Inhalation anthrax is produced by breathing aerosolized spores and is associated with the processing of infected animals' wool, skins, and hair. They can have a biphasic display, beginning with a mild illness including coughing, fever, and tiredness, then resulting in a rapid development of pneumonia, severe hypoxia, and dyspnea (Bower et al., 2022).

15.6 Vector-Borne Transmission

This is the spread of infectious pathogens via a carrier, usually an insect like a mosquito, tick, or flea. Several biotoxins can enter the body via this route, most commonly through the bite of an infected vector. The tick-borne encephalitis virus (TBEV) corresponds within the *Flavivirus* genus and the family Flaviviridae. It is closely linked to other tick-borne flaviviruses, such as the sheep louping sick virus and the human Omsk hemorrhagic fever virus (Michelitsch et al., 2019).

TBEV is spread by saliva when hard ticks feed. The virus replicates initially at the tick bite site and then infects the adjacent lymph glands that drain the area. Other organs associated with the reticulo-endothelial system, such as the spleen, bone marrow, and liver, may become polluted, resulting in encroachment of the brain and spinal cord. This causes inflammation and degradation, as well as cellular dysfunction of neurons (Pustijanac et al., 2023). Throughout their lives, these ticks graze on a variety of small animals, birds, and big mammals. However, tiny rodents are the principal animal reservoirs for the virus and humans are unintentional hosts who have a small part in epidemiology (Phipps and Johnson, 2022).

The infection, Leishmaniasis, is brought on by an intracellular parasite that is transmitted to people by being bitten by a sandfly, namely *Lutzomyia* and *Phlebotomus*. Particularly, the transmission was characterized as an experimental mistake (Hoyos et al., 2016). It is one of the seven most significant tropical diseases, posing a severe global health threat with a wide range of clinical symptoms and a possibly deadly consequence. The causal agent is an obligate unicellular protozoan with two life stages: a promastigote, which serves as the infection vector and feeds on the vertebrate host's blood. Its second stage is an amastigote, which dwells in the host's phagocytic cells (Wetzel et al., 2016). This can be identified by a localized increase in temperature as well as edema. An erythematous, innocuous papule forms at the location of the infection. After 2 days, it transforms into a vesicle, then a pustule, and once it ruptures, either by itself or as a result of scratching, it produces a circular ulcer. These ulcers can last anywhere from 3–5 months to 15–20 years. If the lesion is not secondarily infected, it does not cause pain. In some cases, lymphadenopathy, poor general health, lymphedema, and fever may occur. Once the mucosae of the nasopharynx and oropharynx are involved, painful nodules might induce blocked airways. Such medical variety is especially challenging to treat; it has no spontaneous remission, so the sickness can persist for up to 20 years (Torres-Guerrero et al., 2017).

15.7 Water-Borne Transmission

These are poisons that can spread through polluted water. Microorganisms (cyanobacteria), once referred to as blue-green algae, are Gram-negative bacteria that inhabit terrestrial as well as aquatic settings. Their growth is influenced by chemical and physical variables. In marine settings, calm, sunny weather combined with the availability of nutrients such as nitrogen and phosphorus can result in huge cyanobacterial blooms. Given that cyanobacteria may create a wide range of bioactive compounds, including cyanotoxins, whatever toxin naturally present inside such cyanobacterial cells may accumulate, reaching amounts that could damage people and animals (Svirčev et al., 2019). While livestock represents the majority of known cyanobacterial intoxications, cyanobacterial toxins have caused disease and mortality in human populations, including outbreaks of gastroenteritis, hepatomegaly, and pneumonia-like symptoms (Metcalf et al., 2021). One hundred people died at a hemodialysis clinic, and more than a quarter were determined to have been exposed to liver-damaging microcystins by intravenous infusion of water that had been poorly cleansed and had originated from a lake identified as having cyanobacterial blooms. During the poisoning incident, a few people who came into contact with the improperly disinfected water complained of neurological symptoms such as tinnitus, vertigo, fainting, dizziness, and vision issues (Jochimsen et al., 1998).

15.8 Factors Influencing Transmission

Climate change, land use and agricultural practices, and food safety and handling are various factors that could impact the spreading of biotoxins in humans. Temperature, precipitation, and humidity all play important roles in the transmission and survival of zoonotic illnesses, and shifts in these environmental variables due to warming temperatures may aid in their spread and survival. Climate change may impact existing infections or create new ones in food due to changes in animal husbandry, transmission, and biotoxin survival, among other factors. Elevated temperatures can accelerate the growth of foodborne bacterial pathogens, leading to an increase in biotoxin cases and may lead to increased demand for irrigation water, raising the danger of biotoxin contamination from manure and sewage (Herrera et al., 2016). It may also greatly impact more than half of all infectious illnesses. This is not just true for currently existing infectious agents as these changes also encourage the formation of novel infectious agents and the reintroduction of previously repressed diseases (Mora et al., 2022). Examples of this include *Campylobacter enteritis, Salmonella,* and *Vibrio,* which are associated with increased temperature and humidity (David et al., 2017; Butsch et al., 2023; Food and Agriculture Organization of the United Nations and World Health Organization, 2020), and parasites such as *Cryptosporidia* and *Giardia* have been linked to extreme weather changes such as flooding (Cacciò and Chalmers, 2016).

Human-induced land use is one of the key causes of a variety of infectious disease epidemics. Land use changes include forest destruction, development of roads, agricultural encroachment, dam construction, irrigation, wetland alteration, mining, urbanization, and other activities. These changes, consequently, cause a cascade of occurrences that accelerate the onset of infectious illnesses (Paul et al., 2018). Globally, there is a strong link between land usage and malaria transmission. In Africa, urbanization has been shown to reduce Anopheles mosquito reproduction. However, varied communities with insufficient environmental management and peri-urban agriculture provide optimal habitats for mosquitos, resulting in increased spreading of malaria because of bigger adult Anopheles populations as well as higher malaria outbreaks compared to other agricultural regions (Chaves et al., 2020).

Food additives are used to increase food's technical performance while preserving its sensory characteristics and are applied throughout the manufacturing, preparation, processing, shape, packing, shipping, and storage. Modern food production requires using chemicals under specific conditions and for acknowledged reasons. Additives are classed depending on their functional capabilities, including colors, preservation agents, antioxidants, emulsifiers, stabilizing agents, regulators, thickeners, gelling agents, acidity, flavor enhancers, sweeteners, polishing agents, modified starches, and moisture retention for packaging and sequestering (Krivohlavek, 2018). Food-contact materials and objects consist of both organic and inorganic macromolecular components. Unwanted migration from food packaging poses a concern to food quality and safety. Over 3000 chemicals may have an impact on food safety which include foodborne diseases (norovirus, *Campylobacter* sp., Salmonella). It can come into touch with food at various phases of the product's storage, preparation, and transportation (Hald et al., 2016).

15.9 Case Studies

15.9.1 Historical Outbreaks

Throughout time, there have been several reports of pathogens or biotoxin outbreaks spreading among humans and taking lives with some tracing back to the Middle Ages. An example is what is known as "ergotism", or ergot poisoning. The substance ergot is a fungal illness caused by the parasite *Claviceps purpurea* that results in black kernels on plants. Consuming infected rye grains with ergot alkaloids, such as contaminated rye bread, has now been known to lead to ergotism (Píchová et al., 2018). Ergot has been suggested to have been the source of strange outbreaks in Europe during the Middle Ages. Symptoms may include mass hysterias and psychosis, which are aggravated by a persistent fear of vengeance or demonic participation. Medical historians understand that ergotism may have caused widespread psychoses and convulsions (Grzybowski et al., 2021). Saint Anthony's fire was also commonly associated with ergotism, although it might also be caused by erysipelas, wound infections, plague, scurvy, or smallpox (Cervellin et al., 2021).

Ciguatera poisoning (CP) is the most frequent not transmissible seafood-borne illness in the world, with an estimated 10,000 to 50,000 cases per year. The earliest documented occurrence of CP occurred in 1601 on the south coast of Mauritius Island. Subsequently, in 1748, when Admiral Boscawen's squadron arrived on the remote Island of Rodrigues, it emerged that 1500 individuals passed away from eating poisoned fish. In 1774, a captain saw a fish poisoning occurrence while anchored in Vanuatu (Pacific Ocean), which was subsequently identified as CP. The first CP occurrence in the Caribbean occurred in 1862 along the Mexican coast, after a French crew traveling into the Gulf of Mexico became ill following consuming parrot fish (Chinain et al., 2021). The yearly incidence rate in French Polynesia was approximately 18/10,000 in 2016 (Yang et al., 2016). From 1996 to 2006, the annual incidence in the French West Indies was 0.3/10,000 and 0.2/10,000 in Guadeloupe and Martinique, respectively (Friedman et al., 2017). But significantly more severe cases have been reported in the same time frame in Caribbean countries like the English Virgin Islands, Montserrat, and Antigua that border the French West Indies. Fewer than 20% of occurrences are thought to be reported (Boucaud-Maitre et al., 2018). Eating Mexican flag cabrilla or starry grouper (*Epinephelus labriformis*) was connected to 25 cases of CP in 1992. In 1993, there was another CFP outbreak when seven crew members of a tuna ship became drunk after consuming garropa (*Epinephelus* sp.) and cabrilla (*Mycteroperca* sp.). Fishermen on El Pardito Island and Punta San Evaristo reported five cases of poisoning following the consumption of fish liver between 1993 and 1997. Diarrhea; nausea; pains in the hands, feet, eyes, and belly; headache; fatigue; desquamation surrounding the lips, brows, and hands; tongue and lip paralysis; and, in one case, convulsions were among the symptoms (Núñez-Vázquez et al., 2018).

Aflatoxicosis (AFB) is a fungal toxin caused by *Aspergillus* spp. that is primarily ignored globally and is caused by eating food tainted with aflatoxins. Up to 40% of instances of carcinoma of the liver in Africa and 28.2% worldwide are caused by the sickness. Major cases usually start with low-grade fever, anorexia, and malaise and proceed to potentially fatal acute hepatitis with convulsions, vomiting, abdominal pain, lung congestion, and ultimately death (Kinyenje et al., 2023). In nations like Tanzania and Kenya, the impact of contaminants like aflatoxin in goods has been significant, leading to acute and chronic exposure of the populace. The issue of aflatoxins particularly in Kenya has drawn attention from various sectors worldwide (Mutegi et al., 2018). Kenya saw two significant human aflatoxicosis outbreaks: the first in 1981, resulting in 12 fatalities, and the second in the 2004–2005 harvest season. Both incidents took place in Kenya's lower east. Aflatoxin B1-lysine adduct concentrations in blood, elevated dietary aflatoxin levels, and positive hepatitis B surface antigen titers have all been connected to hepatocellular carcinoma and aflatoxicosis in Kenyans (Wambui et al., 2016). Tanzania has documented three big incidents in recent years: 2016, 2017, and 2019, with the most recent in 2023 being one of the worst cases (Wuiya et al., 2022). The present epidemic happened over the same season as prior outbreaks, with the only variation being the location. The regions were defined by activities and meteorological conditions promoting the *Aspergillus* fungus's growth. These include maize as a common main diet, significant rains and warm temperatures, and past reports of aflatoxicosis epidemics. Due to the weakened human immune system and decreased resistance to aflatoxin exposure, chronic illness, chronic medication use, and chronic alcohol intake have all been associated with a greater chance of aflatoxicosis (Kinyenje et al., 2023).

15.10 Mechanism of Action

15.10.1 Effect on Human Physiology

Depending on the kind and degree of exposure, biotoxins may include a variety of consequences on how the human body functions once they are absorbed. Saxitoxins damage peripheral nerves, which results in signs associated with shellfish poisoning such as tingling or numbness around the lips. The local absorption of poisons through the buccal mucous membranes is the source of these symptoms. Then, these sensations extended to the neck and face. Frequent signs and symptoms include headaches, nausea, vomiting, diarrhea, stinging in the toes and fingertips, and occasionally temporary blindness (Pratheepa and Vasconcelos, 2017). Most symptoms appear quickly and may last for many days. Severe cases include paraesthesia in the legs and arms; motor weakness; giddiness; confused speech; and cerebellar symptoms such as ataxia, motor incoordination, and dysmetria. Constriction around the neck is the first sign of respiratory problems. Severe poisoning can cause profound muscle paralysis, breathing difficulties, and death within a day after consumption (Morabito et al., 2017). Domoic acid is an excitatory amino acid, neurotransmitter, and neurotoxic to the brain and spinal cord because of its effects on excitatory amino acid receptors as well as synaptic transmission. It works in the same way as kainic acid. Memory loss and gastrotoxicity come from the increased vulnerability of the CA1 and CA3 areas of the hippocampus, which are in charge of learning and memory processing (Radad et al., 2018).

The primary targets of brevetoxins have been shown to be voltage-dependent Na^+ channels. By lowering the action potential threshold and delaying channel closure, these toxins prevent neuronal transmission by increasing the conductance of Na^+ ions and prolonging the depolarization of nerve cells. The impact causes many symptoms, including gastrointestinal and neurological issues (Turner et al., 2015). Within a few hours to a few hours, symptoms such as numbness, tingling, and paraesthesias of the lips, face, and extremities; bronchoconstriction; convulsions; paralysis; diarrhea; vomiting; nausea; reversal of heat and cold sensations; arrhythmias; hypotension; and paralysis may appear (Pierre et al., 2018). Suppression of nerve and muscle transmission causes skeletal tissue and muscle damage in the respiratory system, gastrointestinal tract, and diaphragm, leading to tetrodotoxin poisoning. After intake, toxic effects may manifest within 10 to 45 minutes. While some patients with sudden poisoning may require several days to fully recover, most recover with no lasting effects (Lago et al., 2015). In addition to severe respiratory failure, hypoxia, hypotension, bradycardia, cardiac dysrhythmias, lingual numbness, generalized flaccid paralysis, early motor paralysis, incoordination, slurred speech, aphonia, and fixed/dilated pupils are among the acute symptoms. Both cardiac collapse and respiratory failure are the causes of death in lethal circumstances (Vilariño et al., 2018).

15.11 Target Organs and Systems

The brain and spinal cord, lungs, heart, kidneys, and other organs are only a few of the body parts that biotoxins can affect in different ways. These effects can be specific to a form of biotoxin or could be a common indicator of the effects of these toxins. As most of the toxins discussed had a focus on their role in the nervous system, other parts of the human body will be discussed in this section, such as the hepatic system. Aflatoxins can harm various organs, including the liver, and have been identified as a major contributor to the pathogenesis of liver cirrhosis and hepatocellular carcinoma, with reports linking aflatoxin-contaminated foods to varying degrees of liver injury, including cirrhosis (Mekuria et al., 2020). The damaging impact of aflatoxins on the liver is associated with their activation of metabolism into the free radical AFB1-exo-8,9-epoxide (AFBO) by cytochrome P450 (CYP450) enzymes, which leads to the production of ROS, including superoxide anion, hydroxyl radical (HO), and per hydroxyl radical (HOO–). An imbalance between insufficient antioxidant defenses and excessive ROS formation can lead to oxidative stress, which can harm biological components in cellular systems, including DNA, lipids, and proteins (Saad-Hussein et al., 2019).

Non-alcoholic fatty liver disease (NAFLD) progression has been associated with microcystins. The study discovered that low doses of microcystins given intraperitoneally or orally altered the plasma of exposed animals' liver lipid content, increased obesity, and oxidative stress markers including superoxide dismutase and catalase in addition to glutathione levels (Zhang et al., 2015). According to a different study, long-term low-dose oral exposition to microcystins decreased the longevity rate and increased hepatic damage by causing excess fat deposition in hepatocytes, even at 2.5–4.5 times lower than acceptable limits. Additionally, it was shown that modest dosages of the toxin enhanced the phosphorylation pattern of proteins connected to development, inflammation, and the immune response cycle, as well as genes linked to oxidative stress, cholestasis, and hepatotoxicity (Lad et al., 2022). Microcystins are additionally demonstrated to impact the GI tract, which is where the toxin accumulates the most. The small intestine absorbs microcystins primarily, which results in inflammation, ROS generation, and intestinal death. The duodenum, jejunum, and ileum of mice were examined in this study to examine the harmful effects of intraperitoneal microcystin administration on these GI tracts. The results showed that the apoptotic index was substantially elevated in every region of the small intestine shortly after exposure and remained elevated even 32 hours later. The apoptotic index increased most in the duodenum, then in the jejunum and ileum (Botha et al., 2004). In a separate study, the researchers found that patients who drank from sources with greater microcystin concentrations had a much higher risk of colorectal cancer than patients who drank from clean sources (Zhou et al., 2002).

For many years, *Stachybotrys chartarum*, frequently referred to as "black mold," has been linked for decades to severe pulmonary hemorrhage in the United States. It produces trichothecene mycotoxins, which are known to cause lung inflammation among other things. The moisture from leaks, condensation, penetration, and water damage is what leads to the growth of this mold. Their infection, which was marked by a bloody cough, was more common in infants (Dyląg et al., 2022). Furthermore, it is well known that exposing rats repeatedly to dry, unextracted, but living *S. chartarum* conidia can result in vascular remodeling, immune cell infiltration, and pulmonary inflammation. Four weeks after exposure, a T-helper cell type 2-mediated response was discovered, and by 13 weeks, the majority of the neutrophils, eosinophils, and macrophages in the bronchoalveolar lavage (BAL) fluid were present (Croston et al., 2020).

Shigo toxin is a bacterial toxin produced by *Escherichia coli* that is associated with hemolytic uremic syndrome (HUS), a clinical condition marked by low blood platelet counts, hemolytic anemia, and acute kidney injury (AKI). It is also the main risk factor for AKI in infants. Additionally, it may have deadly effects on the gastrointestinal tract, leading to neurological issues and, in the worst cases, even death. Hemorrhagic colitis symptoms, such as diarrhea and upset stomach, are the first signs of a Shigo toxin infection. Damage to the arteries can result in hemolytic anemia, deep vein thrombosis, and kidney damage (Joseph et al., 2020). Shigo toxin-producing *Escherichia coli* (STEC) invade the colonic epithelium after consuming infected food or drink. Shiga toxins are subsequently released by STEC, causing further damage to the intestinal mucosa's vascular network and resulting in hemorrhagic colitis. After entering the bloodstream and entering the systemic circulation, the toxin can bind to platelets and granulocytes and travel to the kidney along with other intended regions (Lee and Tesh, 2019). Endocytosis can result from this toxin's attachment to the glycolipid globotriaosylceramide (Gb3Cer) on the cell membrane. After that, it moves via the retrograde transport channel to the trans-Golgi network, where its enzymatic domains are released into the cytoplasm, preventing protein synthesis and resulting in damage, apoptosis, ER stress, and inflammation (Liu et al., 2022).

15.12 Prevention and Control Strategies

The transmission of biotoxins and the effects that follow are topics regularly discussed, but a major focus should be put on ways to mitigate or prevent these actions from occurring. Various methods by individuals, companies, and communities have to be put in place to reduce the casualties these toxins can cause.

15.13 Surveillance and Monitoring

Because of the negative consequences that algal blooms may have on biotoxins, numerous approaches have been developed to monitor their spread and growth. Remote sensing has grown in popularity in recent decades as a low-cost approach for tracking the behavior of these algae. One powerful but still-emerging tool for environmental monitoring is the unmanned aerial vehicle (UAV), which presents a desirable and more affordable substitute for routine in-situ field data collection. (Bagaram et al., 2018). Apart from unmanned aerial vehicles, the advancement of compact image sensors presents novel opportunities for environmental use cases. The main parts of UAVs are spectral cameras or imagers, which can be thermal or multispectral and have a big influence on the quality of image data. The accuracy of photogrammetric data depends on the optical performance standards of these sensors, which include zoom lenses, fully automated focusing, and image stabilization (Wu et al., 2019).

Water-quality sensors can help with monitoring, assessment, and research by characterizing high-temporal frequency changes at the sub-daily scale in fundamental water properties and chemical features, such as the presence of toxic algal blooms. Measurements can be conducted at a frequency of seconds and documented across time intervals of months or years. The data can be used to characterize water-quality impairment at different times per hour or day, and it is typically collected weekly or monthly at a given location for periods of a year or less, or in short-term surveys spanning a few days to a few weeks, and it is used as assessment instruments and early warning systems for notifying against these toxin-producing algae (Myers, 2019).

15.14 Public Health Measures

The public has to be notified and well informed about these biotoxins and the ways to prevent their transmission. Public awareness and sensitization through the media and campaigns are great ways to notify people about how best to protect themselves and their families from a potential infection. Regulatory authorities from various nations must guarantee that monitoring systems are reliable and kept up to speed with the growing number of novel biotoxins, as well as food industry operator inspections. Enhancing transdisciplinary collaborative activities to implement eco-innovation sustainable solutions is critical to improving seafood safety, as are creative toxicological methodologies for evaluating seafood safety. Improved toxin detection technologies and enhanced toxin monitoring initiatives will also help to reduce human consumption of seafood pollutants. Customers will be better able to comprehend the danger and the need for safe actions as a result of this (Choudhury et al., 2022). Testing of these foodborne toxins is an essential method to reduce their transmission. During foodborne botulism outbreak investigations, it is advised that foods be examined for preformed neurotoxins as well as the neurotoxigenicity of isolates. In the lack of live microorganisms, conventional procedures are still applied. Suspicious food products are often examined utilizing conventional cultural approaches (Singh et al., 2015). This is also done for other toxins such as staphylococcal enterotoxins, ricin, and seafood toxins.

Efforts must be taken to educate clients about the risks involved with seafood consumption, as well as correct handling practices. In Kenya, exposure to aflatoxin is high due to a lack of information about adequate grain storage techniques and insect infestation. Mycotoxin exposure in spices and herbs was also not well known, and raising awareness of the issue should be a priority. As much interest and attention has been focused only on cereals and nuts, frequent training on the contamination by mycotoxin is necessary, as well as enhanced efforts to promote awareness and educate both makers and users of herbs and spices (Wakhungu et al., 2023).

15.15 Conclusion

The many pathways of biotoxin transmission to humans present a complicated picture, stressing the necessity for a diversified preventative strategy. Ingesting contaminated food or water is a recognized risk, especially for biotoxins generated by dangerous algae or bacteria. However, the peril does not end there. The inhalation of airborne toxins, such as those created by mold or from certain agricultural activities, can potentially be hazardous. Furthermore, biotoxins can be absorbed directly via the skin when in touch with plants, insects, or even marine animals. Venomous organisms, such as spiders and snakes, jellyfish, and stingrays, directly inject biotoxins, which can have a variety of health consequences.

Knowing how these transmissions occurred via examinations of historical epidemics spanning many decades of civilization and how they were found has helped modern medical historians understand how to effectively regulate the spread. It was also vital to assess the impact of their spread on human physiology, especially organs that include the lungs, liver, kidney, and more.

Understanding the various transmission pathways is critical for creating effective preventative methods. Targeted actions, such as properly handling food and water purification and using suitable protective gear while handling potentially hazardous goods, can greatly minimize exposure risk. Furthermore, public education initiatives can enhance knowledge of biotoxin hazards in everyday settings, allowing people to make educated decisions. Recognizing the many ways in which biotoxins may enter the human body allows us to work toward a future in which these hazardous compounds represent less of a threat to our health.

References

Anderson, P.D. (2012). Bioterrorism: Toxins as Weapons. *Journal of Pharmacy Practice*, 25(2), pp.121–129.

Averin, A.S., Сергеевич, A.A., Utkin, Y.N. and Николаевич, У.Ю. (2021). Cardiovascular Effects of Snake Toxins: Cardiotoxicity and Cardioprotection. *Acta Naturae*, [online] 13(3), pp.4–14.

Bagaram, M.B., Giuliarelli, D., Chirici, G., Giannetti, F. and Barbati, A. (2018). UAV Remote Sensing for Biodiversity Monitoring: Are Forest Canopy Gaps Good Covariates? *Remote Sensing*, 10(9), pp.1397–1397.

Beatty, P.R., Puerta-Guardo, H., Killingbeck, S.S., Glasner, D.R., Hopkins, K. and Harris, E. (2015). Dengue Virus NS1 Triggers Endothelial Permeability and Vascular Leak That Is Prevented by NS1 Vaccination. *Science Translational Medicine*, 7(304), p.304ra141.

Benkerroum, N. (2020). Chronic and Acute Toxicities of Aflatoxins: Mechanisms of Action. *International Journal of Environmental Research and Public Health*, [online] 17(2).

Boadu, O., Gombolay, G.Y., Caviness, V.S. and El Saleeby, C.M. (2018). Intoxication From Accidental Marijuana Ingestion in Pediatric Patients. *Pediatric Emergency Care*, 36, Publish Ahead of Print.

Botha, N., van de Venter, M., Downing, T.G., Shephard, E.G. and Gehringer, M.M. (2004). The Effect of Intraperitoneally Administered Microcystin-LR on the Gastrointestinal Tract of Balb/c Mice. *Toxicon*, 43(3), pp.251–254.

Boucaud-Maitre, D., Vernoux, J.-P., Pelczar, S., Daudens-Vaysse, E., Aubert, L., Boa, S., Ferracci, S. and Garnier, R. (2018). Incidence and Clinical Characteristics of Ciguatera Fish Poisoning in Guadeloupe (French West Indies) Between 2013 and 2016: A Retrospective Cases-Series. *Scientific Reports*, 8(1).

Bower, W.A., Hendricks, K.A., Vieira, A.R., Traxler, R.M., Weiner, Z., Lynfield, R. and Hoffmaster, A. (2022). What Is Anthrax? *Pathogens (Basel, Switzerland)*, [online] 11(6), p.690.

Breijyeh, Z., Jubeh, B., Bufo, S.A., Karaman, R. and Scrano, L. (2021). Cannabis: A Toxin-Producing Plant with Potential Therapeutic Uses. *Toxins*, [online] 13(2).

Butsch, C., Beckers, L.-M., Nilson, E., Frassl, M.A., Brennholt, N., Kwiatkowski, R.E. and Söder, M. (2023). Health Impacts of Extreme Weather Events—Cascading Risks in a Changing Climate. *PubMed*, [online] 8(Suppl 4), pp.33–56.

Cacciò, S.M. and Chalmers, R.M. (2016). Human Cryptosporidiosis in Europe. *Clinical Microbiology and Infection*, [online] 22(6), pp.471–480.

Cervellin, G., Longobardi, U. and Lippi, G. (2021). One Holy Man, One Eponym, Three Distinct Diseases: St. Anthony's Fire Revisited. *Acta Bio Medica: Atenei Parmensis*, [online] 92(1), p.e2021008.

Chaves, L.S.M., Fry, J., Malik, A., Geschke, A., Sallum, M.A.M. and Lenzen, M. (2020). Global Consumption and International Trade in Deforestation-Associated Commodities Could Influence Malaria Risk. *Nature Communications*, 11(1).

Chen, N., Xu, S., Zhang, Y. and Wang, F. (2018). Animal Protein Toxins: Origins and Therapeutic Applications. *Biophysics Reports*, 4(5), pp.233–242.

Chinain, M., Gatti, C.M.I., Darius, H.T., Quod, J.-P. and Tester, P.A. (2021). Ciguatera Poisonings: A Global Review of Occurrences and Trends. *Harmful Algae*, 102, p.101873.

Choudhury, S., Medina-Lara, A., Daniel, N. and Smith, R. (2022). Seafood Safety: A Need for Greater Awareness. *Journal of Public Health Research*, 11(3), p.227990362211240.

Costa, P.R., Marques, A. and Diogène, J. (2019). Marine Biotoxins and Seafood Poisoning. *Toxins*, 11(10), p.558.

Croston, T.L., Lemons, A.R., Barnes, M.A., Goldsmith, W.T., Orandle, M.S., Nayak, A.P., Germolec, D.R., Green, B.J. and Beezhold, D.H. (2020). Inhalation of *Stachybotrys chartarum* Fragments Induces Pulmonary Arterial Remodeling. *American Journal of Respiratory Cell and Molecular Biology*, 62(5), pp.563–576.

David, J.M., Pollari, F., Pintar, M., Nesbitt, A., Butler, A.J. and Ravel, A. (2017). Do Contamination of and Exposure to Chicken Meat and Water Drive the Temporal Dynamics of Campylobacter Cases? *Epidemiology and Infection*, 145(15), pp.3191–3203.

Dorner, B. and Rummel, A. (2015). Preface Biological Toxins—Ancient Molecules Posing a Current Threat. *Toxins*, 7(12), pp.5320–5321.

Dyląg, M., Spychała, K., Zielinski, J., Łagowski, D. and Gnat, S. (2022). Update on Stachybotrys Chartarum—Black Mold Perceived as Toxigenic and Potentially Pathogenic to Humans. *Biology*, 11(3), p.352.

Falach, R., Sapoznikov, A., Gal, Y., Israeli, O., Leitner, M., Seliger, N., Ehrlich, S., Kronman, C. and Sabo, T. (2016). Quantitative Profiling of the in Vivo Enzymatic Activity of Ricin Reveals Disparate Depurination of Different Pulmonary Cell Types. *Toxicology Letters*, 258, pp.11–19.

Food and Agriculture Organization of the United Nations and World Health Organization. (2020). *Risk Assessment Tools for Vibrio parahaemolyticus and Vibrio vulnificus Associated with Seafood.* [online] *apps.who.int*. Food and Agriculture Organization of the United Nations. Available at: https://apps.who.int/iris/handle/10665/330867.

Franke, H., Scholl, R. and Aigner, A. (2019). Ricin and Ricinus Communis in Pharmacology and Toxicology-from Ancient Use and 'Papyrus Ebers' to Modern Perspectives and 'Poisonous Plant of the Year 2018'. *Naunyn-Schmiedeberg's Archives of Pharmacology*, 392(10), pp.1181–1208.

Friedman, M., Fernandez, M., Backer, L., Dickey, R., Bernstein, J., Schrank, K., Kibler, S., Stephan, W., Gribble, M., Bienfang, P., Bowen, R., Degrasse, S., Flores Quintana, H., Loeffler, C., Weisman, R., Blythe, D., Berdalet, E., Ayyar, R., Clarkson-Townsend, D. and Swajian, K. (2017). An Updated Review of Ciguatera Fish Poisoning: Clinical, Epidemiological, Environmental, and Public Health Management. *Marine Drugs*, [online] 15(3), p.72.

Fry, B.G., Roelants, K., Champagne, D.E., Scheib, H., Tyndall, J.D.A., King, G.F., Nevalainen, T.J., Norman, J.A., Lewis, R.J., Norton, R.S., Renjifo, C. and de la Vega, R.C.R. (2009). The Toxicogenomic Multiverse: Convergent Recruitment of Proteins into Animal Venoms. *Annual Review of Genomics and Human Genetics*, [online] 10, pp.483–511.

Glasner, D.R., Puerta-Guardo, H., Beatty, P.R. and Harris, E. (2018). The Good, the Bad, and the Shocking: The Multiple Roles of Dengue Virus Nonstructural Protein 1 in Protection and Pathogenesis. *Annual Review of Virology*, [online] 5(1), p.227.

Glasner, D.R., Ratnasiri, K., Puerta-Guardo, H., Espinosa, D.A., Beatty, P.R. and Harris, E. (2017). Dengue Virus NS1 Cytokine-Independent Vascular Leak Is Dependent on Endothelial Glycocalyx Components. *PLOS Pathogens*, 13(11), p.e1006673.

González, C., Ballesteros-Mejia, L., Díaz-Díaz, J., Toro-Vargas, D.M., Amarillo-Suarez, A.R., Gey, D., León, C., Tovar, E., Arias, M., Rivera, N., Buitrago, L. S., Pinto-Moraes, R.H., Sano, I.S., Decaëns, T., González, M.A., Kitching, I.J. and Rougerie, R. (2023). Deadly and Venomous Lonomia Caterpillars Are More Than the Two Usual Suspects. *PLOS Neglected Tropical Diseases*, 17(2), p.e0011063.

Grzybowski, A., Pawlikowska-Łagód, K. and Polak, A. (2021). Ergotism and Saint Anthony's Fire. *Clinics in Dermatology*, 39(6).

Hald, T., Aspinall, W., Devleesschauwer, B., Cooke, R., Corrigan, T., Havelaar, A.H., Gibb, H.J., Torgerson, P.R., Kirk, M.D., Angulo, F.J., Lake, R.J., Speybroeck, N. and Hoffmann, S. (2016). World Health Organization Estimates of the Relative Contributions of Food to the Burden of Disease Due to Selected Foodborne Hazards: A Structured Expert Elicitation. *PLOS One*, 11(1), p.e0145839.

Herrera, M., Anadón, R., Iqbal, S.Z., Bailly, J.D. and Ariño, A. (2016). Climate Change and Food Safety. *Food Safety*, [online] pp.149–160.

Herzig, V., Cristofori-Armstrong, B., Israel, M.R., Nixon, S.A., Vetter, I. and King, G.F. (2020). Animal Toxins—Nature's Evolutionary-Refined Toolkit for Basic Research and Drug Discovery. *Biochemical Pharmacology*, [online] 181.

Hoyos, C.L., Cajal, S.P., Juarez, M., Marco, J.D., Alberti D'Amato, A.M., Cayo, M., Torrejón, I., Cimino, R.O., Diosque, P., Krolewiecki, A.J., Nasser, J.R. and Gil, J.F. (2016). Epidemiology of American Tegumentary Leishmaniasis and Trypanosoma Cruzi Infection in Northwestern Argentina. *BioMed Research International*, 2016, pp.1–8.

Huang, E., Pillai, S.K., Bower, W.A., Hendricks, K.A., Guarnizo, J.T., Hoyle, J.D., Gorman, S.E., Boyer, A.E., Quinn, C.P. and Meaney-Delman, D. (2015). Antitoxin Treatment of Inhalation Anthrax: A Systematic Review. *Health Security*, [online] 13(6), pp.365–377.

Hurley, W., Wolterstorff, C., MacDonald, R. and Schultz, D. (2014). Paralytic Shellfish Poisoning: A Case Series. *Western Journal of Emergency Medicine*, [online] 15(4), pp.378–381.

Jalink, M. (2020). Ocular Complications of Spitting Cobra Venom. *Indian Journal of Ophthalmology*, 68(11), p.2632.

Janik, E., Ceremuga, M., Saluk-Bijak, J. and Bijak, M. (2019). Biological Toxins as the Potential Tools for Bioterrorism. *International Journal of Molecular Sciences*, [online] 20(5).

Jochimsen, E.M., Carmichael, W.W., An, J., Cardo, D.M., Cookson, S.T., Holmes, C.E.M., Antunes, M.B., de Melo Filho, D.A., Lyra, T.M., Barreto, V.S.T., Azevedo, S.M.F.O. and Jarvis, W.R. (1998). Liver Failure and Death After Exposure to Microcystins at a Hemodialysis Center in Brazil. *New England Journal of Medicine*, 338(13), pp.873–878.

Joseph, A., Cointe, A., Mariani Kurkdjian, P., Rafat, C. and Hertig, A. (2020). Shiga Toxin-Associated Hemolytic Uremic Syndrome: A Narrative Review. *Toxins*, 12(2), p.67.

Kinyenje, E.S., Kishimba, R., Mohamed, M., Mwafulango, A., Eliakimu, E. and Kwesigabo, G. (2023). Aflatoxicosis Outbreak and Its Associated Factors in Kiteto, Chemba and Kondoa Districts, Tanzania. *PLOS Global Public Health*, [online] 3(8), p.e0002191.

Krivohlavek, A. (2018). Food Safety, Standards and Norms Against Bioterrorism: Food Safety and Hazards. *Defense Against Bioterrorism*, pp.239–248.

Kularatne, S.A.M. and Senanayake, N. (2014). Venomous Snake Bites, Scorpions, and Spiders. *Handbook of Clinical Neurology*, 120, pp.987–1001.

Lad, A., Breidenbach, J.D., Su, R.C., Murray, J., Kuang, R., Mascarenhas, A., Najjar, J., Patel, S., Hegde, P., Youssef, M., Breuler, J., Kleinhenz, A.L., Ault, A.P., Westrick, J.A., Modyanov, N.N., Kennedy, D.J. and Haller, S.T. (2022). As We Drink and Breathe: Adverse Health Effects of Microcystins and Other Harmful Algal Bloom Toxins in the Liver, Gut, Lungs and Beyond. *Life*, [online] 12(3), p.418.

Lago, J., Rodríguez, L., Blanco, L., Vieites, J. and Cabado, A. (2015). Tetrodotoxin, an Extremely Potent Marine Neurotoxin: Distribution, Toxicity, Origin and Therapeutical Uses. *Marine Drugs*, [online] 13(10), pp.6384–6406.

Lebeau, G., Lagrave, A., Ogire, E., Grondin, L., Seriacaroupin, S., Moutoussamy, C., Mavingui, P., Hoarau, J.-J., Roche, M., Krejbich-Trotot, P., Desprès, P. and Viranaicken, W. (2021). Viral Toxin NS1 Implication in Dengue Pathogenesis Making It a Pivotal Target in Development of Efficient Vaccine. *Vaccines*, [online] 9(9), p.946.

Lee, M.-S. and Tesh, V.L. (2019). Roles of Shiga Toxins in Immunopathology. *Toxins*, [online] 11(4), p.212.

Liu, Y., Thaker, H., Wang, C., Xu, Z. and Dong, M. (2022). Diagnosis and Treatment for Shiga Toxin-Producing Escherichia Coli Associated Hemolytic Uremic Syndrome. *Toxins*, [online] 15(1), p.10.

Mahato, D.K., Lee, K.E., Kamle, M., Devi, S., Dewangan, K.N., Kumar, P. and Kang, S.G. (2019). Aflatoxins in Food and Feed: An Overview on Prevalence, Detection and Control Strategies. *Frontiers in Microbiology*, 10.

Malik, K., Kommana, S., Paul, J. and Krakauer, M. (2020). Synthetic Cannabinoid-Induced Ocular Self-Injury. *Orbit*, 40(4), pp.326–328.

Mekuria, A.N., Routledge, M.N., Gong, Y.Y. and Sisay, M. (2020). Aflatoxins as a Risk Factor for Liver Cirrhosis: A Systematic Review and Meta-Analysis. *BMC Pharmacology and Toxicology*, 21(1).

Metcalf, J.S., Tischbein, M., Cox, P.A. and Stommel, E.W. (2021). Cyanotoxins and the Nervous System. *Toxins*, [online] 13(9), p.660.

Michelitsch, A., Wernike, K., Klaus, C., Dobler, G. and Beer, M. (2019). Exploring the Reservoir Hosts of Tick-Borne Encephalitis Virus. *Viruses*, 11(7), p.669.

Mora, C., McKenzie, T., Gaw, I.M., Dean, J.M., von Hammerstein, H., Knudson, T.A., Setter, R.O., Smith, C.Z., Webster, K.M., Patz, J.A. and Franklin, E.C. (2022). Over Half of Known Human Pathogenic Diseases Can Be Aggravated by Climate Change. *Nature Climate Change*, [online] 12(12).

Morabito, S., Silvestro, S. and Faggio, C. (2017). How the Marine Biotoxins Affect Human Health. *Natural Product Research*, 32(6), pp.621–631.

Mutegi, C.K., Cotty, P.J. and Bandyopadhyay, R. (2018). Prevalence and Mitigation of Aflatoxins in Kenya (1960-to Date). *World Mycotoxin Journal*, 11(3), pp.341–357.

Myers, D.N. (2019). Innovations in Monitoring with Water-Quality Sensors with Case Studies on Floods, Hurricanes, and Harmful Algal Blooms. *Separation Science and Technology*, pp.219–283.

Nelsen, D.R., Nisani, Z., Cooper, A.M., Fox, G.A., Gren, E.C.K., Corbit, A.G. and Hayes, W.K. (2013). Poisons Toughens, and Venoms: Redefining and Classifying Toxic Biological Secretions and the Organisms That Employ Them. *Biological Reviews*, 89(2), pp.450–465.

Núñez-Vázquez, E.J., Almazán-Becerril, A., López-Cortés, D.J., Heredia-Tapia, A., Hernández-Sandoval, F.E., Band-Schmidt, C.J., Bustillos-Guzmán, J.J., Gárate-Lizárraga, I., García-Mendoza, E., Salinas-Zavala, C.A. and Cordero-Tapia, A. (2018). Ciguatera in Mexico (1984–2013). *Marine Drugs*, [online] 17(1).

Oliveira Alves, A. and Filho, F.B. (2017). An Unpleasant Encounter with Termites. *The Journal of Pediatrics*, 182, pp.396–396.e1.

O'Neill, K., Musgrave, I.F. and Humpage, A. (2016). Low Dose Extended Exposure to Saxitoxin and Its Potential Neurodevelopmental Effects: A Review. *Environmental Toxicology and Pharmacology*, 48, pp.7–16.

Parak, M., Asgari, A., Nourian, Y.H. and Ghanei, M. (2024). A Review of Poisoning with Various Types of Biotoxins and Its Common Clinical Symptoms. *Toxicon (Oxford)*, p.107629.

Paul, P., Kangalawe, R.Y.M. and Mboera, L.E.G. (2018). Land-Use Patterns and Their Implication on Malaria Transmission in Kilosa District, Tanzania. *Tropical Diseases, Travel Medicine and Vaccines*, 4(1).

Phipps, L.P. and Johnson, N. (2022). JMM Profile: Tick-Borne Encephalitis Virus. *Journal of Medical Microbiology*, 71(5).

Píchová, K., Pažoutová, S., Kostovčík, M., Chudíčková, M., Stodůlková, E., Novák, P., Flieger, M., van der Linde, E. and Kolařík, M. (2018). Evolutionary History of Ergot with a New Infrageneric Classification (Hypocreales: Clavicipitaceae: Claviceps). *Molecular Phylogenetics and Evolution*, 123, pp.73–87.
Pierre, O., Misery, L., Talagas, M. and Le Garrec, R. (2018). Immune Effects of the Neurotoxins Ciguatoxins and Brevetoxins. *Toxicon: Official Journal of the International Society on Toxinology*, [online] 149, pp.6–19.
Pratheepa, V. and Vasconcelos, V. (2017). Binding and Pharmacokinetics of the Sodium Channel Blocking Toxins (Saxitoxin and the Tetrodotoxins). *Mini-Reviews in Medicinal Chemistry*, 17(4), pp.320–327.
Pustijanac, E., Buršić, M., Talapko, J., Škrlec, I., Meštrović, T. and Lišnjić, D. (2023). Tick-Borne Encephalitis Virus: A Comprehensive Review of Transmission, Pathogenesis, Epidemiology, Clinical Manifestations, Diagnosis, and Prevention. *Microorganisms*, [online] 11(7), pp.1634–1634.
Radad, K., Moldzio, R., Al-Shraim, M., Al-Emam, A. and Rausch, W.-D. (2018). Long-Term Neurotoxic Effects of Domoic Acid on Primary Dopaminergic Neurons. *Toxicology in Vitro*, 52, pp.279–285.
Rajabizadeh, M., Van Wassenbergh, S., Mallet, C., Rücklin, M. and Herrel, A. (2020). Tooth-Shape Adaptations in Aglyphous Colubrid Snakes Inferred from Three-Dimensional Geometric Morphometrics and Finite Element Analysis. *Zoological Journal of the Linnean Society*, [online] 191.
Rossetto, O. and Montecucco, C. (2019). Tables of Toxicity of Botulinum and Tetanus Neurotoxins. *Toxins*, 11(12), p.686.
Roxas Duncan, V.I. (2011). Of Beans and Beads: Ricin and Abrin in Bioterrorism and Biocrime. *Journal of Bioterrorism & Biodefense*, s2(1).
Saad-Hussein, A., Moubarz, G., Mohgah, S.A., Wafaa, G.S. and Aya, H.M. (2019). Role of Antioxidant Supplementation in Oxidant/Antioxidant Status and Hepatotoxic Effects Due to Aflatoxin B1 in Wheat Miller Workers. *Journal of Complementary and Integrative Medicine*, 16(4).
Singh, A.K., Garber, E., Principato, M.C., Hall, S. and Sharma, S.K. (2015). Biotoxins and Food Safety. *Toxicology*, pp.185–210.
Stoll, A., Shenton, D.P., Green, A.C. and Holley, J.L. (2023). Comparative Aspects of Ricin Toxicity by Inhalation. *Toxins*, [online] 15(4), p.281.
Svirčev, Z., Lalić, D., Bojadžija Savić, G., Tokodi, N., Drobac Backović, D., Chen, L., Meriluoto, J. and Codd, G.A. (2019). Global Geographical and Historical Overview of Cyanotoxin Distribution and Cyanobacterial Poisonings. *Archives of Toxicology*, 93(9), pp.2429–2481.
Tkachev, A.V., Tkacheva, O.L., Zubova, T.V., Pleshkov, V.A. and Smolovskaya, O.V. (2020). Effect of Mycotoxins on the Spermatozoa and Embryos of Animals. *Advances in Animal and Veterinary Sciences*, 8(s3).
Tohmé, M.J. and Delgui, L.R. (2021). Advances in the Development of Antiviral Compounds for Rotavirus Infections. *MBio*, 12(3).
Torres-Guerrero, E., Quintanilla-Cedillo, M.R., Ruiz-Esmenjaud, J. and Arenas, R. (2017). Leishmaniasis: A Review. *F1000Research*, [online] 6(1), p.750.
Troeger, C., Khalil, I.A., Rao, P.C., Cao, S., Blacker, B.F., Ahmed, T., Armah, G., Bines, J.E., Brewer, T.G., Colombara, D.V., Kang, G., Kirkpatrick, B.D., Kirkwood, C.D., Mwenda, J.M., Parashar, U.D., Petri, W.A., Riddle, M.S., Steele, A.D., Thompson, R.L. and Walson, J.L. (2018). Rotavirus Vaccination and the Global Burden of Rotavirus Diarrhea Among Children Younger Than 5 Years. *JAMA Pediatrics*, [online] 172(10), p.958.

Turner, A.D., Higgins, C., Davidson, K., Veszelovszki, A., Payne, D., Hungerford, J. and Higman, W. (2015). Potential Threats Posed by New or Emerging Marine Biotoxins in UK Waters and Examination of Detection Methodology Used in Their Control: Brevetoxins. *Marine Drugs*, [online] 13(3), pp.1224–1254.

Vilariño, N., Louzao, M.C., Abal, P., Cagide, E., Carrera, C., Vieytes, M.R. and Botana, L.M. (2018). Human Poisoning from Marine Toxins: Unknowns for Optimal Consumer Protection. *Toxins*, [online] 10(8).

Visciano, P., Schirone, M., Berti, M., Milandri, A., Tofalo, R. and Suzzi, G. (2016). Marine Biotoxins: Occurrence, Toxicity, Regulatory Limits and Reference Methods. *Frontiers in Microbiology*, 7.

Wakhungu, C.N., Okoth, S., Wachira, P. and Otieno, N.A. (2023). Prevalence of Aflatoxin B1 in Marketed Herbs and Spices in Nairobi County Kenya: Consumer Awareness, Practices, and Associated Health Risks. *Journal of Agriculture and Food Sciences*, 20(2), pp.31–61.

Wambui, J.M., Karuri, E.G., Ojiambo, J.A. and Njage, P.M.K. (2016). Application of Probabilistic Modeling to Quantify the Reduction Levels of Hepatocellular Carcinoma Risk Attributable to Chronic Aflatoxins Exposure. *Nutrition and Cancer*, 69(1), pp.1–13.

Wetzel, D.M., Rhodes, E.L., Li, S., McMahon-Pratt, D. and Koleske, A.J. (2016). The Src Kinases Hck, Fgr, and Lyn Activate Arg to Facilitate IgG-mediated Phagocytosis and Leishmania Infection. *Journal of Cell Science*, [online] 129(16), pp.3130–3143.

Whitfield, S., Griffiths, G., Jenner, D., Gwyther, R., Stahl, F., Cork, L., Holley, J., Green, A. and Clark, G. (2017). Production, Characterisation and Testing of an Ovine Antitoxin Against Ricin; Efficacy, Potency and Mechanisms of Action. *Toxins*, 9(10), p.329.

Wu, D., Li, R., Zhang, F. and Liu, J. (2019). A Review on Drone-Based Harmful Algae Blooms Monitoring. *Environmental Monitoring and Assessment*, 191(4).

Wuiya, C.Z., Silayo, V.C.K., Nyamete, F. and Majubwa, R.O. (2022). Assessment of Farmer's Awareness in Harvesting and Postharvest Handling Practices for Management of Aflatoxins on Maize in Morogoro Region. *International Journal of Agriculture, Environment and Bioresearch*, 7(5), pp.36–49.

Yang, Z., Luo, Q., Liang, Y. and Mazumder, A. (2016). Processes and Pathways of Ciguatoxin in Aquatic Food Webs and Fish Poisoning of Seafood Consumers. *Environmental Reviews*, 24(2), pp.144–150.

Zhang, F., Lee, J., Liang, S. and Shum, C. (2015). Cyanobacteria Blooms and Non-Alcoholic Liver Disease: Evidence from a County Level Ecological Study in the United States. *Environmental Health*, 14(1).

Zhang, X., Kuča, K., Dohnal, V., Dohnalová, L., Wu, Q. and Wu, C. (2014). Military Potential of Biological Toxins. *Journal of Applied Biomedicine*, 12(2), pp.63–77.

Zhou, L., Yu, H. and Chen, K. (2002). Relationship Between Microcystin in Drinking Water and Colorectal Cancer. *PubMed*, 15(2), pp.166–171.

16

Emerging Applications of Biotoxin Detection in Food

Prity Das, Arundhuti Chatterjee, Sharon Bose, and Sandip Mondal

16.1 Introduction

Biotoxins, as their name suggests, can be broken down to two words: bio, meaning living, and toxin, meaning poisonous. From this, we can clearly state that biotoxins are naturally produced chemical substances or entities that are produced by bacteria, fungi, and plants in general as a defense mechanism that stops the producer from being consumed (Singh, Garber et al. 2015; Janik, Ceremuga et al. 2019). Biotoxins are classified into the following groups (Figure 16.1).

Microalgal phytotoxins are those toxins that are produced in the bodies of microbes. These are further subcategorized as:

1. Cyanobacteria: these include saxitoxins, gonyautoxins, and anatoxins, which work by neurotoxic and hepatotoxic mechanisms.
2. Dinoflagellates: these include saxitoxins, gonyautoxins, and okadaic acid palytoxins, which work by the neurotoxic and hepatotoxic mechanisms.
3. Diatoms: these only include domoic acid, which is neurotoxic and acts on ionotropic glutamate receptors (Rhodes, Selwood et al. 2006).

Mycotoxins, or fungal biotoxins, include aflatoxins, trichothecenes, stachybotrytoxins, and ergot alkaloids, which work by inhibiting the actions of the CNS system and protein synthesis.

- Bacterial toxins include cholera toxin, tetanus neurotoxin, and *Staphylococcus aureus* enterotoxins (SEs).
- Plant toxins include ricin, abrin, and alkaloids like atropine, which inhibit protein synthesis and block acetylcholine receptors.
- Fish toxins include tetrodotoxin, which is neurotoxic (Paterson 2006).

 DOI: 10.1201/9781003500605-19

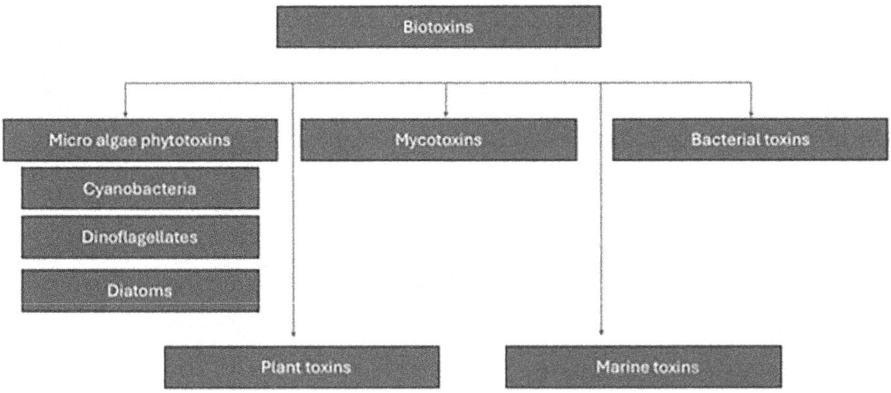

FIGURE 16.1
Classification of biotoxin.

While biotoxins do not affect the food in which they're present, because they act as a defense mechanism, they act as their predators or, in our case, consumers. Ackee fruit: Hypoglycin A is a stable toxin found here due to improper harvest. This may result in vomiting, coma, and death. Blue-green algae contains microcystins, which cause gastrointestinal distress. Honey, or mad honey, usually contains grayanotoxins; this causes nausea, vomiting, or dizziness. Mushroom toxins are well known to be present in most types of wild mushrooms; this may lead to nausea or diarrhea (Morabito, Silvestro et al. 2018).

Biotoxins present in food can have significant impacts on both human health and the ecosystem.

1. Longer-term effect on humans
   - Chronic health conditions: neurological disorders, hepatic disorders, immune suppression, and even cancer.
   - Developmental effects: early exposure during pregnancy may cause severe issues for fetal health and its deployment.
   - Cumulative effects: the buildup of toxins in the body has adverse effects in later years.

2. Impact on the ecosystem
   - Biodiversity loss—the decline of sensitive species—disruption of climate is what causes the formation of toxins in the first place.
   - Altered ecosystem dynamics—toxic algal blooms, fish toxin breaking out, biomagnification of toxins—can harm a huge part of the ecosystem.

- Economic consequences—fishery, tourism, and aquaculture are all affected due to biotoxin disruption (Ababouch 2014; Morabito, Silvestro et al. 2018).

Understanding and detecting biotoxins in food is crucial for mitigating their adverse effects and protecting both human health and the environment.

16.2 Biotoxin Detection Tests for Food

While biotoxins are necessary for the producer's body, they can have the opposite effect on humans who consume them. The accumulation of biotoxins in the human body can lead to foodborne illness, which can be life-threatening in the long run. Therefore, detecting and analyzing biotoxins in food is critical for the population's well-being.

The presence of biotoxins in food has been known for a long time, but due to a lack of information and technology, people were unable to prevent the illnesses they caused. In the 19th century, Louis Pasteur's work on food contamination and spoilage was revolutionary. Later, Belgium bacteriologist Emily Pierre Marie Van Ermengem introduced the mouse lethality test, which became popular. Today, immunoassay, polymerase chain reaction (PCR), mass spectroscopy, and new technologies such as biosensors (which provide on-site results) are used to detect biotoxins. A public health agency tests and monitors the amount of biotoxins present in food to ensure the safety and regulation of food consumption.

The biotoxin detection tests are discussed in the following.

16.2.1 Mouse Bioassay, or Mouse Lethality Test

The mouse lethality test (Figure 16.2) aids in determining the exposure to toxicity due to diarrheal shellfish poison (DSP) and the amount of paralytic shellfish poison (PSP toxin). We can observe the mortality and morbidity rate of the toxin in the given population or subjects, for example, boNT potency (botulinum toxin obtained from *Clostridium botulium* bacteria); the limit is $1LD_{50}$ (Notermans, Stam et al. 2014).

In this test, the subjects, mice, are taken and injected with the collected sample (which might contain biotoxin) via the intraperitoneal route (IP). The mice are observed until they die. To confirm that the mice have died due to a particular toxin, further tests are conducted. In the case of botulinium toxin (which is a type of biotoxin), we check the type of botulinium toxin that caused the toxicity in the subject's body.

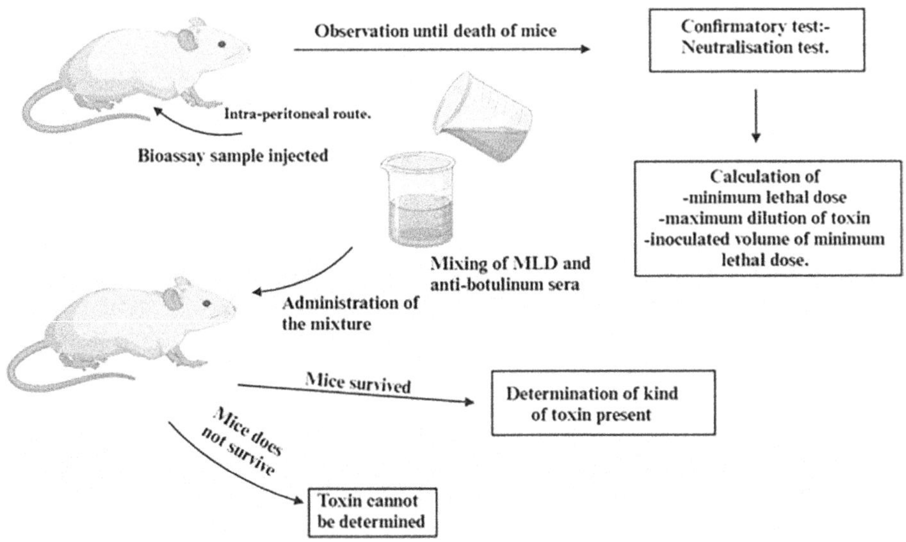

FIGURE 16.2
Mouse bioassay.

At first, the minimum lethal dose (MLD) is calculated, along with the calculation of the maximum dilution of the toxin (the reason for the subject's or mouse's death) and the inoculated volume containing the lethal minimum dose (LMD). Meanwhile, different anti-botulinum sera are obtained that have the capability to neutralize the toxin. Then the minimum lethal dose is mixed with each of the anti-botulinum sera (previously obtained). All mice are then injected with the mixture of MLD and anti-toxin sera in equal volume to monitor the survival of the subjects. So it can be concluded that the mice who survive the tests are capable of neutralizing the toxin. As a result, the anti-sera and toxin are compatible, and the anti-botulinum sera type allows us to determine the type of toxin that was present in the given sample and caused toxicity among the mice.

Botox contains Onabotulinum toxinA, a purified neurotoxin protein derived from the bacterium *Clostridium botulinum* (Solomon and Lilly 2001).

The main drawback of this method is that toxic profiling cannot be obtained. The interference of the matrix has the potential to cause errors in the experiment. The most specific point is that the whole experiment is against laboratory ethics (animal protection from scientific subjects) (Robson, Toscano et al. 2022).

16.2.2 Cell-Based Bioassay

The cell-based bioassay (CBA) possesses distinct capabilities for detecting toxicity, assessing drug efficacy, and accurately determining protein function. It also has the ability to understand the pathophysiology of any particular disease state (Solzin, Eppler et al. 2023).

The sample is taken, which will be tested with a particular cell line where the biotoxin will be tested (if the biotoxin is known, then the cell selection can preferably be particular for a better result and observation). The selected cell line is then cultivated and exposed to the particular biotoxin. As a result of cellular responses that can be observed, there can be variable results from this particular experiment, such as alteration of morphological features after being exposed to the toxin, cell viability, apoptosis and necrosis induction, inflammatory responses (ELISA and PCR measure the level), gene expression, and the protein level. After this comes the data analysis part. Based on the data, the dose-response relationship curve is determined. The accuracy and reliability of the assay are checked to report the result at the end (Arkin, Glicksman et al. 2012), such as a mouse neuroblastoma (Neuro-2a) cell-based assay for detecting saxitoxin, a potent marine biotoxin produced by certain species of dinoflagellates.

16.2.3 Tissue Culture-Based Bioassay

The tissue culture-based bioassay (TCBA) has better prospects of interacting with the organ cell to provide more relevant results and can help in the determination of the morphological structure of the organ and its changes due to the presence of the foreign compound (toxicity). The effect of biotoxin on complex structures can be observed more vividly.

A sample is taken, which will be tested on a particular tissue of an organ, or a very thin slice of an organ is taken, which will be cultured and exposed to the specific sample. The rest of the test is the same as the cell-based bioassay (Masi, Spagni et al. 2021).

The TCBA differs from the cell-based bioassay in several ways.

1. More complex than the CBA.
2. Interaction with the organ, cell, and tissue is better defined and easier to understand.
3. The morphological structure of the tissue and the alteration due to biotoxin (if any alteration is taking place) can be identified and studied in a more constructive way.

Compared to CBA, TCBA is more relevant for interpretation in the human body (Langer 2016).

16.2.4 Microscopic Analysis

Microscopic analysis has the advantage of determining the structure of the biotoxin, though not all biotoxins have definite structures. Morphological

TABLE 16.1
Microscopic Analysis

Process and Instrument	Type of Biotoxin	Example	References
Gram staining	Bacterial	Botulium toxin obtained from *Clostridium botulium* bacteria. Gram positive in nature. Under light microscopy, it retains its color.	(Tiwari and Nagalli 2023)
Fluorescent dye	Specific toxin	Aflatoxin obtained from *Aspergillus flevus* fungi. Appropriate wavelength is needed to see under the microscope.	(Rai, Bhattarai et al. 2021)
Dark field microscopy	Cholera toxin	Cholera toxin obtained from *vibrio cholerea*. It appears bright under dark field microscopy.	(Benenson, Islam et al. 1964)

characteristics can also be specified and classified as needed (characteristic features such as size, shape, color retention property, etc.) (McNamara, Difilippantonio et al. 2005).

The preparation of a sample begins at the source. The sample is then diluted for a better result. The diluted sample is then used for the microscopy.

Identification is done through analysis (Table 16.1). In this part, all the various magnifications on the sample, along with the documentation and comparison with other samples and standards, are done. For confirmation, a PCR test is done. The main drawback is that this test cannot detect all biotoxins, as many lack specific structures or features.

16.2.5 Chemical Detection

16.2.5.1 Thin-Layer Chromatography

Thin-layer chromatography (TLC) has the specific potential to separate the components present in the sample on the basis of absorption and polarity. Characterization of the compound (volatility, solubility, absorbance, etc.) is also possible (Al-Harrasi, Bhatia et al. 2022).

Preparation of the stationary phase consist of the mixture of many solvents (one of the major parts for the separation of the compound present in the sample).

Preparation of TLC plate: The TLC plate can be either precoated with silica gel present in the plate, so it can be directly used for the test, or a blank TLC plate can be used, which needs to be prepared by applying and drying silica gel on both sides evenly to create the stationary phase.

A sample is taken in small amounts and put on the baseline of the TLC plate. The stationary phase is already present in the developing chamber, so the TLC plate will be placed vertically on the stationary phase or the mixture of the solvents. The developing chamber is then covered to prevent any possibility of evaporation of the solvents. The capillary movement of the mobile phase is observed until it approximately reaches the top of the plate (near the top). Then the TLC plate is removed and dried (Al-Harrasi, Bhatia et al. 2022). The spot or spots are visualized, such as in the case of alkaloid biotoxin, when it is dipped in the iodine solution to give a distinctive color to identify. Later, analysis and calculation are done.

16.2.5.2 High-Performance Liquid Chromatography

The primary objective of high-performance liquid chromatography (HPLC) (Figure 16.3) is to confirm the identification of the biotoxin along with quantitative analysis (Besbes, Monser et al. 2024). First, the mobile phase is prepared with the specific pH (if the pH is not desired, it will be adjusted according to

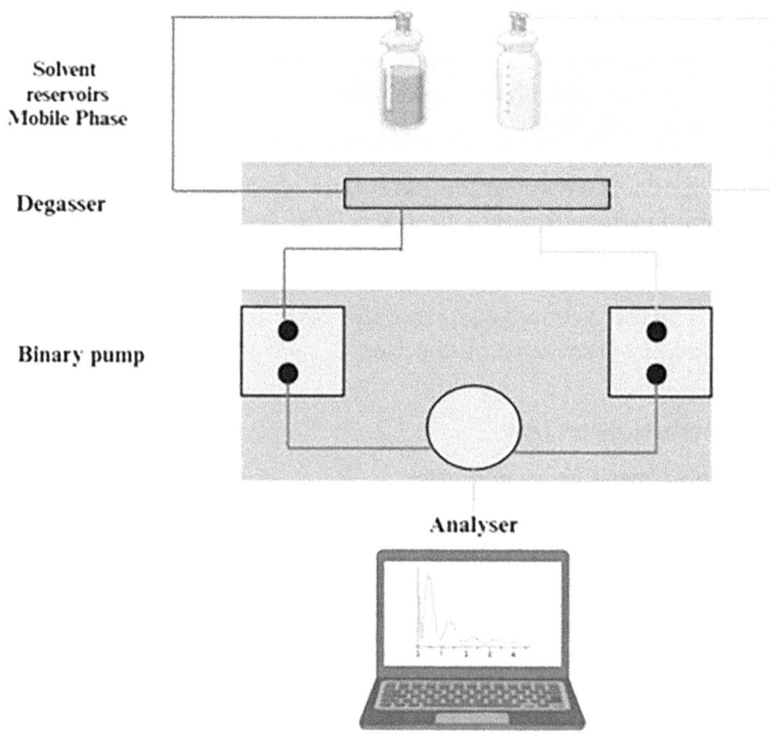

FIGURE 16.3
HPLC instrumentation.

the requirements). The mobile phase is then filtered by a suitable filter under vacuum conditions so that the phase is properly degassed. The HPLC system will be set up (points to be pondered: the HPLC machine setup varies from model to model, so it will be done according to the manual, and there will be a point indicator to indicate the flow of the mobile phase in the column attached to the analyzer; a purge valve will be attached to the mobile phase to remove the bubbles; otherwise, it will cause an error in the result). The standard is run through the HPLC multiple times to maintain its repeatability. The sample is then loaded. The machine is turned on, and the separation process takes place. Chromatograms can be seen on the monitor as a result. Results and observations help in the analysis (Wahi, Cerjak et al. 2009). The things that we obtain from the chromatogram are: retention time, peak areas, peak height, and calibration curve.

16.2.5.3 **Gas Chromatography**

Gas chromatography (GC) has the capability to separate a volatile biotoxin from the given sample (mixed with other components) and detect particular chemical constituents (Wang and Paré 1997).

The sample is vaporized into the gaseous phase and passed through the capillary column. The components of the gas will separate out due to the presence of a stationary phase in the column. Inert gas is propelled into the column. Component separation will take place on the basis of the rate of escape from the column due to boiling point and polarity. The detector detects the time required for each component. The primary disadvantages of this chromatography include the requirement for a pure form of carrier gas and the fact that not all biotoxins are volatile by nature (Al-Bukhaiti, Noman et al. 2017).

16.2.5.4 **Gas Chromatography Coupled with Mass Spectrometry**

The prime objective of this test is the structural identification of biotoxins, which is a more accurate method of identification than gas chromatography and mass spectrometry (Vishwakarma 2021).

The sample is vaporized into the gaseous phase. Then the gas is passed through the capillary column to do GC. The separated components are passed through the interface. The inert gas is removed from the interface to maintain the chromatographic resolution. The pressure is then decreased. Then the gas is passed to the mass spectrometer (MS), where it passes through the heated transfer line to ionize the gas. The positively charged chamber accelerates the ionized gas particles. The presence of a magnetic field in the system causes deflection of the ionized particles. The detector detects the beam of deflection ions, thus obtaining the result (Turner 2022).

16.2.6 Immunochromatography

Immunochromatography can aid in providing a better result, as the method is a combination of immunoassay (mentioned later) and chromatography, with less time required as compared to the processes individually (Watson 2000).

The procedure is based on the principle of ELISA (mentioned later in the immunoassay division) but carried out on the chromatographic paper using capillary action. Here, two layers of antibody are used: one is immobilized on the chromatographic paper, and the other is labeled with the fluorescent dye. The test kit is ready to be used to analyze the sample (biotoxin present). When the liquid (sample) is given, it migrates to the line of fluorescent antibodies and forms an antigen-antibody complex (immune complex). Then the sample further migrates to the immobilized antibody to form an immune complex. The presence of more and more complexes provides coloration. The color suggests the result of the test (Weller 2000).

16.2.7 Immunoassay

Many immunoassay types are popular for biotoxin determination tests, but ELISA stands out as the most sensitive and reliable method, as discussed in the following.

16.2.7.1 Enzyme-Linked Immunoassay

Since ELISA can detect only a specific few marine biotoxins, it can be considered a drawback of the method (Malaysia, Malaysia et al. 2019). In ELISA, first, samples are collected. Specific antibodies are immobilized against biotoxin on the surface of the microtiter and kept overnight. The other unbound sites with milk protein or casein are blocked to prevent non-specific binding. The diluted sample is added to the plate wells. It is incubated so that biotoxins bind with the antibodies. The plate is washed using a buffer solution (to remove unbounded parts). A secondary antibody conjugated to horseradish peroxidase is added. Incubation is done so that secondary antibodies can bind. A substrate is then added so that detectable signals can be obtained, which produces a colored or fluorescent product. The intensity of the signal is measured and compared with a standard curve, and from the graph, the amount of biotoxin present can be quantified (Figure 16.4) (Bidwell 1976).

16.2.8 Spectrophotometry

The main objective of spectrophotometry is the identification of chemical constituents on the basis of their physicochemical properties (Bunaciu, Hoang et al. 2013). A sample of food is taken, and by protein precipitation or solvent extraction, a sample is prepared. The biotoxins are then separated from other compounds using chromatographic techniques. The isolated

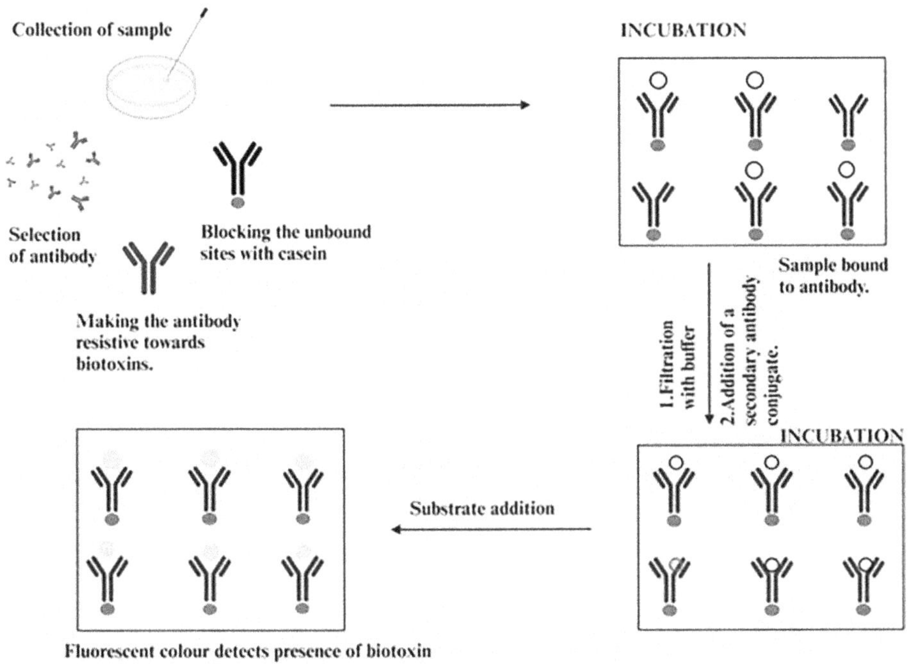

FIGURE 16.4
Mechanism of ELISA.

biotoxins are introduced into a mass spectrometer, where they are converted into ions. Here, the ions are accelerated, and due to the presence of an electric or magnetic field, they separate on the basis of their mass-to-charge ratio. From this, identification of biotoxins can be done with the help of molecular weight (Dadi, Yasir et al. 2022).

16.2.9 Polymerase Chain Reaction

Polymerase chain reaction (PCR) is specifically used for the detection and identification of specific gene sequences as well as for the enhancement of the number of target regions of the DNA (copying) so that it can be analyzed (Patel, Kumar et al. 2022). A sample is taken. DNA/RNA extraction is done from the sample as the PCR analyzes the DNA/RNA sequencing. For DNA/RNA extraction, the necessary reagents or the master mix are taken into PCR tubes and heated at approximately 940°C (thermal cycler). (Sometimes mineral oil is added to prevent evaporation due to heat; this is an optional step.) The heat causes denaturation of the DNA hydrogen bond, resulting in double-stranded or single-stranded DNA. The sample is cooled down to 50–600°C to rebind the denatured bonds (DNA primers anneal with the help of the DNA polymerase enzyme). The purine and pyrimidine bases

(A, G, T, and C) will have separated strands present in the DNA, which will form the extension of the DNA provided in the sample. The temperature cycle of heating up to 940°C and cooling down to 50–600°C will be repeated automatically multiple times (35–40 times), resulting in rapid amplification of the given DNA or RNA sample (extension). The replicas of nucleic acid will be compared to standard nucleotides in separating gel. Then electric current is passed through it to form bands like a ladder of nucleic acids (A, G, T, and C), depending on the molecular size and electric charge present in it. (gel electrophoresis). The newly formed band migrates to the gel's level for identification (end-point PCR) (Khehra, Padda et al. 2023).

qPCR is another type of PCR with a slightly different methodology. But it has more advantages over end-point PCR, such as:

1. More rapid results.
2. Comparatively less time consuming.
3. Gel electrophoresis can be omitted due to the use of fluorescent dye.
4. Specific product amplification is possible (Rieu and Powers 2009).

16.2.10 Biosensors

Biosensors are one of the modern technologies that have gained vast popularity globally in the industrial area due to their integrated approach with a shorter time requirement. This method enables the accurate and precise on-site determination of biotoxins in the sample (Naresh and Lee 2021).

Here, identifying agents are biologically active materials such as enzymes, antibodies, antigens, and cells, which act as signal transducers. The signal is later detected by the sensor, which produces a result (Singh, Kumar et al. 2020).

On the basis of the identifying agent, the biosensors for the identification of the biotoxins are classified (Figure 16.5), along with examples.

The flowchart (Figure 16.5) gives the classification of various types of biosensing tests based on the factors, the first being cell-biosensor, which is used in the determination of bacterial toxins such as botulinum toxin and *S. aureus* toxin. Mass-spectrometry-based biosensors are further subdivided into two types: electrospray ionization, which determines the additive present in the food, and matrix-assisted laser desorption-based biosensors, used for protein toxin identification. A sodium ion channel-based biosensor functions on the mechanism of the sodium ion channel to determine the presence of paralytic shellfish toxins such as saxitoxin and neosaxitoxin. Enzyme-based biosensors work on the principle of enzyme activity. It is further classified as an acetylcholine esterase sensor responsible for identifying the presence of organophosphate pesticides in fruits and vegetables and an HRP (also known as a horseradish peroxide biosensor), which determines the presence of myotoxin metabolites. Immunosensors working through the immunoassay principle are further subdivided into two types of biosensors: first, ELISA biosensors,

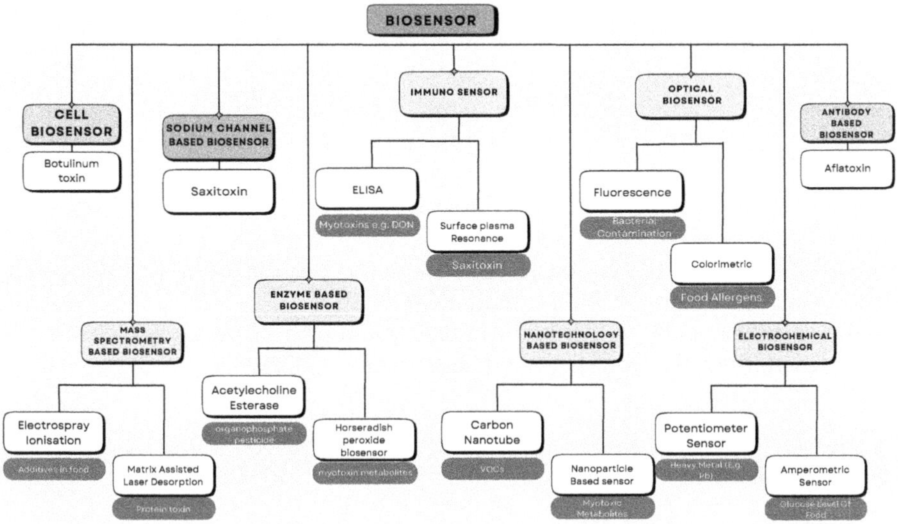

FIGURE 16.5
Classification of biosensors.

determining the presence of mytoxins such as aflatoxin, DON (deoxynivalenol), and ZEN (zearalenone), and second, surface plasma resonance (SPR) is used for the determination of marine biotoxins, namely domoic acid and saxitoxin. Nanotechnology-based biosensors are divided into two subdivisions: carbon nanotube sensors, which determine volatile organic compounds in food packaging, and nanoparticle-based biosensors for determining myotoxin metabolites. Optical biosensors are again classified as fluorescence biosensors to determine bacterial contamination and colorimetric-based biosensors for the presence of food allergens such as gluten, peanuts, milk, and soy. Electrochemical biosensors are conducted as potentiometer sensors for the detection of heavy metals (lead, cadmium, and mercury in seafood), and amperometric biosensors are used for the detection of the percentage of glucose present in food, beverages, juice, and dairy products, as they work on the principle of the glucose oxidase enzyme. Last, antibody-based biosensors work on the principle of the antibody-antigen complex, which determines the presence of aflatoxin (Mehrotra 2016; Alhadrami 2018).

16.2.11 Next-Generation Sequencing

This method is specifically used for the identification of nucleotides, where the sample nucleotide is compared with the previously present standard nucleotide. Here we can also determine the therapeutic pathway along with the diagnosis of genetic disease. Even for prognosis determination, it is also helpful (Prasad, Bhargava et al. 2021).

Sample collection is done first. DNA and RNA extraction from the sample is done in the next step (biotoxin producer present in the sample). DNA extraction is then fragmented into smaller pieces (library preparation). Then, with the help of adapters, the fragments are sequenced for next-generation sequencing (NGS) platform (such as Illumina). The NGS platform prepares the genetic information of the DNA (including the toxin sequencing). The data is then analyzed (toxin detection, identification of the gene where toxin is present, toxin-producer identification, probable effects of the toxin in the body). PCR and assays are done to confirm the identification of the nucleotide in the given sample (Behjati and Tarpey 2013).

The main drawback of this technique is that it only allows for nucleic acid–based toxin identification (Pervez, Hasnain et al. 2022).

16.3 Industrial Applications of Advanced Techniques for Detecting Biotoxins in Food

The food industry is globally one of the leading prospects for the economy. For centuries, food has been an enduring part of our world, and their significance will only continue to grow, both in the immediate future and for generations to come. Also, these industries are the exact places that work as breeding grounds for biotoxins. Therefore, to secure the health of the people and decrease the amount of toxicity in food by ensuring the quality and safety of the food, there are dozens of detection tests followed by the protocol of the Food and Drug Administration (FDA). Depending upon the process, food is classified as in the following figures (Figure 16.6).

First, negligibly processed foods, as the name suggests, require little to no processing to make them easier to digest. They are usually naturally occurring substances that are farmed and used in agriculture. For example, fresh, chilled, vacuum-packed vegetables; fruits and grains; dried fruits; unsalted nuts; roots and tubers; fungi; corn and wheat flour; poultry and dairy products; protein-rich foods such as meat and fish; seafood; and cash crops.

The next category of food is self-preservative in nature; it is not intended to be used as itself but as an additive for the purpose of preservation. This category includes salts, sugars, plant oils, animal fat, and corn starch.

Following this, the classification is divided into processed foods, which are also known as ready-to-go food items. These are usually canned items with added preservatives and a limited shelf life. These food items are also popular due to their sophisticated packaging and transportation benefits. Examples given are canned vegetables, fruits with added sugar, cereals and pulses with added salts, salted meat and fish preserved in oil and salt, cheese, and bread.

Last, the classification categorizes a major part of food as chemically synthesized products. These items have as raw ingredients naturally grown

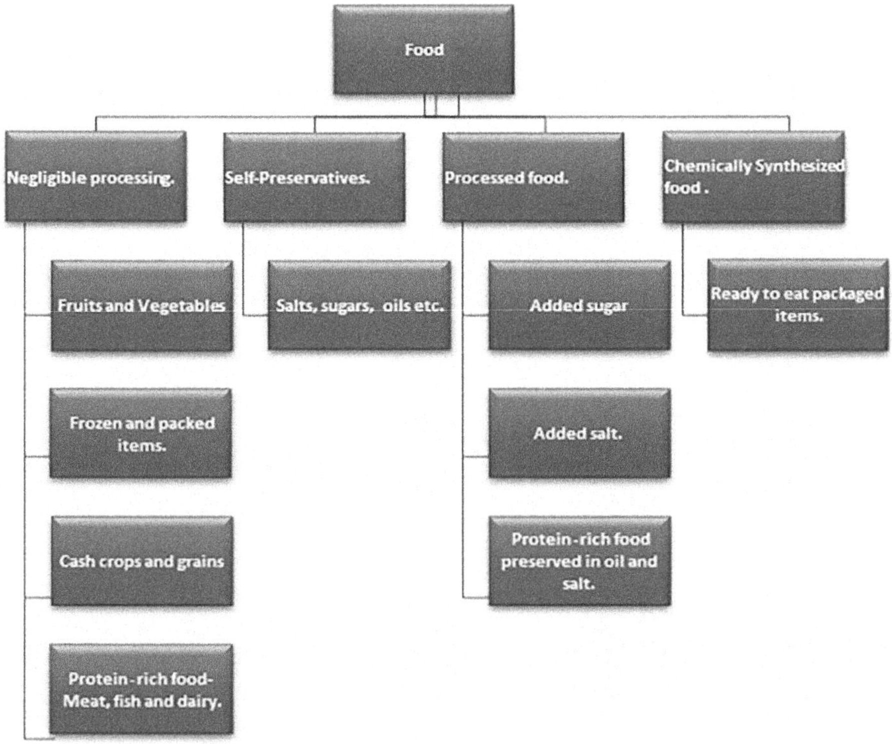

FIGURE 16.6
Classification of food.

items, which are then processed on a large-scale basis in industries, which results in them having almost no nutritional value due to the loss of a considerable amount of whole food. For instance, pre-prepared pizzas have whole wheat, meat, vegetables, and preservatives as raw items. Even though they have ample nutrition individually, once synthesized, they remain nothing but a high-calorie food. A few more examples are soft drinks, energy drinks, ice creams, chocolates, candies, cookies, cakes, mayonnaise, frozen products, cup noodles, instant soups, pies, nuggets, sausages, and hamburgers. Table 16.2 provides tests to detect biotoxins present in different foods.

16.4 Case Studies Related to Biotoxins in Food

Ciguatoxins (CTX) are potent lipophilic toxins that are produced by dinoflagellates belonging to the families Gambeirdiscus and Fukuyoa and are responsible for causing ciguatera fish poisoning (CFP) in humans. CFP is

TABLE 16.2

Test to Detect Biotoxins Present in Different Foods

Category	Sub-Category	Biotoxin	Detection Test	Reference
Negligibly processed food	Fruits and vegetables	Furocoumarins	Inter-laboratory ring test, HPLC, MS	(Dolan, Matulka et al. 2010; Macmaster, Owen et al. 2012; Testa Camillo, Russo et al. 2023)
		Lectins	Latex agglutination test, direct ELISA, ELISA biosensor	(Kaul, Read et al. 1991; Radhakrishnan, Park et al. 2022; World Health Organization 2023)
		Cyanogenic glycoside	HPLC, Guignard sodium picrate test (specific test), colorimetric method	(Cho, Do et al. 2013; Hartanti and Cahyani 2020)
		Glycoalkaloids	HPLC, ELISA	(King 1980; Kodamatani, Saito et al. 2005)
		4-methoxypyridoxine	HPLC, Diazo test	(Ostrovskaya, Ivanov et al. 2019; Gong, Wu et al. 2020)
		Colchicine	MS, liquid chromatography, TLC	(Bodoki, Oprean et al. 2005; Vollmer, Wagmann et al. 2022)
		Muscarine	Hydrophilic interaction liquid chromatography, high-resolution MS	(Chan, Ng et al. 2023; Flament, Gaulier et al. 2024)
		Aflatoxin	HPLC, immunoassay, TLC, MS	(Fernández-Cruz, Mansilla et al. 2010; Namjoo, Salamat et al. 2016; Shabeer, Asad et al. 2022)
		Ochratoxin A	Electrochemical biosensor, immunosensor	(Taylor and Eitenmiller 1986; Wei and Zhang 2018)
		Patulin	Fluorescence assay, HPLC, ELISA, GC-MS	(de Champdore, Bazzicalupo et al. 2007; Sadhasivam, Barda et al. 2021)
		Alternaria toxin	ELISA, GC, MS, TLC, liquid chromatography coupled with UV detector	(Fernández-Cruz, Mansilla et al. 2010; Puvača, Avantaggiato et al. 2022)

Frozen and packed items	Streptococci toxin	Cell-based bioassay, PCR, gram staining	(Weiser 1957; Spellerberg and Brandt 2022)
	Hemolysin BL	CBA, immunoblot assay	(Moravek, Wegscheider et al. 2004)
	Nonhemolytic enterotoxin	Bioluminescence assay, cell-based biosensor, immunosensor	(Rasooly, Do et al. 2020; Reis 2024)
	Cytotoxin k	Immunofluorescence microscopy, CBA, immunoassay	(Fagerlund, Lindbäck et al. 2010; Zhao and Sun 2022)
	Colibactin	Liquid chromatography-MS	(Wehrle, Moravek et al. 2009; Watanabe, Tsunematsu et al. 2023)
Cash crops and grains	Aflatoxin	HPLC, immunoassay, liquid chromatography, MS	(Namjoo, Salamat et al. 2016; Castano-Duque, Winzeler et al. 2023)
	Ochratoxin A	Electrochemical biosensor, immunosensor	(Wei and Zhang 2018; Gurikar, Shivaprasad et al. 2023)
Meat	Harmane	HPLC, fluorescence detection	(Zheng, Wang et al. 2000; Louis, Zheng et al. 2007)
	Ochratoxin A	Electrochemical biosensor, immunosensor	(Wei and Zhang 2018; Vlachou, Pexara et al. 2022)
	Aflatoxin B1	ELISA, HPLC, MS	(Yadav, Singh et al. 2019; Pleadin, Lešić et al. 2021; Yin, Niu et al. 2022)
	Botulinum toxin	MBA, immuno-PCR, MS, PCR, nanobiosensor	(Barr, Moura et al. 2005; Hill, Skerry et al. 2010; Wang, Schill et al. 2020)

(Continued)

TABLE 16.2 *(Continued)*

Test to Detect Biotoxins Present in Different Foods

Category	Sub-Category	Biotoxin	Detection Test	Reference
	Fish and seafood	Paralytic shellfish poisoning	MBA, biosensor, LC	(Santana-Viera and Lara-Martin 2023; Wei, Luo et al. 2023)
		Amnesic shellfish poisoning	LC-MS, LC	(Luckas, Erler et al. 2015)
		Emerging pufferfish poisoning	Hybrid antibody-aptamer assay, MBA	(Shkembi, Skouridou et al. 2021)
		Ciguatoxin	Radio immunoassay, enzyme immunoassay	(Hokama 1985)
		Tetrodotoxin	MS, LC-MS, surface plasmon resonance sensor	(Taylor, Vaisocherová et al. 2011)
		Brevetoxin	ELISA, rapid lateral flow assay	(Tripathi, Upadhyay et al. 2018)
		Azaspiracid	Electrochemical immunosensor, qPCR, immunoassay	(Wietkamp, Tillmann et al. 2019)
		Domoic acid	Immunosensor, ELISA	(Leonardo, Kilcoyne et al. 2018)
		Okadaic acid	ELISA, colorimetric enzymatic assay	(Micheli, Radoi et al. 2004)
		Saxitoxin	Biosensor, ELISA, immunoassay	(Hayat, Barthelmebs et al. 2012; Wharton, Feyereisen et al. 2017)
		Diarrhetic shellfish poisoning	Electrospray ionization, LC-MS	(Suzuki and Yasumoto 2000)
		Neurotoxic shellfish poisoning	MBA, LC-MS, MS	(Watkins, Reich et al. 2008; Fang and Qiu 2023)
	Dairy products	Aflatoxin	HPLC, immunoassay, liquid chromatography, MS	(Namjoo, Salamat et al. 2016; Shabeer, Asad et al. 2022)
		Ochratoxin	Electrochemical biosensor, immunosensor	(Taylor and Eitenmiller 1986; Wei and Zhang 2018)
		Botulinum toxin	MBA, immuno-PCR, MS, PCR	(Hill, Skerry et al. 2010; Wang, Schill et al. 2020)
		Deoxynivalenol (small quantity present)	GC-MS, LC-MS, ELISA	(Olsson, Börjesson et al. 2002; Han, Li et al. 2019)
		Zearalenone (low conc)	Immunochromatography, LC, TLC	(Bu, Bai et al. 2022)

Self-preservative food	Salt	Staphylococcal enterotoxin	Cell-based bioassay, PCR, gram staining	(Hennekinne, Brun et al. 2009)
		Cereulide	Gram staining	(Toh, Moffitt et al. 2004)
		Histamine	Enzymatic assay	(Taylor and Eitenmiller 1986)
	Sugar and starch	Patulin	Fluorescence assay, HPLC, ELISA, GC-MS	(de Champdore, Bazzicalupo et al. 2007; Monteagudo, Torres et al. 2023)
		Ochratoxin A	Electrochemical biosensor, immunosensor	(Taylor and Eitenmiller 1986; Batista, Chalfoun et al. 2003)
		Aflatoxin	HPLC, immunoassay, liquid chromatography, MS	(Gourama and Bullerman 1995; Shabeer, Asad et al. 2022)
		Fumonisins	ELISA, HPLC	(Kamle, Mahato et al. 2019)
	Oil and fat	Ochratoxin A	Electrochemical biosensor, immunosensor	(Taylor and Eitenmiller 1986; Batista, Chalfoun et al. 2003)
		Aflatoxin	HPLC, immunoassay, liquid chromatography, MS	(Gourama and Bullerman 1995; Kanungo and Bhand 2013)
		Fumonisins	ELISA, HPLC	(Kamle, Mahato et al. 2019)
		Cyclopiazonic acid	Spectrophotometry, TLC, HPLC, ELISA	(Lansden 1986; Uka, Moore et al. 2017)
Processed food	Added-sugar food	Patulin	Fluorescence assay, HPLC, ELISA, GC-MS	(Yong 1996; de Champdore, Bazzicalupo et al. 2007)
		Ochratoxin A	Electrochemical biosensor, immunosensor	(Taylor and Eitenmiller 1986; Batista, Chalfoun et al. 2003)
		Aflatoxin	HPLC, immunoassay, liquid chromatography, MS	(Shabeer, Asad et al. 2022; Pisoschi, Iordache et al. 2023)
		Fumonisins	ELISA, HPLC	(Kamle, Mahato et al. 2019)
		Mycotoxin	HPLC, ELISA	(Keskin and Eyupoglu 2023)

(Continued)

TABLE 16.2 *(Continued)*

Test to Detect Biotoxins Present in Different Foods

Category	Sub-Category	Biotoxin	Detection Test	Reference
	Added salt food	Staphylococcal enterotoxin	Cell-based bioassay, PCR, gram staining	(Mehrotra, Wang et al. 2000)
		Cereulide	Gram staining	(Mäntynen and Lindström 1998)
		Mycotoxin	HPLC, ELISA	(Keskin and Eyupoglu 2023)
	Protein rich food preserved in oil and fat	Ochratoxin A	Electrochemical biosensor, immunosensor	(Taylor and Eitenmiller 1986; Batista, Chalfoun et al. 2003)
		Aflatoxin	HPLC, immunoassay, liquid chromatography, MS	(Kanungo and Bhand 2013; Namjoo, Salamat et al. 2016)
		Cyclopiazonic acid	Spectrophotometry, TLC, HPLC, ELISA	(Huang, Dorner et al. 1994; Matsudo and Sasaki 1995)
		Biogenic amines	Semi-quantitative TLC, HPLC	(Santos 1996; Valls, Bello et al. 2002)
Chemically synthesized food	Beverages	Patulin	Fluorescence assay, HPLC, ELISA, GC-MS	(de Champdore, Bazzicalupo et al. 2007; Al-Hazmi 2010)
		Ochratoxin A	Electrochemical biosensor, immunosensor	(Taylor and Eitenmiller 1986; Batista, Chalfoun et al. 2003)
		Biogenic amines	Semi-quantitative TLC, HPLC	(Santos 1996; Costa, Balthazar et al. 2015)
	Frozen products	Deoxynivalenol	GC-MS, LC-MS, ELISA	(Olsson, Börjesson et al. 2002; Han, Li et al. 2019)
		Zearalenone	Immunochromatography, LC, TLC	(Bu, Bai et al. 2022)
		Ergot alkaloids	LC, MS	(Crews 2015)
		Botulinum toxin	MBA, immuno-PCR, MS, PCR	(Hill, Skerry et al. 2010; Wang, Schill et al. 2020)
		Ciguatoxin	Radio immunoassay, enzyme immunoassay	(Hokama 1985)

Ice cream and frozen yogurt	*Bacillus cereus* enterotoxin	Hemolysis test, PCR, agglutination assay	(Mäntynen and Lindström 1998)
	Cyclopiazonic acid	Spectrophotometry, TLC, HPLC, ELISA	(Lansden 1986; Huang, Dorner et al. 1994)
	Patulin	Fluorescence assay, HPLC, ELISA, GC-MS	(de Champdore, Bazzicalupo et al. 2007; Al-Hazmi 2010)
Flour confectionaries	Aflatoxin	HPLC, immunoassay, liquid chromatography, MS	(Namjoo, Salamat et al. 2016; Shabeer, Asad et al. 2022)
	Deoxynivalenol	GC-MS, LC-MS, ELISA	(Olsson, Börjesson et al. 2002; Han, Li et al. 2019)
Sugar confectionaries	Patulin	Fluorescence assay, HPLC, ELISA, GC-MS	(de Champdore, Bazzicalupo et al. 2007; Monteagudo, Torres et al. 2023)
	Ochratoxin A	Electrochemical biosensor, immunosensor	(Batista, Chalfoun et al. 2003; Wei and Zhang 2018)
Chocolate confectionaries	Ochratoxin A	Electrochemical biosensor, immunosensor	(Batista, Chalfoun et al. 2003; Skarkova, Ostry et al. 2013)
	Aflatoxin	HPLC, immunoassay, liquid chromatography, MS	(Namjoo, Salamat et al. 2016; Pisoschi, Iordache et al. 2023)
Ready to eat food	Ochratoxin A	Electrochemical biosensor, immunosensor	(Skarkova, Ostry et al. 2013; Wei and Zhang 2018)
	Aflatoxin	HPLC, immunoassay, liquid chromatography, MS	(Gourama and Bullerman 1995; Shabeer, Asad et al. 2022)
	Fumonisins	ELISA, HPLC	(Kamle, Mahato et al. 2019)

characterized by neurological, gastrointestinal, and cardiovascular disorders. They are named after their geographical source: those found in the Indian Ocean are called I-CTX, those from the Caribbean Sea are called C-CTX, and those from the Pacific Ocean are called P-CTX.

Among these, C-CTX has been emerging in the Caribbean Sea due to environmental factors and the rise in pollution.

Worldwide incidents: world production of seafood demand is rising by the day due to the growing population. This demand is causing increasing pressure on the fishing grounds, leading to imports from which ciguatoxis is endemic. Hence, the disease is widespread in tropical and subtropical marine areas, especially in the Caribbean region, Pacific region, and Indian region, where the risk of getting ciguatera is as high as 25% (Habibi, Uddin et al. 2021).

In Europe, from 1971 to 2007, CFP cases were reported from consuming rabbit fish *(Siganus luridus)*, sauce *(Sarpa salpa)*, and other edible fish in the Mediterranean Sea (Acosta 2015). To curb this, the European Union has adopted policies to ensure food safety.

In conclusion, fishing activity on islands and tropical and subtropical agents pose a severe risk of catching fish with ciguatoxin. Therefore, careful monitoring should be done to mitigate the impacts of climate change and reduce the risk of ciguatoxin attack.

16.5 Future Prospects

Technological advancements have led to the development of more precise and rapid methods for detecting biotoxins, such as high-sensitivity biosensors. As we already know, a number of biotoxin detection tests already exist on the market and are conducted on a large scale. However, a select few stand out due to their superior accuracy, sensitivity, and cost-effectiveness. However, none of the tests appear to cover all of the factors mentioned previously, making them undesirable yet necessary. Therefore, the development of more sensitive biosensors is necessary.

Research aimed at increasing the shelf life of biosensors: As previously discussed, biosensors are typically expensive. Therefore, a short shelf life can lead to significant losses, particularly in industries. Therefore, studies aimed at increasing the shelf-life of biosensors should be made a primary focus (Kumar, Singh et al. 2022).

Microchips in the detection of biotoxins, which are highly specific, have efficacy, and are cost-saving: Recent studies have been emerging to show the influence of microchips in the detection of biotoxins using microfluidic chips and microarrays. These are being pursued due to their efficiency, sensitivity, cost-effective nature, and portability (Zhang, Yu et al. 2014; Man, Liang et al. 2017).

Advancements in the development of aptasensors: The present aptasensors show a very high sensitivity towards all the samples against which they have been tested. Also, they show better results compared to other biotoxin tests, yet only 15 such aptasensors are known; therefore, studies should be conducted based on learning more about their mechanism of action and binding properties, along with their principles, to minimize the negative impact on the mass population. Hence, studies should be encouraged so that marine biotoxins can be detected more accurately using aptasensors (Ye, Liu et al. 2019).

Prompt and instantaneous testing: post-production testing of individual products is both time consuming and may result in product loss. Therefore, there is a growing trend towards portable, accurate, and instantaneous testing due to its immediate result declaration and speedy access (Zhao, Huang et al. 2018).

Biotoxin waste management or treatment should be made compulsory before its disposal. Just because a biotoxin has been detected, it does not mean that the biotoxin will not be affecting the already vulnerable environment. Hence, it is absolutely crucial to conduct treatments on the by-products and waste that are a result of biotoxin detection in such a way that they either do not affect the environment or become environmentally friendly.

16.6 Research Gap

Despite the existence of numerous biotoxin detection tests, none of them meet the criteria of high sensitivity, accuracy, and cost-effectiveness, particularly when conducted on a large scale. Despite conducting experiments in bulk, the confirmation of their by-products and waste disposal methods remains elusive. A study regarding the proper waste management of biotoxin detection tests should be conducted to understand their environmental influence. Any industry must prioritize protecting the environment to avoid contributing to its degradation, especially in the current circumstances. Environmental refining is the primary concern of any nation, as it has a direct influence on biodiversity. Global warming is increasing at an alarming rate, leading to changes or genetic modifications in numerous species. Therefore, we should monitor biotoxin detection tests, their by-products, and waste to prevent any negative impact on the upward growth curve of bio-environmental degradation.

16.7 Conclusion

The current technology has enabled us to broaden our horizons and explore the various new possibilities in biotoxin detection and determination. One of the most relevant tools is the use of biosensors. Through this chapter, we have seen that biosensors are one of the most relevant detection tests or instruments for the detection of biotoxins due to their broad spectrum, which enables us to detect biotoxins both at a large scale and in variety. NGS identifies specific nucleotides and compares them to the standard present, determining the therapeutic pathway along with the detection of diseases. The FDA also adheres to this standard protocol. Advancements from historical techniques like the mouse lethality test to modern methodologies such as immunoassays, PCR, mass spectrometry, and biosensors have significantly improved our ability to detect biotoxins accurately and efficiently. These technologies not only enhance our understanding of biotoxin presence in food but also provide crucial insights into their impacts on human health and ecosystems. The implementation of these advanced detection methods is essential for ensuring food safety and mitigating the adverse effects of biotoxins. The future of biotoxin detection looks encouraging, with the possibility of even more sophisticated and quick testing methods that can be integrated into food safety protocols globally.

References

Ababouch, L. (2014). "Food safety assurance systems: Good practices in fisheries and aquaculture." *Encyclopedia of Food Safety* **4**: 159–167.

Acosta, F. (2015). "Ciguatera, an emerging human poisoning in Europe." *Journal of Aquaculture & Marine Biology* **3**(1).

Al-Bukhaiti, W. Q., A. Noman, A. S. Qasim and A. Al-Farga (2017). "Gas chromatography: Principles, advantages and applications in food analysis." *International Journal of Agriculture Innovations and Research* **6**(1): 1473–2319.

Alhadrami, H. A. (2018). "Biosensors: Classifications, medical applications, and future prospective." *Biotechnology and Applied Biochemistry* **65**(3): 497–508.

Al-Harrasi, A., S. Bhatia, D. Kaushik, T. Behl and S. Chigurupati (2022). "Standardization and quality control of crude drugs." *Recent Advances in Natural Products Science*, CRC Press: 211–234.

Al-Hazmi, N. (2010). "Determination of patulin and ochratoxin A using HPLC in apple juice samples in Saudi Arabia." *Saudi Journal of Biological Sciences* **17**(4): 353–359.

Arkin, M. R., M. A. Glicksman, H. Fu, J. J. Havel and Y. Du (2012). "Inhibition of protein-protein interactions: Non-cellular assay formats." *Assay Guidance Manual [Internet]* **1**: 1–21.

Barr, J. R., H. Moura, A. E. Boyer, A. R. Woolfitt, S. R. Kalb, A. Pavlopoulos, L. G. McWilliams, J. G. Schmidt, R. A. Martinez and D. L. Ashley (2005). "Botulinum neurotoxin detection and differentiation by mass spectrometry." *Emerging Infectious Diseases* **11**(10): 1578.

Batista, L. R., S. M. Chalfoun, G. Prado, R. F. Schwan and A. E. Wheals (2003). "Toxigenic fungi associated with processed (green) coffee beans (Coffea arabica L.)." *International Journal of Food Microbiology* **85**(3): 293–300.

Behjati, S. and P. S. Tarpey (2013). "What is next generation sequencing?" *Archives of Disease in Childhood-Education and Practice* **98**(6): 236–238.

Benenson, A., M. Islam and W. Greenough Iii (1964). "Rapid identification of Vibrio cholerae by darkfield microscopy." *Bulletin of the World Health Organization* **30**(6): 827.

Besbes, N., L. Monser, B. A. Nabli and S. Sadok (2024). Determination of hydrophilic marine biotoxins in bivalve molluscs by liquid chromatography coupled with tandem mass spectrometry (LC-MS/MS). *Journal of Food Composition and Analysis* **130**: 106169.

Bidwell, D. (1976). "The enzyme-linked immunosorbent assay (ELISA)." *Bulletin of the World Health Organization* **54**: 129–139.

Bodoki, E., R. Oprean, L. Vlase, M. Tamas and R. Sandulescu (2005). "Fast determination of colchicine by TLC-densitometry from pharmaceuticals and vegetal extracts." *Journal of Pharmaceutical and Biomedical Analysis* **37**(5): 971–977.

Bu, T., F. Bai, S. Zhao, X. Sun, P. Jia, K. He, Y. Wang, Q. Li and L. Wang (2022). "Dual-modal immunochromatographic test for sensitive detection of zearalenone in food samples based on biosynthetic staphylococcus aureus-mediated polymer dot nanocomposites." *Analytical Chemistry* **94**(14): 5546–5554.

Bunaciu, A. A., V. D. Hoang and H. Y. Aboul-Enein (2013). "Applications of differential spectrophotometry in analytical chemistry." *Critical Reviews in Analytical Chemistry* **43**(3): 125–130.

Castano-Duque, L., E. Winzeler, J. M. Blackstock, C. Liu, N. Vergopolan, M. Focker, K. Barnett, P. R. Owens, H. van der Fels-Klerx and M. M. Vaughan (2023). "Dynamic geospatial modeling of mycotoxin contamination of corn in Illinois: Unveiling critical factors and predictive insights with machine learning." *Frontiers in Microbiology* **14**: 1283127.

Chan, T. Y. C., S. W. Ng, C. K. Chan, H. H. C. Lee and T. W. L. Mak (2023). "Cholinergic mushroom poisoning with a detection of muscarine toxin in urine." *Journal of Medical Cases* **14**(6): 222.

Cho, H.-J., B.-K. Do, S.-M. Shim, H. Kwon, D.-H. Lee, A.-H. Nah, Y.-J. Choi and S.-Y. Lee (2013). "Determination of cyanogenic compounds in edible plants by ion chromatography." *Toxicological Research* **29**: 143–147.

Costa, M. P., C. F. Balthazar, B. L. Rodrigues, C. A. Lazaro, A. C. Silva, A. G. Cruz and C. A. Conte Junior (2015). "Determination of biogenic amines by high-performance liquid chromatography (HPLC-DAD) in probiotic cow's and goat's fermented milks and acceptance." *Food Science & Nutrition* **3**(3): 172–178.

Crews, C. (2015). "Analysis of ergot alkaloids." *Toxins* **7**(6): 2024–2050.

Dadi, M., M. Yasir, M. Dadi and M. Yasir (2022). "Spectroscopy and spectrophotometry: Principles and applications for colorimetric and related other analysis." *Colorimetry* **1**: 81–102.

de Champdore, M., P. Bazzicalupo, L. De Napoli, D. Montesarchio, G. Di Fabio, I. Cocozza, A. Parracino, M. Rossi and S. D'Auria (2007). "A new competitive fluorescence assay for the detection of patulin toxin." *Analytical Chemistry* **79**(2): 751–757.

Dolan, L. C., R. A. Matulka and G. A. Burdock (2010). "Naturally occurring food toxins." *Toxins* **2**(9): 2289–2332.

Fagerlund, A., T. Lindbäck and P. E. Granum (2010). "Bacillus cereus cytotoxins Hbl, Nhe and CytK are secreted via the Sec translocation pathway." *BMC Microbiology* **10**: 1–8.

Fang, L. and F. Qiu (2023). "Determination of neurotoxic shellfish poisoning toxins in shellfish by liquid chromatography-tandem mass spectrometry coupled with dispersive solid phase extraction." *Heliyon* **9**(11).

Fernández-Cruz, M. L., M. L. Mansilla and J. L. Tadeo (2010). "Mycotoxins in fruits and their processed products: Analysis, occurrence and health implications." *Journal of Advanced Research* **1**(2): 113–122.

Flament, E., J. M. Gaulier, N. Paret, N. Jarrier, C. Bruneau, G. Creusat, J. Guitton and Y. Gaillard (2024). "Application to several suspected poisoning cases of a validated analytical method for the determination of muscarine in human biological matrices using liquid chromatography with high-resolution mass spectrometry detection." *Drug Testing and Analysis* **16**(4): 331–338.

Gong, H., C.-E. Wu, G.-J. Fan, T.-T. Li, J.-H. Wang and T. Wang (2020). "Determination of native contents of 4′-O-methylpyridoxine and its glucoside in raw and heated Ginkgo biloba seeds by high-performance liquid chromatography." *Journal of Food Measurement and Characterization* **14**: 917–924.

Gourama, H. and L. B. Bullerman (1995). "Aspergillus flavus and aspergillus parasiticus: Aflatoxigenic fungi of concern in foods and feeds: A review." *Journal of Food Protection* **58**(12): 1395–1404.

Gurikar, C., D. Shivaprasad, L. Sabillón, N. N. Gowda and K. Siliveru (2023). "Impact of mycotoxins and their metabolites associated with food grains." *Grain & Oil Science and Technology* **6**(1): 1–9.

Habibi, N., S. Uddin, M. D. Bottein and M. Faizuddin (2021). "Ciguatera in the Indian Ocean with Special Insights on the Arabian Sea and Adjacent Gulf and Seas: A Review." *Toxins (Basel)* **13**(8).

Han, L., Y.-T. Li, J.-Q. Jiang, R.-F. Li, G.-Y. Fan, J.-M. Lv, Y. Zhou, W.-J. Zhang and Z.-L. Wang (2019). "Development of a direct competitive ELISA kit for detecting deoxynivalenol contamination in wheat." *Molecules* **25**(1): 50.

Hartanti, D. and A. N. Cahyani (2020). "Plant cyanogenic glycosides: An overview." *Farmasains: Jurnal Farmasi dan Ilmu Kesehatan* **5**(1): 1–6.

Hayat, A., L. Barthelmebs and J.-L. Marty (2012). "A simple colorimetric enzymatic-assay for okadaic acid detection based on the immobilization of protein phosphatase 2A in sol-gel." *Applied Biochemistry and Biotechnology* **166**: 47–56.

Hennekinne, J.-A., V. Brun, M.-L. De Buyser, A. Dupuis, A. Ostyn and S. Dragacci (2009). "Innovative application of mass spectrometry for the characterization of staphylococcal enterotoxins involved in food poisoning outbreaks." *Applied and Environmental Microbiology* **75**(3): 882–884.

Hill, B. J., J. C. Skerry, T. J. Smith, S. S. Arnon and D. C. Douek (2010). "Universal and specific quantitative detection of botulinum neurotoxin genes." *BMC Microbiology* **10**: 1–16.

Hokama, Y. (1985). "A rapid, simplified enzyme immunoassay stick test for the detection of ciguatoxin and related polyethers from fish tissues." *Toxicon* **23**(6): 939–946.

Huang, X., J. Dorner and F. S. Chu (1994). "Production of aflatoxin and cyclopiazonic acid by various aspergilli: An ELISA analysis." *Mycotoxin Research* **10**(2): 101–106.

Janik, E., M. Ceremuga, J. Saluk-Bijak and M. Bijak (2019). "Biological toxins as the potential tools for bioterrorism." *International Journal of Molecular Sciences* **20**(5).

Kamle, M., D. K. Mahato, S. Devi, K. E. Lee, S. G. Kang and P. Kumar (2019). "Fumonisins: Impact on agriculture, food, and human health and their management strategies." *Toxins* **11**(6): 328.

Kanungo, L. and S. Bhand (2013). "Fluorimetric immunoassay for multianalysis of aflatoxins." *Journal of Analytical Methods in Chemistry* **2013**(1): 584964.

Kaul, R., J. Read and B. Mattiasson (1991). "Screening for plant lectins by latex agglutination tests." *Phytochemistry* **30**(12): 4005–4009.

Keskin, E. and O. E. Eyupoglu (2023). "Determination of mycotoxins by HPLC, LC-MS/MS and health risk assessment of the mycotoxins in bee products of Turkey." *Food Chemistry* **400**: 134086.

Khehra, N., I. S. Padda and C. J. Swift (2023). *Polymerase Chain Reaction (PCR): StatPearls [Internet]*, StatPearls Publishing.

King, R. R. (1980). "Analysis of potato glycoalkaloids by gas-liquid chromatography of alkaloid components." *Journal of the Association of Official Analytical Chemists* **63**(6): 1226–1230.

Kodamatani, H., K. Saito, N. Niina, S. Yamazaki and Y. Tanaka (2005). "Simple and sensitive method for determination of glycoalkaloids in potato tubers by high-performance liquid chromatography with chemiluminescence detection." *Journal of Chromatography A* **1100**(1): 26–31.

Kumar, V., S. Singh and B. Singh (2022). "Recent advances in biosensors technology to increase shelf life of vegetables." *Annals of Horticulture* **15**(2): 257–262.

Langer, G. (2016). "Implementation and use of state-of-the-art, cell-based in vitro assays." *New Approaches to Drug Discovery* 171–190.

Lansden, J. A. (1986). "Determination of cyclopiazonic acid in peanuts and corn by thin layer chromatography." *Journal of the Association of Official Analytical Chemists* **69**(6): 964–966.

Leonardo, S., J. Kilcoyne, I. A. Samdal, C. O. Miles, C. K. O'Sullivan, J. Diogène and M. Campàs (2018). "Detection of azaspiracids in mussels using electrochemical immunosensors for fast screening in monitoring programs." *Sensors and Actuators B: Chemical* **262**: 818–827.

Louis, E. D., W. Zheng, W. Jiang, K. T. Bogen and G. A. Keating (2007). "Quantification of the neurotoxic β-carboline harmane in barbecued/grilled meat samples and correlation with level of doneness." *Journal of Toxicology and Environmental Health, Part A* **70**(12): 1014–1019.

Luckas, B., K. Erler and B. Krock (2015). "Analysis of marine biotoxins using LC-MS/MS." *Natural Products from Marine Algae: Methods and Protocols* 277–297.

Macmaster, A. P., N. Owen, S. Brussaux, H. Brevard, R. Hiserodt, H. Leijs, N. Bast, B. Weber, G. Loesing and A. Sherlock (2012). "Quantification of selected furocoumarins by high-performance liquid chromatography and UV-detection: Capabilities and limits." *Journal of Chromatography A* **1257**: 34–40.

Malaysia, S., E. Malaysia, Y. S. Choong, G. J. Tye, N. W. H. A. Karim, T. S. Lim, K. M. F. Mustaffa, C. H. Leow, C. Y. Leow and V. Balakrishnan (2019). *Conference Proceedings–4th International Conference on Molecular Diagnostics and Biomarker Discovery: Antibody Technology*. BMC Proceedings, Springer.

Man, Y., G. Liang, A. Li and L. Pan (2017). "Recent advances in mycotoxin determination for food monitoring via microchip." *Toxins* **9**(10): 324.

Mäntynen, V. and K. Lindström (1998). "A rapid PCR-based DNA test for enterotoxic Bacillus cereus." *Applied and Environmental Microbiology* **64**(5): 1634–1639.

Masi, G., G. Spagni, L. Campetella, G. Monte, E. Sabatelli, A. Evoli, C. Papi and R. Iorio (2021). "Assessing the role of a tissue-based assay in the diagnostic algorithm of autoimmune encephalitis." *Journal of neuroimmunology* **356**: 577601.

Matsudo, T. and M. Sasaki (1995). "Simple determination of cyclopiazonic acid." *Bioscience, Biotechnology, and Biochemistry* **59**(3): 355–357.
McNamara, G., M. J. Difilippantonio and T. Ried (2005). "Microscopy and image analysis." *Current Protocols in Human Genetics* **46**(1): 4.4. 1–4.4. 34.
Mehrotra, M., G. Wang and W. M. Johnson (2000). "Multiplex PCR for detection of genes for Staphylococcus aureus enterotoxins, exfoliative toxins, toxic shock syndrome toxin 1, and methicillin resistance." *Journal of Clinical Microbiology* **38**(3): 1032–1035.
Mehrotra, P. (2016). "Biosensors and their applications: A review." *Journal of Oral Biology and Craniofacial Research* **6**(2): 153–159.
Micheli, L., A. Radoi, R. Guarrina, R. Massaud, C. Bala, D. Moscone and G. Palleschi (2004). "Disposable immunosensor for the determination of domoic acid in shellfish." *Biosensors and Bioelectronics* **20**(2): 190–196.
Monteagudo, A. A., A. Torres, F. Chamorro, M. A. Prieto, R. Perez-Gregorio, J. Simal-Gandara and P. Otero (2023). *Rapid Identification of the Mycotoxin Patulin by Gas Chromatography-Mass Spectrometry*. Biology and Life Sciences Forum, MDPI.
Morabito, S., S. Silvestro and C. Faggio (2018). "How the marine biotoxins affect human health." *Natural Product Research* **32**(6): 621–631.
Moravek, M., M. Wegscheider, A. Schulz, R. Dietrich, C. Bürk and E. Märtlbauer (2004). "Colony immunoblot assay for the detection of hemolysin BL enterotoxin producing Bacillus cereus." *FEMS Microbiology Letters* **238**(1): 107–113.
Namjoo, M., F. Salamat, N. Rajabli, R. Hajihoseeini, F. Niknejad, F. Kohsar and H. Joshaghani (2016). "Quantitative determination of aflatoxin by high performance liquid chromatography in wheat silos in Golestan Province, North of Iran." *Iranian Journal of Public Health* **45**(7): 905.
Naresh, V. and N. Lee (2021). "A review on biosensors and recent development of nanostructured materials-enabled biosensors." *Sensors* **21**(4): 1109.
Notermans, S., C. Stam and A. Behar (2014). *Clostridium Detection of Neurotoxins of Clostridium botulinum: Encyclopedia of Food Microbiology* (Second Edition), Academic Press: 481–484.
Olsson, J., T. Börjesson, T. Lundstedt and J. Schnürer (2002). "Detection and quantification of ochratoxin A and deoxynivalenol in barley grains by GC-MS and electronic nose." *International Journal of Food Microbiology* **72**(3): 203–214.
Ostrovskaya, V. M., A. V. Ivanov and D. Y. Marchenko (2019). "Determination of pyridoxine by means of an indicator diazo-test strip." *Open Journal of Analytical and Bioanalytical Chemistry* **3**(1): 001–005.
Patel, N., R. Kumar, C. Savalia, I. Kalyani and J. Solanki (2022). "Public health risk of antibiotic resistant phenotypes and molecular confirmation of staphylococcus aureus isolated from bovine raw milk of South Gujarat." *India* **11**: 327–334.
Paterson, R. R. M. (2006). "Fungi and fungal toxins as weapons." *Mycological Research* **110**(9): 1003–1010.
Pervez, M. T., M. J. U. Hasnain, S. H. Abbas, M. F. Moustafa, N. Aslam and S. S. M. Shah (2022). "[Retracted] a comprehensive review of performance of next-generation sequencing platforms." *BioMed Research International* **2022**(1): 3457806.
Pisoschi, A. M., F. Iordache, L. Stanca, A. I. Petcu, L. Purdoiu, O. I. Geicu, L. Bilteanu and A. I. Serban (2023). "Comprehensive overview and critical perspective on the analytical techniques applied to aflatoxin determination: A review paper." *Microchemical Journal* **191**: 108770.

Pleadin, J., T. Lešić, D. Milićević, K. Markov, B. Šarkanj, N. Vahčić, I. Kmetič and M. Zadravec (2021). "Pathways of mycotoxin occurrence in meat products: A review." *Processes* **9**(12): 2122.

Prasad, A., H. Bhargava, A. Gupta, N. Shukla, S. Rajagopal, S. Gupta, A. Sharma, J. Valadi, V. Nigam and P. Suravajhala (2021). "Next generation sequencing." *Advances in Bioinformatics* 277–302.

Puvača, N., G. Avantaggiato, J. Merkuri, G. Vuković, V. Bursić and M. Cara (2022). "Occurrence and determination of Alternaria mycotoxins alternariol, alternariol monomethyl ether, and tentoxin in wheat grains by QuEChERS method." *Toxins* **14**(11): 791.

Radhakrishnan, A., K. Park, I.-S. Kwak, M. Jaabir and J. Sivakamavalli (2022). "Classification of lectins." *Lectins: Innate Immune Defense and Therapeutics*, Springer: 51–72.

Rai, M., S. Bhattarai and C. M. Feitosa (2021). *Ethnopharmacology of Wild Plants*, CRC Press: 416.

Rasooly, R., P. Do and B. Hernlem (2020). "Quantitative bioluminescence assay for measuring Bacillus cereus nonhemolytic enterotoxin complex." *PLOS One* **15**(9): e0238153.

Reis, M. J. (2024). *Data, Signal and Image Processing and Applications in Sensors II*, MDPI. **24**: 2555.

Rhodes, L., A. Selwood, P. McNabb, L. Briggs, J. Adamson, R. Van Ginkel and O. Laczka (2006). "Trace metal effects on the production of biotoxins by microalgae." *African Journal of Marine Science* **28**(2): 393–397.

Rieu, I. and S. J. Powers (2009). "Real-time quantitative RT-PCR: Design, calculations, and statistics." *The Plant Cell* **21**(4): 1031–1033.

Robson, M. G., W. A. Toscano, Q. Meng and D. A. Kaden (2022). *Risk Assessment for Environmental Health*, CRC Press.

Sadhasivam, S., O. Barda, V. Zakin, R. Reifen and E. Sionov (2021). "Rapid detection and quantification of patulin and citrinin contamination in fruits." *Molecules* **26**(15): 4545.

Santana-Viera, S. and P. A. Lara-Martin (2023). "Analysis of paralytic shellfish toxins in seafood by liquid chromatography: A critical review of the methodologies developed." *Trends in Environmental Analytical Chemistry* **37**: e00190.

Santos, M. S. (1996). "Biogenic amines: Their importance in foods." *International Journal of Food Microbiology* **29**(2–3): 213–231.

Shabeer, S., S. Asad, A. Jamal and A. Ali (2022). "Aflatoxin contamination, its impact and management strategies: An updated review." *Toxins* **14**(5): 307.

Shkembi, X., V. Skouridou, M. Svobodova, S. Leonardo, A. S. Bashammakh, A. O. Alyoubi, M. Campàs and C. K. O'Sullivan (2021). "Hybrid antibody-aptamer assay for detection of tetrodotoxin in pufferfish." *Analytical Chemistry* **93**(44): 14810–14819.

Singh, A. K., E. A. E. Garber, M. C. Principato, S. Hall and S. K. Sharma (2015). "Biotoxins and food safety." *Biological Toxins and Bioterrorism*. P. Gopalakrishnakone, M. Balali-Mood, L. Llewellyn and B. R. Singh. Springer: 185–210.

Singh, S., V. Kumar, D. S. Dhanjal, S. Datta, R. Prasad and J. Singh (2020). "Biological biosensors for monitoring and diagnosis." *Microbial Biotechnology: Basic Research and Applications* 317–335.

Skarkova, J., V. Ostry, F. Malir and T. Roubal (2013). "Determination of ochratoxin A in food by high performance liquid chromatography." *Analytical Letters* **46**(10): 1495–1504.

Solomon, H. M. and T. Lilly (2001). *BAM Chapter 17: Clostridium botulinum*, Food and Drug Administration.
Solzin, J., K. Eppler, B. Knapp, H. Buchner and E. Bluhmki (2023). "Optimising cell-based bioassays via integrated design of experiments (ixDoE)-A practical guide." *SLAS Discovery* **28**(1): 29–38.
Spellerberg, B. and C. Brandt (2022). "Laboratory diagnosis of *streptococcus pyogenes* (group A streptococci)." *Streptococcus Pyogenes: Basic Biology to Clinical Manifestations* [Internet] (Second Edition), University of Oklahoma Health Sciences Center: 1–14.
Suzuki, T. and T. Yasumoto (2000). "Liquid chromatography-electrospray ionization mass spectrometry of the diarrhetic shellfish-poisoning toxins okadaic acid, dinophysistoxin-1 and pectenotoxin-6 in bivalves." *Journal of Chromatography A* **874**(2): 199–206.
Taylor, A. D., H. Vaisocherová, J. Deeds, S. DeGrasse and S. Jiang (2011). "Tetrodotoxin detection by a surface plasmon resonance sensor in pufferfish matrices and urine." *Journal of Sensors* **2011**(1): 601704.
Taylor, S. L. and R. R. Eitenmiller (1986). "Histamine food poisoning: Toxicology and clinical aspects." *CRC Critical Reviews in Toxicology* **17**(2): 91–128.
Testa Camillo, M. R., M. Russo, A. Trozzi, L. Mondello and P. Dugo (2023). "Quantification of coumarins, furocoumarins and polymethoxyflavones in hydroalcoholic fragrances by supercritical fluid chromatography-tandem mass spectrometry." *Journal of Essential Oil Research* **35**(5): 461–470.
Tiwari, A. and S. Nagalli (2023). *Clostridium botulinum Infection*. StatPearls [Internet], StatPearls Publishing.
Toh, M., M. Moffitt, L. Henrichsen, M. Raftery, K. Barrow, J. Cox, C. Marquis and B. Neilan (2004). "Cereulide, the emetic toxin of Bacillus cereus, is putatively a product of nonribosomal peptide synthesis." *Journal of Applied Microbiology* **97**(5): 992–1000.
Tripathi, P., N. Upadhyay and S. Nara (2018). "Recent advancements in lateral flow immunoassays: A journey for toxin detection in food." *Critical Reviews in Food Science and Nutrition* **58**(10): 1715–1734.
Turner, D. (2022). "GC-MS principle, instrument and analyses and GC-MS/MS." *Technology Networks-Analysis and Separations* 1–5.
Uka, V., G. G. Moore, N. Arroyo-Manzanares, D. Nebija, S. De Saeger and J. Diana Di Mavungu (2017). "Unravelling the diversity of the cyclopiazonic acid family of mycotoxins in Aspergillus flavus by UHPLC triple-TOF HRMS." *Toxins* **9**(1): 35.
Valls, J. E., R. A. Bello and M. S. Kodaira (2002). "Semiquantitative analysis by thin-layer chromatography (TLC) of biogenic amines in dried, salted and canned fish products." *Journal of Food Quality* **25**(2): 165–176.
Vishwakarma, S. (2021). "Principle." *Instrumentation, and Applications of Gas Chromatography-Mass Spectrometry (GC-MS)* **10**.
Vlachou, M., A. Pexara, N. Solomakos and A. Govaris (2022). "Ochratoxin A in slaughtered pigs and pork products." *Toxins* **14**(2): 67.
Vollmer, A. C., L. Wagmann and M. R. Meyer (2022). "Toxic plants—detection of colchicine in a fast systematic clinical toxicology screening using liquid chromatography-mass spectrometry." *Drug Testing and Analysis* **14**(2): 377–381.
Wahi, I. R. P., H. H. Cerjak, G. Sauthoff and V. Buck (2009). "Thermo fisher scientific UHPLC enables enhanced resolution separations of complex drug mixtures." *International Journal of Materials Research (Formerly Z. Metallkd.)* **100**(10): 1471.

Wang, Y., K. M. Schill, H. C. Fry and T. V. Duncan (2020). "A quantum dot nanobiosensor for rapid detection of botulinum neurotoxin serotype E." *ACS Sensors* **5**(7): 2118–2127.

Wang, Z. and J. J. Paré (1997). "Gas chromatography (GC): Principles and applications." *Techniques and Instrumentation in Analytical Chemistry*, Elsevier. **18:** 61–91.

Watanabe, K., Y. Tsunematsu and M. Sato (2023). *Detection Method and Detection Probe for Colibactin and Colibactin-Producing Bacteria*, Google Patents.

Watkins, S. M., A. Reich, L. E. Fleming and R. Hammond (2008). "Neurotoxic shellfish poisoning." *Marine Drugs* **6**(3): 431–455.

Watson, I. (2000). "Clinical diagnosis: chromatography." *Encyclopedia of Separation Science* 2484–2490.

Wehrle, E., M. Moravek, R. Dietrich, C. Bürk, A. Didier and E. Märtlbauer (2009). "Comparison of multiplex PCR, enzyme immunoassay and cell culture methods for the detection of enterotoxinogenic Bacillus cereus." *Journal of Microbiological Methods* **78**(3): 265–270.

Wei, L.-N., L. Luo, B.-Z. Wang, H.-T. Lei, T. Guan, Y.-D. Shen, H. Wang and Z.-L. Xu (2023). "Biosensors for detection of paralytic shellfish toxins: Recognition elements and transduction technologies." *Trends in Food Science & Technology* **133**: 205–218.

Wei, M. and W. Zhang (2018). "The determination of ochratoxin A based on the electrochemical aptasensor by carbon aerogels and methylene blue assisted signal amplification." *Chemistry Central Journal* **12**: 1–8.

Weiser, H. (1957). "Bacteriology of precooked frozen foods." *Journal of Food Protection* **20**(2): 33–35.

Weller, M. G. (2000). "Immunochromatographic techniques: A critical review." *Fresenius' Journal of Analytical Chemistry* **366**: 635–645.

Wharton, R. E., M. C. Feyereisen, A. L. Gonzalez, N. L. Abbott, E. I. Hamelin and R. C. Johnson (2017). "Quantification of saxitoxin in human blood by ELISA." *Toxicon* **133**: 110–115.

Wietkamp, S., U. Tillmann, D. Clarke and K. Toebe (2019). "Molecular detection and quantification of the azaspiracid-producing dinoflagellate Amphidoma languida (Amphidomataceae, Dinophyceae)." *Journal of Plankton Research* **41**(2): 101–113.

World Health Organization (2023). *Toxicological Evaluation of Certain Veterinary Drug Residues in Food: Prepared by the Ninety-Fourth Meeting of the Joint FAO/WHO Expert Committee on Food Additives (JECFA)*, World Health Organization.

Yadav, S. K., M. Singh and S. Ponmariappan (2019). "ELISA based detection of botulinum neurotoxin type 'F'in red meat and canned fish." *Defence Life Science Journal* **4**: 226–230.

Ye, W., T. Liu, W. Zhang, M. Zhu, Z. Liu, Y. Kong and S. Liu (2019). "Marine toxins detection by biosensors based on aptamers." *Toxins* **12**(1): 1.

Yin, S., L. Niu and Y. Liu (2022). "Recent progress on techniques in the detection of aflatoxin B1 in edible oil: A mini review." *Molecules* **27**(19): 6141.

Yong, R. K. (1996). *Immunological Detection of Molds, Including Mycotoxin Producers, in Foods*, Purdue University.

Zhang, Z., L. Yu, L. Xu, X. Hu, P. Li, Q. Zhang, X. Ding and X. Feng (2014). "Biotoxin sensing in food and environment via microchip." *Electrophoresis* **35**(11): 1547–1559.

Zhao, L., Y. Huang, Y. Dong, X. Han, S. Wang and X. Liang (2018). "Aptamers and aptasensors for highly specific recognition and sensitive detection of marine biotoxins: Recent advances and perspectives." *Toxins* **10**(11): 427.
Zhao, Y. and L. Sun (2022). "Bacillus cereus cytotoxin K triggers gasdermin D-dependent pyroptosis." *Cell Death Discovery* **8**(1): 305.
Zheng, W., S. Wang, L. F. Barnes, Y. Guan and E. D. Louis (2000). "Determination of harmane and harmine in human blood using reversed-phased high-performance liquid chromatography and fluorescence detection." *Analytical Biochemistry* **279**(2): 125–129.

17

Availability of Biotoxins in Foods: Animal and Plant Sources

Peace Abiodun Olajide, Victoria Olufunmi Adeyemo-Eleyode, Babatunde Oluwafemi Adetuyi, Charles Chinazaekpele Chidume, Oluwatosin Adefunke Adetuyi, and Gaber El-Saber Batiha

17.1 Introduction

The term "biotoxins" describes substances or byproducts that are harmful to humans, animals, or microbes. They are typically found in pathogenic substances, bacteria, viruses, fungi, rickettsiae, protozoa, and other organisms that can cause illness or even death (Bradley et al., 2001). Their poisonous reaction can range from a mild one (like that of ergot alkaloid), an acute one (like that of Shiga toxin), to one that is nearly instantaneous (like that of botulinum toxin) (Veldhoen et al., 2008; Simpson, 2004). Biotoxin contaminations have the potential to spread rapidly throughout the entire world, endangering animal and human health as well as having an impact on both domestic and international trade. The FAO, EU, USA, and other nations have set increasingly stringent maximum residue limits for biotoxins due to their serious risks.

17.2 Plant Toxins

Within the class of phytotoxins known as plant toxic proteins, eukaryotic cells are unable to produce new proteins. Toxins in this class are glycoproteins, which are composed of two subunits joined by a disulfide bond to create a dimer and have molecular weights of about 60 kDa. One of the subunits is lectin with carbohydrate binding sites (B-chain), which works with selective N-glycosidase (A-chain) to modify the 28S rRNA-60S ribosomal subunit (Hartley & Lord, 2004). Plant seeds are the source of the initial recognition of the lectin protein group, which binds to certain sugars. There are certain

DOI: 10.1201/9781003500605-20

connections between lectins and toxins, even though lectins are generally not extremely poisonous (Wang & Xu, 2000). They might potentially function as immunotoxins and recognition markers in cellular differentiation. Due to its inhibition of protein synthesis, only A-chain is hazardous. The removal of adenine from positions 4 and 324 of 28S rRNA by the A-chain catalytically inactivates the 60S ribosomal subunit. Numerous plants have been found to have ribosome-inactivating proteins (RIPs), some of which are extremely poisonous when combined with B-chain. Toxin-carrying A-chains are transported across cell membranes by the B-chain, which attaches to cell surface receptors. Before the A-chain is internalized by the cell and stops protein synthesis, it is not active (Stirpe, 2004). Approximately 2000 polysomes can be disabled per minute by each poison molecule, which is sufficient to eventually kill the cell. Ricine, abrin, modessin, viscumin, and volkensin are the most well-known examples of this class of toxic plant proteins (Olsnes, 2004; Patockaa & Stredab, 2002).

17.3 Ricin

The protein known as ricin is generated by the *Ricinus communis* castor oil plant. Although it originated in tropical Africa, it has since spread to temperate and subtropical regions. The toxin ricin, which is found in large concentrations in the seeds, makes the entire plant toxic. Additionally, the seeds contain ricinoleic acid triglyceride, a purgative oil. For generations, folk medicine has utilized the seeds as a means of treating many illnesses.

The substance that makes *R. communis* seeds poisonous is called ricin (Rutenber & Robertus, 1991). For many years, ricin has been recognized as a toxin due to the mortality of livestock. A kid may die from one to three seeds, an adult may get poisoned from two to four seeds, and an adult may die from eight seeds. A human lethal dosage is around 1 μg/kg (Clark, 1997). When given parenterally, ricin is far more effective because the alimentary tract largely eliminates it. Known as an N-glycosidase, the globular protein comprising 267 amino acids is responsible for the poisonous activity of ricin's A-chain. Eight alpha helices and eight beta sheets make up the protein known as the A-chain (Katzin et al., 1991; Morris & Wool, 1994). With 262 amino acid residues, the B-chain is categorized as a lectin (Katzin et al., 1991). The two galactose binding sites on the B chain have a propensity for binding to galactosides and are attracted to glycoproteins that have galactose on their cell surface (Rutenber & Robertus, 1991). A disulfide bond connecting residues 4 of the B-chain and 259 of the A-chain connects the two glycoproteins (Montfort et al., 1987). A glycoprotein, ricin binds specifically to mannose receptors on reticuloendothelial system cells. N-linked oligosaccharides rich in mannose make up its side chains, which are carbs. Asparagines 95 and 135 of the B-chain and asparagines 10 and 236 of the A-chain are the precise locations with the ability to bind high mannose carbohydrate chains of ricin.

The A-chain's ability to deactivate the cell's ribosomes is essentially what causes the harmful effects of ricin. Based on its binding to structures at the cell surface containing mannose, galactose, or both, the B-chain is thought to help the A-chain enter the cell (Olsnes & Kozlov, 2001). In this manner, the protein is internalized, entering the cell as a vesicle-bound complex of toxin-binding sites. The ricin B-chain assists the A-chain in escaping by binding to the endosomal membrane and letting the A-chain pass through. The disulfide bond is then broken, resulting in the B-chain's separation from the A-chain. This delivers the A-chain to the cytoplasm, where the Golgi apparatus picks it up and moves it to the endoplasmic reticulum [14].

At the endoplasmic reticulum, ricin depletes adenine from specific RNA sequences on the 28S ribosomal subunit, hence rendering the cell ribosomes inactive (Lord et al., 1994). A single A-chain molecule has the power to disable every ribosome in a cell, halting protein synthesis and ultimately leading to cell death. The toxin's specificity for eukaryotic ribosomes should be noted. The hairpin loop on the 28S rRNA that houses the tetranucleotide loop GAGA is the most plausible target for ricin on the ribosome; nonetheless, it is thought that the ribosome conformation is essential for the protein's recognition (Lord et al., 1994). Ricine is therefore not a protein that is unique to nucleotide sequences.

Ricine is the only toxin that is found in substantial quantities in nature. It is the byproduct of castor oil, and the method of isolating ricin is simple and reasonably priced. This toxin may appeal to developing nations due to its inexpensive cost and ease of manufacturing. Toxin warfare has a terrible allure for countries or terrorist groups that lack the funds to purchase nuclear weapons and other cutting-edge means of death. This is because biological and toxic weapons are inexpensive, simple to produce, and easy to hide. If utilized properly, even tiny amounts could result in severe harm and suffering for a great number of people (Patočka, 1998). Part of the reason ricin is so important as a possible poison for biological warfare is its accessibility. Every year, a million metric tons of castor beans are processed to produce castor oil, with 5% of the bean weight being ricin. Additionally, the toxin exhibits high toxicity and stability across multiple exposure pathways, including the respiratory route (Patočka, 2001a, 2001b).

In a biological warfare scenario, ricin is expected to be released as a toxic cloud. Furthermore, it might be administered intraperitoneally to specific individuals as a terrorist or sabotage tool. Furthermore, ricin is stable and simple to make. When ricin enters the body, it kills whatever cells it comes into touch with, which is why it has toxic consequences. If a person inhales a sufficient quantity of ricin, breathing difficulties and circulatory system consequences should result in death within 36–48 hours. It is anticipated that ingesting ricin will result in internal bleeding, the death of important organs, and the individual's death. Victims with injected ricin die from severe organ failure.

Predicted symptoms are derived from studies conducted on animals and inadvertent human exposures that did not result in death. The symptoms would most likely differ based on whether ricin was injected, swallowed, or inhaled. The typical symptoms of ricin exposure include coughing, chest tightness, breathing difficulties, nausea, and muscle aches about three hours after inhalation. After that, there would be a serious inflammation of the lungs and airways, more trouble breathing, cyanosis, and, in 36 to 48 hours, death due to a collapse of the circulatory and respiratory systems. When someone consumes ricin, they are expected to experience internal bleeding in their stomach and intestines, failure of their liver, spleen, and kidneys, and eventually pass away due to the collapse of their circulatory vessels. There wouldn't be any specific impacts on the lungs or airways. When someone injects ricin, the surrounding muscles and lymph nodes die visibly, and the person's essential organs are likely to fail and eventually die (Patočka & Středa, 2003).

17.4 Viscumin

The principal pharmacologically active ingredient of mistletoe (*Viscum album*) extract, known as viscumin or mistletoe lectin I, ML I, was found to be poisonous to members of the RIP family in the late 1980s (Krauspenhaar et al., 1999). It functions through the same mechanism as ricin and is similarly harmful. Like ricin, viscumin attaches itself to its cell of interest via the A chain's enzymatic activity, which inhibits the cell's ability to produce proteins. When a target cell experiences a disturbance, it triggers a cellular response to stress that releases cytokines and, if viscumin concentrations are too high, starts cell death. The majority of the interactions between the A- and B-subunits are hydrophobic.

17.5 Abrin

Abrus precatorius (also known as rosary pea) seeds contain a strong poison known as abrin. Sharon and Lis (1972) described its application as a research instrument (Sharon & Lis, 1972). There are two types of abrin: abrin a and abrin b. Two chains—an A-chain and a B-chain—make up each. The A and B chains are joined by a disulfide bond that is formed between Cys247 of the A-chain and Cys8 of the B-chain. There are three folding domains and 251 residues in the A-chain. The A-chain depletes sites 4 and 324 of 28S rRNA of adenine, hence catalytically inactivating 60S ribosomal subunits and preventing protein synthesis. A lectin that is specific to galactose, the B-chain, helps abrin attach to cell membranes (Chen et al., 1992; Sandvig et al., 1976).

Both variants of abrin have a B-chain with 268 amino acid residues, of which 256 are identical. Based on a comparison of their sequences with the ricin B-chain, it is shown that the abrin B-chain and the ricin B-chain have two saccharide-binding sites that were identified during the crystallographic study (Kimura et al., 1993). Moreover, 60% of the residues in the ricin B-chain and the abrin B-chain are complementary.

Since abrin's method of action is the same as ricin's (Patočka, 2001a, 2001b), mice exposed to abrin are 75 times more toxic than those exposed to ricin (0.04 μg/kg versus 3 μg/kg). Both ricin and abrin intoxications require the same diagnosis, clinical manifestations, course of therapy, safeguards, prevention, and other measures (Olsnes et al., 1978; Patočka, 2001a, 2001b).

17.6 Modeccin

Adenia digitata, an African succulent plant, yields the lectin modeccin from its roots. It functions similarly to ricin (Olsnes et al., 1982), acting on similar pathways (Olsnes et al., 1978; Refsnes et al., 1977). The plant is not as widely available as abrin or even ricin because it doesn't appear to have any major applications as a food or medication. The seed does appear to be widely accessible, though. Modeccin subunits were designated modeccin 4B after they were isolated and refined from Adenia digitata roots using a technique called affinity chromatography on Sepharose 4B (Gasperi-Campani et al., 1978). They consist of a B subunit (mol. wt. 31,000), which attaches to cells, and an A subunit (mol. wt. 26,000), which prevents the creation of proteins. Following Sepharose 6B's acid treatment, an additional type of modeccin that Sepharose 4B was unable to maintain was purified using affinity chromatography. This form is now known as modeccin 6B. Modeccin 6B is made up of two subunits with molecular weights of 27,000 and 31,000 that are connected by a disulfide bond. Its molecular weight is identical to that of modeccin 4B. The subunits could not be separated because of their strong insolubility without sodium dodecyl sulphate. In comparison to modeccin 4B, modeccin 6B exhibits a minor reduction in toxicity to animals, lacks erythrocyte agglutination, and demonstrates a greater potency in inhibiting protein synthesis in a rabbit reticulocyte lysate. At a dosage of 0.31 μg/ml, it can achieve 50% inhibition (Barbieri et al., 1980).

17.7 Volkensin

Volkensin is a lectin that is extracted from *Adena volkensii,* popularly referred to as the kilyambiti plant. It operates similarly to ricin in terms of toxicity and by the same method of ribosome-inactivating protein (Chambery et al., 2004).

This poisonous, quite ugly succulent plant is native to Africa and doesn't seem to be very interesting. Despite this, it has demonstrated potential as an investigative chemical in the field of neurology because of its ability to be taken up and transported by particular types of neurons. There can be pressure on the research community to create commercial sources (Patočka & Středa, 2003).

17.8 Animal Toxins

A vast range of protein poisons are produced by several distinct animal sources, such as frogs, spiders, snakes, scorpions, slugs, and sea anemones. Only the poisonous principle of sea snails in the genus *Conus*, or conotoxins, is included on the Australian Group's control list.

17.9 Conus Toxins (Conotoxins)

The sea snails of the genus *Conus*, which hunt fish, create these poisonous peptides. A concoction of toxic substances secreted by the snails causes the fish that is being attacked to become paralyzed (Lewis, 2004). Members of the Conidae family have long been prized for their unusual and exquisitely decorated shells. Cone shells have just recently gained interest as a fascinating subject for scientific study. Marine snails called cone shells can be found all over the world in reef habitats. With the use of their special venoms, they immobilize other marine life as prey. They may also pose a threat to people. There are 30 recorded cases of humans being envenomated by fish-eating cone shells, several of which were fatal (Fegan & Andresen, 1997).

Every species has a different venom composition, and even individual snails within a species have different venom compositions that have all developed to best paralyze their prey. Small peptide toxins with a length of 12–30 amino acid residues are the active ingredients in venom. Because of many disulfide bridges, their conformations are extremely tight. These disulfide bridge motifs aid in the definition of several conotoxin structural groups. There are currently tens of conotoxins identified, which are categorized into four groups. With just two disulfide bridges, alpha-conotoxins are the shortest. The peptide chains of mu, omega, delta, and kappa conotoxins are characterized by the presence of three disulfide bridges connecting distinct cysteine residues (Ohizumi & Matsunaga, 2001).

The alpha, omega, and mu-conotoxins are the paralyzing elements of the venom that have been the subject of current studies. Though they all work by

TABLE 17.1

Certain *Conus* Toxin Types and Their Biological Targets

Alpha	**Mu**	**Omega**
Receptors for nicotinic acetylcholine. The result is a paralyzing effect akin to curare.	Channels for sodium. Saxitoxin and tetrodotoxin similarly target this area, and their effects are comparable.	Calcium channels connected to the neuromuscular junction's nerve impulse transmission.
Delta	**Kappa**	**Conantokins**
Channels for sodium. They decelerate the sodium channel's inactivation, in contrast to mu conotoxins.	Channels for potassium. Because they create tremors by blocking the "shaker" potassium channel, they are often referred to as shaker peptides.	NMDA receptors for glutamate. This inhibits nerve signals whose neurotransmitter of choice is glutamic acid instead of acetylcholine.

blocking neural communication, these conotoxins do so by focusing on various parts of the process. While mu-conotoxins target voltage-gated sodium channels, alpha-conotoxins target nicotinic ligand-gated channels, and omega-conotoxins target voltage-gated calcium channels (Table 17.1).

Conus venoms also contain another class of peptides called conantokins, which are the first peptide antagonists to target glutamate receptors, the main excitatory receptors in the vertebrate central nervous system. The N-methyl-D-aspartate (NMDA) receptor subtype of glutamate receptors, which are ligand-gated calcium channels, is specifically inhibited by conantokins. The biological effects of conantokins are fairly remarkable and have not been well studied to date (Castellin & Porok, 2000).

The lethality of individual conotoxins in mammals might differ significantly, even within the same class. While some omega conotoxins that cause tremors are fatal at low concentrations, others in the same group are not. Nevertheless, they are only hazardous when given intracranially (into the brain) to rats and mice. For mice, deadly dosages of certain alpha conotoxins can be as low as 25 µg/kg. Given that the dosage needed to kill a mouse in 20 minutes is used to calculate toxicity, there's a chance this estimate of toxicity is excessive. Cone snail venom is a complex cocktail of peptides, and its combined toxicity may be far more harmful than the sum of its parts because of the synergistic interaction of the poisons targeting different sections of neural function. Cone snails have been reported to kill humans in some cases.

17.10 Conclusion

In summary, meals derived from both plant and animal sources may contain biotoxins, which pose a serious risk to human health. Strict rules and efficient monitoring systems are necessary to detect and reduce the hazards of biotoxin contamination in the food supply chain. We can protect public health and consumer safety by putting comprehensive preventive and control measures in place. This highlights the significance of ongoing research and industry partnerships to address this pressing issue.

References

Barbieri, L., Zamboni, M., Montanaro, L., Sperti, S., & Stirpe, F. (1980). Purification and properties of different forms of modeccin, the toxin of Adenia digitata: Separation of subunits with inhibitory and lectin activity. *Biochemical Journal, 185*(1), 203–210.

Bradley, K. A., Mogridge, J., Mourez, M., Collier, R. J., & Young, J. A. (2001). Identification of the cellular receptor for anthrax toxin. *Nature, 414*(6860), 225–229.

Castellin, F. J., & Porok, M. (2000). Conantokins inhibitors of ion flow through the N-methyl-D-aspartate receptor channels. *Current Drug Targets, 1*(3), 219–235.

Chambery, A., Di Maro, A., Monti, M. M., Stirpe, F., & Parente, A. (2004). Volkensin from Adenia volkensii Harms (kilyambiti plant), a type 2 ribosome-inactivating protein: Gene cloning, expression and characterization of its A-chain. *European Journal of Biochemistry, 271*(1), 108–117.

Chen, Y. L., Chow, L. P., Tsugita, A., & Lin, J. Y. (1992). The complete primary structure of abrin-a B chain. *FEBS Letters, 309*(2), 115–118.

Clark, K. (1997). *The chemical weapons convention: Chemical and toxin warfare agents and disarmament*. Royal Military College of Science, Cranfield University.

Fegan, D., & Andresen, D. (1997). Conus geographus envenomation. *The Lancet, 349*(9066), 1672.

Gasperi-Campani, A., Barbieri, L., Lorenzoni, E., Montanaro, L., Sperti, S., Bonetti, E., & Stirpe, F. (1978). Modeccin, the toxin of Adenia digitata: Purification, toxicity, and inhibition of protein synthesis in vitro. *Biochemical Journal, 174*(2), 491–496.

Hartley, M. R., & Lord, J. M. (2004). Cytotoxic ribosome-inactivating lectins from plants. *Biochimica et Biophysica Acta (BBA)-Proteins and Proteomics, 1701*(1–2), 1–14.

Katzin, B. J., Collins, E. J., & Robertus, J. D. (1991). Structure of ricin A-chain at 2.5 Å. *Proteins: Structure, Function, and Bioinformatics, 10*(3), 251–259.

Kimura, M., Sumizawa, T., & Funatsu, G. (1993). The complete amino acid sequences of the B-chains of abrin-a and abrin-b, toxic proteins from the seeds of Abrus precatorius. *Bioscience, Biotechnology, and Biochemistry, 57*(1), 166–169.

Krauspenhaar, R., Eschenburg, S., Perbandt, M., Kornilov, V., Konareva, N., Mikailova, I., . . . Betzel, C. (1999). Crystal structure of mistletoe lectin I from viscum album. *Biochemical and Biophysical Research Communications, 257*(2), 418–424.

Lewis, R. J. (2004). Conotoxins as selective inhibitors of neuronal ion channels, receptors, and transporters. *IUBMB Life, 56*(2), 89–93.

Lord, J. M., Roberts, L. M., & Robertus, J. D. (1994). Ricin: Structure, mode of action, and some current applications. *The FASEB Journal, 8*(2), 201–208.

Montfort, W., Villafranca, J. E., Monzingo, A. F., Ernst, S. R., Katzin, B., Rutenber, E., . . . Robertus, J. D. (1987). The three-dimensional structure of ricin at 2.8 A. *Journal of Biological Chemistry, 262*(11), 5398–5403.
Morris, K. N., & Wool, I. G. (1994). Analysis of the contribution of an amphiphilic alpha-helix to the structure and the function of ricin A chain. *Proceedings of the National Academy of Sciences, 91*(16), 7530–7533.
Ohizumi, Y., & Matsunaga, K. (2001). Chemical structures and the mechanism of action of peptide toxins from cone shells. *Tanpakushitsu Kakusan koso, Protein, Nucleic Acid, Enzyme, 46*(4 Suppl), 449–454.
Olsnes, S. (2004). The history of ricin, abrin, and related toxins. *Toxicon, 44*(4), 361–370.
Olsnes, S., Haylett, T., & Sandvig, K. (1982). The toxic lectin modeccin. In *Methods in enzymology* (Vol. 83, pp. 357–362). Academic Press.
Olsnes, S., & Kozlov, J. V. (2001). Ricin. *Toxicon, 39*(11), 1723–1728.
Olsnes, S., Sandvig, K., Eiklid, K., & Pihl, A. (1978). Properties and action mechanism of the toxic lectin modeccin: Interaction with cell lines resistant to modeccin, abrin, and ricin. *Journal of Supramolecular Structure, 9*(1), 15–25.
Patočka, J. (1998). Toxicological characteristic of ricin (Article in Czech). *Voj Zdrav Listy, 67*, 166–168.
Patočka, J. (2001a). Abrin and ricin-two dangerous poisonous proteins. *ASA Newsletter, 85*, 205–208.
Patočka, J. (2001b). The toxins of cyanobacteria. *Acta Medica (Hradec Kralove), 44*(2), 69–75.
Patočka, J., & Středa, L. (2003). Plant toxic proteins and their current significance for warfare and medicine. *Journal of Applied Biomedicine, 1*, 141–147.
Patockaa, J., & Stredab, L. (2002). A brief review of natural nonprotein neurotoxins. *ASA Newsletter, 89*(2), 16–24.
Refsnes, K., Haylett, T., Sandvig, K., & Olsnes, S. (1977). Modeccin—a plant toxin inhibiting protein synthesis. *Biochemical and Biophysical Research Communications, 79*(4), 1176–1183.
Rutenber, E., & Robertus, J. D. (1991). Structure of ricin B-chain at 2.5 Å resolution. *Proteins: Structure, Function, and Bioinformatics, 10*(3), 260–269.
Sandvig, K., Olsnes, S., & Pihl, A. (1976). Kinetics of binding of the toxic lectins abrin and ricin to surface receptors of human cells. *Journal of Biological Chemistry, 251*(13), 3977–3984.
Sharon, N., & Lis, H. (1972). Lectins: Cell-agglutinating and sugar-specific proteins: Lectins provide new tools for studying polysaccharides, glycoproteins, and cell surfaces, and for cancer research. *Science, 177*(4053), 949–959.
Simpson, L. L. (2004). Identification of the major steps in botulinum toxin action. *Annual Review of Pharmacology and Toxicology, 44*, 167–193.
Stirpe, F. (2004). Ribosome-inactivating proteins. *Toxicon, 44*(4), 371–383.
Veldhoen, M., Hirota, K., Westendorf, A. M., Buer, J., Dumoutier, L., Renauld, J. C., & Stockinger, B. (2008). The aryl hydrocarbon receptor links TH17-cell-mediated autoimmunity to environmental toxins. *Nature, 453*(7191), 106–109.
Wang, K. Y., & Xu, Q. (2000). Lectins and toxins. *Sheng wu hua xue yu Sheng wu wu li xue bao Acta Biochimica et Biophysica Sinica, 32*(3), 201–205.

18

Extraction Techniques of Biotoxins in Food

Anjaneyulu Musini, P Gnana Deepu, Jogipeta Harihara, Kathroju Harikrishna, and Mariyam Fatima

18.1 Introduction

Biotoxins are toxic compounds naturally produced by living organisms. While these toxins do not harm the organisms themselves, they can be harmful to other creatures, including humans, when consumed. Biotoxins are a crucial issue for food safety, as they can harm both consumers and livestock, causing health issues. These natural toxins contaminate various food sources, such as plants like cassava and almonds, potatoes, tomatoes, cereals, dried fruits, and shellfish, posing significant risks to human health when consumed. These toxins have serious health consequences, including allergic responses, neurological diseases, gastrointestinal abnormalities, respiratory symptoms, and even death (Singh et al., 2015; Natural Toxins in Food, 2023). Biotoxins are especially important in food safety because of their broad and possibly serious health consequences. Preventing foodborne illness requires strict safety practices and regulations to ensure food safety.

Specific biotoxins, such as cyanogenic glycosides and mycotoxins, pose risks due to their presence in everyday foods. For example, cyanogenic glycosides are found in plants like cassava and almonds, solanines and chaconine in potatoes and tomatoes, mycotoxins in cereals and dried fruits, and algal toxins in shellfish (Natural Toxins in Food, 2023), which can lead to mild symptoms like stomachaches and diarrhea to more severe conditions like paralysis and long-term neurological damage.

Developing effective strategies, such as implementing stringent food testing protocols, enhancing agricultural practices, and regulating food processing, is crucial to reducing the impact of biotoxins on public health, and ensuring food safety and quality in production and supply.

 DOI: 10.1201/9781003500605-21

18.1.1 Significance of Biotoxins in Food Production, Consumption, and Public Health

- Food Production: Biotoxins can affect the entire food production chain, from agriculture to processing and distribution. Contaminated crops or animal products can lead to economic losses and pose risks to farm workers and consumers (Natural Toxins in Food, 2023).
- Consumption: Consuming food contaminated with biotoxins can result in foodborne illnesses such as gastrointestinal disturbances, neurological disorders, and respiratory symptoms, with both immediate and long-term health consequences.
- Public Health: Biotoxins pose a public health challenge, as they can lead to widespread outbreaks and are hard to control in the food supply (Makinde et al., 2023).

18.1.2 General Characteristics and Properties of Biotoxins

Biotoxins possess a range of characteristics and properties that make them uniquely potent:

High Specificity and Potency: Biotoxins are highly specific, often targeting particular cellular receptors or enzymes. For instance, botulinum toxin inhibits neurotransmitter release, causing muscle paralysis, while tetrodotoxin blocks sodium channels in nerve cells, preventing nerve signal transmission.

Structural Diversity: The molecular structures of biotoxins are incredibly diverse, ranging from small molecules like alkaloids to large proteins and enzymes. This structural diversity enables a variety of ways in which biotoxins can interact with the body, such as disrupting cellular functions or interfering with vital processes.

Biological Activity: Biotoxins can affect cell activity, protein synthesis, and communication among cells. They can disrupt cell membranes, impede protein synthesis, modify cellular signaling pathways, and interfere with neurotransmission. This biological action frequently results in severe symptoms such as paralysis, respiratory failure, or organ destruction, which can appear quickly, ranking some biotoxins among the most dangerous poisons known (Singh et al., 2015).

Environmental Persistence and Bioaccumulation: Biotoxins generated by marine dinoflagellates may accumulate in the food chain. Shellfish that eat poisonous algae build poisons in their tissues, which can be dangerous to humans when consumed. This bioaccumulation can have serious ecological and health repercussions, such as red tides, which cause mass fish death and human poisoning.

Therapeutic and Biotechnological Applications: Despite their toxicity, biotoxins offer therapeutic potential for treating ailments such as muscular spasms and cosmetic issues. Botulinum toxin, for example, is administered in small, regulated dosages to treat muscular spasms and cosmetic concerns. Furthermore, biotoxin discoveries have accelerated advances in medicine development, pest control, and cellular mechanism research.

18.2 Types of Biotoxins

Biotoxins are diverse groups of naturally occurring toxins produced by different organisms, and their presence in food can pose serious health risks. Understanding, the various types of biotoxins is crucial for effective food safety management, and their effects are essential for developing strategies to mitigate their impact on public health and ensure the safety and quality of food (Singh et al., 2015).

18.2.1 Classification of Biotoxins

Biotoxins are classified based on their origin, chemical nature, and mechanism of action. Some of the types of biotoxins are discussed in the following (Singh et al., 2015). Table 18.1 presents the types, sources, health effects, and examples of various biotoxins, while Figure 18.1 illustrates the different categories of biotoxins.

18.2.1.1 Mycotoxins

Mycotoxins are toxic compounds produced by fungi (molds) that grow on food crops, commonly found in food items such as contaminated grains, cereals, nuts, spices, and other agricultural products. Exposure to mycotoxins can lead to acute poisoning, immune deficiencies, and long-term health effects such as cancer and liver damage. The most prevalent mycotoxins include aflatoxins, ochratoxin A, patulin, and zearalenone, each associated with specific health risks such as liver damage and carcinogenicity.

Examples of Mycotoxins:

- Aflatoxins—Produced by *Aspergillus* species; commonly found in peanuts, corn, and tree nuts, are potent carcinogens and can cause liver damage.
- Ochratoxins—Produced by *Aspergillus* and *Penicillium* species; found in cereals, coffee, and dried fruits, can cause kidney damage and are potential carcinogens.

TABLE 18.1
Types of Biotoxins

Type of Toxins	Source	Health Effects	Examples	References
Mycotoxins	Contaminated grains, nuts, spices, and other agricultural products.	Acute poisoning, immune deficiencies, and long-term health effects such as cancer and liver damage.	• Aflatoxins • Ochratoxins • Fumonisins	
Marine biotoxins	Shellfish (such as mussels, clams, oysters, scallops, etc.), algal blooms.	Neurological and gastrointestinal symptoms.	• Saxitoxins • Ciguatoxins • Domoic acid	(Marine Biotoxins, n.d.) (Dillon et al., 2021)
Plant toxins	Various plant species.	Mild digestive disturbances to severe poisoning and death.	• Lectins • Cyanogenic glycoside • Solanine	(Phycotoxins, n.d.)
Bacterial Toxins	*Bacillus cereus*, *Clostridium botulinum*, and *Staphylococcus aureus*	Food poisoning, severe foodborne illnesses, with symptoms ranging from mild gastrointestinal distress, vomiting, and diarrhea to severe life-threatening conditions like botulism.	• Botulinum toxin • Staphylococcal enterotoxin • *Bacillus cereus* toxin	(Detection of Bacterial Toxins in Food, n.d.; Makinde et al., 2023)

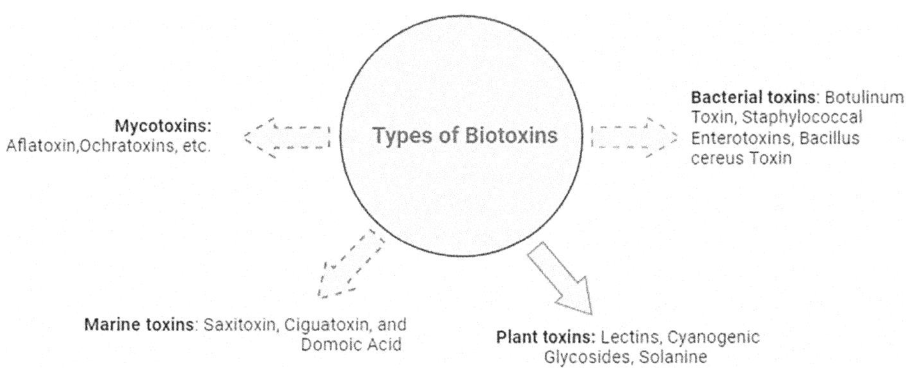

FIGURE 18.1
Types of biotoxins.

- Fumonisins—Produced by *Fusarium* species; found in corn and corn-based products, can cause liver and kidney toxicity and are linked to esophageal cancer.

18.2.1.2 Marine Biotoxins

Marine biotoxins are toxins produced by certain types of marine algae (phytoplankton) and can accumulate in seafood. These are primarily associated with shellfish (such as mussels, clams, oysters, scallops, etc.) and other seafood contaminated by harmful algal blooms. Exposure to marine biotoxins can cause neurological and gastrointestinal symptoms, and in severe cases, can be fatal. Toxins, such as ciguatoxins and tetrodotoxin, can cause serious health issues including neurological disorders and paralysis. The increasing prevalence of harmful algal blooms due to environmental changes underscores the importance of monitoring and managing these toxins in seafood (Marine Biotoxins, n.d.; Dillon et al., 2021).

Examples of Marine Biotoxins

- Saxitoxins—found in contaminated shellfish, cause paralytic shellfish poisoning (PSP); symptoms include numbness, paralysis, and respiratory failure.
- Ciguatoxins—found in tropical reef fish (e.g., barracuda, king mackerel), cause ciguatera fish poisoning (CFP); symptoms include nausea, vomiting, and neurological effects such as tingling and temperature sensitivity.
- Domoic Acid—found in shellfish, causes amnesic shellfish poisoning (ASP); symptoms include gastrointestinal distress and memory loss.

18.2.1.3 Plant Toxins

Plants produce various toxins as defense mechanisms against predators and environmental stress. These naturally occurring compounds found in certain plants can be toxic to humans if consumed. Common plant toxins include solanines, chaconine, and cyanogenic glycosides in everyday foods like potatoes and cassava. Ingestion of raw or improperly processed plant parts can cause a range of health effects, from mild digestive disturbances to severe poisoning and death.

Examples of Plant Toxins

- Lectins—Found in beans and legumes; can cause gastrointestinal distress and inhibit nutrient absorption if not properly cooked.

- Cyanogenic Glycosides—Found in cassava, almonds, and stone fruits; can release cyanide, leading to respiratory failure and death if consumed in large quantities.
- Solanine—Found in green or sprouted potatoes; can cause nausea, vomiting, and neurological symptoms.

18.2.1.4 Bacterial Toxins

Bacterial biotoxins are produced by pathogenic bacteria such as *Bacillus cereus*, *Clostridium botulinum*, and *Staphylococcus aureus*, either as part of their metabolism or upon cell death. Exposure to bacterial toxins can cause food poisoning and severe foodborne illnesses, with symptoms ranging from mild gastrointestinal distress, vomiting, and diarrhea to severe life-threatening conditions like botulism (Singh et al., 2015; Makinde et al., 2023).

Examples of Bacterial Toxins

- Botulinum Toxin—Produced by *Clostridium botulinum*; found in improperly canned or preserved foods. Causes botulism, characterized by paralysis and respiratory failure.
- Staphylococcal Enterotoxins—Produced by *Staphylococcus aureus*; found in improperly stored meat, dairy, and bakery products. Cause staphylococcal food poisoning, with symptoms like nausea, vomiting, and diarrhea.
- *Bacillus cereus* Toxin—Produced by *Bacillus cereus*; found in rice, pasta, and starchy foods. Causes vomiting and diarrhea.

18.3 Extraction Techniques

The extraction of biotoxins is a vital step in the investigation and characterization of harmful chemicals produced by living organisms. The extraction procedure involves separating, concentrating, and purifying biotoxins from complicated compounds to allow for accurate identification and quantification. It is essential to optimize extraction conditions to achieve optimal biotoxin recovery, as insufficient extraction might result in misleading negative findings. Furthermore, the analytical technique utilized for biotoxin analysis must be considered during the extraction process to guarantee compatibility and accuracy in findings. Overall, a complete understanding of the extraction process is essential for accurate analysis and characterization of dangerous chemicals. Proper extraction procedures have a significant influence on the reliability and validity of biotoxin study outcomes (Martins et al., 2023).

18.3.1 Objectives and Factors Influencing Biotoxin Extraction

18.3.1.1 Objectives of Biotoxin Extraction

Basic objectives for the extraction of biotoxins include:

- To isolate or separate biotoxins from food and food products
- To increase the concentration of biotoxins for easier detection and analysis
- To remove impurities

18.3.1.2 Factors Influencing Extraction Efficiency

Factors influencing the extraction efficiency of biotoxins include:

- Matrix Complexity: The composition of the sample matrix can significantly affect the extraction efficiency. Complex matrices such as food, soil, and biological tissues can contain fats, proteins, and other substances that complicate the extraction process.
- Physicochemical Properties of Biotoxins: Properties such as solubility, polarity, stability, and volatility of biotoxins influence the choice of extraction methods.

Other factors impacting extraction efficiency include the extraction solvent, extraction time, and temperature. These criteria must be considered while establishing an extraction procedure to achieve the best possible recovery of biotoxins from the sample matrix.

18.3.2 General Steps in Biotoxin Extraction

The biotoxin extraction process involves several key steps: sample preparation, extraction, purification, biotoxin separation, detection, and quantification. Sample preparation includes initial steps to ready the sample for analysis, such as homogenization and drying.

18.3.2.1 Sample Preparation

- Homogenization is crucial in the sample preparation process as it helps to evenly mix and break down the sample for accurate analysis. Common methods of homogenization include grinding, blending, and sonicating.
- Drying plays a vital role in sample preparation by removing moisture from the sample, which is essential for achieving optimal extraction results. Methods such as air drying, oven drying, and freeze drying

are commonly employed for this purpose. It is important to ensure that the sample is properly homogenized and dried to reduce variations in analytical results. Proper sample preparation procedures have a significant influence on the accuracy and reliability of subsequent analyses.

18.3.3 Extraction

An overview of the extraction of biotoxins is provided in Table 18.2, and a comparative analysis of traditional and modern techniques is provided in Table 18.3.

TABLE 18.2

Extraction Techniques of Biotoxins

Extraction Techniques	Principle	Application
Liquid-liquid extraction	Partitioning biotoxins between immiscible solvents.	Effective for hydrophobic toxins.
Solid-phase extraction	Adsorption onto solid sorbents (e.g., cartridges, disks).	Selective, rapid, and automated.
Supercritical fluid extraction	Uses supercritical CO_2 as a solvent.	Marine toxins and mycotoxins.
QuEChERS	Salting-out liquid-liquid extraction followed by dispersive solid-phase extraction (d-SPE) for cleanup.	Pesticides and mycotoxins.
Immunoaffinity chromatography	Antibodies immobilized on a solid phase to selectively bind biotoxins.	Mycotoxins and marine biotoxins.

TABLE 18.3

Comparative Analysis of Traditional Techniques and Modern Techniques

Comparative Analysis	Traditional Techniques	Modern Techniques
Efficiency and selectivity	Effective but time consuming.	Faster, more selective, and environmentally friendly.
Sample preparation	Longer preparation times.	Reduced sample preparation steps.
Overall performance	Established but resource intensive.	Efficient, precise, and suitable for high-throughput analysis.

18.3.3.1 Traditional Extraction Techniques

Traditional biotoxin extraction methods have played an important role in maintaining food safety, particularly in monitoring seafood for paralytic shellfish poisoning toxins. The mouse bioassay, a technique developed over 50 years ago, is commonly used for testing biotoxins. In this procedure, mice are injected with an acid extract of shellfish, and the time to death is measured. Highly poisonous extracts are diluted such that death occurs within 5 to 15 minutes. Despite being widely used, this method has faced criticism due to ethical concerns and the requirement to maintain a specific mouse colony, making it labor intensive and less favorable in contemporary environments (Dias et al., 2022).

Other traditional extraction techniques include the following.

18.3.3.1.1 Liquid-Liquid Extraction (LLE)

It involves the separation of a solute between two immiscible liquid phases, typically an aqueous phase and an organic solvent. The differential solubility of the biotoxin in these phases enables its separation from the food matrix. During LLE, the food sample is homogenized and diluted with water or an appropriate buffer. Organic solvents like chloroform or ethyl acetate are added to the sample and vigorously shaken or vortexed to facilitate the transfer of the biotoxin into the organic phase. The mixture is allowed to settle, and the phases are separated by centrifugation or gravity. The organic phase, containing the extracted biotoxin, is collected for further analysis. This technique is simple, cost effective, and widely applicable. However, the solvents used can be hazardous, leading to potential emulsification and necessitating multiple steps for complete recovery (Libretexts, 2023).

Examples:

Aflatoxins: extracted from grains and nuts using chloroform or methanol-water mixtures.

Domoic acid: extracted from shellfish using methanol or acetone.

18.3.3.1.2 Solid-Phase Extraction (SPE)

It utilizes a solid adsorbent material to selectively retain the biotoxin from a liquid sample, allowing impurities to be washed away and the biotoxin to be eluted in a purified form. In this process, the SPE cartridge or disk is conditioned with a solvent to activate the adsorbent surface. Later, the liquid sample is allowed to pass through the cartridge, allowing the biotoxin to adsorb onto the solid phase, while the solvent is washed away with the cartridge to remove unbound impurities. Later, the biotoxins are eluted from the solid phase using a solvent with a high affinity for the toxin. This technique offers high selectivity, can concentrate the analyte, and reduces matrix interferences. However, it necessitates specific cartridges for different biotoxins

(The Role of Solid Phase Extraction (SPE) in a Food and Beverage Laboratory, 2023; Food Safety and Solid Phase Extraction, 2023).

Examples:

Ochratoxin A: extracted from coffee and wine using C18 or polymeric SPE cartridges.

Saxitoxins: Extracted from shellfish using ion-exchange SPE cartridges.

18.3.3.1.3 Precipitation Methods

This method involves the addition of a reagent that causes the biotoxin or interfering substances to precipitate out of the solution, allowing for their removal by centrifugation or filtration. In this method, precipitating agents such as salts or organic solvents are added to the sample to create a mixture. Later, the mixture is mixed gently and centrifuged to separate the precipitate. The biotoxins that are present in the supernatant are collected for further analysis. This method is straightforward, cost effective, and efficient for eliminating proteins and other large molecules.

Examples:

Mycotoxins: extracted from cereals using acetonitrile for protein precipitation.

Bacterial Toxins: Extracted from food matrices using ammonium sulfate precipitation.

18.3.3.2 Modern Extraction Techniques

18.3.3.2.1 Supercritical Fluid Extraction (SFE)

SFE uses supercritical carbon dioxide to efficiently extract biotoxins from food. In this process, the food sample is homogenized and placed in the extraction vessel. Carbon dioxide is brought to supercritical conditions (above its critical temperature and pressure) and passed through the sample. The supercritical fluid, containing dissolved biotoxins, is depressurized to separate the biotoxins. This method is eco-friendly, eliminates the need for harmful solvents, and is ideal for sensitive compounds.

Examples:

Extraction of domonic acid from mussels and aflatoxins from peanuts using supercritical CO_2 with ethanol as a co-solvent.

18.3.3.2.2 QuEChERS

QuEChERS (quick, easy, cheap, effective, rugged, and safe) is a method that uses liquid-liquid extraction with added salts, followed by solid-phase extraction for purification. In this process, the homogenized sample is mixed with acetonitrile and a salt mixture to induce phase separation. The organic phase is separated using centrifugation and is subjected to dispersive SPE using adsorbents to remove impurities. This method is quick and affordable, uses little solvent, and can be used with different sample types.

Examples:

Extraction of multiple mycotoxins (aflatoxins, deoxynivalenol, and zearalenone) from wheat samples.

18.3.3.2.3 Immunoaffinity Chromatography (IAC)

IAC uses antibodies on a solid surface to specifically capture biotoxins from a sample. The captured toxins are released using a particular solvent. In this process, the IAC column is conditioned with a buffer. The sample is allowed to pass through the column, where biotoxins bind to the antibodies present in the column. The column is washed to remove unbound impurities and biotoxins are eluted using a buffer or solvent.

Examples:

Extraction of brevetoxins from shellfish.

18.3.4 Purification of Biotoxins

The purification of biotoxins is an essential step during the extraction of biotoxins, as the extracted biotoxins are in the form of compounds along with impurities and other chemicals.

Filtration: Particulate matter is removed/ purified through filtration.

Centrifugation: Biotoxins, when centrifuged, separate based on their density.

Chromatographic Techniques: Techniques like high-performance liquid chromatography (HPLC) or gas chromatography (GC) are used to separate the biotoxin from the remaining impurities.

18.3.5 Separation of Biotoxins

18.3.5.1 Chromatographic Methods

Liquid chromatography-mass spectrometry (LCMS) is recognized for its excellent sensitivity and selectivity, making it a powerful tool for detecting multiple toxins simultaneously. It has become the cornerstone for the separation of biotoxins in food safety analysis. The integration of LC with mass spectrometry enhances the ability to resolve coeluting compounds by their molecular masses, which is crucial for the accurate identification of various biotoxins (De Girolamo et al., 2022).

Gas chromatography (GC) is a pivotal technique in the analysis of volatile substances, where compounds are separated based on their volatility in a gas phase. In GC, a sample is vaporized and carried through a column by an inert gas such as helium or nitrogen. The separation occurs as different compounds interact variably with the column's stationary phase, allowing for distinct elution times. This method is especially effective for analyzing complex mixtures and can be coupled with mass spectrometry (GCMS) to enhance specificity and sensitivity in detecting trichothecenes9, a group of mycotoxins (Gas Chromatography, 2023).

High-performance liquid chromatography is another critical chromatographic technique used extensively for the detection of mycotoxins and other biotoxins in food and feed. HPLC operates under high pressure, which allows the use of smaller particle sizes for the stationary phase, leading to better separation and shorter analysis times. The technique often employs UV/diode array and fluorescence detection to identify and quantify single or structurally related mycotoxins. The integration of mass spectrometry with HPLC and ultra-HPLC systems has significantly advanced the field, enabling the simultaneous detection of multiple mycotoxins at very low concentrations in complex matrices.

Moreover, the growing affordability of high-resolution mass spectrometry (HRMS) systems, such as orbitrap MS and TOF MS, has broadened the scope of biotoxin analysis, enabling the screening and quantification of both known and unknown compounds in complex food matrices.

18.3.5.2 Electrophoretic Techniques

Electrophoretic techniques offer an alternate means of separating biotoxins, particularly for quick screening applications. Techniques like capillary electrophoresis (CE) employ a narrow-fused silica capillary instead of typical electrophoretic gels, allowing for fine control of sample migration at high voltage. This approach is very useful for managing tiny sample quantities and performing high-resolution separations. Despite its promise, CE has seen limited use in toxin analysis, but continuing research shows it may become a more significant tool in the area. Challenges such as the manufacture of fluorescent derivatives and the requirement for specific detection systems such as laser fluorescence detectors have been identified; however, they are being solved through technical developments.

18.3.6 Detection and Quantification

18.3.6.1 Mass Spectrometry

Mass spectrometry (MS) is a powerful analytical tool for identifying and quantifying biotoxins in food. This approach delivers great sensitivity and specificity, which is critical for food safety and quality management. Inductively coupled plasma mass spectrometry (ICPMS) and tandem mass spectrometry (MS/MS) are modern methods that improve selectivity. ICPMS, for example, entails digesting the sample with techniques such as acid digestion or microwave digestion to solubilize analytes, which are subsequently ionized and identified. MS may also be used with immunoaffinity chromatography (IACMS) to increase the isolation and identification of food toxins such as mycotoxins and pesticides, with antibody-based columns providing great selectivity (Ahuja et al., 2023).

18.3.6.2 UV/Visible Spectroscopy

UV/visible spectroscopy is a simple and cost-effective analytical method used to assess food quality. It works based on light absorption by sample compounds, which is measured over a range of wavelengths. This approach is very beneficial for quantitatively analyzing food components and detecting specific biotoxins. The interaction of UV and visible light with various chemicals allows for the quantification of their content in the food matrix. Modern UV/vis spectrophotometers can handle a wide range of sample types, including solids, liquids, and gases, and can do quantitative analyses with minimum sample preparation (Power et al., 2019).

These spectroscopic methods, coupled with mass spectrometry, are essential for accurately detecting and quantifying biotoxins in food, and they contribute considerably to public health safety by monitoring and controlling possible foodborne risks.

18.4 Practical Applications

18.4.1 Implementation in Food Industry

The prevention of foodborne illness hinges on the effective implementation of food safety programs, which include proper handling procedures, good sanitation, and hygiene, along with the application of standard food analysis techniques at each step of food processing. Workers in food industries and public services play a pivotal role in ensuring a safe food supply. To support these efforts, government regulations and recommendations are designed and managed by various agencies, ensuring that the composition and quality of food are safe for consumers.

Despite rigorous safety measures, a limited number of foodborne illness cases are attributed to toxin poisoning. Toxins, whether derived from bacteria, plants, or seafood, are lethal and their severity varies based on their interaction with target sites. These include botulinum neurotoxins, staphylococcal enterotoxins, saxitoxins, and tetrodotoxins, which pose significant health risks.

In developed countries, an estimated 5–10% of the population is affected by foodborne illness, with even higher rates in developing countries. This underscores the critical need for continuous improvement and implementation of robust food safety practices.

In the realm of analytical screening and confirmation of natural biotoxins, challenges persist. Techniques such as immunoassays, thin-layer chromatography (TLC), and liquid chromatography with UV fluorescence detection (LCUV/FL) are commonly employed. Moreover, the use of mass detection technologies like ACQUITY QDa for routine multi toxin screening is highlighted for its benefits, providing a comprehensive overview of common mycotoxins and regulated levels in various food commodities.

A specific method demonstrated for screening regulated mycotoxins in wheat using ultraperformance liquid chromatography-tandem mass spectrometry (UPLCMS/MS) showcases the advanced capabilities in quantitative confirmatory methods, which adhere to stringent validation requirements per European Union legislation. These advancements in food toxin analysis are crucial for enhancing food safety and protecting public health, making it easier for new users to understand and apply these methods in different industry settings.

18.5 Future Directions

18.5.1 Innovations in Extraction

Recent advancements in the field of biotoxin detection are steering toward the development of novel, state-of-the-art biosensor technologies. These innovations are not only enhancing the sensitivity and accuracy of marine biotoxin testing but are also tailored to meet the practical necessities of end users, particularly in regulatory environments. The trend towards making biosensors smaller and more portable helps in onsite and real-time detection of marine biotoxins with less sample volume and processing steps. This advancement supports field monitoring and early warning systems, crucial for managing biotoxin outbreaks effectively (Waters Corporation—Food Qc Safety Research, 2015).

18.5.2 Trends in Biotoxin Detection

Integrating nanotechnology into biosensor designs is revolutionizing the detection of marine biotoxins, providing exceptional sensitivity and selectivity. Nanoparticles and nanocomposites are being increasingly utilized to improve biosensor performance, which is pivotal in the precise and rapid detection of biotoxins. Furthermore, the application of surface functionalization techniques has enhanced the specificity and stability of these biosensors, enabling the immobilization of biomolecules such as antibodies and aptamers onto sensor surfaces.

Moreover, the growing trend of integrating biosensors with the Internet of Things (IoT) and data analytics platforms is transforming biotoxin monitoring. This integration allows for real-time data analysis and continuous surveillance of marine environments, ensuring timely responses to toxin events. Additionally, the development of multiplexed detection capabilities in biosensors, capable of identifying multiple toxins simultaneously, is reducing analysis time and costs, thereby enhancing comprehensive monitoring of marine environments.

The future of biotoxin detection in food safety is also witnessing a surge in the development and improvement of rapid point-of-site testing (POST) methods. These methods are designed to be sensitive, measurable, accurate, and real-time (SMART), catering specifically to the needs of novice users and aiming for international acceptance and validation. The current lack of diverse commercial testing kits for marine toxin analysis highlights the importance of ongoing developments in this field, focusing on multiplexing capabilities and rapid point-of-site testing to influence future market trends (Zhu et al., 2024).

These future directions highlight a shift towards more sophisticated, user-friendly, and efficient methods of biotoxin detection, ensuring that new users can easily grasp and apply these technologies in various contexts, thereby enhancing food safety and public health.

18.6 Conclusion

The challenges associated with detecting and managing the risks of biotoxins in food are multifaceted, ranging from the variability of toxin concentrations in individual shellfish to the difficulties in predicting harmful algal blooms. Current monitoring methods, such as visual confirmation of water discoloration and traditional mouse bioassays, are often reactive and time consuming. These methods require enhancement to address the rapid and accurate detection needs essential for public health safety.

Furthermore, the lack of comprehensive data on the biology and ecology of harmful algae complicates the development of predictive models for algal blooms. This limitation underscores the necessity for long-term, routine monitoring, and research to gather essential data that can inform more effective regulatory and monitoring strategies.

Given these challenges, there is an urgent global need to develop and adopt rapid, reliable, and sensitive detection methods for marine toxins. Techniques such as liquid chromatography-mass spectrometry have been identified as promising due to their high selectivity and low limits of detection. Furthermore, the ability of biosensors to detect multiple toxins simultaneously is a major advancement in the field.

To support these technological advancements, the establishment of an accessible database containing comprehensive information on marine toxins, including their chemical properties, sources, and regulatory limits, would be invaluable. This resource would speed up the development of new analytical methods and help standardize testing procedures across various regions.

Effectively addressing these issues requires researchers, regulatory bodies, and industry stakeholders to work together to improve current methodologies and introduce new technologies for proactive and preventive management of biotoxin risks in food.

References

Ahuja, Vishal, Amanpreet Singh, Debarati Paul, Diptarka Dasgupta, Petra Urajová, Sounak Ghosh, Roshani Singh, Gobardhan Sahoo, Daniela Ewe, and Kumar Saurav. "Recent Advances in the Detection of Food Toxins Using Mass Spectrometry." *Chemical Research in Toxicology* 36, no. 12 (December 7, 2023): 1834–1863. https://doi.org/10.1021/acs.chemrestox.3c00241.

De Girolamo, Annalisa, Vincenzo Lippolis, and Michelangelo Pascale. "Overview of Recent Liquid Chromatography Mass Spectrometry-Based Methods for Natural Toxins Detection in Food Products." *Toxins* 14, no. 5 (May 4, 2022): 328. https://doi.org/10.3390/toxins14050328.

Detection of Bacterial Toxins in Food. (n.d.). https://www.rapidmicrobiology.com/test-method/detection-of-bacterial-toxins-in-food.

Dias, Daniela B., Raphaela Fritsche-Guenther, Friederike Gutmann, Georg N. Duda, Jennifer Kirwan, and Patrina S. P. Poh. "A Comparison of Solvent-Based Extraction Methods to Assess the Central Carbon Metabolites in Mouse Bone and Muscle." *Metabolites* 12, no. 5 (May 18, 2022): 453. https://doi.org/10.3390/metabo12050453.

Dillon, Michael, Maja A. Zaczek-Moczydlowska, Christine Edwards, Andrew D. Turner, Peter I. Miller, Heather Moore, April McKinney, Linda Lawton, and Katrina Campbell. "Current Trends and Challenges for Rapid SMART Diagnostics at Point-of-Site Testing for Marine Toxins." *Sensors* 21, no. 7 (April 3, 2021): 2499. https://doi.org/10.3390/s21072499.

Food Safety and Solid Phase Extraction—An Essential Guide for Switching from a Manual to an Automated Protocol. (January 5, 2023). https://www.gilson.com/default/learninghub/post/food-safety-and-solid-phase-extraction-an-essential-guide-for-switching-from-a-manual-to-an-automated-protocol.html.

Gas Chromatography. *Chemistry LibreTexts*. (August 29, 2023). https://chem.libretexts.org/Bookshelves/Analytical_Chemistry/Supplemental_Modules_(Analytical_Chemistry)/Instrumentation_and_Analysis/Chromatography/Gas_Chromatography.

Libretexts. "Liquid-Liquid Extraction." *Chemistry LibreTexts* (August 29, 2023). https://chem.libretexts.org/Bookshelves/Analytical_Chemistry/Supplemental_Modules_(Analytical_Chemistry)/Analytical_Sciences_Digital_Library/Contextual_Modules/Sample_Preparation/02_Liquid-Liquid_Extraction.

Makinde, Oluwadamilola M., Michael Sulyok, Rasheed A. Adeleke, Rudolf Krska, and Chibundu N. Ezekiel. "Bacteriological Quality and Biotoxin Profile of Ready-to-Eat Foods Vended in Lagos, Nigeria." *Foods* 12, no. 6 (March 13, 2023): 1224. https://doi.org/10.3390/foods12061224.

Marine Biotoxins. (n.d.). https://www.fao.org/4/y5486e/y5486e07.htm.

Martins, Rodrigo, Ana Barbosa, Bárbara Advinha, Hélia Sales, Rita Pontes, and João Nunes. "Green Extraction Techniques of Bioactive Compounds: A State-of-the-Art Review." *Processes* 11, no. 8 (July 26, 2023): 2255. https://doi.org/10.3390/pr11082255.

Natural Toxins in Food. (March 10, 2023). https://www.who.int/news-room/fact-sheets/detail/natural-toxins-in-food.

Phycotoxins. *WUR* (n.d.). https://www.wur.nl/nl/onderzoek-resultaten/onderzoeksinstituten/food-safety-research/analysing-food-and-feed/natural-toxins/phycotoxins.htm.

Power, A.C., J. Chapman, S. Chandra, and D. Cozzolino. *Ultraviolet-visible spectroscopy for food quality analysis*. Elsevier eBooks, 91–104 (2019). https://doi.org/10.1016/b978-0-12-814217-2.00006-8.

The Role of Solid Phase Extraction (SPE) in a Food and Beverage Laboratory. (February 1, 2023). https://www.gilson.com/default/learninghub/post/the-role-of-solid-phase-extraction-spe-in-a-food-and-beverage-laboratory.html.

Singh, A.K., E.A.E. Garber, M.C. Principato, S. Hall, and S.K. Sharma. "Biotoxins and Food Safety." In: Gopalakrishnakone, P., Balali-Mood, M., Llewellyn, L., and Singh, B.R. (eds) *Biological toxins and bioterrorism: Toxinology*. Springer, 185–210 (2015). https://doi.org/10.1007/978-94-007-5869-8_20.

Waters Corporation—Food Qc Safety & Research. "An Integrated Strategy for Natural Biotoxin Analysis—Waters Corporation—Food Safety." *SlideShare* (February 11, 2015). https://www.slideshare.net/slideshow/an-integrated-strategy-for-natural-biotoxin-analysis-waters-corporation-food-safety/44540804.

Zhu, Xiangwei, Yufa Zhao, Long Wu, Xin Gao, Huang Huang, Yu Han, and Ting Zhu. "Advances in Biosensors for the Rapid Detection of Marine Biotoxins: Current Status and Future Perspectives." *Biosensors* 14, no. 4 (April 19, 2024): 203. https://doi.org/10.3390/bios14040203.

19

Exploring the Origin and Epidemiology of Biotoxins in Foods and Feeds: An Updated Perspective

Victoria Olufunmi Adeyemo-Eleyode, Babatunde Oluwafemi Adetuyi, Peace Abiodun Olajide, Charles Chinazaekpele Chidume, Felix Oladele Okunlola, Peter Gbenga Oni, and Ayobami Ifeoluwa Awe

19.1 Introduction

Biotoxins which can also be referred to as biological toxins are chemical substances (toxins) produced by animal, plants and microorganisms (algae, fungi, bacteria among others). These toxins protect its producers and have health effects on consumers (Wilson and Ho, 2021). All international bodies (World bank, World Health Organization- WHO, UNICEF, United Nations, FAO among others) support access to enough safe and nutritious food because food security, food safety and nutrition are closely linked (Munialo and Mellor, 2023; Al Alnabi et al., 2022). However, at different cases pathogens or toxins of biological origin are consumed in foods or feeds resulting to food borne diseases (Pires et al., 2020). About ten percent of the world population fall ill after consuming contaminated food and or drink each resulting to loss of 33 million health life years and 420, 000 deaths (Lee and Yoon, 2021). The presence of biotoxins in dry foods cannot be underestimated; there must be an efficient committee on management strategies to prevent food contaminants from entering food chain. Biotoxins can also be referred to as natural toxins; as they serve as defense for the producers and poison for the consumers and or source thus express their value with beneficial and deleterious effects. The detrimental effects include food intoxication as a cause of death to all life forms that have contact with them (Clark et al., 2020). Seafoods, cereals, fruits, vegetables, ready-to-eat foods, single cell proteins, crops and meat stock has been reported to contains biotoxins from microbes (microbial toxins or micro-toxins), plants(phytotoxins) and animals (zootoxins), with incidence via food contamination including food spoilage during food storage, processing, handling, plant growth and so on (Salaheieh, 2023; Choi, 2023) (Figure 19.1 and 19.2).

DOI: 10.1201/9781003500605-22

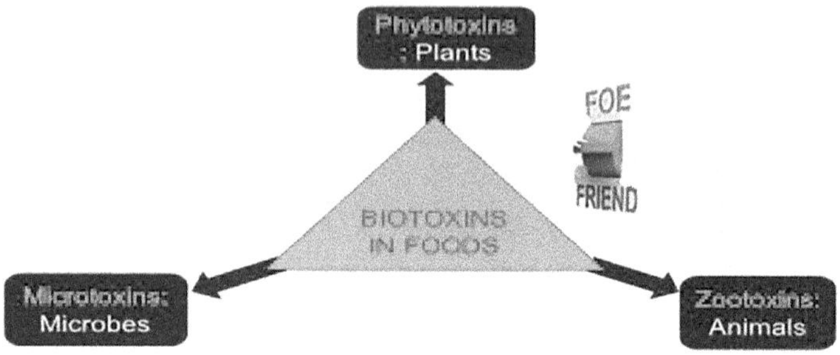

FIGURE 19.1
Biotoxin in foods

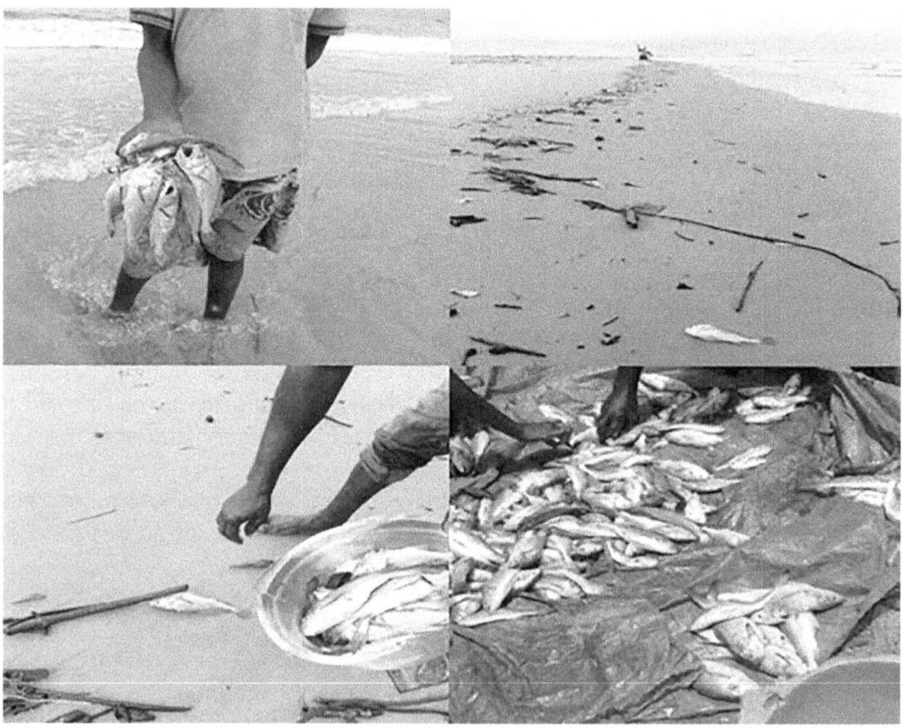

FIGURE 19.2
Influence of anthropogenic factors (oil spills) on water bodies in Niger Delta, Nigeria

The five main food groups are starchy foods, fat, dairy, protein, fruits and vegetables under the seven classes of foods as carbohydrates, proteins, fats, vitamins, minerals, dietary fiber and water. Globally, biotoxins are consumed unknowingly, these are subdivided into three based on their origin: zootoxins, phytotoxins and microtoxins (microbial toxins: mycotoxins, algal toxins, bacteria toxins and more) (Awuchi et al., 2021). Severity of toxins is based on dose and molecular size, this is in accordance to cultural belief saying "everything is toxic". The molecular size and dose of toxins are the two factors that separates non-toxic from toxic (for example, drinking 5 liters of water in 2 hrs.). Thereby, excessive consumption of good things is harmful to our health which may results to conditions in severe pains and even deaths (Dolan et al., 2010).

Polluting substances can gain entry inside foods from the environment resulting to spoilage and or contaminations by pathogen or biotoxins; symptoms or long-term effects in human beings and animals when all these enters the body (via foods/drinks/feeds) via different routes are inevitable (Ewim et al., 2023; Tang et al., 2023; Yadav et al., 2015; Alshannaq and Yu, 2017). Beneficial microbes, animal and plant nutrients are not solely the materials present in foods as toxins are inclusive (Yadav et al., 2015). They may be separated during food processing, proper food preparation, sanitation and hygiene (Tang et al., 2023). All these biotoxins in accordance to Centers for Disease Control and Prevention (CDC) (CDC, 2022); originates from microbes, plants and animals. Plant toxin (phytotoxin) examples are colchicine, ricin, abrin; seafoods' as major animal toxin source includes tetrodotoxin, ciguatoxin, brevetoxin. While some are from microbes (algae, fungi or bacteria) contamination or spoilage (botulin, aflatoxin, enterotoxins, saxitoxins, trichothecene). Quality control implanted and adopted food industries workers through government policies is sufficient to end this harmful menace. The health implication of foodborne illness ranges from immediate smarting symptoms to swift deaths of individuals and animals. This is a global concern to reduce dangers associated with consumption of unsafe food items. Some coastal aerosols particles are inhalable particle-bound marine biotoxins (Stein and Bulboaca, 2017; Yu et al., 2022). Microbial toxins account for over fifty percent of the know biotoxin (Stein and Bulboaca, 2017). It is now therefore individual and collaborative efforts to ensure foods and or feeds safety, through these measures: (1) discard unpresentable or discolored food, in particular contaminated or mouldy foods (tampered packaged foods such as canned foods, sealed foods among others); these in against traditional knowledge and belief in underdeveloped and developing countries as the upper part of the mouldy foods will be scraped off while where the fungal hyphae will be consumed unknowingly; (2) consume only identified (nonpoisonous) wild plants, single cell proteins, mushrooms and more; (3) not to assume that if something is 'natural' it is automatically safe; (4) to discard any food that have unacceptable sensory properties (offensive taste, appearance, texture, flavor or smell). Livings organisms are ever-present hence, biotoxins are always present in different foods or feeds and their effects depend on the source, dose and time.

Some individuals have food prohibitions based on their genetic make-up; food allergies (milk, fish, shellfish, cereals, tree nuts, wheat, peanuts, animal proteins and soybeans); Phenylketonuria (PKU disease); Lactose intolerance;

Disaccharide intolerance; Trimethylaminuria (fish odor syndrome); Favism; Gluten intolerance; Galactosemia; Ornithine transcarbamylase deficiency (OTD) among others. Consumption of prohibited food by individuals with these defects append indigestion, bloating, diarrhea, hepatomegaly, cirrhosis, renal failure, seizures, mental retardation, Infant mortality and so on. Other effects of food and drug interactions or food- food interactions may result to additive, synergistic and antagonistic effect for effective nutritional diets for all (Uduwana et al., 2023; Chen et al., 2022; Zhou et al., 2020). The antagonistic effect of some foods with a specific drug results in an abated effect of the drug and the additive effect to enhance the drug action, an example is garlic and ketonazole.

19.2 Factors that Influence the Availability of Biotoxins in Foods

Adequate temperature and time control throughout food preparation, processing, cooling, and storage is necessary to guarantee food safety and high quality. The physical, chemical, and microbiological properties of each type of food, such as water activity, pH, shelf life, nature, and the initial population of microorganisms present there, must all be taken into account in order to achieve a good control the establishment of contamination and or infection. The use of sewage for irrigation and manure as natural fertilizer are two dangerous agricultural practices that provide the greatest risk of contamination in primary production globally. These practices go against the core principle of avoiding biotoxin contamination of raw materials at all costs. Depending on the procedures used at different stages, there are varied dangers of contamination. (Fukuda, 2015; Jevšnik et al., 2007; Lee et al., 2015; Liu et al., 2022; Anniballi et al., 2002; Xu et al., 2021; Silva Jr, 2007; Kafetzopoulos et al., 2013; Rajkovic et al., 2020; Huang et al., 2014; Kalaitzidou et al., 2021).

Exponential growth of microbes in food during transportation must be under control against biotoxins production and proliferation of pathogenic microorganisms. Significant variables to consider during food transportation includes containers/packaging material types, temperature, direct exposure to sunlight, humidity, and airflows. Another measure is the information consumers guidelines about proper handling of prepackaged foods (handling, storage and preparation information). Predominantly, microorganisms, all the more explicitly microbes, can multiply under any various circumstances. Although bacteria can adapt to various conditions that promote their growth. These circumstances incorporate food macromolecules contents. Information on optimal conditions can influence bacteria proliferation, bacterial infections, and food contamination. Foods nutrients are required for microbial growth and those that can restrain their microbial multiplications (antimicrobial macromolecules in foods), this makes food varieties an obvious objective for the microorganisms to develop, hence, transient. To diminish the breakdown of food and to forestall foodborne diseases (FBDs), both extrinsic and intrinsic factors of a specific foods must be controlled (Kalaitzidou et al., 2021).

19.3 Extrinsic Parameters

Relative humidity, temperature, oxygen availability, with the presence and activities of other microbes are the environmental factors. Each of these factors influence the microbial growth rate as microorganisms (microbes) have an optimal, minimum and maximum temperature range to grow. Therefore, temperature determines not only the microbial types and the proliferation rate. Thermal treatment (moist or dry heat) may be employed as a preservation or sterilization (method to control microbial activity) in foods/feeds and for foods or feeds equipment's/raw material and utensils (Lee et al., 2015). Transient microbes presence could create an environment that can inhibit or be lethal for other pathogens and microtoxins {or example; mycotoxins, botulin (negative effect -), bacteriocins, antimicrobial metabolites- organic acids, lactic acid (+)}. Bacteriocins, nicins and other secondary metabolites produced by microbes are of importance as antibiotics or used as foods/feeds bio-preservatives. Bacteriocins created by Gram-positive microorganisms are organically dynamic proteins with bactericidal activity. Some bacteriocins created by these microscopic organisms repress an assortment of pathogenic microbes in foods/feeds including, *Bacillus cereus, Clostridium perfringens, Listeria monocytogens, Escherichia coli, A. hydrophila,* and *Staphylococcus aureus* and so on.

Other significant measures are the utilization of food safeguarding strategies, which can be physical or substance. Inside the actual strategies, there are the customary or modern sanitization, lack of hydration, safeguarding in adjusted air, and light. To keep a satisfactory quality assurance and control inorder to limit the gamble of feeds/foods contamination, microbial markers can be utilized; these markers don't address a potential wellbeing risk, in any case, an enormous number of them demonstrate lacks in cleanliness and sterile nature of food items; it likewise prompts a decline in the time span of usability and could be connected with the presence of pathogenic microorganisms. The super microbial markers are oxygen consuming mesophilic, which are coliforms (Enterococci, *E. coli*), *S. aureus* and lactic corrosive microorganisms. When the gamble factors are distinguished, it is important to lay out a framework that permits to forestall and diminish every one of them; to do this, a technique with logical premise and efficient profile has been laid out, this is known as Risk Examination and Basic Control Point (Hazard Analysis and Critical Points-HACCP). A scientific approach ought to confirm the type of microbes or toxins produced by them and quantity present in an environment; that can be a possible source of contamination to set an effective strategies (Lee et al., 2015; Liu et al., 2022; Anniballi et al., 2002; Xu et al., 2021; Silva Jr, 2007; Kafetzopoulos et al., 2013).

CDC expresses the rundown of poisons in food items (CDC, 2022), various sorts of poisons, for example, bacterial, parasitic toxins, algal toxins, fungal toxins (mycotoxins), green growth or plant poisons, as well as metals, poisonous synthetic compounds (cadmium, copper, zinc, lead, copper, and pesticides), or actual impurities that can cause sicknesses in humans and animals; these can cause the notable "foodborne illnesses" (CDC, 2022; Uduwana et al., 2023). Foodborne illnesses can be arranged into two gatherings: harming and contamination. Harming is brought about by the admission of compound or natural poisons, biotoxins can be tracked down in food, while microorganisms are absent. Disease is brought about by the admission of food containing practical microbes. Moreover, a harmful disease (toxicoinfection: such as cholera infection among others), is brought about by eating food with microbes that proceed to produce toxin in the host (animals or humans) resulting to illness. Relative mugginess (RH) in the climate is another significant element that help water activity (Aw) inside food. This outward element influences microbial development and must be affected by temperature. Oxygen accessibility and presence of different gases in the climate for food safeguarding and different practices corresponding to food varieties; this large number of elements are significant as they are continually entwined, a few microorganisms have an outright prerequisite for oxygen, while others fill in all out shortfall of it, and others might develop regardless of the available oxygen level. Microbes that require free oxygen are called vigorous or aerobic microbes, while those that flourish with little or no oxygen are called anaerobic; and those that develop both in presence or nonappearance of free oxygen are known as facultative microorganisms. Carbon dioxide is the main environmental gas that is utilized to control food microorganisms. Alongside oxygen, it is utilized in bundled food with altered environment. Ozone is one more environmental gas with antimicrobial properties, and for a really long time, it has been utilized as a specialist to stretch time span of usability of particular kinds of food. Despite the fact that being viable against various microorganisms, it is an exceptionally oxidizing specialist; subsequently, it can't be utilized in that frame of mind for foods or feeds containing high level of lipid, because it influence rancidity. Typically, ozone levels of 0.15–5.00 ppm in the air restrain the development of certain microorganisms that deteriorate feed/food (Silva Jr, 2007; Kafetzopoulos et al., 2013; Rajkovic et al., 2020; Huang et al., 2014; Kalaitzidou et al., 2021).

19.4 Intrinsic Parameters

These natural factors include water activity, pH- hydrogen ion concentration, oxidation-decrease potential, antimicrobial compounds present in food/feed, biological structures, supplements, and restraining substances. Water action or water activity (Aw) It is characterized as how much water accessible for the development of microorganisms; proliferation of microbes reduce when water activity additionally decline. This is connected with relative moistness (RH) mathematically, hence: RH = 100 × Aw. Microorganisms have fundamental wholesome necessities, the majority of them need outer wellsprings of carbon, nitrogen, energy, minerals; while some require the presence of a particular nutrient for optimum growth As a rule, organisms have the most minimal supplement necessity, trailed by Gram-negative microbes, then yeasts lastly, Gram-positive microorganisms, which have the most noteworthy prerequisites (CDC, 2022). The antagonistic impact of pH with two parts of the microbial cell-working of its catalysts and supplements transportation to the cell. The cytoplasmic layer of microorganisms is somewhat impermeable to H+ and OH– particles; its fixation in the cytoplasm remains sensibly steady, regardless of the wide varieties that might happen in the pH of its encompassing. At the point when microorganisms are in a climate beneath or over the nonpartisan level, their capacity to multiply relies upon their capacity to change the natural pH to a more fitting reach, since key parts like DNA or ATP require an impartial medium (Liu et al., 2022; Anniballi et al., 2002). The pH for the ideal development of most microorganisms is near lack of bias. Yeasts can fill in a corrosive climate and flourish in a middle reach (4.0–4.5), in spite of the fact that they get by in values somewhere in the range of 1.5 and 8.5. Organisms endure a wide reach (0.5–11.0), yet their development is by and large higher in an acidic pH (excessively corrosive for yeasts and other microbes). By and large, natural products such as wine (2.9–4.2), fresh or fermented sauerkraut (3.3–3.6), vinegars (2.4–3.4) and so on have pH values lower than those required for microbial growth especially bacteria (fungi can strive in acidic environment), so they can for the most part be deteriorated by organisms and yeasts. Seafood's and some meats possess pH (hydrogen ion concentration) values equivalent to 5.6, thus encourage deterioration by microbial (Lee et al., 2015; Liu et al., 2022; Anniballi et al., 2002; Xu et al., 2021). Bacterial development is typically multiplied ideally at pH esteems near the nonpartisan level (Xu et al., 2021).

19.5 Animal Toxins in Foods

The bio-origin of animal toxins is from the substrate that animal feeds on and contamination of water bodies (seafoods) including naturally produced toxins by animals for predation and defence; all these are referred zootoxins. In some animals, toxins through feeding activity may not be distributed evenly across different parts of the tissue, but concentrated at a particular animal organ or tissue (Stein and Bulboaca, 2017). Examples includes catfish, octocpus (e. g. *Hapalochlaena lunulata*), shellfish, mussel (e. g. *Perna viridis*), frogs, lizards, insects etc. All these animal products are from captive ponds, domestication, wildlife and natural water bodies. Almost all seafoods are carnivorous and feed on some animals that naturally produce toxins (e.g. dinoflagellates). The type of toxins presents in animal food products depends on if they are aquatic, terrestrial or amphibians; as a high number of biotoxins are from aquatic animals causing animal toxins outbreaks. Anthropogenic (oil spills, charcoal burning) and natural sources are also involved for bioaccumulation of biotoxins in seafoods. Majority of animal toxins are from seafoods, and historically those on the food chain peak have high concentrations of biotoxins such as mackerel (Scomberomorus spp.), bonito (Sarda spp.), halibut (Hippoglossus spp.), marlin among others. Most of these seafoods are transported all over the world (Dolan et al., 2010; Yu et al., 2022; Uduwana et al., 2023; Chen et al., 2022) (Table 19.1).

19.6 Plant Toxins in Foods

The bio-origin of plant toxins is from the chemical substances in soil from wastes, herbicides, pesticides, microbes, chemical reactions in plants or produced by plant itself. They are referred to as secondary metabolites. Phytotoxins serves for defensive purposes and they may be toxic animals, humans and plants themselves. Those produced by plants are Terpenes (T), Alkaloids (A) and Phenolics (P) classes- T: nicotine, caffeine, cocaine, morphine, ephinedrine A: taxor, resin, limonoid, saponins; P: furanocoumarin, tannin, thousands of essential oils have been discovered. Examples of phytotoxins-containing foods listed as natural toxins source include cassava, sorghum bamboo (WHO, 2023; Sotiropoulou et al., 2016; Bachmann et al., 1998; Selmar et al., 2015) (Table 19.2)

19.7 Microtoxins and Other Biotoxins in Foods

Microtoxins are toxins produced by microbes, the toxins produced by fungi are referred to as mycotoxins; those produced by bacterial are subdivided

TABLE 19.1

Effect of Animal Toxins on Human's Health

Foods: Animal	Continent	Toxin Present	Health Effects	Ref.
Oil fish/Cocco, Escolar (naturally occur; not from microbes)	In most developed countries	Gempylotoxin (Escolar oil)	Massive consumption of fish containing it, together with the fish's low melting point and indigestibility, results in oily diarrhea (keriorhoea)	(Tete and Kuete, 2014; Baralla et al., 2017; CFS, 2022; Yoshinaga-Kiriake et al., 2021)
Animal- based Meats with naturally occurring biotoxins for defence and feeding (sea snail or whelk)	Globally	Tetramine	upon neurotoxin ingestion, symptoms like ophthalmagia, dizziness, migraine, ataxy, stomach ache, fingers prickling, vomiting and watery stool	(Mekarunothai et al., 2024; Njinga et al., 2023; Yoshinaga-Kiriake et al., 2021; Kim et al., 2009)
Fishes (caused by dinoflagellate Gambier-discus toxicus). High CTX concentrations could are present in snapper, barracuda, grouper and jacks	Worldwide	Ciguatoxins (CTX)	nausea, vomiting, and diarrhea within two to six hours, which are succeeded by neurologic manifestation like lack of sensation in a specific region and whole, aches in the muscles and joints, headaches, tingling, heart failure, hyperpiesia, cloudy vision, and immobility. In few cases, Ciduatera fish poisoning is lethal	(Li et al., 2023)
Dinoflagellate *Karenia brevis* produce toxin in fish		Brevetoxins	Unlike PSP, there is no deaths reported from NSP neurotoxic shellfish poisoning (NSP), Abdominal discomfort, nausea, dizziness, restlessness, widespread muscle fatigue, ataxy, chills, migraine, myalgia, cold/hot temperature range reversal, and progressive paralysis are among the symptoms that typically appear two to four hours after consumption of contaminated shellfish. Severe poisoning could cause convulsions, dilated pupils, and bradycardia.	(Dolan et al., 2010; Ungureanu et al., 2023; Adetutu et al., 2023)
Ingesting biotoxin contaminated molluscan shellfish produced from these three genera: Gymnodium, Alexan-drium, and Pyrodinium	Globally	Saxitoxins (heterocyclic guanidines)	Outbreaks of Paralytic shellfish poisoning (PSP) have occurred worldwide. May results to deaths. The initial phase of this toxin activity in humans is the systema nervosum periphericum and the toxicity symptoms include nerve weakness.	(Jevšnik et al., 2007; Lee et al., 2015; Liu et al., 2022; Anniballi et al., 2002; Xu et al., 2021; Silva Jr, 2007; Kafetzopoulos et al., 2013; Rajkovic et al., 2020; Huang et al., 2014)

(Continued)

TABLE 19.1 *(Continued)*

Effect of Animal Toxins on Human's Health

Foods: Animal	Continent	Toxin Present	Health Effects	Ref.
Milk (contaminated by Bigelowia spp., Ageratina *altissima* etc.)	USA	Tremetol	Milk sickness	(Huang et al., 2014; Ding et al., 2017; Schrenk et al., 2023)
Freshwaters fishes (*Clarias gariepinus*, *Oreochromis niloticus*, *Euthynnus alletteratus*, *Tilapia brevimanus*)	Nigeria	Heavy metals (HMs)- (Pb, Fe, Mn, As, Cd, Ni, Co, Cr, Zn, Cu)	Tissue damage in animals and humans	(Kalaitzidou et al., 2021; Shahsavan et al., 2017; Nkosi et al., 2021)
Honey (contaminated by sheeps, oleander etc.)	Globally	Grayanotoxins	Mad honey disease	(Baralla et al., 2017; CFS, 2022; Yoshinaga-Kiriake et al., 2021)
Frozen and canned fishes (*Scomber scombrus*, tuna)	In most developing countries	HMs (Pb, Fe, Mn, As, Cd, Ni, Co, Cr, Zn, Cu)	Tissue damage in animals and humans	(Yoshinaga-Kiriake et al., 2021; Kim et al., 2009; Li et al., 2023; Asakawa et al., 2019)
Game animals (buffaloes, auks, predator birds, water fowls)	Globally	HMs (Pb, Fe, Mn, As, Cd, Ni, Co, Cr, Zn, Cu)	Tissue damage in animals and humans	(Kim et al., 2009; Li et al., 2023; Kamle et al., 2022)
Octopus	Globally	Tetrodotoxin	Muscles paralysis, body weakening, respiratory arrest and or even death	(Kim et al., 2009; Li et al., 2023; Kamle et al., 2022)
Red wines, spoiled scombroid fishes (mackerel, saury and so on).	Globally	Biogenic amines group: Histamine, tyramine, Putresine, spermine, sperimidine and cadaverine (immunogen)	Fatigue¸ Hives/dermatitis, Headaches or migraines, Nasal congestion or sinus issues Erythema (redness) and more	(Dolan et al., 2010)
During food processing and or preservation (spices, animal protein, beverages among other)	Globally (humans' factors)	Nitrosamines (human carcinogens)	Cancer and similar effects	(Dolan et al., 2010)
Food processing (coffee, vegetable proteins etc.)	Globally	Chloropropanols	Kidney effects probably as a result of long-term exposure.	(Dolan et al., 2010)

Food processing (margarines, spreads, shortenings and frying oil)	Globally (humans' factors)	Trans fatty acids (TFAs)	These toxins are formed through liquid oil hydrogenation or bacterial hydrogenation. High intake of TFAs result influence the establishment coronary artery disease.	(Dolan et al., 2010)
Food processing (canned/ jar foods, baby foods etc.)	Globally	Furan (mutagen)	cytotoxicity and hepatocarcinogenicity	(Dolan et al., 2010)
Food processing	Globally	Polycyclic aromatic hydrocarbons	Long term effects such as tumor or cancer	(Dolan et al., 2010)
Food processing	Globally	Acrylamide	Muscle paralysis, unsteadiness and so on	(Dolan et al., 2010)
Food processing	Globally	Heterocyclic aromatic amines	Long term effects such as tumor or cancer	(Dolan et al., 2010)
Storage (potatoes)	Globally (humans' factors)	Glycoalkaloids (solanine and chaconine)	Long term effects such as tumor or cancer	(Dolan et al., 2010)

TABLE 19.2

Effect of Phytotoxins on Human's Health

Foods: Plants	Continent	Toxin Present	Health Effects	Ref.
Cassava, Oak moss and so on	Globally	Prussic acid	Humans: tropical ataxic neuropathy resulting to demyelin-ization of the optic, auditory, and peripheral nerve cells	(Dolan et al., 2010)
Contaminated Grains (from the environment)	China, Dakota	Selenium	Humans: toxicity manifestation incudes hair loss, loss of nail and body structure deformation.	(Dolan et al., 2010)
Sage, clary, tansy, wormwood	USA, Spain, Denmark & Portugal and other countries	β-Thujone	Humans: Central nervous systems effects characterized by tonic-clonic or solely clonic convulsions	(Dolan et al., 2010)
Hypericum perforatum	Globally	Hypericin	Humans: photosensitization, and at high continuous doses, some liver damage may occur Grazing animals: restlessness, skin irritation, hind limb weakness, panting, confusion, depression, mania and hyperactivity	(Dolan et al., 2010)
Baked products, whole wheat flours, whole rye flours	Globally	Amylase inhibitors	occupational toxicity known as —baker's asthma disease, food allergen, weight loss control	(Dolan et al., 2010)
Food crops (vegetables, fruits and so on), Medicinal plants	Globally	HMs (Pb, Fe, Mn, As, Cd, Ni, Co, Cr, Zn, Cu)	Carcinogenic	(Dolan et al., 2010)
Plants (French beans)	In some countries	Phaseolotoxin	Phenotypic changes in plants	(Bachmann et al., 1998)
Edible tubers, fruits (cauliflower, eggplants, potatoes, tomatoes, peppers) and tobacco	Globally	Nicotine	Increased risk to gastrointestinal, respiratory and cardiovas-cular disorders, neurodegenerative diseases (Parkison disease and so on)	(Selmar et al., 2015; Koleva, 2011)
Unripe wild tomatoes, potatoes and eggplants	Globally	Tomatine	Abdominal pain, weakness, vomiting and so on	(Koleva, 2011)
Energy drinks, chocolates, tea etc.	Globally	Caffeine	In large doses, it causes sleep disorder, anxiety, high blood pressure, headache etc.	(Kalisz et al., 2023)

Teas (*Illicium* spp.)	Globally	Anethole	Illnesses ranged from serious neurological effects, such as seizures, to vomiting, jitteriness and rapid eye movement.	(Lal et al., 2022)
Pepper, carrot, mace, nutmeg etc.	Globally	Myristicin	Carcinogen, genotoxic	(Dolan et al., 2010; Ewim et al., 2023; Gotz et al., 2022; Tito et al., 2022)
Legumes (beans), carbohydrates and grains	Globally	Lectins (ricin, phytohaemagglutinin)	Anti-nutrition components, deaths (useful in bioterroism)	(Adamcova et al., 2021)
Milk, honey, Herbs, legumes (cereals) etc.	Globally	Pyrrolizidine alkaloids	Ingestion of food containing this toxin through accidental contamination of foodstuffs, once in the body system, pyeeoles may develop in the liver then, disseminate to the lungs and cause pulmonary hypertension or vasculature.	(Casado et al., 2022)
Milk, Unripe fruits (Ackee etc.)	USA, Jamaica and other Caribbean nations	Hypoglycin A	Jamaican vomiting sickness syndrome (Symptoms of poisoning following 6 to 48 hours of ingestion and incorporate sleepiness, continued regurgitating, thirst, wooziness, fever or free entrails. Depletion of the strong and sensory systems, breakdown, extreme lethargies, and demise).	(Gonzalez et al., 2018; Engel et al., 2023)
Parsley, spinach, broccoli, cocoa, etc	Globally	Oxalic acid	Calcium insolubility through binding to it cause bioaccumulation of oxalates resulting to decreased bone repair and development, kidney stones, renal toxicity, vomiting, diarrhea, convulsions, coma and impaired blood clotting	(Clark et al., 2019; Dolan et al., 2010; Chakraborty et al., 2013)
Cucumber, pumpkins Zucchini etc. (biotoxins level are increased I them due to drough, soil pH, high temperature, low soil fertility). Source from cucurbitacin-containing pecticides.	Globally	Cucurbitacins (most common bitter compuund)	Stomach cramps and diarrhea	(Dolan et al., 2010)
Fruits and vegetables such as blueberries, black currants, red beets, Brussels sprouts and red cabbage as fish, crab, clams and in some other seafoods	Globally	Anti-thiamine compounds (thiaminase)	This antivitamins cause thiamine deficiency and it may lead to weakness and weight loss. Severe thiamine deficiency produces beri-beri: a disease characterized by anorexia, cardiac enlargement, and muscular weakness leading to ataxia.	(Dolan et al., 2010)

(Continued)

TABLE 19.2 *(Continued)*

Effect of Phytotoxins on Human's Health

Foods: Plants	Continent	Toxin Present	Health Effects	Ref.
Spices, Herbal teas, clover, tonka bean, woodruffetc.		Coumarins	promotes bleeding, and may be regarded as been responsible for liver damage, fatalities by hemorrhaging in animals and humans (laboratory rats, cattle rearing) due to long term effects	(Dolan et al., 2010; Gotz et al., 2022; Tito et al., 2022; Adamcova et al., 2021)
Consumption of large amounts of Tofu, bean curd etc.-Grains and seeds (legumes, nuts, and other plants)		Phytic acid	Phytate inhibit digestive enzymes such as trypsin, pepsin, α-amylase and ß-glucosidase., while phytate-mineral complexes are insoluble in the intestinal tract, reducing mineral bioavailability. Thus, mineral deficiencies or decreased protein and starch digestibility may result from ingestion of foods containing high amounts of phytate could.	(Dolan et al., 2010)
Herbs tea, cinnamon, nutmeg, camphor, sassafras	Globally	Safrole (present in aromatic oils)- carcinogen	Weight loss, cancer and other related health effects; are also influenced by anthropogenic factors	(Dolan et al., 2010; Kalisz et al., 2022; Lal et al., 2022; Gotz et al., 2022; Tito et al., 2022; Adamcova et al., 2021; Casado et al., 2022; Gonzalez et al., 2018; Engel et al., 2023; Chakraborty et al., 2013; Barbosa et al., 2019)

into four (neurotoxins, endotoxins, exotoxins, cytotoxins), protozoan toxins and those produced by harmful algal bloom (Algal toxins). It can be referred to as microbial toxins, microtoxins or microbiotoxins. There is an increase of the geographical and temporal distribution of harmful algae that results to harmful algal blooms (HABs). Other microbial groups (fungi and bacteria) are involved in biotoxin generation in foods. Examples of HABs microalgae includes *Alexandrium catenella, A. catenella* Pyrodinium bahamense var. compressum (PBC) among others. Warmer seawater temperatures, duration, and water bodies biological and chemical contamination is responsible for this increase in bio-absorption of toxins level by seafoods. The temperature ranges from 18 ◦C to 21 ◦C for 2 days; the study reported by Barbosa et al. (2019) showed a rise in first day based on temperature variance and the toxicity level doubled on the second day. Toxigenic algae are part of the source of biotoxins found in seafoods, other foods and water with maximum acceptable limit by WHO of toxic substances (Microcystin-LR) in tank water that may use for drinking is 0.5 1.0 microgram/cubic decimeter (Tito et al., 2022). Bacterial toxins are food safety hazards causing a reasonable percentage of all reported foodborne outbreaks in Europe and other countries.

Microbes are known to be ubiquitous thereby they are the highest biotoxins producing in number, types and growth rates. With over five hundred mycotoxins known and continuous discovery of new ones. This vast distribution of natural toxins in foods such as cereals, nuts, and dried fruits pose a danger to animal and human health conditions. A few bacterial classifications can deliver poisons straightforwardly in the food, however different kinds can create them whenever they have colonized the digestive tract. Among the microbes associated with foodborne Diseases (FBDs) that are additionally viewed as toxigenic are *Aspergillus* flavus, *Salmonella* spp., *Vibrio parahaemolyticus, Vibrio cholerae, Staphylococcus aureus, Clostridium botulinum, Clostridium perfringens,* Microcytis species, Oscillatoria species, *Bacillus cereus, Listeria monocytogenes, Trypanosome species, Climacostomum virens* among others (Buonanno and Ortenzi, 2010; Makinde et al., 2023; Al-Hussieny, 2022; Wang et al., 2018; Chen et al., 2019; Nawaf, 2023). Foodborne infection, food intoxication and food toxicoinfetion which may result to acute diarrhea syndromes, fever and even death from dehydration can be avoided, especially in children under the age of 5 and in immunocompromised people (Figure 19.3). Some toxins may develop as result of time-temperature opportunity during storage to produce certain such as histamine among others and also encourage the proliferation and establishment of a transient flora that is toxigenic or toxins through improper food processing (Chen et al., 2019; Nawaf, 2023; Eckley et al., 2022) (Table 19.3).

TABLE 19.3

Effect of Microtoxins on Human's Health

Foods: Microbes	Continent	Toxin Present	Health Effects	Ref.
Grains and its products, animal proteins (poultry, pork, red meat and seafoods), Chicken eggs, Seafoods (shellfish, sea fan corals, clams, scallops, mussels): fungi (*Aspergillus sydowii*, y *Aspergillus fumigatus*, *A. flavus*, *Penicillium waksmanii*, *Trichoderma* spp., and *Cladosporium* spp.); bacteria (*Vibrio tasmaniensis*) and algae	Globally	Mycotoxins (Aflatoxins, sydowinin A or B, alamethicin, sydowinol, patulin, gliotoxin, peptaibol, griseofulvin); algal toxins (okadaic acid, domoic acid, saxitoxin, carbamoyl toxins)	gastrointestinal side effects of spewing, stomach issue, the runs, and neurological side effects of migraine, momentary cognitive decline, cerebrum harm, and most severe cases result to death	(Al-Hussieny, 2022; Wang et al., 2018; Chen et al., 2019; Nawaf, 2023; Eckley et al., 2022)
Industrially processed foods (Biscuits, Shawarma, Bread) contaminated by *Gibberella zeae*, *Fusarium* spp. Also present in animal feeds	Specific locations	Mycotoxins (Zearalenone, Vomitoxin/Deoxynivalenol)	Gastroenteritis with long term effects may result to colon cancer	(Wang et al., 2018; Chen et al., 2019; Nawaf, 2023; Eckley et al., 2022; Tacconi et al., 2023; CFS, 2018; Costa et al., 2019; Deng et al., 2023; Zgouridou et al., 2022; Bryant, 2022)
Seafoods and canned foods (anthropogenic and natural sources)	Environmental actions (pesticides, herbicides and industrial effluents), and bacteria action (anaerobically)	Methyl mercury	mad hatter syndrome, influence the establishment of spoilage microbes and pathogens	(Al-Hussieny, 2022; Eckley et al., 2022)
Dog fish etc.	Enteric bacteria action	Trimethylamine oxide	Acts as a neurotoxin which may results to cancer	(Tacconi et al., 2023)
Dairy, Milk, meat, versatile ready to eat food products, rice, pasta, raw and unprocessed food (*Bacillus cereus* strains)	Globally	emetic toxin, cereulide, Amylovorin, Rhizobiotoxine Tabtoxin and diarrheal enterotoxins	symptoms, which include nausea, vomiting, and sometimes abdominal cramps and/or diarrhea that usually resolve within 24 hr. Fatalities have been reported	(Makinde et al., 2023; CFS, 2018)

Edible ice	Globally	Coliform bacteria	Diarrhea, vomting among others	(CFS, 2018)
Fish, vegetables, fruits, salads and processed refrigerated foods. (*Clostridium botulinum*, as well as some strains of *C. argentinense*, C. baratii, C. butyricum, C. sporogenes, and C. novyi: including serotypes)	Globally	Neurotoxins (botulin etc.)	Convulsion and death; if not immediately treated	(Deng et al., 2023)
Meats and poultry products as a result of temperature abuse during the cooking, cooling, or holding of foods (*C. perfringens*)	Second most common foodborne illness in developed countries (e.g. United States)	several toxins that mediate a number of histotoxic and enterotoxic diseases in humans and animals	Abdominal cramps, diarrhea etc.	(Zgouridou et al., 2022; Bryant, 2022; Yan et al., 2020)
meat and meat products, poultry and egg products, milk and dairy products, salads, bakery products, particularly cream-filled pastries and cakes, and sandwich fillings (*Staphylococcus aureus*)	Incidentally pathogenic isolates from nonhuman contact.	staphylococcal enterotoxins (SEs)	Emesis (vomiting etc.) ethic may results to death	(Hayashi et al., 2018; Bimerew et al., 2023; Visciano and Schirone, 2022; Adekoya et al., 2019)
Indigenous/Artisanal foods (Eko, Kokoro, Adun) contaminated by *Gibberella zeae*, *Fusarium* spp.	Sub-Saharan Africa	Fumonisins, Aflatoxins, Ochratoxins		(Visciano and Schirone, 2022; Adekoya et al., 2019; Janik et al., 2019; OSTC, 2011; CDC, 2022; Teshome et al., 2022; Feng et al., 2015)

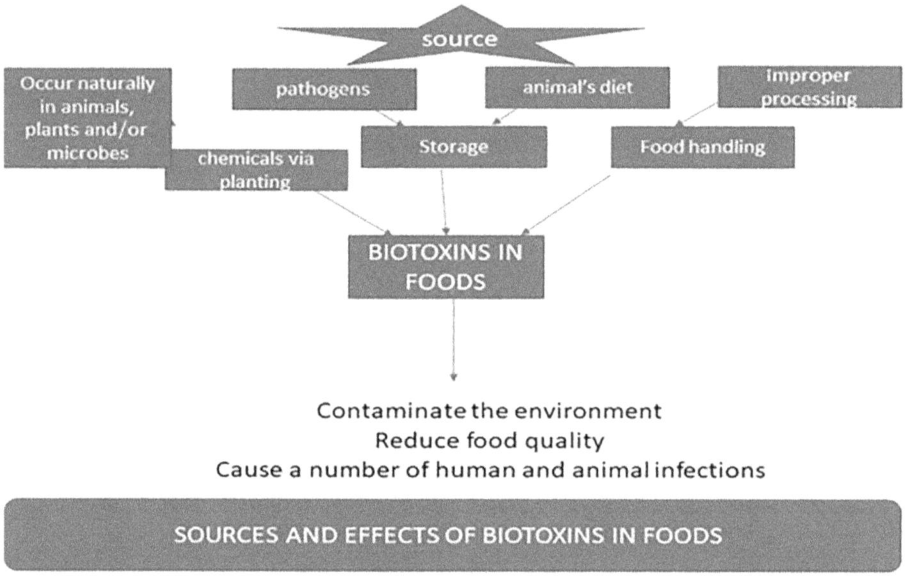

FIGURE 19.3
Effects and sources of biotoxins in foods (Table 19.1–19.3)

19.8 Control of Biotoxins in Foods

Surveillance system on water bodies, raw materials, and finished products must be in existence. Water treatment should be done periodically due to microbial growth nature and effect of environmental waste disposals into water bodies; these include chlorination, activated charcoal treatment among others, water treatment using ozone have been the most effective; this ozone method of removal of algal toxins in water can be employed in beverages and other companies. The Standard Organization of Nigeria (SON) and other statutory bodies mandates the labeling of any product that contains substances that may cause allergies, proteins produced from these offending foods, or unintentional additions or tastes. While any highly refined oil made from a common food allergy (such as peanut or soybean oil) or any food ingredient is exempt from labeling due to a legal notice or petition process (Dolan et al., 2010; Eckley et al., 2022; Gotz et al., 2022).

Bryant (2022) proposed limit to product substitution (such as fish mislabeled sample number), intermittent use of mycotoxin binder (activated charcoal) in animal feeds, discourage feeding animals with spoiled foods, educational programs on biotoxins and their associative factors. It is necessary for epidemiologist and medical practitioners to know the etiology, prevalence, source and incidence of the pathogens causing foodborne diseases (FBDs) that circulate in their regions; not only to know the morbidity and mortality rate, but also to provide the population with the treatment (appropriate medical attention and care needed to limit the spread and effect of the pathogen causing FBDs) and a lasting preventive measure.

19.9 Case Report of Biotoxins in Foods

Every district has explicit financial qualities, this impact occurrence and the death pace of FBDs related. The Shigella genera possesses the first spot in quite a while in all locales; with different result of contamination. Microbes are the gathering that causes FBDs, trailed by certain cestodes and helminthes; in any case, In African locales, cestodes, and helminths are the gathering that causes FBDs on the grounds that wellbeing and financial circumstances limit legitimate food taking care of. Also, the pervasiveness of microorganisms in these nations is higher than in evolved nations (Teshome et al., 2022; Visciano and Schirone, 2022; Tete and Kuete, 2014). For instance, in most developed countries, Salmonella, Clostridium, and Campylobacter species account for foodborne infection or diseases cases; their primary and secondary sources include domesticated animals and homegrown creatures, with improper food processing, preparation and storage thereby increasing morbidity and mortality (Visciano and Schirone, 2022; Wang et al., 2018; Stein and Bulboaca, 2017).

Biotoxins intoxications occurring recurrently every year due to mistaken consumption of a particular plant species (physical similarities), contamination during plant harvest, cultural initiation and as medicinal plants. The prevalent microbes that cause food poisoning differs from one countries to another although, *S. aureus* is the consistently prevalent with reports indicate that *S. aureus* is responsible for up to 41% of food contamination outbreaks. Despite the fact that it can affects individuals of all ages, the reach with the most elevated occurrence goes from 20 to 49 years old, where up to 48% of the cases can be concentrated. The fundamental food items connected with food contamination brought about by *S. aureus* are chicken and eggs, cakes, pastas, sauces, milk, and its inferred items. Universally, the biggest cases by ETEC (Enterotoxigenic *Escherichia coli*) in number is about 240 million, and *Shigella* spp is approximately 200 million cases; notwithstanding cases of EPEC, other virulent strains of E. coli and other pathogens are reported and fatal. Altogether, more than 40% of the cases and passings brought about by foodborne diseases (FBDs) affecting youngsters younger than 5 years of age, immunocompromised patients and aged people. Food contamination brought about by *B. cereus* can happen any season; it doesn't present a characterized geological dispersion, and in light of the fact that it is normally tracked down in the climate due to their ability to produce spores that can withstand adverse conditions, its distribution in various types of food occurs easily, especially in those of plant origin such as cereals and rice. Reports about food poisoning outbreaks caused by *Bacillus cereus* are underestimated due to the lack of diagnostic tools; however, globally, there are figures where food poisoning caused by this pathogen occupies from 1 to 17.5% of the total cases of food poisoning caused by bacteria (Teshome et al., 2022; Wang et al., 2018; Stein and Bulboaca, 2017). A young farmer in Ethiopia was reportedly affected due to BOAA from chicken/ grass pea; this is still endemic in India, Ethiopia and Bangladesh. Most plants that possess hallucination properties (Amarathus, jimson weed) may have similar effects. Although *Lathyrus sativus* was known to be cause of epidemic in North Africa, Middle East, Asia and Indian subcontinent as dose, gender and other factors influence the establishment of infection and or disease (Tacconi et al., 2023; Tang et al., 2023). Pinnatoxins (PnTXs) was first isolated from *Pinna attenuta* (bivalve mollusk) in 1990 with seven toxin analogues (A, B, C, D, E, F and G) concurrently isolated up till today. First report of aflatoxin recovered from yam chips, cassava and maize products sold in southwestern, Nigeria, Benin republic and other African countries (Ungureanu et al., 2023; Shahsavani et al., 2017; Silva, 2007). Saxitoxin in Putterfish was reported in USA, likewise, there was a first report of seafood poisoning (GTX 1–4) in Spain produced by *Aspergillus minutum*. Fermented foods are the best and reliable food processing but biotoxins have also been reported in fermented foods because of improper storage (raw materials and or food products), inappropriate starter culture and processing conditions (Yadav et al., 2015; Xu et al., 2021; Böhme et al., 2012). This alternate the rise in fermented foods and products consumption because they are generally safe probiotics while most of these fermented foods possess pharmacological properties. Aflatoxins and other mycotoxins have been detected in indigenous alcoholic beverages in Nigeria and South Africa (Böhme et al., 2012). Various cases of biogenic amines and histamine in fermented and non-fermented foods (Yadav et al., 2021; Xu et al., 2015).

Biotoxins is a global concern as food is also a necessity for humans and animals, first case report of algal toxin was reported in Malaysia (2013, 2014) which eventually result to death in around Sabah and Pahang territories. Risk occurrence of biotoxins in dry animal foods increases due to their composition (grains and vegetables) (Ungureanu et al., 2023). The economic influence of animal in each country cannot be overemphasized for food security and dissemination (exportation). Yan et al. (2020) report natural occurrence of deoxynivalenol and its derivatives from maize and wheat marketed in China. Food intoxication brought about by *C. botulinum* is less incessant and the epidemiological data about it is scant; episodes of food contamination brought about by this microbe normally incorporate individuals from one family, that is to say, they don't include an enormous number of people and the primary driver of such flare-ups is the utilization of canned food at home. Food contamination brought about by *Clostridium* species (*C. perfringens* and or *C. botulinum*) happens whenever of the year, yet it is more regular somewhat recently of the year. It doesn't present a topographical circulation; in certain nations like the US, the flare-ups brought about by this microorganism possess the second spot in foodborne sicknesses. For the most part, this sort of episodes influences an enormous number of people as most cases are brought about by the admission of animal protein; the defilement of meat and other food items is from dungs or contaminated hands and utensils (WHO, 2023; Wilson, 2021).

19.10 Economic Importance of Biotoxins in Foods

Sourcing of good raw materials by industries will minimize the spread of pathogens and their toxins. These biotoxins in foods are responsible for a number of plant and animal diseases; humans left over foods or wastes from animal feeds can be reconstituted as fertilizers for plant and affect plants or otherwise used as another animal feeds resulting in development of an infection in those animals. Some of the biotoxins are utilized in bioterrorism using foods and drinks as vehicles. For foods that required storage, they reduce the quality and quantity during storage. All these affect the economy of a geographical location in diverse ways (Visciano and Schirone, 2022; Wang et al., 2018). Some of these natural toxins serves as a dependable product in food preservations for example; essential oils (EOs) are naturally present in every aspect of a plant, which includes stem, seeds, strip, bark, blooms, and entire plants. They are utilized in the majority of nations because of their and pharmacological properties thus, their use as food additives, perfumes among others (Salaheieh, 2023; CFS, 2022; Silva, 2007).

The use of artificial chemicals may result in intoxication, cancerous development, degenerative disorders and hypersensitive reactions. EOs and other plants macromolecules (extracts) have gain global interest by food manufacturers due to their ability in controlling the growth of pathogens and or biotoxins, reduce antimicrobial resistance and food safety. Biotoxins are useful macromolecules in epidemiological and ecological studies because about six most danger biotoxins considered as biological warfare agents (bioterrorism): botulinum toxin, staphylococcal enterotoxins, *Clostridum perferinges,* ricin, abrin and T-2 toxin can be transmitted among living organisms (humans and animals) through food, water and feeds (Feng et al., 2015; Böhme et al., 2012; Grass et al., 2013).

19.11 Conclusion

Surveillance system on biotoxins should be employed in control for all food products (human and animals' consumption) especially those that will be exported. This chapter is to influence research works to detect the presence of phytotoxins, mycotoxins and other hidden biotoxins in foods, water bodies among others. Moreso, their synergistic effects. All foods-related companies should follow food safety guidelines in their state or territories in support with World Health Organizations (WHO) and other agencies to support this view. A specific protocol at all levels in foods handling must be done properly from storage and processing (preparation/cooking). Industrial use of antioxidants from plants in preservation must gain more acceptance in all society over the chemical preservatives which have numerous side effects.

Although most of this biotoxins are beneficial in various fields (cancer therapy) based on the active ingredients and some have been declared safe to be consumed directly. Quality extraction of useful components may be done on extremely toxic one. In laboratory, presently there are biotechnological approach in biological characterization of biotoxins but the gold standard animal bioassays. Other analytical techniques used for detection of biotoxins in foods for control and monitoring grounds are immunoassays, culture, nano-sensor based techniques and chromatography.

References

Adamcova, A., Laursen, K. H., and Ballin, N. Z. 2021. Lectin activity in commonly plant-based foods: Calling for method harmonization and risk assessment. *Foods*, 10, 11, 2796.

Adekoya, I., Obadina, A., Olorunfemi, M., Akande, O., Landschoot, S., De Saeger, S., and Njobeh, P. 2019. Occurrence of bacteria and endotoxins in fermented foods and beverages from Nigeria and South Africa. *International Journal of Food Microbiology*, 305.

Adetutu, A., Adegbola, P. I., and Aborisade, A. B. 2023. Heavy metal concentrations in four fish species from the Lagos lagoon and their health implications. *Heliyon*, 9, 12, e21689.

Al Alnabi, D. I. B., Al-Shawi, S. G., Al-Younis, Z. K., Swadi, W. A., Yousif, A. Y., Hafsan, H., and Mahmudiono, T. 2022. Heavy metal in the soil-grain-food path: An overview of the role of mycotoxins in potential hazards associated with animal products. *Food Science and Technology*, 42.

Al-Hussieny, A. A. 2022. *Algae toxins and their treatment*. IntechOpen.

Alshannaq, A., and Yu, J.-H. 2017. Occurrence, toxicity, and analysis of major mycotoxins in food. *International Journal of Environmental Research and Public Health*, 14, 6, 632.

Anniballi, F., Fenicia, L., Franciosa, G., and Aureli, P. 2002. Influence of pH and temperature on the growth of and toxin production by neurotoxigenic strains of Clostridium butyricum type E. *Journal of Food Protection*, 65, 8, 1267–1270.

Asakawa, M., Matsumoto, T., Umezaki, K., Kaneko, K., Yu, X., Gomez-Delan, G., Tomano, S., Noguchi, T., and Ohtsuka, S. 2019. Toxicity and toxin composition of the greater blue-ringed octopus Hepalaochlaena lunulate from Ishigaki Island, Okinawa prefecture, Japan. *Toxins (Basel)*, 11, 5, 245.

Awuchi, C. G., Ondari, E. N. Ogbonna, C. U., Upadhyay, A. K., Baran, K., Odilichukwu, C., Okpala, R., Korzeniowska, M., and Guine, R. P. F. 2021. Mycotoxins affecting animals, foods, humans, and plants: Types, occurrence, toxicities, action mechanisms, prevention and detoxification strategies: A revisit. *Foods*, 10, 6, 1279.

Bachmann, A. S., Matile, P., and Slusarenko, A. J. 1998. Inhibition of ornithine decarboxylase activity by phaseolotoxin: Implications for symptom production in halo blight of French bean. *Physiological and Molecular Plant Pathology*, 53, 5–6, 287–299.

Baralla, E., Varoni, M. V., Sedda, T., Pasciu, V., Floris, A., and Demontis, M. P. 2017. Microcystins presence in mussels (*Mytilus galloprovincialis*) and two productive mediterranean's Lagoons (Sardina, Italy). *BioMed Research International*, 3769245.

Barbosa, V., Santos, M., Anacleto, P., Maulvault, A. L., Pousao-Ferreira, P., Costa, P. R., and Marques, A. 2019. Paralytic shellfish toxins and ocean warming: Bioaccumulation and ecotoxicological responses in juvenile gilthead seabream (*Sparus aurata*). *Toxins (Basel)*, 11, 7, 408.

Bimerew, M., Gebremeskel, T., Beletew, B., Ayalneh, M., Ayaliew, W., and Wodaje, M. 2023. Prevalence of neurolathriysm and its associated factors in grass pea cultivation areas of Dawunt district, North-Eastern Ethiopia; 2022: A community based multilevel analysis. *BMC Neurology*, 23, 357.

Böhme, K., Fernández-No, I. C., Barros-Velázquez, J., Gallardo, J. M., Cañas, B., and Calo-Mata, P. 2012. Species identification of food spoilage and pathogenic bacteria by MALDI-TOF mass fingerprinting. In: Kapiris, K., editor. *Food quality*. IntechOpen, pp. 27–47.

Bryant, C. J. 2022. Plant-based animal product alternatives are healthier and more environmental sustainable than animal products. *Future Foods*, 6, 100174.

Buonanno, F., and Ortenzi, C. 2010. The protozoan toxin climacostol and its derivatives: Cytotoxicity studies on 10 species of free-living ciliates. *Versita Biologia*, 65, 4, 675–680.

Casado, N., Morante-Zarcero, S., and Sierra, I. 2022. The concerning food safety issue of pyrrolizidine alkaloids: An overview. *Trends in Food Science & Technology*, 120, 123–139.

Centre for Disease Control (CDC). 2022. *Bioterrorism agents/diseases (by category)*. CDC. Accessed on February 4, 2024.

Centre for Disease Control (CDC). 2022. *Biotoxin-emergency preparedness & response*. CDC. Accessed on February 4, 2024.

Centre for Disease Control (CDC). 2022. *National biomonitoring program*. CDC. Accessed on February 4, 2024.

Centre for Disease Control and Prevention. 2022. *Health practices on cruise ships: Training for employees* [Internet]. Available from: https://www.cdc.gov/nceh/vsp/training/videos/environadd.htm.

Centre for Food Safety (CFS). 2018. *Food safety focus*. Centre for Food Safety. Accessed on February 1, 2024.

Centre for Food Safety (CFS). 2022. *Natural toxins in foods (safe food for all)*. Centre for Food Safety. Accessed on January 12, 2024.

Chakraborty, N., Ghosh, R., Ghosh, S., Narula, K., Tayal, R., Datta, A., and Chakraborty, S. 2013. Reduction of oxalate levels in tomato fruit and consequent metabolic remodeling following overexpression of a fungal oxalate decarboxylase. *Plant Physiology*, 162, 1, 354–378.

Chen, S., Zhang, X., Yan, Z., Hu, Y., and Yibo, L. 2019. Development and application of immunoaffinity column purification and ultrahigh performance liquid chromatography-tandem mass spectrometry for determination of domoic acid in shellfish. *Toxins*, 11, 83.

Chen, X., Li, H., Zhang, B., and Deng, Z. 2022. The synergistic and antagonistic antioxidants interactions of dietary phytochemical combinations. *Critical Reviews in Food Science and Nutrition*, 62, 20, 5658–5677.

Choi, L. 2023. Review of food poisoning outbreaks related to local food premises and food businesses. *Centre for Food Safety*, 200, 1.

Clark, G. C., Casewell, N. R., Elliot, C. T., Harvey, A. L., Jamieson, A. G., Strong, P. N., and Turner, A. D. 2019. Friends and foes? Emerging impacts of biological toxins. *Trends in Biochemical Sciences*, 44, 4, 365–379.

Costa, P. R., Marques, A., and Diogène, J. 2019. Marine biotoxins and seafood poisoning. *Toxins*, 11, 558.

Deng, Y., You, L., Wang, X., Wu, W., Kuca, K., Wu, Q., and Wei, W. 2023. Deoxynivalenol: Emerging toxic mechanisms and control strategies, current and future perspectives. *Journal of Agricultural and Food Chemistry*, 71, 29, 10901–10915.

Ding, L., Qiu, J., and Li, A. 2017. Proposed biotransformation pathways of new metabolites of paralytic shellfish toxins based in field and experimental mussel samples. *Journal of Agricultural and Food Chemistry*, 65, 5494–5502.

Dolan, L. R., Matulka, R. A., and Burdock, G. A. 2010. Naturally occurring food toxins. *Toxins*, 2, 2289–2332.

Eckley, C. S., Luxton, T. P., Knightes, C. D., and Shah, V. 2022. Methylmercury production and degradation under light and dark conditions in the water column of the hells canyon reservoirs, USA. *Environmental Toxicology Chemistry*, 40, 7, 1829–1839.

Engel, A. M., El-Khatib, A. H., Klevenhusen, F., Weiss, M., Aboling, S., Sachse, B., Schafer, B., Weigel, S., Pieper, R., and Fischer-Tenhagen, C. 2023. Detection of d hypoglycin A and MCPrG metabolites in the milk and urine of pasture dairy cows after intake of Sycamore seedlings. *Journal of Agricultural and Food Biochemistry*, 71, 28, 10751–10760.

Ewim, D. R. E., Orikpete, O. F., Scott, T. O., Onyebuchi, C. N., Onukogu, A. O., Uzougbo, C. G., and Onunka, C. 2023. Survey of wastewater issues due to oil spills and pollution in Niger Delta area of Nigeria: A secondary data analysis. *Bulletin of the National Research Centre*, 47, 116.

Feng, L., Chen, X., Liu, S., Zhou, Z., and Yang, R. 2015. Two family outbreak of botulism associated with the consumption of smoked ribs in Sichuan Province, China. *International Journal of Infectious Diseases*, 30, 74–77.

Fukuda, K. 2015. Food safety in a globalized world. *Bulletin of the World Health Organization*, 93, 212.

Gonzalez, M. S., Hyde, C., Lovera, I., and Piercy, R. J. 2018. Detection of equine atypical myopathy-associated hypoglycin A in plant material: Optomisation and validation of a novel LC-MS based method derivitisation. *PLOS One*, 13, 7, e0199521.

Gotz, M. E., Sachse, B., Schafer, B., and Eisenreich, A. 2022. Myristicin and elemicin: Potentially toxic alkenbenzenes in foods. *Foods*, 11, 13, 1988.

Grass, J. E., Gould, L. H., and Mahon, B. E. 2013. Epidemiology of foodborne disease outbreaks caused by Clostridium perfringens, Unites States, 1998–2010. *Foodborne Pathogens and Disease*, 10, 2, 131–136.

Hayashi, A., José Dorantes-Aranda, J., Bowman, J. P., and Hallegraeff, G. 2018. Combined cytotoxicity of the phycotoxin okadaic acid and mycotoxins on intestinal and neuroblastoma human cell models. *Toxins*, 10, 526.

Huang, L., Wang, J., Chen, W. C., Li, H. Y., Liu, J. S., Jiang, T., and Yang, W-D. 2014. P-glycoprotein expression in *Perna viridis* after exposure to *Prorocentrum lima*, a dinoflagellate producing DSP toxins. *Fish Shellfish Immunology*, 39, 254–262.

Janik, E., Ceremuga, M., Sluk-Bijak, J., and Bijak, M. 2019. Biological toxins as the potential tools for bioterrorism. *International Journal of Molecular Sciences*, 20, 5, 1181.

Jevšnik, M., Hlebec, V., and Raspor, P. 2007. Consumers' awareness of food safety from shopping to eating. *Food Control*, 19, 8, 737–774.

Kafetzopoulos, D. P., Psomas, E. L., and Kafetzopoulos, P. D. 2013. Measuring the effectiveness of the HACCP food safety management system. *Food Control*, 33, 2, 505–513.

Kalaitzidou, M. P., Nannou, C. I., Lambropoulou, D. A., Papageorgiou, K. V., Theodoridis, A. M., Economou, V. K., Giantsis, I. A., Angelidis, P. G., Kritas, S. K., and Petridou, E. J. 2021. First report of detection of microcystins in farmed Mediterranean mussels Mytilus galloprovincialis in Thermailos gulf in Greece. *Journal of Biological Research*, 28, 1, 8.

Kalisz, O., Studzinska, S., and Bocian, S. 2023. A determination of the content in dietary supplements according to green chemistry principles. *Foods*, 12, 13, 2474.

Kamle, M., Mahato, D. R., Gupta, A., Pandhi, S., Sharma, B., Dhawan, K., Vasundhara, Mishra, S., Kumar, M., Tripathi, A. D., and Rasane, P. 2022. Deoxynivalenol: An overview on occurrence, chemistry, biosynthesis, health effects and its detection, management and control strategies in food and feed. *Microbiology Research*, 13, 2, 292–314.

Kim, J. H., Lee, K. J., Suzuki, T., Kim, C. M., Lee, J. Y., Mok, J. S., and Lee, T. S. 2009. Identification of tetramine, a toxin in whelks, as the cause of a poisoning incident in Korea and the distribution of tetramine in fresh and boiled whelk (Neptunea intersculpta). *Journal of Food Protection*, 72, 9, 1935–1940.

Koleva, I. I. 2011. Alkaloids in the human food chain: Natural occurrence and possible adverse effects. *Molecular Nutrition & Food Research*, 56, 1, 30–52.

Lal, M., Begum, T., Godi, R., Sarma, N., Munda, S., Pandey, S. K., Baruah, J., Tamang, R., and Saikia, S. 2022. Anethole rish *Clauswna heptaphylla* (Roxb.) Wight & Arn., essential oil pharmacology and genotoxic efficiencies. *Scientific Reports*, 12, 9978.

Lee, H., and Yoon, Y. 2021. Etiological agents implicated in foodborne illness worldwide. *Food Science of Animal Resources*, 41, 1, 1–7.

Lee, S. J., Si, J., Yun, H. S., and Ko, G. 2015. Effect of temperature and relative humidity on the survival of foodborne viruses during food storage. *Applied and Environmental Microbiology*, 81, 6, 2075–2081.

Li, Q., Mahmudiono, T., Mohammadi, H., Nematollahi, A., Hoseinvandtabar, S., Mehri, F., Hasanzadeh, V., Limam, I., Fakhri, Y., and Thai, V. N. 2023. Concentration ciguatoxins in fillet of fish: A global systemic review and meta-analysis. *Heliyon*, 9, 8, e18500.

Liu, D., Zhang, C., Pu, Y., Chen, S., Liu, L., Cui, Z., and Zhong, Y. 2022. Recent advances in pH- responsive freshness indicators using natural food colorants to monitor freshness. *Foods*, 11, 13, 1884.

Makinde, O. M., Sulyok, M., Adeleke, R. A., Krska, R., and Ezekiel, C. N. 2023. Bacteriological quality and biotoxin profile of ready-to-eat foods vended in Lagos, Nigeria. *Foods*, 12, 6, 1224.

Mekarunothai, A., Bacher, M., Buathong, R., Intarasam, S., Tayana, N., Kongkiatpaiboon, S., Charoenrat, T., and Napiroon, T. 2024. B-sitosterol isolated from the leaves of Tremia orientalis (Cannabaceae) promotes viability and proliferation of BF-2 cells. *PeerJ*, 12, e16774.

Munialo, C. D., and Mellor, D. D. 2023. A review of the impact of social disruptions on food security and food choice. *Food Science and Nutrition*, 12, 1, 13–23.

Nawaf, A. 2023. Mycotoxin source and its exposure causing mycotoxicosis. *Bioinformation*, 19, 4, 348–357.

Njinga, R. L., Adebayo, A. S., and Olufemi, A. P. 2023. Bioaccumulation of heavy metals in water and organs of Tilapia brevimanus and Euthynnus alletteratus from a coaster water in Southwestern Nigeria. *Environmental Sciences Europe*, 35, 85.

Nkosi, D. V., Bekker, J. L., and Hoffman, L. 2021. Toxic metals in wild ungulates and domestic meat animals slaughtered for food purposes: A systemic review. *Foods*, 10, 11, 2853.

Ohio Section Technology Committee (OSTC). 2011. *White paper on algal toxin treatment, environmental protection agency*. OSTC, pp. 1–6.

Pires, S. M., Thomsen, S. T., Nauta, M., Poulsen, M., and Jakobsen, L. S. 2020. Food safety implications of transitions toward sustainable healthy diets. *Food and Nutrition Bulletin*, 41, 2, 104–124.

Rajkovic, A., Jovanovic, J., Monteiro, S., Decleer, M., Andjelkovic, M., Foubert, A., Beloglazova, N., Tsilla, V., Sas, B., Madder, A., De Saeger, S., and Uyttendaele, M. 2020. Detection of toxins involved in foodborne diseases caused by gram-positive bacteria. *Comprehensive Reviews in Food Science and Food Safety*, 19, 1605–1657.

Salaheieh, N. 2023. *More than 400 products including breakfast sandwiches and fruit cup recalled due to possible Listeria contamination*. Repot on CNN. Accessed on February 5, 2024.

Schrenk, D., Bignami, M., Bodin, L., Chipman, J. K., del Mazo, J., Grasl-Kraupp, B., Hogstrand, C., Hoogenboom, L. R., Leblanc, J.-C., Nebbia, C. S., Nielsen, E., Ntzani, E., Petersen, A., Sand, S., Schwerdtle, T., Vleminckx, C., Duseemud, B., Hart, A., Mulder, P., Viviani, B., Anastassiadou, M., Cacio, C., Riolo, F., and Wallace, H. 2023. Risks for human health related to the presence of grayanotoxins in certain honey. *European Food Safety Authority Journal*, 21, 3, e07866.

Selmar, D., Engelhardt, U. H., Hansel, S., Thrane, C., Nowak, M., and Kleinwachter, M. 2015. Nicotine uptake by peppermint plalants as a possible source in plant derived products. *Agronomy for Sustainable Development*, 35, 1185–1190.

Shahsavani, A., Fakhri, Y., Ferrante, M., Keramati, H., Zandsalimi, Y., Bay, A., Pouya, S. R. H., Moradi, B., Bahmani, Z., and Khaneghah, A. M. 2017. Risk assessment of heavy metals bioaccumulation: Fished shrimps from the Persian gulf. *Toxins Reviews*, 34, 4, 322–330.

Silva Jr, E. A. 2007. *Manual of hygienic control in food service systems*. Varela, vol. 623, 6th ed. ISBN:8585519533.

Sotiropoulou, N. S. D., Kokkini, M. K., Megremi, S. F. P., Daferera, D. J., Skotti, E. P., Kimbaris, A. C., Polissiou, M. G., and Tarantilis, P. A. 2016. Determination of A- and B- Thujone in wormwood and sage infusions of Greek flora and estimation of their average toxicity. *Current Research in Nutrition and Food Science*, 4.

Stein, R. A., and Bulboaca, A. E. 2017. Mycotoxins. *Foodborne diseases*, 3rd ed. London: Academic Press, 2017.

Tacconi, E., Palma, G., Biase, D. D., Luciano, A., Barbieri, M., de Nigris, F., and Bruzzese, F. 2023. Microbial effect on trimethylalamine N-oxide production: From cancer to fitness- A practical preventing recommendation and therapies. *Nutrients*, 15, 3, 563.

Tang, X., Zuo, J., Yang, C., Jiang, J., Zhang, Q., Ping, J., and Li, P. 2023. Current trends in biosensors for biotoxins (mycotoxins, marine toxins, and bacterial food toxins): Principles, application, and perspective. *TrAC Trends in Analytical Chemistry*, 165, 117144.

Teshome, E., Forsido, S. F., Rupasinghe, H. P. V., and Olika-Keyata, E. 2022. Potentials of natural preservatives to enhance food safety and shelf life: A review. *Scientific World Journal*, 9901018.

Tete, G. N., and Kuete, V. 2014. Acute and substance toxicities of African medicinal plants. *Toxicological Survey of African Medicinal Plants*, 63–98.

Tito, J. C. R., Luna, L. M. G., Noppe, W. N., and Hubert, I. A. 2022. First report on microcystin-LR in water reservoirs of Eastern Cuba, and environmental trigger factors. *Toxins*, 14, 3, 209.

Uduwana, S., Abeynayake, N., and Wickramasinghe, I. 2023. Synergistic, antagonistic, and additive effects on the resultant antioxiadant activity in infusions of green tea with bee honey and Citrus limonum extracts as additives. *Journal of Agriculture and Food Research*, 12, 100571.

Ungureanu, E. L., Mocanu, A. L., Stroe, C. A., Duta, D. E., and Mustatea, G. 2023. Assessing Health risks associated with heavy metals in food: A bibliometric analysis. *Foods*, 12, 21, 3974.

Visciano, P., and Schirone, S. 2022. Update on biogenic amines in fermented and non-fermented beverages. *Foods*, 11, 3, 353.

Wang, L., Zhang, Q., Yan, Z., Tan, Y., Runyue, Z., Yu, D., Yang, H., and Wu, A. 2018. Occurrence and quantitative risk assessment of twelve mycotoxins in eggs and chicken tissues in China. *Toxins*, 10, 11, 477.

Wilson, B. A., and Ho, M. 2021. The biosecurity threat posed by biological toxins. *Biological Toxins and Bioterroism*, 141–183.

World Health Organization (WHO). 2023. *Fact sheets: Natural toxins in food*. WHO. Accessed on February 1, 2024.

Xu, X., Li, T., Ji, Y., Jiang, X., Shi, X., and Wang, B. 2021. Origin, succession, and control of biotoxin in wine. *Frontiers in Microbiology*, 12, 703391.

Yadav, A., Kumar, R., and Pande, A. K. 2015. Some common food toxins and their effect on human health. *Journal of the Kalash Science*, 3, 3, 1–6.

Yan, P., Liu, Z., Liu, S., Yao, L., Liu, Y., Wu, Y., and Gong, Z. 2020. Natural occurrence of deoxynivalenol and its acetylated derivatives in Chinese maize and wheat collected in 2017. *Toxins*, 12, 200.

Yoshinaga-Kiriake, A., Ishizaki, S., and Nagashima, Y. 2021. Tetramine contents in the salivary glands from 16 species of marine carnivorous gastropods collected along Japanese coasts. *Shokuhin Eiseigaku Zasshi*, 62, 6, 203–208.

Yu, S., Zhou, X., Hu, P., Chen, H., Shen, F., Yu, C., Meng, H., Zhang, Y., and Wu, Y. 2022. Inhalable particle-bound marine biotoxins in a coastal atmosphere: Concentration levels, influencing factors and health risk. *Journal of Hazardous Materials*, 434, 128925.

Zgouridou, A., Tripidaki, E., Giantsis, I. A., Theodorou, J. A., Kalaitzidou, M., Raitsos, D. E., Lattos, A., Mavropoulou, A. M., Sofianos, S., Karagiannis, D., and Chaligiannis, I. 2022. The current situation and potential effects of climate change on the microbial load of marine bivalves of the Greek coastlines: An integrative review. *Environmental Microbiology*, 24, 3, 1012–1034.

Zhou, S., Huang, G., and Chen, G. 2020. The antagonistic activity of H1 receptor antagonists as medicinal foods. *Trends in Food Science & Technology*, 105, 1–16.

20

Emerging Trends in Cyanotoxins: Unravelling Threats and Discovering Benefits in Food Safety

Charles Chinazaekpele Chidume, Peace Abiodun Olajide, Victoria Olufunmi Adeyemo-Eleyode, Babatunde Oluwafemi Adetuyi, Oluwatosin Adefunke Adetuyi, and Ayobami Ifeoluwa Awe

20.1 Introduction

Cyanobacteria, the earliest photosynthetic gram-negative microorganisms, play a pivotal role in global ecosystems. With an estimated global biomass of about a billion tons, they actively contribute to essential ecological processes like the carbon and nitrogen cycles (Munoz et al., 2021; Kulabhusan & Campbell, 2021).

Freshwater habitats, comprising lakes, rivers, and reservoirs, are ecologically vital, regulating the world's temperature and serving as crucial resources for human socioeconomic well-being. However, various human activities, such as improper sewage treatment, agricultural runoff, excessive fertilizer use, and eutrophication, have adversely impacted freshwater ecosystems, leading to an overabundance of algae and cyanobacteria (Kulabhusan & Campbell, 2021).

Despite the ecological significance of cyanobacteria, under specific conditions, they can undergo rapid multiplication, resulting in nuisance blooms, a phenomenon exacerbated by eutrophication and climate change (Munoz et al., 2021).

Anthropogenic eutrophication has caused cyanobacterial blooms to occur more frequently and in increasing quantities worldwide in recent decades, endangering the quality of water (Munoz et al., 2021). Cyanotoxins are dangerous secondary metabolites that are produced by these blooms. They have different chemical compositions, such as alkaloids, cyclic peptides, and non-protein amino acids, and range in toxicity. Water sources may get contaminated by cyanotoxins, which could affect food production, drinking water supply, recreational activities, and irrigation (Munoz et al., 2021; Plaas & Paerl, 2020). A condition known as "anthropogenic eutrophication"

DOI: 10.1201/9781003500605-23

occurs when the quality of the water declines for a variety of reasons, including increased nitrogen and phosphorus levels brought on by urbanization and the treatment of industrial wastewater discharged into rivers and lakes (Rocha et al., 2023).

The growing frequency of cyanotoxins in water bodies worldwide has raised concerns for human and animal health, particularly in agriculture and aquaculture. Drinking water in various regions, including the United States, Australia, Europe, and Africa, has shown elevated levels of cyanotoxins over the past two decades. These toxins, associated with gastrointestinal, respiratory, and inflammatory symptoms, pose acute health risks, and prolonged exposure has been linked to an elevated risk of various malignancies (Munoz et al., 2021; Kulabhusan & Campbell, 2021; Zhang et al., 2022).

Despite the World Health Organization's recommendations leading to regulations in certain countries, the risks associated with cyanotoxins remain significant due to their high toxicity, resistance to conventional water treatment, and chemical diversity (Ruibal-Conti et al., 2019; Munoz et al., 2021). Cyanotoxins can cause a variety of health problems when they enter the human body by the skin, inhalation, or ingestion.

Exposure to cyanobacterial blooms that produce cyanotoxins in recreational and drinking water sources can lead to several disease conditions, including headaches; dizziness; fever; hypoxia; cyanosis; paralysis; vomiting; diarrhea; weakness; serious oral inflammation and digestive problems; skin, eye, nose, and throat irritation; asthma-like symptoms; muscle tremors; nausea; tingling in the fingertips and toes; respiratory or cardiac arrest; and vomiting. Depending on the types and amounts of cyanotoxins, the exposure routes, the individual's weight, and the age of the afflicted persons, the effects of cyanotoxins may manifest minutes to days after exposure (Svirčev et al., 2019).

Cyanotoxin exposure over an extended period may be one of the factors contributing to the development of carcinogenesis (Svirčev et al., 2019).

This chapter comprehensively explores the diverse landscape of cyanotoxins, covering their types, sources, health risks, detection methods, and mitigation strategies.

20.2 Types of Cyanotoxins

Many secondary metabolites that are either harmful or non-toxic can be produced by cyanobacteria. Among the non-toxic ones include phytohormones, siderophores, and UV protection substances such as mycosporine (Rocha et al., 2023).

Regarding the dangerous ones, certain species of bloom-forming cyanobacteria create cyanotoxins, which can be fatal if ingested or come into contact with contaminated water (Rocha et al., 2023). Cyanotoxins affect the skin, neurological system, and the liver and digestive system (Hernandez et al., 2022).

Cyanotoxins can be classified into different types according to which physiological systems, organs, tissues, or cells are primarily affected. These include;

1. Hepatotoxins, including *nodularins* (NOD), *anabaenopeptin* (AB), *microcystins* (MCs), and *cylindrospermopsin* (CYN);
2. Neurotoxins comprising *β-N-methylamino-l-alanine* (BMAA), *saxitoxins* (STX), and *anatoxin-a* (ATX);
3. Irritating toxins such as *lipopolysaccharides*; and
4. Dermatotoxins.

However, cyanobacteria from many genera produce the same kind of poisons. For instance, *Microcystins* which are the subject of substantial research owing to their widespread effects, are produced by different cyanobacteria like *nostoc, microcystis, plankothrix,* and *anabaena*. Moreover, even within a single species, cyanobacteria can have both toxic and non-toxic variants (Kulabhusan & Campbell, 2021; Rocha et al., 2023).

20.2.1 Hepatotoxins

Numerous cyanotoxins that are known to impact the liver, including *cylindrospermopsin, nodularin,* and *microcystin,* have been connected to tumor promotion and possible carcinogenesis. These hepatotoxins, especially *microcystins,* are produced by cyanobacteria species such as *Aphanizomenon, Dolichospermum* (often called *Anabaena*), *Fischerella, Microcystis, Nostoc, Oscillatoria, Planktothrix, Syne-chococcus,* and *Trichodesmium* (Sini et al., 2021).

20.2.2 Microcystins

More than 279 congeners of *microcystins* are produced by several cyanobacteria species, including *Aphanizomenon, Dolichospermum (ex Anabaena), Nostoc, Limnothrix, Phormidium, Oscillatoria, and Planktothrix*. The first cyanobacterium from which MCs were isolated was *Microcystis aeruginosa*, from which their full structural characterization was obtained in 1984. With the amino acid Adda (3-amino-9-methoxy-2,6,8-trimethyl-10-phenyl-4,6-decadienoic acid) present in their structure, MCs are non-ribosomal processed cyclic heptapeptides (Abdallah et al., 2021).

MCs inhibit the protein serine/threonine phosphatases PP1 and PP2A, which is how they operate as tumor promoters and possible human carcinogens. One such MC is the extremely poisonous MC-leucine arginine (MC-LR). The cytoskeleton, lipid peroxidation, oxidative stress, apoptosis, defective

DNA repair, and cellular proliferation are among the cellular pathways that are altered as a result of this inhibition, which results in intracellular protein hyperphosphorylation (Sini et al., 2021).

While MCs pose a little threat to humans when they collect in the livers of fish and other aquatic inedible animals, they can potentially cause intoxication when they build up in the muscles of fish and other invertebrates (Abdallah et al., 2021).

20.2.3 Nodularins

Nodularins, another class of cyclic pentapeptide cyanotoxins, inhibit protein phosphatase 1 and 2A, resulting in hepatotoxic effects. Synthesized by the genera *Nodularia and Nostoc*, NODs share structural similarities with MCs but are truncated according to the gene cluster sequence. There are currently ten different forms of NODs based on the amino acid Adda. They exhibit some tumor-promoting characteristics similar to MCs (Sini et al., 2021; Catherine et al., 2016).

NODs—in particular, *Nodularin-R*—have been found in several places across the world, including North America, Australia, the Baltic Sea, and Europe. Although there isn't much solid proof that NODs bioaccumulate in crops, a few reports have shown that they are present in developing countries (Abdallah et al., 2021).

20.2.4 Cylindrospermopsin

With congeners like 7-epi-CYN and 7-deoxy-CYN, *cylindrospermopsin* is a tricyclic guanidine moiety linked with hydroxymethyl uracil. Produced by the genera *Umezakia, Aphanizomenon, Lyngbya, Oscillatoria, Phormidium, Planktothrix,* and *Raphidiopsis* (also known as *Cylindrospermopsis*), CYN is recognized for its cytotoxic, genotoxic, immunotoxic, and perhaps carcinogenic effects in the liver (Dong et al., 2023; Blahova et al., 2021).

Up to 90% of all CYN is detected as an extracellular or free toxin, in contrast to MCs, which are found in smaller amounts. Water quality management is made more difficult by the toxin's resistance to standard water treatment techniques, high solubility, and remarkable stability in aquatic environments. CYN inhibits the production of glutathione and proteins, leading to oxidative stress and DNA damage (Hercog et al., 2020; Abdallah et al., 2021).

20.2.5 Anabaenopeptins

The cyclic peptides known as *anabaenopeptins* are produced by several taxa, including *Microcystis, Planktothrix, Nodularia,* and *Anabaena*. They have over 96 congeners that have not received much research. Some ABs inhibit exopeptidases or serine proteases, but specific amino acids within ABs can block protein phosphatases PP1 and PP2A (Hernandez et al., 2022).

20.2.6 Neurotoxins

Toxins produced by cyanobacteria and microalgae function via different molecular mechanisms. A possible involvement of cyanotoxins in human neurodegenerative disorders is suggested by the *neurotoxin β-N-methylamino-Lalanine* (L-BMAA), which was found in the brain and CSF fluid of patients suffering from Alzheimer's and Lou Gehrig's diseases (Sini et al., 2021).

Cyanobacterial neurotoxins are categorized into three main classes based on how they work: *saxitoxins* (which include compounds such as carbamate, N-sulfocarbonyl, and decarbamyl); *anatoxins* (such as *anatoxin-a, homoanatoxin-a,* and *guanitoxin*); and L-BMAA and its isomers (*2,4-diaminobutyric acid, 2,4-DAB,* and *aminoethylglycine, AEG*).

20.2.7 Saxitoxin

Saxitoxin and its 57 variants constitute the class of paralytic shellfish toxins (PSTs). STX, a well-researched and highly potent natural neurotoxin, was structurally elucidated in 1971. It features a tricyclic system, 3,4-perhydropurine, including two guanidinium groups. By blocking sodium channels in the central nervous system (CNS) after passing across the blood-brain barrier, STX functions as a reversible voltage-gated sodium channel blocker and produces paralytic effects (Sini et al., 2021; Du et al., 2019).

One of the deadliest poisons, STX, has been employed in chemical warfare in the past. Globally, STXs are responsible for about 2000 instances of paralytic shellfish poisoning annually, with a 15% fatality rate (Du et al., 2019).

According to Food and Drug Administration guidelines, shellfish should have no more than 80 μg of STXs per 100 g. Synthetic trichomonads, which can accumulate in shellfish and endanger human consumption, are produced by cyanobacteria. *Anabaena, Aphanizomenon, Cuspidothrix, Cylindrospermopsis, Dolichospermum, Fischerella,* and *Gehlerinema* are among the genera that can produce STX (Du et al., 2019).

Understanding the molecular processes behind STX toxicity is crucial, particularly for populations with prolonged low-dose exposure through a seafood diet in coastal regions (Sini et al., 2021).

When voltage-gated sodium channel isoform Nav1.9 is present, exposure to STXs reduces the development of axons in cultured primary murine motoneurons and neuronal cell lines (PC12 and SH-SY5Y). Remarkably, pharmacological stimulation of NaV1.9 may provide a possible pathway for promoting axon regeneration and maintenance in neurodegenerative diseases such as spinal muscular atrophy (SMA), where deficits in synapse maintenance are central (Sini et al., 2021).

20.2.8 Anatoxin-a

Water-soluble cyanotoxins, such as *anatoxin-a* and its structural homolog *homoanatoxin-a,* are lethal neurotoxins that are produced by several cyanobacterial species, including *Dolichospermum, Aphanizomenon,* and *Anabaena* (Valadez-Cano et al., 2023; Wood et al., 2018; Sini et al., 2021).

Blooms harboring *anatoxins* are commonplace across the world. The alkaloid anatoxin-a functions as an agonist on the postsynaptic terminals of motor neurons and the central nervous system (CNS) via binding to nicotine acetylcholine receptors (nAChRs) (Rodgers et al., 2018; Bruno et al., 2016).

Isolated in the 1970s from the freshwater cyanobacteria *Anabaena flos-aquae, anatoxin-a* can become lethal when concentrations are high enough to paralyze the neurological system. These neurotoxins, however, have a short half-life and are unstable, breaking down quickly into harmless compounds, especially in environments with high pH and light (Du et al., 2019; Bruno et al., 2016).

Although *anatoxin-a* has been connected to numerous animal poisoning cases across the globe and has been shown, at least *in vitro,* to induce inflammation and death in immune and brain cells, there isn't enough proof at this time to conclude that it has negative effects on the brain. Thus, any link between *anatoxin* exposure and neurodegeneration needs to be further investigated (Sini et al., 2021).

20.2.9 L-BMAA

First isolated from *Cycascircinalis* seeds, L-BMAA is present in nearly every known category of cyanobacteria, including symbionts (e.g., *Nostoc*), free-living cyanobacteria (e.g., *Anabaena, Microcystis*), marine diatoms (e.g., *Navicula, Skeletonema*), and dinoflagellates (e.g., *Gymnodinium*), constituting one of the most diverse elements of biodiversity (Rodgers et al., 2018).

L-BMAA is made up of a methylamino side chain, an amino group, and a carboxyl group that contains carbon. N-2-aminoethylglycine (AEG), β-amino-N-methyl alanine (BAMA), and 2,4-diaminobutyric acid (2,4-DAB) (Du et al., 2019) are the three structurally significant isomers of L-BMAA.

Despite some differing opinions, a growing amount of experimental evidence points to a substantial correlation between L-BMAA and neurodegenerative disorders that progress slowly, including AD, PD, ALS, and the Guam islands' ALS/Parkinsonism dementia complex (ALS/PDC) (Sini et al., 2021).

L-BMAA is neurotoxic, and while several toxicity mechanisms have been suggested, it is still unclear how it contributes to neurotoxicity and neurodegeneration. This amino acid is non-lipophilic and non-essential; it can exist in both free and bound forms inside proteins (Buratti et al., 2017; Du et al., 2019).

20.2.10 Dermatotoxins

20.2.11 Aplysiatoxins

The marine cyanobacteria *Lyngbya majuscula* produces dermatoxic alkaloids called aplysiatoxins in tropical and subtropical climates. *3,4-dihydroxyvaleric acid and 4,6,6,10,12-pentamethyl-3,7,9,11,15-tetraoxy-15-phenylpentadecanoic acid* make up the bislactone structure of these compounds (Zhang et al., 2020). Through PKC activation, *aplysiatoxins, such as oscillatoxin A, 31-noroscillatoxin B, 3-methoxydebromo-aplysiatoxin, anhydro-aplysiatoxin, debromoaplysiatoxin, and oscillatoxin,* induce contact dermatitis. Furthermore, they can activate latent HIV-1 provirus production and serve as effective tumor promoters in mouse skin carcinogenesis, according to recent research (Du et al., 2019).

20.2.12 Lyngbyatoxins

Lyngbyatoxins are dermatoxic alkaloids that were isolated from a Hawaiian shallow-water species of *Lyngbya majuscula.* They are distinguished by a connected linalyl side group at C-7 to an indolactam ring. Marine cyanobacteria produce vesicatory and extremely inflammatory chemicals called lingbyatoxins, which include *Lyngbyatoxin A-C, 12-epi-lyngbyatoxin A, 2-oxo-3(R)-hydroxy-lyngbyatoxin A, 2-oxo-3(R)-hydroxy-13-N-desmethyllyngbyatoxin A, and 2,3-seco-2,3-dioxolyngbyatoxin A*. They are poisonous to sea turtles, irritate human skin, and are strong tumor promoters that activate protein kinase C (PKC) (Demay et al., 2019; Du et al., 2019; Nisha Nandhini et al., 2023).

20.2.13 Lipopolysaccharides

Often referred to as *lipoglycans* and *endotoxins, lipopolysaccharides* (LPS) are big molecules made up of a lipid and a polysaccharide. The outer membrane protein makes up over 75% of the surface area of cyanobacterial cell walls. The main cause of LPS's negative effects is its fatty acid component, Lipid-A, which irritates both human and animal tissues and causes allergic reactions (Kehr & Dittmann, 2015; Swartzendruber et al., 2022; Skočková et al., 2023). While it is believed that all cyanobacteria and gram-negative bacteria produce LPS, certain cyanobacteria like *Agmenellum, Anabaena, Anacystis, Microcystis, Oscillatoria, Phormidium, Schizothrix,* and *Spirulina* are known to produce this toxin (Du et al., 2019; Skočková et al., 2023). Cyanobacterial LPS has been associated with various human illnesses, including fever, allergies, headaches, gastrointestinal problems, respiratory disorders, and skin conditions. Although skin contact with cyanobacterial LPS triggering rashes lacks substantial evidence, these toxins play an indirect role in exacerbating hepatotoxic liver injury and affecting the biotransformation and toxicity of cyanotoxins (Du et al., 2019; Skočková et al., 2023) (Table 20.1).

TABLE 20.1

Types of Cyanotoxins and Associated Health Effects (Kulabhusan & Campbell, 2021; Mutoti et al., 2022)

Cyanotoxins	Classification	Transient Health Effect	Deleterious Health Impact
Microcystins	Hepatotoxins	Pneumonia, dermatitis, swelling and bleeding in the liver, and stomach discomfort	Carcinogenic, liver failure resulting in death
Anatoxins	Neurotoxins	Pulmonary disease, burning sensations, and discomfort	Cardiac arrest
Cylindrospermopsins	Hepatotoxins	Pneumonia, dermatitis, diarrhea, inflammation and bleeding of the liver	Anorexia, chronic liver disease resulting in death, and malaise
Nodularins	Hepatotoxins	Similar effects as microcystins	Similar effects as microcystins
Saxitoxin	Neurotoxins	Discomfort, numbness, sleepiness, confused speech, and respiratory paralysis that can be fatal	Paralysis of the muscles; breathing difficulties; and numbness in the mouth, throat, and extremities
β-N-methylamino-lalanine	Neurotoxins	Language difficulties, disorientation (easily getting lost), emotional fluctuations, motivational decline, and behavioral problems	Cancer and neurological disease
Lyngbyatoxins	Dermatotoxin	Inflammation of the skin	Kidney injury and severe dermatitis
Lipopolysaccharides	Lipopolysaccharides	Skin irritation and abdominal ache	Hypertension, disseminated intravascular coagulation, heart disease, fever, leucopenia, and organ failure

20.3 Global Impact of Cyanotoxins on Aquatic Food Products

Bioaccumulation of cyanotoxins poses a severe threat to various aquatic products, including seafood, aquatic goods, food animals, and crops, leading to the consumption of high toxin concentrations even when initially present in minimal amounts (J. Lee et al., 2017). The production of cyanotoxins by cyanobacterial blooms seriously jeopardizes the well-being of both terrestrial and aquatic ecosystems.

The accumulation of cyanotoxins in both aquatic and terrestrial settings lessens the grazing pressure that zooplankton and other predators exert on cyanobacteria. By accumulating in plants, seeping into groundwater, and adhering to soil, the poisons spread and put human and animal health at risk through ingestion, inhalation, and skin contact (J. Lee et al., 2017).

Hardy et al. discovered that fish from lakes experiencing toxic blooms had saxitoxins and microcystins in their liver, gut, and muscle tissue. They also found that fish samples had levels of up to 0.83 µg/g of *saxitoxins*, 71.6 µg/g of *microcystins*, and 0.768 µg/g of *anatoxin-a*, which suggests a high risk of cyanotoxin exposure (Hardy et al., 2015). Bioaccumulation varies among organs, with the liver and intestines having the highest levels and the muscles having the lowest levels (J. Lee et al., 2017).

The aquatic food chain allows cyanotoxins to enter the human body through bioaccumulation, as shown by Preece et al. At the top of this food chain, fish are highly exposed to cyanotoxins because they breathe and eat, which causes them to accumulate in organs such as the gills, muscles, liver, stomachs, and kidneys (Preece et al., 2017).

Numerous studies globally, including in China, Brazil, Africa, Asia, and Latin America, have identified cyanotoxins in various seafood, highlighting the negative effects on human health (Svirčev et al., 2019; Abdallah et al., 2021). Microcystin (MC) concentrations in the muscles of Nile tilapia studied in Egypt were found to be several times higher than the preliminary Tolerable Daily Intake (TDI) (Abdallah et al., 2021).

O. niloticus in Uganda showed high MC contamination in muscle tissues, with variations in *Microcystin* types in different geographical locations (Simiyu et al., 2018). Three species of table-sized fish from Ethiopia (African sharp-tooth catfish, common carp, and Nile tilapia) were analyzed to determine whether they contained *cylindrospermopsin and microcystins*. The results indicated that while all edible parts, specifically the muscles, were free from contamination, traces of contamination were observed in the liver samples. Notably, three variants of *microcystins* were identified in the contaminated liver samples (Zewde et al., 2018).

In various studies, the seasonal variations and distribution patterns of microcystins, namely MC-LR, MC-YR, and MC-RR, were investigated about commonly consumed Chinese aquatic species, such as mussels (*Corbicula fluminea*), bighead carp (*Aristichthys nobilis*), silver carp (*Hypophthalmichthys molitrix*), and shrimp (*Palaemon modestus* and *Macrobrachium nipponensis*). Samples were taken from Chaohu Lake and Taihu Lake. The study reported significant seasonal differences from the period of June to December correlating *microcystin* concentrations with cyanobacterial blooms. The detected *microcystin* level in edible parts of the various aquatic species was found to be above the permissive level of MC-LR, thus its negative effect during consumption.

Also, the study found that the various aquatic species, Silver carp muscles, bighead carp muscles, shrimp muscles, and mussel feet exceeded the permitted WHO tolerable daily intake level by 16%, 25%, 31%, and 54% respectively (Abdallah et al., 2021).

A study conducted in Edirdir, Turkey, revealed the concentration of *microcystins* in edible fish which varied from 0.36 to 17.54 µg/kg dry weights with higher concentration in the liver and muscles as assessed by ELISA. Higher MC levels were also observed using LC-PDA on re-analysis (Abdallah et al., 2021; Gurbuz et al., 2016). Subsequently, utilizing LC-MS/MS, *Cylindrospermopsin* was found in Lake Iznik, Turkey (Akcaalan et al., 2014).

Investigation of seafood, particularly carp and catfish, revealed variable concentrations of MCs in muscles, with higher MC levels in catfish than carp particularly for some MC variants such as MC-RR detected by LC-MS/MS, emphasizing species specificity (Singh et al., 2014).

Experimental studies in Thailand detected higher levels of MC-LR in prawns compared to Nile tilapia, surpassing provisional tolerable daily intake (TDI) (Abdallah et al., 2021). Another study in Vietnam analyzed apple snails (*Pomacea canaliculata*) for eight MC variants and NODs using LC-MS/MS. The muscular part of apple snails showed the presence of the MC-dmLR variant in three samples. The study suggested that because the viscera of these snails had ten times greater quantities of MC-dmLR, the viscera should be completely removed before food is processed (Pham et al., 2017; Trung et al., 2018).

A link between renal function impairment and exposure to microcystin-LR (MC-LR) was found in an observational study involving 5493 individuals in the southwest region of China, indicating possible health hazards (Abdallah et al., 2021).

Analysis of one of the most prevalent fish species in Brazil, *Geophagus brasiliensis*, showed *microcystin* concentrations below advised thresholds for human consumption. The depuration of MCs in *G. brasiliensis* following exposure for 7, 15, 30, and 90 days was examined in the same study, which discovered that MCs were still identifiable in muscles three months later (de Morais Calado et al., 2018). In Brasilia-FD, Brazil, consumers of silver carp are open to consumption of extreme amounts of mercury, especially during the dry winter season when levels might exceed the suggested provisional tolerable daily intake by 240 times (Oliveira et al., 2013). A study observed that redbreast tilapia (*Tilapia rendalli*), found in Rio de Janeiro, bioaccumulates microcarcinogens in their muscles at a rate 42 times higher than that advised. It is noteworthy that, when exposed to the same concentration of metals during a hazardous bloom, this species' bioaccumulation seems to be lower than that of Nile tilapia (Abdallah et al., 2021).

High MC levels in liver samples of Nile tilapia were observed to cause high mortalities in a study in North East Brazil. The World Health Organization's (WHO) preliminary tolerable daily intake was surpassed by fish muscle and crustacean samples. These results emphasize the possible dangers of MC exposure in aquatic species, emphasizing the need for monitoring to guarantee food safety and differences in bioaccumulation patterns (Díez-Quijada et al., 2019; de Mello et al., 2020; WHO, 2003).

In Latin American countries such as Mexico and Brazil, among others, *cylindrospermopsin* and *saxitoxins* are prominent cyanotoxins present in various seafoods including edible fish species (Abdallah et al., 2021). A study investigated the level of *nodularin* accumulation in crustaceans such as *Palaemonetes argentines* samples from the San Roque Reservoir in Argentina. The toxin was identified by LC-MS/MS up to three weeks after exposure, suggesting its toxicity due to the presence of NOD (Galanti et al., 2013).

There are several ways that cyanotoxins might get into aquatic goods, such as through tainted feeds, direct contact with contaminated water, and biological concentration in the food chain (Mutoti et al., 2022).

Every year, the global fin market exchanges between 26 and 73 million sharks. A study conducted by Neil Hammerschlag and Deborah Mash of the University of Miami Medical School investigated if shark tissues contained the neurotoxic amino acid *β-methylamino-L-alanine* (BMAA), which is generated by cyanobacteria. This study revealed BMAA levels in shark fins which were similar to the range found in the brains of humans who died from neurodegenerative diseases (Mutoti et al., 2022).

For people who eat aquatic cuisine, the buildup of cyanotoxins is a worry. *Microcystins* have been found in red swamp crayfish (*Procamburus clarkii*), *Palemon modestus*, and *Macrobrachium nipponensis*, three species of freshwater shrimp. Furthermore, it was discovered that *saxitoxins* were present in sea pearl oysters (*Pinctada maxima*), and *cyanospermopsin* was present in bivalve hemolymphs, viscera, gonads, and feet. *Bellamya aeruginosa*, a freshwater snail, showed evidence of MC in its gonad, foot, gill, and hepatopancreas. It is noteworthy that most toxins concentrate in inedible parts, highlighting the significance of removing the gonads, digestive tract, and hepatopancreas before eating to reduce the likelihood of intoxication (Mutoti et al., 2022).

20.3.1 Negative Effects of Cyanotoxins in Food Products

Even in cases when initial ambient toxin concentrations are low, the accumulation of cyanotoxins in a variety of food sources, such as plants and livestock, can lead to the consumption of large amounts of these toxins (Mutoti et al., 2022).

There are several ways that food can expose people orally to cyanobacteria and cyanotoxins: contaminated water, vegetables and crops that are planted with water that contains cyanobacteria and cyanotoxins, dairy goods and meat from animals that consume water or eat feed, and dietary supplements that contain cyanobacteria (Codd et al., 2020).

Toxins from cyanotoxin-contaminated water are absorbed by plants, affecting growth and crop yields without causing immediate lethality. When water overflows into the soil, poisons may be retained and cause bioaccumulation in non-blooming periods (J. Lee et al., 2017).

Research shows that leafy crops that are cultivated with water polluted with toxins, can accumulate up to 27% of *microcystin*. Lettuce, extensively studied due to its high consumption, displayed bioaccumulation of microcystins, reaching levels as high as 248 µg/g (Mutoti et al., 2022).

Cultivated tomatoes and peppers in Guatemala, demonstrated the potential to bioaccumulate MC-RR in fruits and seeds when planted with water from Lake Amatitlán (Mutoti et al., 2022).

Exposure frequency and duration determine how much of a poison accumulates. Prolonged exposure or repeated irrigation with contaminated water can lead to the bioaccumulation of cyanotoxins in plants.

Over 15 days, an experiment found that when lettuce was irrigated with water polluted with MC-LR and MC-RR at varying concentrations, the cyanotoxins began to accumulate in the plant. Notably, MC-LR had a greater absorption factor than MC-RR, and this difference grew as MC exposure increased. The investigation also looked at CYN's bioaccumulation and depuration in arugula and lettuce (Mutoti et al., 2022). Beans and other vegetables show similar observations of cyanotoxin accumulation. Due to the larger exposure dose in grains and the fact that they are stapled foods in many countries, cytotoxin accumulation in grains including maize, rice, soybean, and wheat is especially alarming (J. Lee et al., 2017).

Previous research on flour made from *Cycas micronesica* seeds revealed that it contains an environmental neurotoxin. It has been discovered that cyanad seeds, especially those from *Guam cycas micronesica,* contain BMAA, a neurotoxic amino acid generated in coralloid roots by the endosymbiotic cyanobacterium *Nostoc*. According to reports, *Pteropus mariannus* has 10,000 times greater amounts of the BMAA, indicating that it bioaccumulates extensively. It has been reported that BMAA consumption is associated with neurodegenerative disorders such as amyotrophic lateral sclerosis (ALS) and that BMAA has been found in the brains of *Chamorros.* It is thought that dietary ingestion of BMAA leads to its misincorporation into brain proteins, which in turn causes gradual neurodegeneration (Mutoti et al., 2022).

Microcystins have been shown, in a study by S. Lee et al. (2017), to accumulate in agricultural plants that are watered with contaminated water. Carrots and lettuce had the next-highest MC-LR accumulation rates, after green beans. Plants' absorption of water is greatly influenced by aspects associated with their roots.

Since agricultural soil can serve as a possible reservoir for cyanotoxins, it is imperative to address the accumulation and persistence of these toxins in this environment. According to a study, there may be a human exposure pathway through the accumulated MC in fresh produce. This highlights the significance of identifying this pathway as a public health risk in locations where irrigation waters are contaminated with cyanobacteria (S. Lee et al., 2017).

20.3.2 Negative Effect of Cyanotoxins in Drinking Water

Human health is seriously threatened by the formation of hepatotoxins, neurotoxins, dermatotoxins, and cytotoxins by many cyanobacterial bloom genera, such as *Anabaena, Cylindrospermopsis, Microcystis, Nodularia,* and *Plaktothrix*. These toxins have the potential to contaminate not only recreational water but also drinking water and seafood supplies. Consequently, the formation of harmful cyanobacterial blooms has become a pressing global public health concern, necessitating attention and mitigation efforts on a worldwide scale (J. Lee et al., 2017).

Both raw and inadequately treated drinking water may include cyanobacteria and cyanotoxins if the raw water source has a cyanobacterial population (Codd et al., 2020).

Drinking cyanotoxin-contaminated water is a common pathway for cyanotoxin ingestion. Contamination is likely to occur during the breakdown of cyanotoxins, especially when collecting water from surface sources during cyanobacterial blooms. Numerous cases worldwide, spanning all continents, have reported the presence of cyanobacterial toxins in both treated and untreated water.

When comparing areas that use treated water from sources that do not support blooms to those that use groundwater, there has been a notable rise in the incidence of human primary liver cancer in those that use drinking water from reservoirs with yearly cyanobacterial blooms that contain MCs. The hepatitis B and hepatitis C viruses did not appear to be correlated with any other risk factors, such as liver cirrhosis (Codd et al., 2020).

There are increased dangers to human health when drinking water with high levels of cyanotoxins or when consuming even modest doses of these toxins frequently. This underscores the critical importance of addressing and monitoring water quality to mitigate these health concerns on a global scale (Mutoti et al., 2022).

Consumption of toxic cyanobacteria that have not been sufficiently cleaned from raw waters or high quantities of dissolved cyanotoxins as a result of a cyanobacterial bloom being lysed by natural or artificial processes can both have acute or short-term negative consequences (Codd et al., 2020).

Using the globally accepted risk assessment procedure, the WHO has examined the potential health effects of cyanotoxins in drinking water on humans. Based on this, the WHO determined a preliminary guideline value (GV) of 1μg/l for the overall MC-LR concentration in drinking water (Codd et al., 2020).

The World Health Organization has also looked into the potential health effects on humans that may arise from bathing activities that expose people to cyanobacterial cells and cyanotoxins. The WHO has also issued preliminary recommendations for reducing the risk of skin irritation and more serious effects (WHO, 2003; Plaas & Paerl, 2020). However, there are several shortcomings with the current WHO guidelines for bathing waters.

20.3.3 Benefits of Cyanotoxins in Food Safety and Human Health

Blue-green algae, sometimes referred to as cyanobacteria, offer a practical way to deal with issues including water pollution, soil toxicity, and global warming. Through phytoremediation, these bacteria have proven their capacity to successfully lower the concentration of hazardous chemicals in industrial wastewater, minimizing possible harm before release into natural water bodies. Because of their unique capacity to fix atmospheric nitrogen, cyanobacteria are useful as biofertilizers in agriculture. Cyanobacteria fertilizers replace chemical nitrogen-based fertilizers, lowering agricultural production costs while simultaneously lowering environmental dangers. They are used in a variety of industries, such as biofuel production, biocontrol agents, fodder, and biofortification, demonstrating their adaptable potential for sustainable solutions across a range of industries (Malyan et al., 2020; Falfushynska et al., 2023). Their established role as diazotrophs, proficiency in diverse soil ecologies, and competitive ability with native flora make them beneficial. They are often used as inoculants to enhance soil fertility, improve soil structure, and boost crop yields, especially in rice cultivation (Falfushynska et al., 2023; Zhang et al., 2022).

Exciting possibilities arise from identifying and developing cyanobacterial toxins for controlling agricultural insect pests. For instance, the application of a soil-based inoculum containing *Anabaena cylindrica, Anabaena oryzae, Nostoc muscorum,* and *Tolypothrix tenuis,* combined with 72 kg Nha-1, significantly reduced natural infestations of indica rice by the stem borer *Chilo agamemnon* and leaf miner *Hydrellia prosternalis.* Additionally, the biomass extract of the cyanobacterium *Nostoc* demonstrated a substantial reduction in the weight of cotton bollworm larvae, *Heliocoverpa armigera,* a polyphagous insect pest (Falfushynska et al., 2023).

Screening programs at the Indian Agricultural Research Institute identified cyanobacterial strains producing bionematocidal compounds. Culture filtrates of *Synechococcus nidulans* exhibited nematocidal activity against plant-parasitic nematodes such as *Meloidogyne incognita, M. graminicola, Heterodera cajani, H. avenae,* and *Rotylenchulus reniformis,* prevalent pests in northern India (Falfushynska et al., 2023).

Moreover, the biomass extract of the filamentous cyanobacterium *Nostoc* demonstrated inhibitory effects on fungi like *Armillaria* sp., *Penicillium expansum, Rosellinia* sp., and *Sclerotinia sclerotiorum.* This inhibition was observed at a concentration of 0.25 g of dry biomass per liter of inoculated medium, showcasing the potential of cyanobacteria in managing fungal plant pathogens, contributing to agricultural sustainability (Falfushynska et al., 2023).

Also, cyanobacteria and microalgae are globally utilized as food supplements due to their health benefits, providing essential vitamins and exhibiting properties like anti-tumor and antibacterial effects. Human intake of cyanobacteria is often voluntary, driven by their rich protein content, particularly in species like *Spirulina, Nostoc,* and *Aphanizomenon flos-aquae.*

Blue-green algae supplements (BGAS) derived from cyanobacteria, offering detoxification, mood elevation, energy boost, weight loss, and increased alertness, are popular in many industrialized countries. These supplements, available in various forms such as pills, capsules, and powders, are easily accessible without the need for consultation or a doctor's prescription, contributing to the perception of their safety for consumption at high dosages over extended periods (Mutoti et al., 2022).

These algae offer various dietary advantages, containing protein, vitamin C, vitamin E, and essential minerals. Consumed for purposes such as weight loss, immune system enhancement, and cholesterol control, blue-green algae have demonstrated positive effects on allergies, depression, and various medical conditions. While studies support the nutritional value of these algae, there is a lack of research validating claims related to blue-green algae supplements (Mutoti et al., 2022).

20.4 Various Detection Mechanisms for Cyanotoxins in Food and Food Products

Numerous techniques for cyanobacteria identification and quantification have been developed to protect the quality of food and water while also guaranteeing human health. The detection and quantification of cyanotoxins are facilitated by the use of widely used techniques such as liquid chromatography-mass spectrometry (LC-MS) and enzyme-linked immunosorbent assay (ELISA). These techniques are essential for preserving the precision and dependability of cyanobacterial presence assessments, which supports efficient protocols for ensuring the security of water and food supplies (Miglione et al., 2021).

The United States Environmental Protection Agency (USEPA) has formally adopted ELISA, which is included in "Method 546", and (LC-MS), which is described in "Method 544", as accepted techniques because of their effectiveness. These techniques offer recommended procedures for finding *nodularins* and total *microcystins* in water samples, underscoring their significance in ensuring accurate and standardized assessments of cyanotoxins in water and contributing to overall efforts to maintain water quality and safeguard public health (Miglione et al., 2021).

ELISA is a common technique for analyzing cyanotoxins, providing semi-quantitative estimations of toxin quantities. It is quick and affordable and doesn't require highly specialized workers. However, it may lack precision in quantifying distinct variations of toxins, prompting the need for physicochemical approaches for more precise results (Du et al., 2019).

The mouse bioassay, once the "gold standard" for *saxitoxin* assessment, has been improved and standardized for rapid and precise readings. However, immunoassays that rely on antibody interactions are now frequently employed for STX detection due to their effectiveness. Hydrophilic interaction liquid chromatography (HILIC) and LC-MS are adopted for selective reaction monitoring, enhancing the analysis of STXs (Du et al., 2019). When heightened sensitivity and differentiation of congeners within a toxin group are needed, liquid chromatography-mass spectrometry is preferred. In contrast, ELISA is commonly used for total toxin quantification, being more cost effective and time efficient. The choice between the two methods depends on specific analysis requirements and available resources (Miglione et al., 2021).

As an alternative to conventional assays, biosensors provide a quick, easy, and effective way to identify a variety of contaminants, including natural poisons. This shift towards biosensors reflects a move towards more accessible and streamlined methods in the realm of toxin detection, overcoming limitations associated with established methods (Miglione et al., 2021).

In environmental monitoring, biosensors have mostly replaced traditional poison detection techniques. Biosensors and analytical tools for analyte detection can produce specific quantitative or semi-quantitative analytical results. With the use of a transducer and a bioreceptor, biosensors can transform physiological chemical data into a visual signal that a detector can pick up on (Cunha et al., 2018).

Utilization of decentralized electrochemical biosensors presents a significant opportunity for on-field applications in the detection of natural toxins like cyanotoxins. Comprehensive evaluations published recently indicate that during the past ten years, there has been an increasing interest in the development of electrochemical biosensors for the detection of algal toxins (Miglione et al., 2021; Elshafey et al., 2015).

Numerous biosensor techniques, such as colorimetric, electrochemical, fluorescence, and plasmonic methods, have been used to detect cyanotoxins. Due to their special qualities, including compactness, compatibility with portable readers (such as the smartphone-powered potentiostat by PalmSens), and resistance to interference from colored or opaque matrices, electrochemical biosensors have emerged as being especially well suited for decentralized monitoring. Electrochemical platforms for handheld monitoring have seen a considerable improvement in sensitivity and specificity due to the combination of nanomaterials and synthetic recognition probes like as aptamers (Miglione et al., 2021).

Eissa et al. (2014), for example, created a voltammetric aptasensor that can identify MC-LR in fish samples and tap water, with a detection limit of 1.9 pM and excellent specificity. Lebogang used monoclonal antibodies attached to sepharose beads in a micro-immunocolumn to automate the detection of MC-LR in freshwater samples using an amperometric flow ELISA technique called VersAFlo (Lebogang et al., 2017). Utilizing *anatoxin-a* inhibitory effect on cholinesterase enzyme activity, inhibition-based enzymatic biosensors represent an additional strategy for *anatoxin-a* detection. Elshafey used aptasensors, which are specialized receptors based on aptamers, to detect *cylindrospermopsin* in freshwater samples using an unlabeled, highly sensitive aptasensor (Elshafey et al., 2015).

Biosensors are currently not developed enough to completely replace LC-MS and other conventional, laboratory-based methods. But for preliminary screenings, they can be an invaluable supplementary toolkit. The possibility for on-site natural toxin detection, including cyanotoxins, using electrochemical biosensors, highlights their importance in enhancing monitoring strategies, even though they may not entirely replace established laboratory methods (Miglione et al., 2021). Despite this heightened interest, it is crucial to acknowledge that research on these targets, particularly from a biosensor perspective, remains a niche area.

20.5 Conclusion

Numerous cyanobacterial toxins result from the diversity of cyanobacteria. This chapter offers a comprehensive investigation of the risks and possibilities associated with cyanotoxins in food safety. Further effort is necessary to narrow the knowledge gap in this subject, even though the scientific community has achieved tremendous progress in several areas relating to the synthesis, analysis, bioaccumulation, biodegradation, and toxic consequences of cyanobacterial toxins. This might entail developing and approving new analytical methods for the simultaneous assessment of multiple cyanotoxin categories and the variations in those categories in different food matrices from developing countries. Furthermore, more investigation is needed to look into the existence of cyanotoxins in different food plants and shellfish, especially in countries with limited data.

References

Abdallah, M. F., Van Hassel, W. H., Andjelkovic, M., Wilmotte, A., & Rajkovic, A. (2021). Cyanotoxins and food contamination in developing countries: Review of their types, toxicity, analysis, occurrence and mitigation strategies. *Toxins, 13*[11], 786.

Akcaalan, R., Köker, L., Oğuz, A., Spoof, L., Meriluoto, J., & Albay, M. (2014). First report of cylindrospermopsin production by two cyanobacteria (Dolichospermum mendotae and Chrysosporum ovalisporum) in Lake Iznik, Turkey. *Toxins, 6*[11], 3173–3186.

Blahova, L., Sehnal, L., Lepsova-Skacelova, O., Szmucova, V., Babica, P., Hilscherova, K., . . . Blaha, L. (2021). Occurrence of cylindrospermopsin, anatoxin-a and their homologs in the Southern Czech Republic-taxonomical, analytical, and molecular approaches. *Harmful Algae, 108*, 102101.

Bruno, M., Ploux, O., Metcalf, J. S., Mejean, A., Pawlik-Skowronska, B., & Furey, A. (2016). Anatoxin-A, homoanatoxin-A, and natural analogues. *Handbook of Cyanobacterial Monitoring and Cyanotoxin Analysis*, 138–147.

Buratti, F. M., Manganelli, M., Vichi, S., Stefanelli, M., Scardala, S., Testai, E., & Funari, E. (2017). Cyanotoxins: Producing organisms, occurrence, toxicity, mechanism of action and human health toxicological risk evaluation. *Archives of Toxicology, 91*, 1049–1130.

Catherine, A., Bernard, C., Spoof, L., & Bruno, M. (2016). Microcystins and nodularins. *Handbook of Cyanobacterial Monitoring and Cyanotoxin Analysis*, 107–126.

Codd, G. A., Testai, E., Funari, E., & Svirčev, Z. (2020). Cyanobacteria, cyanotoxins, and human health. *Water Treatment for Purification from Cyanobacteria and Cyanotoxins*, 37–68.

Cunha, I., Biltes, R., Sales, M. G. F., & Vasconcelos, V. (2018). Aptamer-based biosensors to detect aquatic phycotoxins and cyanotoxins. *Sensors, 18*[7], 2367.

Demay, J., Bernard, C., Reinhardt, A., & Marie, B. (2019). Natural products from cyanobacteria: Focus on beneficial activities. *Marine Drugs, 17*[6], 320.

de Mello, K., Taniwaki, R. H., de Paula, F. R., Valente, R. A., Randhir, T. O., Macedo, D. R., . . . Hughes, R. M. (2020). Multiscale land use impacts on water quality: Assessment, planning, and future perspectives in Brazil. *Journal of Environmental Management, 270*, 110879.

de Morais Calado, S. L., Santos, G. S., Leite, T. P. B., Wojciechowski, J., Junior, M. N., Bozza, D. C., . . . de Assis, H. C. S. (2018). Depuration time and sublethal effects of microcystins in a freshwater fish from water supply reservoir. *Chemosphere, 210*, 805–815.

Díez-Quijada, L., Prieto, A. I., Guzmán-Guillén, R., Jos, A., & Cameán, A. M. (2019). Occurrence and toxicity of microcystin congeners other than MC-LR and MC-RR: A review. *Food and Chemical Toxicology, 125*, 106–132.

Dong, H., Aziz, M. T., & Richardson, S. D. (2023). Transformation of algal toxins during the oxidation/disinfection processes of drinking water: From structure to toxicity. *Environmental Science & Technology, 57*[35], 12944–12957.

Du, X., Liu, H., Yuan, L., Wang, Y., Ma, Y., Wang, R., . . . Zhang, H. (2019). The diversity of cyanobacterial toxins on structural characterization, distribution and identification: A systematic review. *Toxins, 11*[9], 530.

Eissa, S., Ng, A., Siaj, M., & Zourob, M. (2014). Label-free voltammetric aptasensor for the sensitive detection of microcystin-LR using graphene-modified electrodes. *Analytical Chemistry, 86*[15], 7551–7557.

Elshafey, R., Siaj, M., & Zourob, M. (2015). DNA aptamers selection and characterization for development of label-free impedimetric aptasensor for neurotoxin anatoxin-A. *Biosensors and Bioelectronics, 68*, 295–302.

Falfushynska, H., Kasianchuk, N., Siemens, E., Henao, E., & Rzymski, P. (2023). A review of common cyanotoxins and their effects on fish. *Toxics, 11*[2], 118.

Galanti, L. N., Amé, M. V., & Wunderlin, D. A. (2013). Accumulation and detoxification dynamic of cyanotoxins in the freshwater shrimp Palaemonetes argentinus. *Harmful Algae, 27*, 88–97.

Gurbuz, F., Uzunmehmetoğlu, O. Y., Diler, Ö., Metcalf, J. S., & Codd, G. A. (2016). Occurrence of microcystins in water, bloom, sediment and fish from a public water supply. *Science of the Total Environment, 562*, 860–868.

Hardy, F. J., Johnson, A., Hamel, K., & Preece, E. (2015). Cyanotoxin bioaccumulation in freshwater fish, Washington State, USA. *Environmental Monitoring and Assessment, 187*[11], 1–15.

Hercog, K., Štern, A., Maisanaba, S., Filipič, M., & Žegura, B. (2020). Plastics in cyanobacterial blooms—genotoxic effects of binary mixtures of cylindrospermopsin and bisphenols in HepG2 cells. *Toxins, 12*(4), 219.

Hernandez, B. Y., Biggs, J., Zhu, X., Sotto, P., Nagata, M., Mendez, A. J. P., & Paulino, Y. (2022). Environmental exposure to cyanobacteria hepatotoxins in a Pacific Island community: A cross-sectional assessment. *Microorganisms, 10*[8], 1607.

Kehr, J. C., & Dittmann, E. (2015). Biosynthesis and function of extracellular glycans in cyanobacteria. *Life, 5*[1], 164–180.

Kulabhusan, P. K., & Campbell, K. (2021). Recent trends in the detection of freshwater cyanotoxins with a critical note on their occurrence in Asia. *Trends in Environmental Analytical Chemistry, 32*, e00150.

Lebogang, L., Jantra, J., Hedström, M., & Mattiasson, B. (2017). Electrochemical flow-ELISA for rapid and sensitive determination of microcystin-LR using automated sequential injection system. *Sensors, 17*[7], 1639.

Lee, J., Lee, S., & Jiang, X. (2017). Cyanobacterial toxins in freshwater and food: Important sources of exposure to humans. *Annual Review of Food Science and Technology, 8*, 281–304.

Lee, S., Jiang, X., Manubolu, M., Riedl, K., Ludsin, S. A., Martin, J. F., & Lee, J. (2017). Fresh produce and their soils accumulate cyanotoxins from irrigation water: Implications for public health and food security. *Food Research International, 102*, 234–245.

Malyan, S. K., Singh, S., Bachheti, A., Chahar, M., Sah, M. K., Kumar, A., . . . Kumar, S. S. (2020). Cyanobacteria: A perspective paradigm for agriculture and environment. In *New and future developments in microbial biotechnology and bioengineering* (pp. 215–224). Elsevier.

Miglione, A., Napoletano, M., & Cinti, S. (2021). Electrochemical biosensors for tracing cyanotoxins in food and environmental matrices. *Biosensors, 11*[9], 315.

Munoz, M., Cirés, S., de Pedro, Z. M., Colina, J. Á., Velásquez-Figueroa, Y., Carmona-Jiménez, J., . . . Casas, J. A. (2021). Overview of toxic cyanobacteria and cyanotoxins in Ibero-American freshwaters: Challenges for risk management and opportunities for removal by advanced technologies. *Science of the Total Environment, 761*, 143197.

Mutoti, M., Gumbo, J., & Jideani, A. I. O. (2022). Occurrence of cyanobacteria in water used for food production: A review. *Physics and Chemistry of the Earth, Parts A/B/C, 125*, 103101.

Nisha Nandhini, S., Divya, K. G., & Stalin, N. (2023). Isolation of toxin producing cyanobacteria from aquatic samples with lyngbya. In *Protocols for cyanobacteria sampling and detection of cyanotoxin* (pp. 113–117). Springer Nature.

Oliveira, N. B., Schwartz, C. A., Bloch, C., Paulino, L., & Pires, O. R. (2013). Bioacumulation of cyanotoxins in Hypophthalmichthys molitrix (silver carp) in Paranoá Lake, Brasilia-DF, Brazil. *Bulletin of Environmental Contamination and Toxicology, 90*, 308–313.

Pham, T. L., Shimizu, K., Dao, T. S., & Motoo, U. (2017). First report on free and covalently bound microcystins in fish and bivalves from Vietnam: Assessment of risks to humans. *Environmental Toxicology and Chemistry, 36*[11], 2953–2957.

Plaas, H. E., & Paerl, H. W. (2020). Toxic cyanobacteria: A growing threat to water and air quality. *Environmental Science & Technology, 55*[1], 44–64.

Preece, E. P., Hardy, F. J., Moore, B. C., & Bryan, M. (2017). A review of microcystin detections in Estuarine and Marine waters: Environmental implications and human health risk. *Harmful Algae, 61*, 31–45.

Rocha, M. F., Magalhães-Ghiotto, G. A. V., Bergamasco, R., & Gomes, R. G. (2023). Cyanobacteria and cyanotoxins in the environment and water intakes: Reports, diversity of congeners, detection by mass spectrometry and their impact on health. *Toxicon*, 107589.

Rodgers, K. J., Main, B. J., & Samardzic, K. (2018). Cyanobacterial neurotoxins: Their occurrence and mechanisms of toxicity. *Neurotoxicity Research*, *33*, 168–177.

Ruibal-Conti, A. L., Ruiz, M. A., Rodriguez, M. I., Lerda, D., & Romero, M. D. (2019). Assessment of specific antibodies as biological indicators of human chronic exposure to microcystins. *Ecotoxicology and Environmental Safety*, *175*, 236–242.

Simiyu, B. M., Oduor, S. O., Rohrlack, T., Sitoki, L., & Kurmayer, R. (2018). Microcystin content in phytoplankton and in small fish from eutrophic Nyanza Gulf, Lake Victoria, Kenya. *Toxins*, *10*[7], 275.

Singh, S., & Asthana, R. K. (2014). Assessment of microcystin concentration in carp and catfish: A case study from Lakshmikund Pond, Varanasi, India. *Bulletin of Environmental Contamination and Toxicology*, *92*, 687–692.

Sini, P., Dang, T. B. C., Fais, M., Galioto, M., Padedda, B. M., Lugliè, A., . . . Crosio, C. (2021). Cyanobacteria, cyanotoxins, and neurodegenerative diseases: Dangerous liaisons. *International Journal of Molecular Sciences*, *22*[16], 8726.

Skočková, V., Vašíček, O., Sychrová, E., Sovadinová, I., Babica, P., & Šindlerová, L. (2023). Cyanobacterial harmful bloom lipopolysaccharides induce pro-inflammatory effects in immune and intestinal epithelial cells in vitro. *Toxins*, *15*[3], 169.

Svirčev, Z., Lalić, D., Bojadžija Savić, G., Tokodi, N., Drobac Backović, D., Chen, L., . . . Codd, G. A. (2019). Global geographical and historical overview of cyanotoxin distribution and cyanobacterial poisonings. *Archives of Toxicology*, *93*, 2429–2481.

Swartzendruber, J. A., Del Toro, R. M., Incrocci, R., Seangmany, N., Gurr, J. R., Mayer, A. M., . . . Swanson-Mungerson, M. (2022). Lipopolysaccharide from the cyanobacterium Geitlerinema sp. induces neutrophil infiltration and lung inflammation. *Toxins*, *14*[4], 267.

Trung, B., Dao, T. S., Faassen, E., & Lürling, M. (2018). Cyanobacterial blooms and microcystins in Southern Vietnam. *Toxins*, *10*[11], 471.

Valadez-Cano, C., Reyes-Prieto, A., Beach, D. G., Rafuse, C., McCarron, P., & Lawrence, J. (2023). Genomic characterization of coexisting anatoxin-producing and non-toxigenic Microcoleus subspecies in benthic mats from the Wolastoq, New Brunswick, Canada. *Harmful Algae*, *124*, 102405.

Wood, S. A., Biessy, L., & Puddick, J. (2018). Anatoxins are consistently released into the water of streams with microcoleus autumnalis-dominated (cyanobacteria) proliferations. *Harmful Algae*, *80*, 88–95.

World Health Organization. (2003). *Guidelines for safe recreational water environments: Coastal and fresh waters* (Vol. 1). World Health Organization.

Zewde, T. W., Johansen, J. A., Kifle, D., Demissie, T. B., Hansen, J. H., & Tadesse, Z. (2018). Concentrations of microcystins in the muscle and liver tissues of fish species from Koka reservoir, Ethiopia: A potential threat to public health. *Toxicon*, *153*, 85–95.

Zhang, H. H., Zhang, X. K., Si, R. R., Shen, S. C., Liang, T. T., Fan, T. T., . . . Han, B. N. (2020). Chemical and biological study of novel aplysiatoxin derivatives from the marine cyanobacterium Lyngbya sp. *Toxins*, *12*(11), 733.

Zhang, W., Liu, J., Xiao, Y., Zhang, Y., Yu, Y., Zheng, Z., . . . Li, Q. (2022). The impact of cyanobacteria blooms on the aquatic environment and human health. *Toxins*, *14*[10], 658.

21

Mycotoxins in Feed and Feeding: Promising Detoxification Strategies and Mechanism of Action

Moyosore Joseph Adegbeye, Babatunde Oluwafemi Adetuyi, Valiollah Palangi, Olalekan Blessing Balogun, Anem I. Igirigi, and Sardaman Sardaman

21.1 Introduction

Plant-based sources fulfill most nutritional needs for both humans and livestock. Animal-derived proteins, such as meat, milk, and eggs, undergo vital transformations facilitated by enzymes and microbes in the gastrointestinal tract. During pre- and post-harvest periods, crops are attacked by various fungi (*Aspergillus, Fusarium, Penicillium*) or saprophytic molds, leading to contamination by mycotoxins such as aflatoxin, ochratoxins, ergot, fumonisins, trichothecenes, deoxynivalenol, patulin, citrinin, and zearalenone. Such mycotoxin contamination has significant health and economic implications for both producers and consumers. Moreover, mycotoxins can reduce palatability and nutrient content in feed ingredients, leading to spoilage and posing risks to food security (Bryden, 2012). Mycotoxins are commonly found in agricultural products such as maize, millet, wheat, sorghum, soybean, groundnut cake, and crop by-products. Additionally, mycotoxin contamination may extend to derived products, exemplified by a brewer's dry grain, a by-product of brewing. The livestock industry in Nigeria faces challenges due to inadequate processing and storage of feed items like cassava peels and groundnut cake. This poor storage system gives room for the growth of fungi, which produce mycotoxin.

So, the livestock feed industry uses additives to absorb and mitigate toxins, addressing mycotoxin challenges and promoting animal health (Bryden, 2012). Knowledgeable farmers use binders like BIOMIN and Alltech to reduce mycotoxins in feed, actively promoting animal health. Additionally, various materials, such as zeolites, bentonite, and clays, can adsorb mycotoxins (Jard et al., 2011; Bryden, 2012). Contaminated grains can also be detoxified through physical, chemical, and biological methods (Kabak et al., 2006). Although

DOI: 10.1201/9781003500605-24

chemical methods can be effective, they carry risks of chemical residues, potential toxicity, and increased fungal resistance to antifungals in feed and food. Accessible, affordable, non-toxic, and eco-friendly methods are needed to prevent contamination by toxigenic fungi and their metabolites, minimizing impacts on both humans and animal consumers (Amobonye et al., 2023). It is widely believed that nature has provided each region of the world with natural resources—plants, organisms, and minerals—to address common challenges. This is evident in how wild animals naturally respond to health challenges. This review aims to inform researchers, farmers, and industry stakeholders about new, affordable methods with both on-farm and industrial potential for reducing mycotoxin concentrations. It also examines the mechanisms by which these additives alleviate mycotoxin effects.

21.2 Climate Change and Mycotoxins

Greenhouse gas mitigation and mycotoxin reduction are closely linked, both being significant in animal production. This relationship is interwoven because greenhouse gas emissions (e.g., CH_4, NO_2, etc.) and environmental pollution occur during crop production processes involving CO_2, nitrogen, and phosphorus. Anthropogenic greenhouse gas emissions, such as methane and nitrous oxide, have the capability to warm the climate about 25 and 298 times more than CO_2. Atmospheric methane concentration has grown rapidly between 2014 and 2017, particularly in the tropics and subtropics, with rates ranging from about 8 parts per billion to more than 15 parts per billion/year (Nisbet et al., 2019).

Reports indicate prolonged drought, irregular rainfall, and rising temperatures (UNCCD Press Release, 2015; FAO-IPCC, 2017). Across continents, Africa, the Americas, and Asia experienced the highest levels of drought, while Asia, the Americas, and Europe recorded the most extreme temperatures in 2017 (CRED, 2018). Climate change influences pathogen distribution and intensity (Ostfeld and Brunner, 2015). Crops stressed by drought or insect activity are vulnerable to fungal invasion (Bryden, 2007). Since the end of World War II, European crop harvests have been notably affected by heat waves and unusual temperature increases (Arora et al., 2018).

Climate change causes high temperatures, excessive rainfall, storms, and variations in plant nutritive value and water availability, reducing resilience and increasing susceptibility to fungal infection. Mycotoxin production potentials and toxigenic fungal growth have been aggravated by interacting factors (Bebber et al., 2013; Medina et al., 2017), with continuous and increasing contamination levels in many regions owing to climate change (Battilani et al., 2016; Bandyopadhyay et al., 2016). In tropical climatic sub-Africa, for example, fungal contamination by *Fusarium* and *Aspergillus* (Liew and Mohd-Redzwan,

2018; Kagot et al., 2019) may be heightened by conditions such as temperature, drought, and alteration in rainfall, whereas *Penicillia* are common in temperate areas (Denli and Perez, 2010). Climate change may also increase the susceptibility of fodder crops, processed products, inedible by-products, and stored feedstuffs to contamination by mycotoxins such as aflatoxins (Saminathan et al., 2018). Climate change is expected to increase contamination in areas where mycotoxins are not usually found and areas considered safe due to prolonged hot and dry climate conditions, such as reported in Serbia (Medina et al., 2015) and Hungary (Dobolyi et al., 2013), which are in Europe. Similarly, climate change may raise mycotoxin contamination in agrarian countries in Latin America, such as Argentina and Brazil. Major crop and livestock producers in Asia, including China and India, are also at risk.

21.3 Mycotoxin Consumption and Consequences

Mycotoxins are metabolites produced primarily by *Aspergillus, Penicillium, Fusarium, Alternaria,* and *Cladosporium* genera (Bryden, 2012; Liew and Mohd-Redzwan, 2018). These substances can be highly harmful to animals when ingested through feed and to humans when ingested through food, and they can also be transferred into the human food chain through animal-derived protein. Poverty, ignorance, lack of awareness, unhealthy food processing, and lack of limiting regulations are the major causes of consuming food, feed, and animal protein that are contaminated with mycotoxins, as shown in Figure 21.1.

Many African countries lack regulations for controlling and monitoring mycotoxins, despite high contamination levels, unlike their European Union counterparts (Kagot et al., 2019). These issues affect many African nations, contributing to higher risks of mycotoxin exposure. Unfortunately, mycotoxin contamination is a universal issue, affecting people across all regions and demographics. Regions like Asia, America, Europe, and Australia are also affected by mycotoxin contamination. Nevertheless, regulation and good health care systems could reduce the incidence and help those in developed countries who are affected. Unfortunately, this is often not the case in many developing nations in Africa and parts of Asia.

21.3.1 Mycotoxin Effects on Animal Health

Livestock health, production, and welfare are endangered by mycotoxin contamination. Cattle, sheep, goats, pigs, poultry, rabbits, and equines (Spronck, 2012) are all affected by mycotoxins. They are implicated in anorexia, increased pro-inflammatory cytokines, and serum liver function enzyme concentration. Also, digestive enzymes such as lipase, trypsin, and amylase,

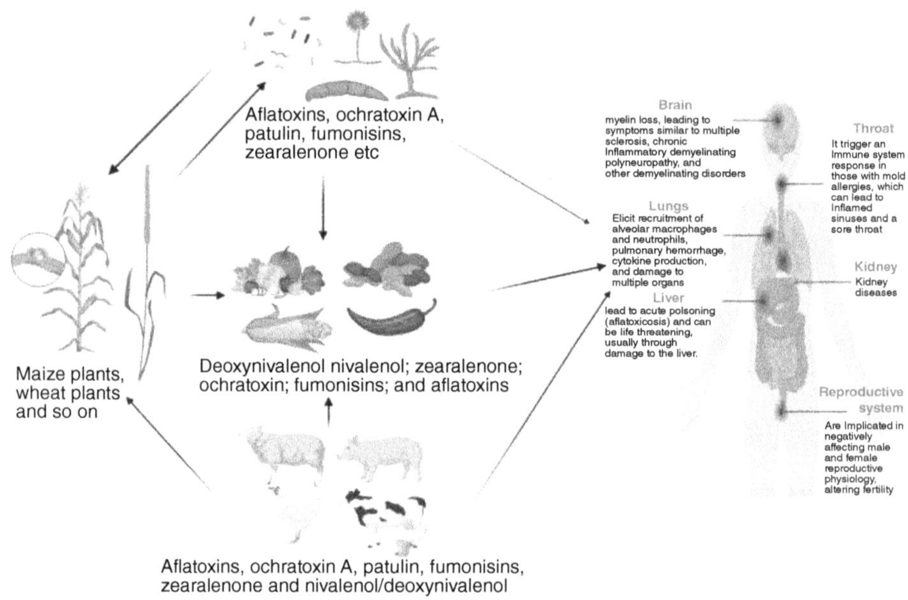

FIGURE 21.1
Overview of the sources, metabolites, and effects of mycotoxins on humans.

tissue circulation of vitamins and minerals, and concentrations of bile salts have been observed to decrease during aflatoxicosis (Osborne et al., 1982; Surai, 2002). Ammonia buildup in litter has been observed in non-ruminants due to increased water intake stimulation (Bryden, 2012) in birds. Similarly, oral lesions have been observed in poultry when trichothecene is ingested (Brake et al., 2000). Exposure to mycotoxin also affects metabolism and distribution of nutrients. In swine, a wide range of diseases are associated with mycotoxins, including pseudo-pregnancy, low conception rate, agalactia, stillbirth, blood in the urine and feces, and immunosuppression (Fink-Gremmels and Malekinejad, 2007).

Ruminants are less affected by mycotoxin than nonruminants. It is mainly attributed to the ability of rumen microbes, mainly protozoa, to metabolize various mycotoxins quickly (Kiessling et al., 1984; Zebeli and Metzler-Zebeli, 2012; Schaumberger, 2015). While this is true, the increased production demands and modern feeding systems of a high-grain concentrated diet compromise gut health (both the foregut and hindgut) by depressing gut pH and causing microbial shifts that may predispose ruminants to mycotoxin absorption, resulting in morbidity and even death (Faniyi et al., 2019). Furthermore, Fantinati (2018) reported that ruminants are predisposed to mastitis and laminitis, decreased milk production, aflatoxin milk residue, hepatocellular injuries, gastroenteritis, diarrhea, immune dysfunction, kidney lesion, low testicular development and sperm count, and ovarian cysts as a result of varying mycotoxins. For example, in India, improper storage of rice straw by farmers led to fungal (*Aspergillus flavus* and *Pencillium notatum*) contamination, which caused mycotoxicosis and resulted in necrosis, weakness, emaciation, and edema and gangrene in the legs, tail, and ear of cattle (Reddy et al., 2016).

21.3.2 Animal-Derived Product Contamination

Mycotoxin metabolism directs its excretion through urine and feces, poultry eggs, and mammalian milk (EFSA, 2009; Adegbeye et al., 2020). These livestock-derived products and other crop-based food products serve as sources of human aflatoxin intake (Prandini et al., 2009). Despite ruminants' ability to detoxify mycotoxin, milk still contains more residue than eggs. There is about 0.3 µg/kg of AFB1 residue in an egg for every 10 mg/kg of AFB_1 (equivalent to 10,000 µg AFB1/kg). This is about 0.003% in egg, compared to turnover of 0.3–2.2% AFB_1 in mammalian milk and in 0.05% for FB1 and T2-toxin (EFSA, 2009). It is therefore crucial to prevent mycotoxins from entering the food chain or being absorbed by the intestine. Furthermore, it has been shown that aflatoxin M1, a metabolite of AFB_1, is more toxic after ingestion than AFB_1 itself (Allcroft et al., 1967). Other co-contaminants of aflatoxin can be found in meat, milk, and eggs (Bryden et al., 2004).

21.3.3 Animal Product Consumers

Mycotoxin contamination is prevalent in developing nations and those affected by climate change. Mycotoxins possess the capacity to induce hepatic carcinogenesis, elicit inflammatory responses, and cause immunosuppression (Iqbal et al., 2013; L. Zhang et al., 2016). Aflatoxin M1 has been detected in human and bovine milk (Mulunda et al., 2013), indicating that the metabolized form of mycotoxins in ruminants may be more abundant and hazardous than the parent toxin. Human exposure to mycotoxins may occur through the consumption of animal products or contaminated food, predisposing consumers to foodborne aflatoxin B1. Children breastfed by mothers who consume contaminated diets or bovine milk containing mycotoxins face health risks as a result of the growing emphasis on prolonged breastfeeding (Adegbeye et al., 2020). Given the increasing human population, evolving dietary habits, and rising demand for milk and milk products, unchecked mycotoxin consumption or contamination could pose imminent challenges. Addressing mycotoxin consumption in mammals and preventing its entry into the food chain is a pressing concern.

21.4 Mode of Action

There have been many studies that have used botanical additives, clay, and chemical methods to reduce mycotoxin growth and concentration both *in vitro* and *in vivo*, with a common conclusion of alleviation. However, with the advancement in technology, interdisciplinary technological transfer and application is becoming easier in the field of agriculture. Because of this we now understand that there are molecular, transcriptional, and cytoplasmic structures and physical alterations that occur when additives are used. The effect of *Balanites aegyptiaca* on aflatoxin concentration reduction has been attributed to the antimicrobial activity due to the presence of phenolic antioxidants and saponin present in it. Cinnamaldehyde has been shown to influence ochratoxin (OTA) production by disrupting cell wall integrity, causing leakage of cytoplasmic content, destruction of mitochondria, cell organelles, fragmentalization of the nuclear membrane, and downregulation of OTA biosynthesis regulatory genes such as pks gene, nrps, laeA, veA, and velB (Wang et al., 2018).

The mechanism of action of unripe banana peel, *Pyracantha koidzumii* leaves, and aloe vera powder on aflatoxin may be attributed to the zeta potential difference between them. There is an electrostatic interaction between AFB_1, the phyto-sorbent, and the polar molecules on its surface (Akar et al., 2009; Zavala-Franco et al., 2018). This physical interaction is responsible for its adsorption from the gut. Proanthocyanidin extracts protected birds by decreasing serum inflammatory cytokines, like tumor necrosis factor-alpha, interferon-gamma, interleukin-1 beta, and interleukin 6 and 10, inhibiting splenic tissue pro-inflammatory cytokines, reducing phosphorylation of NF-κB (p65), and increasing Nrf2 gene expression (Rajput et al., 2019). Extract of hyssop (*Micromeria graeca*) reduced AFB_1 production by decreasing AFB_1 cluster gene expression of aflR, aflS, aflT, and other 23 genes involved in AFB_1 synthesis (El Khoury et al., 2017). The effect of curcumin on AFB_1-induced birds was alleviated by increasing hepatic antioxidant levels, reducing lipid peroxidation, reducing hepatic mRNA levels, or reducing the Cytochrome P450 isozyme responsible for bioactivating AFB_1 into exo-AFB1–8,9-epoxide (AFBO) and increasing serum and liver antioxidant levels (N.-Y. Zhang et al., 2016).

In livestock production, probiotics and prebiotics are used for their non-nutritional benefits, such as improving gut morphology, increasing gut microbes, and adsorbing toxins. Fructo-oligosaccharide's (difructose anhydride III) effect on zearalenone was evidenced by high serum Pi concentration and intestinal ion transport and improved intestinal barrier integrity (Toda et al., 2018), which prevented its absorption into the bloodstream. Actinobacterial strains were able to reduce OTA production by reducing its gene expression (acOTApks, acOTAhal, and acOTAnrps) (El Khoury et al., 2018). *Streptomyces roseolus* reduced aflatoxin production by decreasing the expression of two transcriptional factors (aflR and aflS) and interrupting biosynthesis of the pathway of AFB_1 through norsolorinic acid synthesis (Caceres et al., 2018). It was found that *Bacillus subtilis* ANSB060 exhibited antioxidant activity in ducks by increasing serum and liver T-SOD and GSH-Px levels, as well as reducing mycotoxin residue in the liver (L. Zhang et al., 2016). *Lactobacillus bulgaricus* and *Lactobacillus rhamnosus* in mice induced with aflatoxin downregulated proinflammatory responses such as serum IL-1β, TNF-α, and IL-6;

decreased NF-κB p65 transcriptional activity; and increased serum IFN-γ levels (Chen et al., 2019).

The use of yeast in livestock production improves feed utilization, toxins absorption, and performance. Low-fermenting yeast (*Lachancea thermotolerans*) reduced *A. parasiticus* growth due to the presence of its metabolite 2-phenylethanol, which suppresses genes involved in aflatoxin synthesis (Khan et al., 2004).

Clay is usually of non-nutritional benefit to birds. However, some of these clays can bind or absorb mycotoxins. Modified palygorskite alleviated the effect of fusarium by increasing intestinal barrier function gene expression, such as mucin 2 and zonula occludens-1, claudin-2, secretory immunoglobulin A, superoxide dismutase, and lower diamine oxidase (Cheng et al., 2018). Similarly, Thai bentonite clay binds to AFB_1 because the heat treatment helps to increase the interlayer spaces, which modified the structure of phyllosilicate clay to increase its adsorption efficacy and cation exchange capacity (Phillips et al., 1995; Onal and Sarikaya, 2008; Sakizci et al., 2009). The interactions between π-electrons of aromatic molecules and the large exterior surface area are the basis for which activated carbon fiber (ACF) decreased ochratoxin concentration (EL Khoury et al., 2018).

21.5 Alleviation/Mitigation Strategies

With over 50 years of mycotoxin-mitigation research (Hassan and Zhou, 2018), understanding of employing microorganisms, botanicals, clay, and other benign biosynthesized materials has advanced to address these toxins. Unfortunately, many control strategies have remained confined to laboratory and experimental settings, lacking momentum for practical field application (Chilaka et al., 2017; Wagacha et al., 2008). To be acceptable and sustainable, strategies for *in vivo, in vitro,* or storehouse mycotoxin control must prioritize safety and environmental friendliness. There is a crucial need to develop methods effective in the field, in storage facilities, and *in vivo* to prevent toxigenic fungal growth and subsequent mycotoxin production. Utilizing natural compounds like plant seeds, gels, extracts, modified clays, crop waste, essential oils, seed bioactive extracts, and affordable non-nutritive adsorptive materials could play a pivotal role in achieving these objectives.

21.5.1 Phytogenic Additives

21.5.1.1 Botanical Additives

Prevention strategies could depend on the use of phytogenic substances like plant extracts or essential oils. In the right amount, essential oils derived from plants have antimicrobial properties and could benefit consumers (animal and human). Cinnamaldehyde is a phyto-based compound obtained from the cinnamon plant. Wang et al. (2018) using 0.4, 1.0, and 1.6 mmol/L of cinnamaldehyde, inhibited ochratoxin production by 82, 98.7 and 100%, respectively, compared to the control, which had 1.90 ng/mm^2 OTA concentration. Exposure of *A. ochraceus* growth was inhibited completely after 1-day exposure to 1.6 mmol/L of cinnamaldehyde, while others doses limited mycelia growth by 41%–56.48% after 8 days of exposure. Cinnamaldehyde caused morphological alteration such as the mycelia tip becoming elongated and easy to break, hyphae shrinkage, loss of linearity and depressions on the hyphae surface, and disruption in cell wall and reducing cell wall thickness. Hyssop (*Micromeria graeca*) is an herb that belongs to the Lamiaceae family. El Khoury et al. (2017), using aqueous extracts (5, 10, 12.5, and 15 mg/mL) of hyssop, decreased aflatoxin production from *A. flavus* strain NRRL 62477. High concentrations such as 10 mg/ml caused 99.2% reduction, while 15 mg/ml reduced it beyond the detection level. Similarly, aflatoxin production from *A. flavus* strains E28 and E71 was inhibited by more than 70% using 10 mg/ml. There was severe repression by 8.4–468-fold of about 24 out of 27 genes involved in the AFB_1 enzymatic cascade of converting norsolorinic acid into AFB_1 synthesis; however, transcriptional gene expression showed that mtfA and veA were overexpressed. Therefore, the reduction in aflatoxin production could be attributed to the downregulation of aflR, which leads to the overexpression of mtfA, resulting in the inhibition of AFB_1 production (Zhuang et al., 2016).

Decreasing the bioavailability of mycotoxins using adsorbing agents in feed will reduce their uptake in the intestine and its distributions to the blood, target organs, and even animal products. Zavala-Franco et al. (2018) evaluated the efficacy of unripe banana peel (*Musa sapientum* L. var. paradisiaca), *Pyracantha koidzumii* leaves, and aloe vera powder in a model simulating the gastrointestinal tract of poultry using a 100 µg/kg AFB_1-contaminated diet at different pH values such as pH~5.2, pH~1.7, and pH~6.7 for crop, proventriculus, and intestinal sections, respectively. The zeta potential was –5.9 mV, –12.7 mV, and –20.9 mV for aloe vera powder, banana peel, and *Pyracantha* leaves, respectively. After simulation, banana peel, *Pyracantha* leaves, and aloe powder decreased bioavailable AFB_1 by 28, 46, and 69%, respectively. Thus, these commonly available materials could be included in the diet of poultry. Additionally, their low cost, availability, accessibility, eco-friendliness, and lack of competition make them highly sustainable options for animal production, benefiting livestock farmers of various capacities and scales.

21.5.1.2 Bioactives/Phytocomponents

Grape seeds are regarded as waste products from the wine and grape industry. Their disposal may cause environmental pollution in some countries that do not practice circular agriculture. Grape seed contains bioactive compounds like proanthocyanidin, polymerized and polyphenolic flavonoids (El-Ashmawy et al., 2007; Zhen et al., 2014), epicatechin, and gallocatechin

(Shi et al., 2003). These phytochemicals could protect against aflatoxin-induced liver damage by activating the Nrf2 signaling pathway (Hayes et al., 2010). Oloruntola et al. (2023) reported that walnut kernel powder and Jacobinia leaf powder lessened aflatoxin B1 effect on broiler's health. Rajput et al. (2019) evaluated the impact of grape seed proanthocyanidin (GSPE) on AFB_1-induced broilers. One (1) mg AFB_1/kg–contaminated corn and 1 mg AFB_1/kg + 250 mg GSPE/kg were fed alongside a basal diet. Proanthocyanidin protected the birds against AFB_1 by alleviating oxidative stress damage through increased antioxidation and Nrf2 signaling pathways (Jiang et al., 2016), which has a cytoprotective resistant effect to oxidative stress (Otterbein and Choi, 2000; Haines et al., 2012). Oloruntola et al. (2024) reported that dietary 0.5 g/kg *C. annuum* pericarp and seed powder supplementation mitigate aflatoxin B1 effects and stabilized growth and immune status in broiler chickens. Therefore, grapeseed extract and *Capsicum annuum* induced an anti-inflammatory response and improved the immune system in broilers against aflatoxin.

Among plant components, polyphenols are antioxidants that prevent lipid derivatives from oxidizing (Adegbeye et al., 2018). Due to the antioxidant activity of polyphenol in curcumin, livestock can benefit from its use. Curcumin is a natural polyphenolic compound from turmeric and could alleviate aflatoxicosis due to its antioxidant property. In Zhang et al. (2016), addition of 150 mg/kg of curcumin to the diet of 100 μg AFB_1/kg-induced birds increased hepatic antioxidation (glutathione peroxidase, superoxide dismutase, and catalase) and reduced lipid peroxidation (MDA) and DNA damage (8-OHdG), while the opposite occurred in AFB_1-induced birds. Furthermore, curcumin reduced the bioactivation of AFB_1 into highly reactive exo-AFB1–8,9-epoxide (AFBO)—by cytochrome P450 isozyme—CYP1A1, CYP1A2, CYP2A6, and CYP3A4. Cytochrome CYP450 enzymes play a key role in bioactivation of AFB_1 into the highly toxic AFBO (Diaz et al., 2010). Therefore, curcumin may be added to the diet with respect to mycotoxin alleviation. Olarotimi et al. (2023) also reported that dietary addition of *Sida acuta* leaf meal was beneficial and significantly reduced inflammatory cytokine and oxidative damage biomarkers as well as enhanced anti-inflammatory cytokines, thereby promoting the health status of the cocks fed AFB_1-contaminated rations.

Hermetic storage, one of the available mitigation technologies for mycotoxin, is too expensive for small-scale farmers and developing countries (Okello et al., 2010). To improve the safety of food and feed, we need alternative strategies. Plants in the *Brassicaceae* family produce isothiocyanates from glucosinolates, and these compounds exhibit antimicrobial activity (Adegbeye et al., 2018) with dose-dependent action (Dufour et al., 2012). A small-scale silo system demonstrated that allyl isothiocyanate (AITC) inhibited cereal contamination by *A. flavus* (corn) and *P. verrucosum* (wheat and barley) within 60 days by reducing *A. flavus* and *P. verrucosum* populations (Quiles et al. 2019). Ochratoxin A (OTA) production in wheat and barley was reduced by

90.0% and 99.5% at day 30 and 78.2% and 92.0% at day 60, respectively. However, aflatoxin production in corn contaminated with *A. flavus* was reduced beyond detection levels. Hence, applying AITC to cereal storage could mitigate mycotoxin production. According to Zhang (2004), Luciano and Holley (2009), and Quiles et al. (2019), the electrophilic central carbon atom in the N.C.S group enables isothiocyanate to bind to the amino and thiol groups of amino acids, peptides, and proteins that contain OTA-amino groups and aflatoxin-carboxylic groups.

21.5.2 Clay Treatment

It is extremely important to apply feed additives that limit intestinal absorption of bioavailable toxins in order to ensure animal health and safety of animal-derived products (Sadarman et al., 2021). Although clay such as zeolites and aluminosilicate-containing clays has the ability to adsorb mycotoxins, the indiscriminate adsorption of some vitamins and minerals and the release of heavy metals or dioxins (Abad et al., 2002) have brought some questions about its usage. Yet, observation of decreased toxicity in clay-based animal feeds has stimulated the development of clay additives (Jaynes and Zartman, 2011). Several companies, including BIOMIN and Alltech, manufacture toxin binders that are used in livestock feed. However, not many farmers are well informed or can afford it. Adding clay to feedstuffs as a toxin binder can help reduce contamination in small-holder livestock and reduce mycotoxin problems. There have been many adsorptive clays used with varying results, including kaolin, mica, talc, pyrophyllite, kaolinite, illite, chlorite, smectite, and montmorillonite. The varying result stems from the differences in toxin absorption, which is influenced by the cation exchange capacity on the surface of the clay and its cohesion and adhesion capability, selection, and specific surface area (Phillips et al., 1995; Pimpukdee et al., 2004). In a study carried out by Wongtangtintan et al. (2014), it was found that heating clay (of a variety of sizes—40, 60, 100, and 200 m) increased aflatoxin B1 adsorption by Thai bentonites (containing montmorillonite). Mycotoxin levels decreased by at least 49% when the temperature was raised from 25°C upward. In 40, 60, 100, and 200 m sizes, 92–97% of absorption was increased by applying heat between 600 and 700°C.

Fusariums can affect animal health by altering intestinal morphology and barrier functions. This is because they function as a barrier against toxins and regulate small molecule transport and epithelial cell permeability (Martens et al., 2018). The use of adsorbent materials helps to prevent the absorption of mycotoxins into the intestine, thereby relieving animals of the toxic influence. Clays such as zeolite, kaolinite, and montmorillonites are important adsorptive materials. However, the adsorption capacity of nonpolar/less polar mycotoxins molecules such as fusarium is poor because they have negatively charged hydrophilic surfaces (Vila-Donat et al., 2018). In comparison to nonpolar mycotoxin molecules, palygorskite (Pal) has a weak affinity for magnesium-rich silicate clay minerals (Cheng et al., 2018). It is therefore possible that modification would increase its affinity to mycotoxin. According to Cheng et al. (2018), modified palygorskite (MPAL) was used in broiler feed contaminated with *Fusarium* mycotoxins at a dosage of 1 g/kg. Providing MPAL increased immunological parameters such as bursal of fabicius weight as well as jejunal and ileal secretory immunoglobulin A levels. It also increased ileal superoxide dismutase and decreased jejuna malondialdehyde. In addition, diamine oxidase decreased, while jejunal and ileal villous height increased. The expression of intestinal barrier function genes in the jejunum, such as mucin 2 and zonula occludens-1, increased by 40 and 43.54%, respectively. Ileal claudin-2 was upregulated by 58.76%. An increase in secretory immunoglobulin A indicates limited accessibility of pathogenic bacteria and mucosal antigens to the mucosal barrier (Corthesy, 2013). Lower diamine oxidase indicates that MPAL improved intestinal integrity and prevented mucousa damage by mycotoxin (Wolvekamp and de Bruin, 1994), while lower malondialdehyde and increased superoxide dismutase indicate limited production of free radical and lower lipid peroxidation, respectively. *Zonula occludens*-1 and the transmembrane protein claudins (Lerner and Matthias, 2015) are important components of the intestinal mucosa barrier. Thus, the improvement in intestinal barrier gene expression indicated that MPAL prevented the compromise of tight junction integrity that would have increased its absorption into the bloodstream. As a result, MPAL reduces mycotoxin absorption through gut structure improvement, gut integrity preservation, and immunosuppression prevention.

21.5.3 Microbial/Biocontrol Agents

Generally, biocontrol agents are selected because they are incapable of producing aflatoxins. However, some strains of both aflatoxic and non-aflatoxigenic *Aspergillus* may produce other toxic metabolites, including cyclopiazonic acid, aspertoxin, aflatrem, kojic acid, leporin C, and sterigmatocystin, which could have a negative impact on consumers (Okoth et al., 2018; Kagot et al., 2019). Therefore, innovative biocontrol agents that are nontoxic and deemed safe to use are urgently needed.

21.5.3.1 Prebiotics and Probiotics

21.5.3.1.1 Yeast

Piotrowska and Masek (2015) experiment showed that yeast products, dried brewery yeast and its cell wall adsorbed 41.63 and 57.83% of ochratoxin A. Yeast cell wall adsorbs mycotoxins through hydrogen and ionic bonding or hydrophobic interactions (Huwig et al., 2001). Antagonistic yeast function against toxic fungi by varying mechanisms like biofilm formation, release of oxidants, and competition of nutrients (Liu et al., 2013). Exposure of *A. parasiticus* and *Fusarium graminearum* to low yeast fermenting (*Lachancea thermotolerans*) volatile organic compound derivatives in colonized media plugs resulted in 82% reduction in aflatoxin synthesis and 93% decrease in deoxynivalenol (DON) synthesis, respectively, (Zeidan et al. 2018). As low as 7 cfu of yeast was required to initiate an antagonistic effect of yeast volatile organic compound on fungal colony size and DON synthesis. It required between 200 and 398 cfu of yeast to completely inhibit DON synthesis. Surprisingly, supplementation above 400 cfu of yeast kickstarted DON synthesis by *F. graminearum* again. Thus, precision is needed. Inactivated yeast (*Lachancea thermotolerans*) cell wall removed 82% of ochratoxin OTA at pH 7 and 71% at pH 5. This indicates that yeast efficacy could be pH dependent. Due to weak hydrogen and van der Waals bonds, inactivated yeast cell walls have a greater ability to adsorb mycotoxins (Jouany et al., 2005). This could be used as a harm-reducing strategy in livestock nutrition to reduce intestinal absorption of mycotoxins.

Health benefits can be achieved by using prebiotics and non-digestible oligosaccharides. These oligosaccharides improve gut morphology and integrity; and modulate immune responses of epithelial cells (Akbari et al., 2017). Difructose anhydride III (DFA III) belongs to oligosaccharides (fructose) category and could be a novel prebiotic. Toda et al. (2018) study on zearalenone-exposed cattle fed rice straw supplemented with fructo-oligosaccharide (DFA III) reduced urinary excretion of zearalenone and its metabolites, α-ZOL and β-ZOL. After supplementation, total zearalenone excretion from cattle was reduced by 69.71% and 51% on days 9 and 14, respectively. This reduction in urinary excretion implies high chance of lower residue in milk. It may be related to improved protective effect of additives on intestinal barrier integrity and tight junctions of intestinal epithelium cells.

21.5.3.1.2 Lactobacilli

Probiotics, administered to animals, provide beneficial effects such as enhanced microbial proliferation, improved feed utilization, and enhanced gut morphology, leading to improved animal production. In a study by Chen et al. (2019), *Lactobacillus bulgaricus* and *Lactobacillus rhamnosus* were used against AFB_1-induced hepatitis in mice. Mice were exposed to AFB_1 alone (control), AFB_1 with 10 mg of *L. bulgaricus* (L1), and AFB_1 with 10 mg of *L. rhamnosus* (L2) at a dosage of 300 µg/kg AFB_1. AFB_1-exposed mice exhibited severe hepatic swelling and disarranged hepatic lobule structure, while supplementation with lactobacilli alleviated pathological changes and limited hepatic histopathological damage. Liver function enzymes (ALT, AST) were reduced in the lactobacilli-treated group and increased in the AFB_1-treated group. Serum inflammatory responses were upregulated in the AFB_1 group but downregulated in the *L. bulgaricus* and *L. rhamnosus* treated mice. Lactobacilli supplementation decreased NF-κB p65 transcriptional activities, while AFB_1 increased them. In vitro, *L. bulgaricus* and *L. rhamnosus* effectively decreased AFB_1-induced IL-1β, TNF-α, and NF-κB p65 levels. The regulation of NF-κB and downregulation of proinflammatory cytokines suggest that lactobacilli exert anti-inflammatory responses, reducing chronic inflammation and controlling tissue damage in vital metabolic organs like the liver. Thus, *Lactobacillus bulgaricus* and *Lactobacillus rhamnosus* could serve as a novel preventive strategy for aflatoxicosis.

21.5.3.1.3 Bacillus Strains

Bacillus spp. secrete diverse bioactive metabolites, capable of pathogenic control (Ongena and Jacques, 2008; Hamdache et al., 2011). The use of non-toxigenic antagonistic fungal strains such as rice-associated bacilli strains could be a way out. Five rice-associated bacilli (RAB) (4R, 4S, 6, 14R, and 24) inhibited more than 60% *Aspergillus flavus* growth (Chalivendra et al., 2018). The RAB4R inhibit fungal growth by lysing *A. flavus* hyphal tips. Furthermore, 4R strain provided strong anti-mycotoxigenic activities in maize contaminated with Tox4. Other RAB strains used in the study such as 5, 14S, 17R, 19, and 23S inhibited norsorolinic—an aflatoxin precursor—by at least 80%. Norsorolinic is a precursor of aflatoxin, which is converted after multiple enzyme reaction (Kovac et al., 2018). Thus, using rice-associated bacilli could be a potent fungistatic and strong anti-mycotoxigenic against the effect of *A. flavus* strains, but further in vivo study is needed to confirm its efficacy. Ducks are unable to efficiently metabolize aflatoxin, which makes them highly susceptible to its negative effect (Dalvi, 1986). Besides, the liver—involved in all metabolic functions (Faniyi et al., 2019)—is a major target organ for aflatoxins. Therefore, detoxifying aflatoxin and/or protecting the liver from its damage is paramount. *Bacillus subtilis* may be used as it is considered safe in China (L. Zhang et al., 2016). L. Zhang et al.'s (2016) study supplemented the diet of aflatoxin-contaminated duck with *Bacillus subtilis* ANSB060 at a dosage of 60% moldy maize (22.44 μg/kg aflatoxin level) control and control + added 500 g/t, 1000 g/t, and 2000 g/t of *Bacillus subtilis* ANSB060, respectively. *Bacillus subtilis* ANSB060 supplementation resulted in increased serum total superoxide dismutase by a range of 12.05–13.17%, liver total superoxide dismutase by 15.44–24.16%, and glutathione peroxidase increased by 19.89–26.23%. Aflatoxin residue in animal products such as eggs and milk is a serum food quality concern among policy makers/consumers. It is dangerous because it leads to a gradual accumulation/effect in the body when consumed regularly/consistently and could lead to chronic health issues. AFB_1 residue in the liver of duck was reduced by 41.67–58.33%, while AFM1 residue was reduced by 40–50%, so supplementing *Bacillus* could help reduce mycotoxin residue in livestock organs/products and alleviate mycotoxic effects.

21.5.4 Streptomyces

Streptomyces genera can produce a wide-range of bioactive compounds (Shams-Ghahfarokhi et al., 2013; Barka et al., 2016). This indicates that it could be used as a biocontrol agent to prevent mycotoxin production. Solid co-culturing of four strains (ML5, PH1, SN7, and AT36) of actinobacteria belonging to *Streptomyces* genera with *Aspergillus carbonarius*—an OTA-producing species in European vineyards used in El Khoury et al. (2018)—were able to reduce ochratoxin production in solid medium in a range of 67–83%. The SN7 strain led to a drastic reduction in gene expression between 85.6 and 93.1% for acOTAhal, acOTAnrps, and acOTApks. Further study showed AT36 and S7 exhibited high OTA degrading activity by reducing OTA (100 μg/L) beyond the detection level. In another study, Caceres et al.'s (2018) co-culturing of *Streptomyces roseolus* with *Aspergillus flavus* resulted in reduction ($P < 0.0001$) of AFB_1 from 972.8 μg/L to undetectable levels. This may be attributed to the repression of synthetic pathway gene expression. There were morphological changes that resulted in aberrant spore development alongside hyphae and sixfold decrease in transcriptional factors (aflR and aflS).

21.5.5 Activated Carbon Fibers

Activated carbon fibers exhibit exceptionally high adsorption rates and concentrations which is attributed to their narrow pore size distribution (El Khoury et al., 2018; Le Cloirec et al., 1996; Pelekani and Snoeyink, 1999), making them suitable for continuous processes. In a study by El Khoury et al. (2018), ACF samples (AC15, AC20, and D1200) with Brunauer–Emmett–Teller surface areas of 1758, 2032, and 1428 m^2/g, respectively, removed over 80% of ochratoxin A. When tested for ochratoxin A removal in red wine (pH 4.1) and red grape juice (pH 3.7), ACFs adsorbed 25–50% of OTA within 24 hours, with AC20 exhibiting the highest removal rate of 70% after 48 hours. This suggests that activated carbon fibers can eliminate mycotoxins in liquid substances, liquid matrices, or liquid food.

21.6 Conclusion

The food and feed industry has the potential to benefit from the use of natural, low-cost, and eco-friendly materials to mitigate the effects of mycotoxins. In numerous *in vivo* tests, these materials have demonstrated the capacity to adsorb a multitude of toxins. Additionally, these materials play a role in up-regulating the immune system and preserving gut integrity. The use of phytogenic feed additive/bioactive compounds such as aloe vera, unripe banana, turmeric, mustard, cinnamaldehyde and clay treatments such as heated Thai bentonite and modified palygorskite can help to alleviate mycotoxic effects. Moreover, microbial supplementation, including yeast, lactobacilli, and bacilli, holds promise in alleviating the impact of mycotoxins in livestock. Materials like activated carbon fiber are effective in removing mycotoxins from liquid matrices, particularly relevant to the food industry. Volatile compounds of the isothiocyanate family, such as allyl isothiocyanate from mustard seeds, show potential for storage applications, such as in silo systems. Additionally, difructose anhydride III can be introduced into the diet of ruminants, while *Bacillus subtilis* ANSB060 may be utilized in non-ruminants to mitigate the absorption of mycotoxin residues in animal tissues or products. Generally, the alleviation tendencies of additives include an increase in antioxidant activity, prevention of intestinal absorption of mycotoxins, and modification of the immune system, while serum and liver inflammatory responses and proinflammatory cytokines are also suppressed. Further, *in vivo* studies are needed to test the efficacy of these materials on ruminant, monogastric, and other domesticated hindgut fermenters.

References

Abad E, Llerena JJ, Sauló J, Caixach J and Rivera J 2002. Comprehensive study on dioxin contents in binder and anti-caking agent feed additives. *Chemosphere* 46, 1417–1421.

Adegbeye MJ, Elghandour MMY, Faniyi TO, Perez NR, Barbabosa-Pilego A, Zaragoza-Bastida, A and Salem AZM 2018. Antimicrobial and antihelminthic impacts of black cumin, pawpaw and mustard seeds in livestock production and health. *Agroforestry System* 94, 1255–1268 (2020). https://doi.org/10.1007/s10457-018-0337-0

Adegbeye MJ, Reddy PRK, Chilaka CA, Balogun OB, Elghandour MMY, Rivas-Caceres RR and Salem AZM (2020). Mycotoxin toxicity and residue in animal products: Prevalence, consumer exposure and reduction strategies – A review. *Toxicon* 177, 96–108. https://doi.org/10.1016/j.toxicon.2020.01.007

Akar T, Anilan B, Gorgulu A and Akar ST 2009. Assessment of cationic dye biosorption characteristics of untreated and non-conventional biomass, *Pyracantha coccinea* berries. *Journal of Hazardous Materials* 168, 1302–1309.

Akbari P, Braber S, Varasteh S, Alizadeh A, Garssen J and Fink-Gremmels J 2017. The intestinal barrier as an emerging target in the toxicological assessment of mycotoxins. *Archives of Toxicology* 91, 1007–1029.

Allcroft R, Roberts BA and Butler WH 1967. Aflatoxin in milk. *Food and Cosmetic Toxicology* 5, 597–598.

Amobonye A, Aruwa C, Aransiola SA, John O, Alabi TD and Lalung J 2023. Exploring the potential of fungi in the bioremediation of pharmaceutically active compounds. *Frontiers in Microbiology, Microbiotechnology Section* 14, 1207792. https://doi.org/10.3389/fmicb.2023.1207792.

Arora NK, Fatima T, Mishra I, Verma, M, Mishra J and Mishra V 2018. Environmental sustainability, challenges and viable solutions. *Environmental Sustainability* 1, 309–340.

Bandyopadhyay R, Ortega-Beltran A, Akande A, Mutegi C, Atehnkeng J, Kaptoge L, Senghor AL, Adhikari BN and Cotty PJ 2016. Biological control of aflatoxins in Africa, current status and potential challenges in the face of climate change. *World Mycotoxin Journal* 9, 771–789.

Barka EA, Vatsa P, Sanchez L, Gaveau-Vaillant N, Jacquard C, Klenk H-P, Clément C, Ouhdouch Y and van Wezel GP 2016. Taxonomy, physiology, and natural products of actinobacteria. *Microbiology and Molecular Biology Reviews* 80, 1–43.
Battilani P, Toscano P, Fels-Klerx HJ, Moretti A, Leggieri MC and Brera C 2016. Aflatoxin B1 contamination in maize in Europe increases due to climate change. *Scientific Reports* 6, 24328–24340.
Bebber DP, Ramotowski MAT and Gurr SJ 2013. Crop pests and pathogens move polewards in a warming world. *Nature Climate Change* 3, 985–988.
Brake J, Hamilton PB and Kittrell RS 2000. Effects of the tricothecene mycotoxin diacetoxyscirpenol on feed consumption, body weight, and oral lesions of broiler breeders. *Poultry Science* 79, 856–863.
Bryden WL 2007. Mycotoxins in the food chain, human health implications. *Asia Pacific Journal of Clinical Nutrition* 16, 95–101.
Bryden WL 2012. Mycotoxin contamination of the feed supply chain, implications for animal productivity and feed security. *Animal Feed Science and Technology* 173, 134–158.
Bryden WL, Suksupath S, Taylor DJ and Prasongsidh BC 2004. *Poisonous plant and related toxins*. CABI, Glasgow, pp. 134–139.
Caceres I, Snini SP, Puel O and Mathieu F 2018. *Streptomyces roseolus*, a promising biocontrol agent against *Aspergillus flavus*, the main aflatoxin B1 producer. *Toxins* 10, 1–13.
Centre for Research on the Epidemiology of Disasters (CRED) 2018. *Natural disasters in 2017, Lower mortality, higher cost*, p. 50. http://www.cred.be/publications.
Chalivendra S, DeRobertis C, Pineda JR, Ham JH and Damann K 2018. Rice phyllosphere bacillus species and their secreted metabolites suppress *Aspergillus flavus* growth and aflatoxin production in vitro and in maize seeds. *Toxins* 10, 1–16.
Chen Y, Li R, Chang Q, Dong Z, Yang H and Xu C 2019. *Lactobacillus bulgaricus* or *Lactobacillus rhamnosus* suppresses NF-κB signaling pathway and protects against AFB1-induced hepatitis, a novel potential preventive strategy for aflatoxicosis? *Toxins* 11, 1–15.
Cheng Y, Xu Q, Chen Y, Su Y, Wen C and Zhou Y 2018. Modified palygorskite improves immunity, antioxidant ability, intestinal morphology, and barrier function in broiler chickens fed naturally contaminated diet with permitted feed concentrations of fusarium mycotoxins. *Toxins* 10, 482. https://doi.org/10.3390/toxins10110482.
Chilaka CA, De Boevre M, Atanda OO and De Saeger S 2017. The status of Fusarium mycotoxins in sub-Saharan Africa, a review of emerging trends and post-harvest mitigation strategies towards food control. *Toxins* 9, 36–46.
Corthesy B 2013. Multi-faceted functions of secretory IgA at mucosal surfaces. *Frontiers in Immunology* 4, 185–195.
Dalvi R 1986. An overview of aflatoxicosis of poultry, its characteristics, prevention and reduction. *Veterinary Research Communication* 10, 429–443.
Denli M and Perez JO 2010. Ochratoxins in feed, a risk for animal and human health, control strategies. *Toxins* 2, 1065–1077.
Diaz GJ, Murcia HW and Cepeda SM 2010. Cytochrome P450 enzymes involved in the metabolism of aflatoxin B1 in chickens and quail. *Poultry Science* 89, 2461–2469.
Dobolyi C, Sebok F, Varga J, Kocsubé S, Szigeti G, Baranyi N, Szécsi A, Tóth B, Varga M, Kriszt B, Szoboszlay S, Krifaton C and Kukolya J 2013. Occurrence of aflatoxin producing *Aspergillus flavus* isolates in maize kernel in Hungary. *Acta Alimentaria* 42, 451–459.

Dufour V, Alazzam B, Ermel G, Thepaut M, Rossero A, Tresse O and Baysse C 2012. Antimicrobial activities of isothiocyanates against Campylobacter jejuni isolates. *Frontiers in Cellular Infection and Microbiology* 53, 1–13.

El-Ashmawy IM, Saleh A and Salama OM 2007. Effects of marjoram volatile oil and grape seed extract on ethanol toxicity in male rats. *Basic Clinical Pharmacology Toxicology* 101, 320–327.

El Khoury R, Caceres I, Puel O, Bailly S, Atoui A, Oswald IP, El Khoury A and Bailly J-D 2017. Identification of the anti-aflatoxinogenic activity of *Micromeria graeca* and elucidation of its molecular mechanism in *Aspergillus flavus*. *Toxins* 9, 1–15.

El Khoury R, Choque E, El Khoury A, Snini SP, Cairns R, Andriantsiferana C and Mathieu F 2018. OTA prevention and detoxification by actinobacterial strains and activated carbon fibers, preliminary results. *Toxins* 10, 1–16.

European Food Safety Authority EFSA 2009. *Review of mycotoxin-detoxifying agents used as feed additives, mode of action, efficacy and feed/food safety.* Retrieved on 11 April 2019 from http://www.efsa.europa.eu/en/scdocs/doc/22e.pdf.

Faniyi TO, Adegbeye MJ, Elghandour MMY, Pilego AB, Salem AZM, Olaniyi TA, Adediran O and Adewumi MK 2019. Role of diverse fermentative factors towards microbial community shift in ruminants. *Journal of Applied Microbiology* 127, 2–11.

Fantinati P 2018. Ensuring high quality corn storage, should we trust our feed to deliver cows dairy performance? *Ruminant Issue* 57, 1–12.

FAO-IPCC 2017. *Expert meeting on climate change, land use and food security, final meeting report*. FAO, Rome, January 23–25.

Fink-Gremmels J and Malekinejad H 2007. Clinical effects and biochemical mechanisms associated with exposure to the mycoestrogen zearalenone. *Animal Feed Science and Technology* 137, 326–341.

Haines DD, Lekli I, Teissier P, Bak I and Tosaki A. 2012. Role of haeme oxygenase-1 in resolution of oxidative stress-related pathologies, focus on cardiovascular, lung, neurological and kidney disorders. *Acta Physiology* 204, 487–501.

Hamdache A, Lamarti A, Aleu J and Collado IG 2011. Non-peptide metabolites from the genus bacillus. *Journal of Natural Production* 74, 893–899.

Hassan YI and Zhou T 2018. Promising detoxification strategies to mitigate mycotoxins in food and feed. *Toxins* 10, 1–5.

Hayes JD, McMahon M, Chowdhry S and Dinkovakostova AT 2010. Cancer chemoprevention mechanisms mediated through the keap1-Nrf2 pathway. *Antioxidant Redox Signal* 13, 1713–1748.

Huwig A, Freimund S, Käppeli O and Dutler H 2001. Mycotoxin detoxication of animal feed by different adsorbents. *Toxicology Letters* 122, 179–188.

Iqbal SZ, Asi MR and Ariño A 2013. *Aflatoxins: Brenner's encyclopedia of genetics*. Science Direct, London.

Jard G, Liboz T, Mathieu F, Guyonvarc'h A and Lebrihi A 2011. Review of mycotoxin reduction in food and feed, from prevention in the field to detoxification by adsorption or transformation. *Food Additive and Contaminants: Part A Chemistry Analysis Control Exposure Risk and Assessment* 28, 1590–1609.

Jaynes WF and Zartman RE 2011. Influence of soluble feed proteins and clay additive charge density on aflatoxin binding in ingested feeds. In *Aflatoxins—biochemistry and molecular biology* (Ed GG Ramón). IntechOpen, London, pp 1–22.

Jiang YM, Wang Y, Tan HS, Yu T, Fan XM, Chen P, Zeng H, Huang M and Bi HC 2016. Schisandrol b protects against acetaminophen-induced acute hepatotoxicity in mice via activation of the Nrf2/are signaling pathway. *Acta Pharmacologica Sinica* 37, 382–400.

Jouany JP, Yiannikouris A and Bertin G 2005. The chemical bonds between mycotoxins and cell wall components of Saccharomyces cerevisiae have been identified. *Archiva Zootechnica* 8, 26–50.

Kabak B, Dobson ADW and Var I 2006. Strategies to prevent mycotoxin contamination of food and animal feed, a review. *Critical Reviews of Food Science and Nutrition* 46, 593–619.

Kagot V, Okoth S, De Boevre M and De Saeger S 2019. Biocontrol of aspergillus and fusarium mycotoxins in Africa, benefits and limitations. *Toxins* 11, 1–9.

Khan N, Schisler D, Boehm M, Lipps P and Slininger P 2004. Field testing of antagonists of Fusarium head blight incited by Gibberella zeae. *Biological Control* 29, 245–255.

Kiessling K, Pettersson H, Sandholm K and Olsen M 1984. Metabolism of aflatoxin, ochratoxin, zearalenone, and three trichothecenes by intact rumen fluid, rumen protozoa, and rumen bacteria. *Applied Environmental Microbiology* 47, 1070–1073.

Kovac T, Borisev I, Crevar B, Kenjeric FC, Kovac M, Strelec I, Ezekiel CN, Sulyok M, Krska R and Sarkanj B 2018. Fullerol C60OH24 nanoparticles modulate aflatoxin B1 biosynthesis in Aspergillus flavus. *Scientific Reports* 8, 1–8.

Le Cloirec P, Brasquet C and Subrenat E 1996. The adsorption onto fibrous activated carbon applications to water and air treatments. *ACS Division of Fuel Chemistry* 41, 379–381.

Lerner A and Matthias T 2015. Changes in intestinal tight junction permeability associated with industrial food additives explain the rising incidence of autoimmune disease. *Autoimmunology Reviews* 14, 479–489.

Liew WPP and Mohd-Redzwan S 2018. Mycotoxin, its impact on gut health and microbiota. *Frontiers in Cellular Infection Microbiology* 8, 1–17.

Liu G, Yan T, Wang J, Huang Z, Chen X, Jia G, Wu C, Zhao H, Xue B, Xiao L and Tang J 2013. Biological system responses to zearalenone mycotoxin exposure by integrated metabolomic studies. *Journal of Agriculture and Food Chemistry* 61, 11212–11221.

Luciano FB and Holley RA 2009. Enzymatic inhibition by allyl isothiocyanate and factors affecting its antimicrobial action against Escherichia coli O157:H7. *International Journal of Food Microbiology* 131, 240–245.

Martens EC, Neumann M and Desai MS 2018. Interactions of commensal and pathogenic microorganisms with the intestinal mucosal barrier. *Nature Reviews Microbiology* 16, 457–470.

Medina A, Gilbert MK, Mack BM, OBrian GR, Rodríguez A, Bhatnagar D, Payne G and Magan N 2017. Interactions between water activity and temperature on the Aspergillus flavus transcriptome and aflatoxin B1 production. *International Journal of Food Microbiology* 256, 36–44.

Medina Á, Rodríguez A, Sultan Y and Magan N 2015. Climate change factors and Aspergillus flavus, effects on gene expression, growth and aflatoxin production. *World Mycotoxin Journal* 8, 171–179.

Mulunda M, Ngoma L, Nyirenda M, Motsei L and Bakunzi FA 2013. Decade of aflatoxin M1 surveillance in milk and dairy products in developing countries 2001–2011, a review. In *Mycotoxin and food safety in developing countries* (Ed DH Makun). InTechOpen, Rijeka, Croatia, pp 39–60.

Nisbet EG, Manning MR, Dlugokencky EJ, Fisher RE, Lowry D, Michel SE, Myhre CL, Platt SM, Allen G, Bousquet P, Brownlow R, Cain M, France JL, Hermansen O, Hossaini R, Jones AE, Levin I, Manning AC, Myhre G, Pyle JA, Vaughn BH,

Warwick NJ and White JWC 2019. Very strong atmospheric methane growth in the 4 years 2014–2017, implications for the Paris agreement. *Global Biogeochemical Cycles* 33, 318–342.

Okello DK, Kaaya AN, Bisikwa J, Were M and Oloka HK 2010. Management of aflatoxins in groundnuts. In *A manual for processors and traders in Uganda*. National Agricultural Research Organization, Entebbe, Uganda.

Okoth S, De Boevre M, Vidal A, Di Mavungu DJ, Landschoot S, Kyallo M, Njuguna J, Harvey J and De Saeger S 2018. Genetic and toxigenic variability within Aspergillus flavus population isolated from maize in two diverse environments in Kenya. *Frontiers in Microbiology* 9, 57–69.

Olarotimi OJ, Gbore FA, Adu OA, Oloruntola OD and Jimoh OA 2023. Ameliorative effects of Sida acuta and vitamin C on serum DNA damage, pro-inflammatory and anti-inflammatory cytokines in roosters fed aflatoxin B1 contaminated diets. *Toxicon* 236, 107330. https://doi.org/10.1016/j.toxicon.2023.107330.

Oloruntola OD, Ayodele SO, Oloruntola DA, Olarotimi OJ, Falowo AB, Akinduro VO, Gbore FA, Adu OA and Agbede JO 2024. Dietary supplementation of capsicum powder affects the growth, immunoglobulins, pro-inflammatory cytokines, adipokines, meat, and liver histology of aflatoxin B1 exposed broiler chickens. *Toxicon* 240, 107640. https://doi.org/10.1016/j.toxicon.2024.107640.

Oloruntola OD, Ganiyi TO, Bibire OO, Abdulkadir MT, Oloruntola DA, Akinduro VO, Ayebogan KS and Olaoye TP 2023. Effects of aflatoxin-B on performance, blood and antioxidant status of broiler chickens 1 are lessened by walnut kernel powder and Jacobinia leaf powder dietary supplementation. *Annals of Animal and Biological Research* 3(1), 12–21.

Onal M and Sarikaya Y 2008. Thermal analysis of some organoclays. *Journal of Thermal Analysis and Calorimetry* 91, 1261–1265.

Ongena M and Jacques P 2008. Bacillus lipopeptides, versatile weapons for plant disease biocontrol. *Trends in Microbiology* 16, 115–125.

Osborne DJ, Huff WE, Hamilton PB and Burmeister HR 1982. Comparison of ochratoxin, aflatoxin and T-2 toxin for their effects on selected parameters related to digestion and evidence for specific metabolism of carotenoids in chickens. *Poultry Science* 61, 1646–1652.

Ostfeld RS and Brunner JL 2015. Climate change and Ixodes tick-borne diseases of humans. *Philosophical Transactions of the Royal Society of London. Series B, Biological Sciences* 2015, 370.

Otterbein LE and Choi AMK 2000. Heme oxygenase, Colors of defense against cellular stress. *American Journal of Physiology-Lung Cellular and Molecular Physiology* 279, 1029–1037.

Pelekani C and Snoeyink V 1999. Competitive adsorption in natural water, role of activated carbon pore size. *Water Research* 33, 1209–1219.

Phillips TD, Sarr AB and Grant PG 1995. Selective chemisorption and detoxification of aflatoxins by phyllosilicate clay. *Natural Toxins* 3, 204–213.

Pimpukdee K, Kubena LF, Bailey CA and Phillips TD 2004. Aflatoxin induced toxicities and depletion of hepatic vitamin A in young broiler chicks, protection of chicks in the presence of low levels of novasil plus in the diet. *Poultry Science* 83, 737–744.

Piotrowska M and Masek A 2015. Saccharomyces cerevisiae cell wall components as tools for ochratoxin A decontamination. *Toxins* 7, 1151–1162.

Prandini A, Tansini G, Sigolo S, Filippi L, Laporta M and Piva G 2009. On the occurrence of aflatoxin M1 in milk and dairy products. *Food and Chemical Toxicology* 47, 984–991.
Quiles JM, Nazareth TN, Luz C, Luciano FB, Mañes J and Meca G 2019. Development of an antifungal and antimycotoxigenic device containing allyl isothiocyanate for silo fumigation. *Toxins* 11, 137–150.
Rajput SA, Sun L, Zhang N-Y, Khalil MM, Ling Z, Chong L, Wang S, Rajput IR, Bloch DM, Khan FA, Shaukat A and Qi D 2019. Grape seed proanthocyanidin extract alleviates aflatoxin B1-induced immunotoxicity and oxidative stress via modulation of NF-κB and Nrf2 signaling pathways in broilers. *Toxins* 11, 1–15.
Reddy PRK, Reddy AN, Kishore KR, Reddy VP, Reddy PPR, Ramesh R, Singh S and Prathap B 2016. Bovine mycotoxicosis—a remarkable disease in rice growing areas of Indian subcontinent. *International Journal of Natural Sciences* 7, 805–808.
Sadarman E, Erwan E, Irawan A, Sholikin MM, Solfaine R, Harahap RP, Irawan AC, Sofyan A, Nahrowi N and Jayanegara A 2021. Propolis supplementation affects performance, intestinal morphology, and bacterial population of broiler chickens. *South African Journal of Animal Science* 51(4), 477–487.
Sakizci M, Alver BE and Yorukogullari E 2009. Thermal behavior and immersion heats of selected clays from turkey. *Journal of Thermal Analysis and Calorimetry* 98, 249–436.
Saminathan M, Selamat J, Pirouz AA, Abdullah N and Zulkifli I 2018. Effects of nanocomposite adsorbents on the growth performance, serum biochemistry, and organ weights of broilers fed with aflatoxin-contaminated feed. *Toxins* 10, 1–15.
Schaumberger S 2015. The peril of on/off mycotoxin risk management, science and solutions, a magazine of biomin. *Rumin Issue* 25, 1–12.
Shams-Ghahfarokhi M, Kalantari S and Razzaghi-Abyaneh M 2013. Terrestrial bacteria from agricultural soils, versatile weapons against aflatoxigenic fungi terrestrial bacteria from agricultural soils, versatile. In *Aflatoxins—recent advances and future prospects*. InTechOpen, London, pp 23–39.
Shi J, Yu J, Pohorly JE and Kakuda Y 2003. Polyphenolics in grape seeds—biochemistry and functionality. *Journal of Medicinal Food* 6, 291–299.
Spronck L 2012. *Moulds and mycotoxins in animal feeds, implications for equine health and performance.* Dissertation. Utrecht University, Utrecht, The Netherlands, pp 1–31.
Surai PF 2002. Natural antioxidants and mycotoxins. In *Natural antioxidants in avian nutrition and reproduction.* Nottingham University Press, Nottingham, pp 455–489.
Toda K, Uno S, Kokushi E, Shiiba A, Hasunuma H, Matsumoto D, Ohtani M, Yamato O, Shinya U, Wijayagunawardane M, Fink-Gremmels J, Taniguchi M and Takagi M 2018. Fructo-oligosaccharide DFA III feed supplementation for mitigation of mycotoxin exposure in cattle—clinical evaluation by a urinary zearalenone monitoring system. *Toxins* 10, 1–10.
UNCCD Press Release 2015. *Inception meeting of the UNCCD land degradation neutrality project.* http://www.unccd.int/en/mediacenter/MediaNews/Pages/highlightdetail.aspx?HighlightID=355
Vila-Donat P, Marín S, Sanchis V and Ramos AJ 2018. A review of the mycotoxin adsorbing agents, with an emphasis on their multi-binding capacity, for animal feed decontamination. *Food and Chemical Toxicology* 114, 246–259.

Wagacha J and Muthomi J 2008. Mycotoxin problem in Africa, current status, implications to food safety and health and possible management strategies. *International Journal of Food Microbiology* 124, 1–12.
Wang L, Jin J, Liu X, Wang Y, Liu Y, Zhao Y and Xing F 2018. Effect of cinnamaldehyde on morphological alterations of aspergillus ochraceus and expression of key genes involved in ochratoxin A biosynthesis. *Toxins* 10, 1–12.
Wolvekamp MCJ and de Bruin RWF 1994. Diamine oxidase, an overview of historical, biochemical and functional aspects. *Digestive Diseases* 12, 2–14.
Wongtangtintan S, Saipan P, Tengjaroenkul U, Suthimun S and Tengjaroenkul B 2014. Effect of heat treatment on efficacy of Thai bentonite for adsorption of aflatoxin B1 in vitro. *Livestock Research for Rural Development* 26, 1–7. Retrieved on 21 March 2019.
Zavala-Franco A, Hernández-Patlán D, Solís-Cruz B, López-Arellano R, Tellez-Isaias G, Vázquez-Durán A and Méndez-Albores A 2018. Assessing the aflatoxin B1 adsorption capacity between biosorbents using an in vitro multicompartmental model simulating the dynamic conditions in the gastrointestinal tract of poultry. *Toxins* 10, 1–16.
Zebeli Q and Metzler-Zebeli BU 2012. Interplay between rumen digestive disorders and diet induced inflammation in dairy cattle. *Research in Veterinary Science* 93, 1099–1208.
Zeidan R, Ul-Hassan Z, Al-Thani R, Balmas V and Jaoua S 2018. Application of low-fermenting yeast lachancea thermotolerans for the control of toxigenic fungi aspergillus parasiticus, penicillium verrucosum and fusarium graminearum and their mycotoxins. *Toxins* 10, 1–12.
Zhang L, Ma Q, Ma S, Zhang J, Jia R, Ji C and Zhao L 2016. Ameliorating effects of Bacillus subtilis ANSB060 on growth performance, antioxidant functions, and aflatoxin residues in ducks fed diets contaminated with aflatoxins. *Toxins* 9, 1–12.
Zhang N-Y, Qi M, Zhao L, Zhu M-K, Guo J, Liu J, Gu C-Q, Rajput S, Krumm C, Qi D-S and Sun L-V 2016. Curcumin prevents aflatoxin B1 hepatoxicity by inhibition of cytochrome P450 isozymes in chick liver. *Toxins* 8, 1–10.
Zhang Y 2004. Cancer-preventive isothiocyanates, measurement of human exposure and mechanism of action. *Mutation Research* 555, 173–190.
Zhen J, Qu Z, Fang H, Fu L, Wu Y, Wang H, Zang H and Wang W 2014. Effects of grape seed proanthocyanidin extract on pentylenetetrazole-induced kindling and associated cognitive impairment in rats. *International Journal of Molecular Medicine* 34, 391–401.
Zhuang Z, Lohmar JM, Satterlee T, Cary JW and Calvo AM 2016. The master transcription factor mtfA governs aflatoxin production, morphological development and pathogenicity in the fungus Aspergillus flavus. *Toxins* 8, 29–32.

Index

For Product Safety Concerns and Information please contact our EU representative GPSR@taylorandfrancis.com
Taylor & Francis Verlag GmbH, Kaufingerstraße 24, 80331 München, Germany

www.ingramcontent.com/pod-product-compliance
Ingram Content Group UK Ltd.
Pitfield, Milton Keynes, MK11 3LW, UK
UKHW020024200926
475702UK00014B/2051

* 9 7 8 1 0 3 2 8 1 6 2 4 1 *